Food Microbiology

Food Microbiology

WM FOSTER

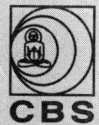

CBS Publishers & Distributors Pvt Ltd

New Delhi • Bengaluru • Chennai • Kochi • Kolkata • Mumbai

Bhopal • Bhubaneswar • Hyderabad • Jharkhand • Nagpur • Patna • Pune
Uttarakhand • Dhaka (Bangladesh) • Kathmandu (Nepal)

**Food
Microbiology**

ISBN: 978-81-239-2829-6

Copyright © Publisher

First Edition: 2016
Reprint: 2019, 2023

Published by **Satish Kumar Jain** and produced by **Varun Jain** for

CBS Publishers & Distributors Pvt Ltd

4819/XI Prahlad Street, 24 Ansari Road, Daryaganj, New Delhi 110 002, India.
Ph: 011-23289259, 23266861

Website: www.cbspd.com
e-mail: delhi@cbspd.com;

Corporate Office: 204 FIE, Industrial Area, Patparganj, Delhi 110 092
Ph: 011-4934 4934   Fax: 011-4934 4935

e-mail: publishing@cbspd.com;
publicity@cbspd.com

Branches

- **Bengaluru:** Seema House 2975, 17th Cross, KR Road, Banasankari 2nd Stage, Bengaluru 560 070, Karnataka, India
  Ph: +91-80-26771678/79   Fax: +91-80-26771680   e-mail: bangalore@cbspd.com
- **Chennai:** 7, Subbaraya Street, Shenoy Nagar, Chennai 600 030, Tamil Nadu, India
  Ph: +91-44-26680620, 26681266   Fax: +91-44-42032115   e-mail: chennai@cbspd.com
- **Kochi:** 42/1325, 1326, Power House Road, Opp KSEB, Power House, Ernakulum Kochi 682 018, Kerala, India
  Ph: +91-484-4059061-65,67   Fax: +91-484-4059065   e-mail: kochi@cbspd.com
- **Kolkata:** 147, Hind Ceramics Compound, 1st Floor, Nilgunj Road, Belghoria, Kolkata-700056, West Bengal, India
  Ph: +033-25633055, 033-25633056   e-mail: kolkata@cbspd.com
- **Lucknow:** Basement, Khushnuma Complex, 7 Meerabai Marg (Behind Jawahar Bhawan),Lucknow-226001, UP, India
  Ph: +0522-4000032   e-mail: tiwari.lucknow@cbspd.com
- **Mumbai:** PWD Shed, Gala no 25/26, Ramchandra Bhatt Marg, Next to JJ Hospital Gate no. 2, Opp. Union Bank of India, Noorbaug, Mumbai-400009, Maharashtra, India
  Ph: 022-66661880/89   e-mail: mumbai@cbspd.com

Representatives

• Hyderabad	0-9885175004	• Jharkhand	0-9811541605	• Nagpur	0-9421945513
• Patna	0-9334159340	• Pune	0-9923910676	• Uttarakhand	0-9716462459

Printed at Glorious Printer, Dilshad Garden, Delhi, India

Preface

Food microbiology is the study of the micro-organisms that inhabit, create, or contaminate food. Of major importance is the study of micro-organisms causing food spoilage. 'Good' bacteria, however, such as probiotics, are becoming increasingly important in food science. In addition, micro-organisms are essential for the production of foods such as cheese, yogurt, other fermented foods, bread, beer and wine. Microbes are single-cell organisms so tiny that millions can fit into the eye of a needle. They are the oldest form of life on earth. Microbe fossils date back more than 3.5 billion years to a time when the earth was covered with oceans that regularly reached the boiling point, hundreds of millions of years before dinosaurs roamed the earth. The field of food microbiology is a very broad one, encompassing the study of micro-organisms which have both beneficial and deleterious effects on the quality and safety of raw and processed foods. Food science is a discipline concerned with all aspects of food-beginning after harvesting, and ending with consumption by the consumer. It is considered one of the agricultural sciences, and it is a field which is entirely distinct from the field of nutrition.

This reference textbook summarises the various aspects of Food Microbiology and is divided into six sections and 25 chapters. Section I deals with food and micro-organisms. Chapter 1 is devoted to basic concepts of food microbiology. The primary tool of microbiologists is the ability to identify and quantitate foodborne micro-organisms. Chapter 2 deals with important micro-organisms in food microbiology. This chapter also discusses general characteristics of mould, their classification and identification. Food contamination can come in the form of bacteria, viruses or parasitic organisms. Considering this chapter 3 focuses on contamination of foods. Chapter 4 concentrates on food spoilage during chemical changes caused by micro-organisms.

Section II discusses principles of food preservation. Chapter 5 acquaints the readers with general principles of food preservation and discusses various preservation processes and growth of micro-organisms. Chapters 6 and 7 are devoted to preservation by use of low and high temperature. Chapter 8 concentrates on preservation by drying which is a method of food preservation that works by removing water from food which inhibits the growth of micro-organisms, and hinders quality decay. Chapter 9 focuses on preservation by radiation which is the process of exposing food to ionising radiation to destroy micro-organisms, bacteria, viruses or insects that might be present in the food. Chapter 10 discusses preservation by food additives, which are added to prevent the deterioration or decomposition of food have been referred to as chemical preservatives.

Section III discusses contamination, preservation, and spoilage of various foods. Chapter 11 deals with contamination, preservation and spoilage of vegetable and fruits. Most of our food consists of agricultural products, which are usually seasonal and spoil quickly. To make food available throughout the year, humans have developed methods to prolong the storage life of products to preserve them. Chapter 12 focuses on contamination, preservation and spoilage of fish and meat. The spoilage of poultry is somewhat different from the spoilage of canned meat. Considering this chapter 13 concentrates on contamination, preservation and spoilage of eggs. Chapter 14 explains contamination, preservation and spoilage of milk products. Various methods and causes of spoilage of milk products are discussed in detail. Chapter 15 is devoted to spoilage of heated canned foods which may spoil due to biological and chemical reasons. Chapter 16 acquaints the readers with miscellaneous foods such as fatty foods, salad dressings, essential oils, bottled soft drinks, spices and other condiments, salt and nutmeats.

Section IV discusses food and enzymes produced by micro-organisms. Chapter 17 concentrates on production of cultures for food fermentations. In simple terms, an organism is cultured or grown under conditions which are typically controlled. Fermentation in food processing typically is the conversion of carbohydrates to alcohols and carbon dioxide or organic acids. Keeping this in mind chapter 18 deals with fermented and microbial foods. Chapter 19 is devoted to miscellaneous fermented food products. The various fermented products discussed are vinegar, cocoa products, coffee, tea, vegetables, etc. Chapter 20 acquaints the readers with food and enzymes from micro-organisms. Enzymes are commonly used in food processing and in the production of food ingredients. Various micro-organisms as food such as single cell protein, fats from micro-organisms, production of other substances added to food, etc. are discussed in detail.

Section V discusses food in relation to disease. Chapter 21 focuses on bacterial agents of foodborne illness. A microbial foodborne illness may result from ingesting a food containing either pathogenic micro-organisms or a toxin or poison is the etiological agent, the illness is called an infection. If a toxin of poison is the causative agent, the illness is called a food intoxication or food poisoning. Chapter 22 deals with nonbacterial agents of foodborne illness. Some foodborne disease outbreaks are not caused by bacteria or their toxins but results from mycotoxins, viruses, rickettsias, parasitic worms or protozoa or from the consumption of food contaminated with toxic substances. The investigation and control of foodborne disease outbreaks are multi-disciplinary tasks requiring skills in the areas of clinical medicine, epidemiology, laboratory medicine, food microbiology, chemistry, food safety and food control, etc. Considering this chapter 23 focuses on the investigation of foodborne disease outbreaks.

Section VI discusses food sanitation and public health. Sanitation is the hygienic means of promoting health through prevention of human contact with the hazards of wastes. Food sanitation refers to the hygienic measures of ensuring food safety. Considering this chapter 24 is devoted to microbiology in food sanitation and describes waste-water sanitation, water microbiology, sewage and waste-water treatment and microbiology of the food products. Chapter 25 deals with food control and discusses need for food control, work of Food and Agricultural Organisation (FAO) of United Nations, and Food and Drug Administration (FDA).

Glossary and index have been provided at the end for quick reference. Diagrams, figures and tables supplement the text. All topics have been covered in a cogent and lucid style to help the reader grasp the information quickly and easily.

It may not be wrong to hold that the present reference textbook of *Food Microbiology* is a complete treatise on this subject. It is essential reading for B. Tech. (Food Technology/Environmental Biotechnology/Microbiology) and students pursuing B.Sc/M.Sc course in Biotechnology and Microbiology. Besides students, this book will prove useful to industrialists and consultants in food processing/food technology.

The reference textbook also caters to the requirement of the syllabus prescribed by various universities for undergraduate and postgraduate courses in the above subjects. It has been prepared with meticulous care, aiming at making the book error-free. Constructive suggestions are always welcome from users of this book.

WM Foster

Contents at a Glance

SECTION V

SECTION VI

Contents

SECTION II

SECTION IV

SECTION V

SECTION I

Food and Micro-organisms

Chapter 1

Basic Concepts of Food Microbiology

INTRODUCTION

Food microbiology is the study of the micro-organisms that inhabit, create or contaminate food. Of major importance is the study of micro-organisms causing food spoilage. 'Good' bacteria, however, such as probiotics, are becoming increasingly important in food science. In addition, micro-organisms are essential for the production of foods such as cheese, yogurt, other fermented foods, bread, beer and wine. Microbes are single-cell organisms so tiny that millions can fit into the eye of a needle. They are the oldest form of life on earth. Microbe fossils date back more than 3.5 billion years to a time when the earth was covered with oceans that regularly reached the boiling point, hundreds of millions of years before dinosaurs roamed the earth.

The field of food microbiology is a very broad one, encompassing the study of micro-organisms which have both beneficial and deleterious effects on the quality and safety of raw and processed foods.

Food science is a discipline concerned with all aspects of food-beginning after harvesting, and ending with consumption by the consumer. It is considered one of the agricultural sciences, and it is a field which is entirely distinct from the field of nutrition.

The primary tool of microbiologists is the ability to identify and quantitate foodborne micro-organisms; however, the inherent inaccuracies in enumeration processess, and the natural variation found in all bacterial populations complicate the microbiologists job. Foodborne illness or food poisoning is caused by consuming food contaminated with pathogenic bacteria, toxins, viruses, prions or parasites. Such contamination usually arises from improper handling, preparation or storage of food. Foodborne illness can also be caused by adding pesticides or medicines to food, or by accidentally consuming naturally poisonous substances like poisonous mushrooms or reef fish. Contact between food and pests, especially flies, rodents and cockroaches, is a further cause of contamination of food.

Some common diseases are occasionally foodborne mainly through the water vector, even though they are usually transmitted by other routes. These include infections caused by Shigella, Hepatitis A, and the parasites Giardia lamblia and Cryptosporidium parvum.

FOOD SPOILAGE

Food spoilage means food becoming unfit for consumption, for example, due to chemical or biological contamination.

Most natural foods have a limited life. Perishable food such as: fish, meat, milk and bread have a short lifespan. Other foods keep a considerably longer time but decompose eventually. There are many

3

causes of food spoilage. Enzymes within some foods bring about their destruction, while chemical reactions such as oxidation and rancidity decompose others — but the main single cause of food spoilage is invasion by micro-organisms such as moulds, yeasts and bacteria.

Micro-organisms are found everywhere, since the conditions which bring about their growth are readily available. Like humans, they prefer a warm, moist environment, a supply of oxygen and food — and because their nutritional requirements are similar to ours, they readily contaminate our food supplies. When food spoilage is caused by the growth of yeasts and moulds it is self-evident: a furry growth covers the food and it becomes soft and often smells bad. Bacterial contamination is more dangerous because very often the food does not look bad: even though severely infected, it may appear quite normal. The presence of highly dangerous toxins and bacterial spores is often not detected until after an outbreak of food poisoning, when laboratory examination and experiments uncover the infecting agent.

Types of Food Spoilage

Physical spoilage

Physical damage to the protective outer layer of food during harvesting, processing or distribution increases the chance of chemical or microbial spoilage. Examples of physical spoilage include:
1. Staling of bakery products and components.
2. Moisture migration between different components.
3. Physical separation of components or ingredients.
4. Moisture loss or gain.

Chemical spoilage

When animal or vegetable material is removed from its natural source of energy and nutrient supply, chemical changes begin to occur which lead to deterioration in its structure. The two major chemical changes which occur during the processing and storage of foods and lead to a deterioration in sensory quality are lipid oxidation (rancidity) and enzymic browning. Chemical reactions are also responsible for changes in the colour and flavour of foods during processing and storage.

Microbial spoilage

These micro-organisms (moulds, yeasts and bacteria) do not cause disease but they spoil food by growing in the food and producing substances which alter colour, texture and odour of the food, making it unfit for human consumption. For example, souring of milk, growth of mould on bread and rotting of fruit and vegetables.

Enzymic Spoilage

Every living organism uses enzymes of many sorts in its bodily functions as part of its normal life cycle. Enzymes are used in creating life. After death, enzymes play a role in the decomposition of once living tissue. For example, the enzymes in a tomato help it to ripen and enzymes produced by the tomato and whatever fungal and bacterial spoilers are on it cause it to decay.

Maillard Browning (Nonenzymic Browning)

This is a browning reaction which occurs during the roasting, baking, grilling and frying of many foods. A chemical reaction takes place between the amino group of a free amino acid or a free amino group on a protein chain and the carbonyl group of a reducing sugar, e.g. glucose. Brown coloured compounds are formed which are responsible for the attractive colour of products such as bread crust, roasted meat, fried potatoes and baked cakes and biscuits. The compounds also give an appetising flavour to the food.

Enzymic browning

When the cells of apples, potatoes and some other fruits and vegetables are cut and exposed to the air, enzymes present in the cells bring about an oxidation reaction; colourless compounds are converted into brown-coloured compounds. Browning does not occur in cooked fruits and vegetables since the enzymes are destroyed by heat. Fruits such as apples, pears, bananas, peaches and avocado are prone to discolouration.

Rancidity

Most fats and oils do not store very well, they develop off flavours and odours known as rancidity. Rancidity is important when considering the shelf life of a food product.

Rancidity is caused by several factors:
1. Absorption rancidity.
2. Oxidative rancidity.
3. Hydrolytic rancidity.

Absorption rancidity

When oils and fats are stored next to strong smelling foods, e.g. onions or garlic or products, e.g. paints, detergents, disinfectants. The smell is absorbed by the fat or oil making it unpleasant to eat.

Oxidative rancidity

Oxygen from the air can oxidise unsaturated fats producing objectionable flavours. This is the most important and common type of rancidity. It involves a 3 phase process: (i) inititiation phase, (ii) propagation phase, and (iii) termination phase.

Hydrolytic rancidity

This is caused by the presence of water, which causes triglycerides to split into glycerol and fatty acids. The rate of hydrolysis in the presence of water alone is negligible but hastens if enzymes (lipases) and micro-organisms (bacteria, moulds and yeasts) are present. It results in the formation of free fatty acids and soaps (salts of free fatty acids). The oil/fat develops a soapy taste/texture. This is a less common type of rancidity but is quite common in emulsion systems such as butter, margarine and cream.

High temperatures, the presence of moisture, oxygen and light are among the factors that speed up rancidity. Different types of fat and oil show varying degrees of resistance to spoilage. Most vegetable oils deteriorate slowly, animal fats deteriorate quicker and marine (fish) oils, which contain a very high proportion of highly unsaturated fatty acids, deteriorate so rapidly that they are useless for edible purposes unless they are refined and hydrogenated.

Importance of Water Activity (a_w) in Microbial Spoilage

Micro-organisms require water to maintain life. The amount of water available in a food can be described in terms of the water activity (a_w). Pure water has an $a_w = 1.0$. The water activity of most fresh foods is 0.99. Water is required by micro-organisms to maintain normal population growth. Removal of water does not kill the microbes but just stops their growth. In order to prevent the growth of micro-organisms in a food the water activity (a_w) of the food must be reduced to 0.6 or below.

Reasons for Preserving Food

Foods are preserved to prolong their shelf life. As soon as animals have been slaughtered and plant foods have been harvested deterioration begins. This involves two main processes:

1. Cells break down due to enzymes present in the food: this process is known as autolysis, meaning 'self destruct'.
2. The disrupted cell structures are vulnerable to the activities of micro-organisms. Micro-organisms cause changes in odour, flavour, colour and texture of food.

For effective food preservation it is necessary to prevent both autolysis and microbial growth.

Reasons for preserving food:

1. Extension of the safe storage life of food.
2. Safety.
3. Acceptability.
4. Nutritive value.
5. Availability.
6. Economic viability.

METHODS OF FOOD PRESERVATION

Freezing and Chilling

Freezing controls the growth of micro-organisms in two ways. The growth rate is reduced due to the low temperatures and water is unavailable because it has been converted to ice. Also, the chemical changes in food are slowed down because of the low temperature. Before freezing foods, inedible parts are removed and it is usual to blanch fruit and vegetables to inactivate enzymes. The number of bacteria is also reduced by blanching.

Commercially, foods are frozen by the quick-freezing process. This method is desirable because ice crystals that form in the food are small; large ice crystals rupture the cell wall and thus change the texture and appearance of food.

Quality of frozen foods

During blanching of fruit and vegetables ascorbic acid (vitamin C) and thiamin (B1) are vulnerable. Nutrients in the form of thaw drip may be lost when foods are thawed—for example, thiamine from meat. Textural changes may occur; soft fruits can become mushy because the cell structure of the fruit collapses.

Chilling

Chilling is a short-term process of preservation. Chilling is based on the principle that microbial activity is reduced in cold storage conditions. At temperatures in the range 0°–5°C the growth of most species of micro-organisms is retarded. Chilled foods are prepared foods which, for reasons of safety or quality, are designed to be stored at or below 8°C for their entire life, e.g. salads. The optimum temperature for storage is 5°C.

Cook chill products are dishes which are cooked and then rapidly chilled between 0°–3°C within 90 minutes. The food is then stored in controlled low temperatures, below 3°C. The product should be reheated thoroughly (to above 72°C for 2 minutes) prior to consumption.

Irradiation

Although irradiation destroys micro-organisms it has no effect on the enzymes in food, so degradation is not prevented. Food irradiation is permitted in some countries. The commercial development of irradiation is limited due to a number of factors such as the cost of equipment, stringent tests needed for safety and the development of undesirable flavours in certain foods.

Heat Treatment

Foods can be preserved by the application of heat in sufficient quantity to kill all micro-organisms and to inactivate enzymes. There are two levels of heat processing:

Pasteurisation

This is heat processing designed to kill pathogenic organisms, and in so doing to kill most spoilage organisms. It is a short-term method of preservation and it extends the storage life of the product a little but makes it bacteriologically safe. This process is used in the pasteurisation of milk for example. Raw milk is heated to 72°C for 15 seconds.

Sterilisation

This is a much more severe heat process aimed to destroy all micro-organisms. Absolute sterility is difficult to obtain as some bacterial spores may survive the process. Commercial sterility is the state achieved in most canning processes, and is heat processing designed to kill virtually all micro-organisms, and most spores, which would be capable of growing during storage. Some organisms can survive the sterilisation process if not processed for enough time or at a high enough temperature, e.g. *Clostridium botulinum*.

Canning

Canning involves the application of heat and aims at destroying micro-organisms and their spores. The heat-treated or sterilised food must be kept in an airtight container to prevent contamination.

Addition of Chemicals

Acids: Such as vinegar are used in pickling. The vinegar prevents the growth of micro-organisms. This is because the food is placed in a low pH solution in which micro-organisms cannot grow.

Permitted chemical preservatives

Preservatives help to reduce or prevent wastage of food through spoilage caused by micro-organisms. Longer shelf life enables a greater variety of products to be kept in store and in the home. Common examples of preservatives include:

Sorbic acid (E200)   Used in soft drinks and processed cheese.
Benzoic acid (E210)   Used in soft drinks.
Sulphur dioxide (E220) Used in dried fruit, dehydrated vegetables, fruit juice, fruit syrup, pickles.
Potassium nitrate (E252) Used in curing bacon, ham and other cured meats.

Fats, oils and foods containing them are subject, over a period of time, to the effects of oxygen in turning the product rancid. Antioxidants are added to such foods to slow down or prevent the process of rancidity (oxidative) and thus extend the shelf life of a product.

Common antioxidants include:

Ascorbic acid (E300)	Used in fruit drinks.
Propyl gallate (E310)	Used in vegetable oils and chewing gum.
Butylated hydroxyanisole (E320)	Used in cheese spread, stock cubes.

Removal of Water

Foods may be preserved by the addition of anti-microbial substances such as:

Salt: Used in the curing of meat such as bacon. The salt or brine (salt solution) reduces the moisture content of the food i.e. it reduces the availability of water (a_w) to micro-organisms. The moisture available to the micro-organism.

Osmosis: The salt solution is more concentrated than the cytoplasm inside the cells of the micro-organism. Therefore, water passes out of the cell and the cell becomes dehydrated. With little moisture, micro-organism growth is retarded.

Sugar: Used in the manufacture of jam and crystallised fruit. The addition of a large quantity of sugar inhibits the growth of micro-organisms by making the water in the fruit cells unavailable. Again, the moisture available to the micro-organism is reduced by osmosis. The high temperature used in jamming also destroys any micro-organism.

Dehydration

Traditionally, foods were dried in the sun. The original processes have advanced considerably, and moisture is now removed by the application of heat in a controlled flow of air.

Methods of drying

1. Sun drying: This method is practical in hot dry climates, but the process is slow and the foods being dried are vulnerable to contamination.
2. Fluidised bed-drying: Warmed air is circulated around the food while it is agitated to stop it from sticking.
3. Spray drying: Spray drying is used for liquids. The liquid is sprayed through fine nozzles into a current of hot air. The water evaporates and leaves behind a fine powder.
4. Roller drying: This is used for pasted foods such as instant breakfast cereals. The paste forms a film on the surface of a heated roller or drum. During the rotation of the roller or drum, the food dries and is finally removed by scrapers.
5. Accelerated freeze-drying (AFD): This involves an initial freezing process which is followed by gradual heating in a vacuum cabinet. During this process ice crystals form and change to vapour without going through the liquid stage (sublimation). The product is porous but differs from its original form. The porous nature of the food makes it suitable for instant rehydration.

Quality of dried foods

Drying alters the cellular structure of food. Retinol (vitamin A), thiamin (B1), ascorbic acid (C), and vitamin E are lost in the drying process. Foods with a high fat content are vulnerable to rancidity and discolouration.

Modified atmosphere packaging (MAP)

MAP is the enclosure of food in a package in which the atmosphere has been changed by altering the proportions of carbon dioxide, oxygen, nitrogen, water vapour and trace gases. The process retards microbial and biochemical activity. Products such as bacon, red meat, poultry and vegetables use this method to increase the shelf life of the product.

Vacuum packing

Foods such as meat or cheese are packed in impermeable plastic material, and the air is sucked out under vacuum. This method prevents the growth of aerobic micro-organisms because of the absence of oxygen.

Permeable packaging

Some types of plastic are semi-permeable and allow the transfer of gases such as oxygen and carbon dioxide and water vapour. This type of material is used for foods such as tomatoes, and is useful because it delays ripening and extends the shelf life by more than a week. Other packaging materials are completely permeable. Sometimes crusty bread is packed in a plastic covering dotted with tiny holes. This type of packaging is advantageous because otherwise trapped moisture would condense and the crust would lose its characteristic crispness.

FOOD SAFETY

Food safety is a scientific discipline describing handling, preparation, and storage of food in ways that prevent foodborne illness. This includes a number of routines that should be followed to avoid potentially severe health hazards. Food can transmit disease from person to person as well as serve as a growth medium for bacteria that can cause food poisoning. Debates on genetic food safety include such issues as impact of genetically modified food on health of further generations and genetic pollution of environment, which can destroy natural biological diversity.

In developed countries there are intricate standards for food preparation, whereas in lesser developed countries the main issue is simply the availability of adequate safe water, which is usually a critical item. In theory food poisoning is 100 per cent preventable.

Key Principles

Five key principles

The five key principles of food hygiene, according to WHO, are:
1. Prevent contaminating food with pathogens spreading from people, pets, and pests.
2. Separate raw and cooked foods to prevent contaminating the cooked foods.
3. Cook foods for the appropriate length of time and at the appropriate temperature to kill pathogens.
4. Store food at the proper temperature.
5. Use safe water and raw materials.

FERMENTATION

Fermentation in food processing typically is the conversion of carbohydrates to alcohols and carbon dioxide or organic acids using yeasts, bacteria, or a combination thereof, under anaerobic conditions. A more restricted definition of fermentation is the chemical conversion of sugars into ethanol. The science of fermentation is known as zymurgy.

Fermentation usually implies that the action of micro-organisms is desirable, and the process is used to produce alcoholic beverages such as wine, beer, and cider. Fermentation is also employed in the leavening of bread, and for preservation techniques to create lactic acid in sour foods such as sauerkraut, dry sausages, kimchi and yogurt, or vinegar (acetic acid) for use in pickling foods.

QUALITY ASSURANCE IN MICROBIOLOGY

Quality assurance (QA) is the total process whereby the quality of laboratory reports can be guaranteed. The term quality control covers that part of QA, which primarily concerns the control of errors in the performance of tests and verification of test results. All materials, equipment and procedures must be adequately controlled. Culture media must be tested for sterility and performance. Each laboratory must have standard operating procedures (SOPs). QA of pre-analytical, analytical and post-analytical stages of microbiological procedures should be incorporated in SOPs. The laboratory must be well lit with dust-free air-conditioned environment. Environmental conditions should be monitored. Supervisory and technical personnel should be well qualified. The laboratory should participate in external and internal quality assurance schemes.

Microbiological investigations are important in the diagnosis, treatment, and surveillance of infectious diseases and policies regarding the selection and use of antimicrobial drugs. It is, therefore, essential that test reports are relevant, reliable, timely, and interpreted correctly. High cost of culture media and reagents, lack of rational approach to the selection and use of microbiological investigations, and a shortage of trained technical staff and clinical microbiologists are important factors in preventing the establishment of essential microbiology services in developing countries.

Chapter 2

Importance of Micro-organisms in Food Microbiology

INTRODUCTION

Moulds (or molds) are fungi that grow in the form of multicellular filaments called hyphae. In contrast, microscopic fungi that grow as single cells are called yeasts. A connected network of these tubular branching hyphae has multiple, genetically identical nuclei and is considered a single organism, referred to as a colony or in more technical terms a mycelium. Moulds do not form a specific taxonomic or phylogenetic grouping, but can be found in the divisions *Zygomycota*, *Deuteromycota* and *Ascomycota*. Some moulds cause disease or food spoilage, others play an important role in biodegradation or in the production of various foods, beverages, antibiotics and enzymes.

There are thousands of known species of moulds which include opportunistic pathogens, saprotrophs, aquatic species, and thermophiles. Like all fungi, moulds derive energy not through photosynthesis but from the organic matter in which they live. Typically, moulds secrete hydrolytic enzymes, mainly from the hyphal tips. These enzymes degrade complex biopolymers such as starch, cellulose and lignin into simpler substances which can be absorbed by the hyphae. In this way, moulds play a major role in causing decomposition of organic material, enabling the recycling of nutrients throughout ecosystems. Many moulds also secrete mycotoxins which, together with hydrolytic enzymes, inhibit the growth of competing micro-organisms.

Moulds reproduce through small spores, which may contain a single nucleus or be multinucleate. Mould spores can be asexual (the products of mitosis) or sexual (the products of meiosis); many species can produce both types. Mould spores may remain airborne indefinitely, may cling to clothing or fur, or may be able to survive extremes of temperature and pressure.

Although moulds grow on dead organic matter everywhere in nature, their presence is only visible to the unaided eye when mould colonies grow. A mould colony does not comprise discrete organisms, but an interconnected network of hyphae called a mycelium. Nutrients and in some cases organelles may be transported throughout the mycelium. In artificial environments like buildings, humidity and temperature are often stable enough to foster the growth of mould colonies, commonly seen as a downy or furry coating growing on food or other surfaces.

Many moulds can begin growing at 4°C (39°F), the temperature within a typical refrigerator or less. When conditions do not enable growth, moulds may remain alive in a dormant state depending on the species, within a large range of temperatures before they die. The many different mould species vary enormously in their tolerance to temperature and humidity extremes. Certain moulds can survive harsh conditions such as the snow-covered soils of Antarctica, refrigeration, highly acidic solvents, and even petroleum products such as jet fuel.

11

Xerophilic moulds use the humidity in the air as their only water source; other moulds need more moisture. Mould has a musty odour.

Cultured moulds are used in the production of foods, including:

1. Cheese (*Penicillium* spp.).
2. Tempeh (*Rhizopus oligosporus*).
3. Oncom (*Neurospora sitophila*).
4. Quorn (*Fusarium venenatum*).
5. Bread.
6. Beer.
7. Some sausages.
8. Soya sauce.

The *koji* moulds are a group of *Aspergillus* species, notably *Aspergillus oryzae*, that have been cultured in eastern Asia for many centuries. They are used to ferment a soyabean and wheat mixture to make soyabean paste and soya sauce. They are also used to break down the starch in rice (saccharification) in the production of *sake* and other distilled spirits. Red rice yeast is a product of the mould *Monascus purpureus* grown on rice, and is common in Asian diets. The yeast contains several compounds collectively known as monacolins, which are known to inhibit cholesterol synthesis.

GENERAL CHARACTERISTICS OF MOULDS

Morphological Characteristics

Morphology means form and structure of moulds is determined by a microscope. The moulds consist of a mass of filaments called Hyphae and mass of these Hyphae is known as Mycelium. Hyphae may be classified as vegetative (growing part) or fertile (production/reproduction) part. The hyphae of most moulds are clear but some are dark or smoky.

By the microscopic examination, gnera of moulds can be identified by the characteristics seen. Moulds are divided into Septate (with cross walls) and Non Septate (without cross walls). Reproduction of moulds are chiefly by asexual spores. The moulds which form sexual spores are termed as perfect. The 'Fungi Imperfecti' (Septate) have only asexual spore. The Non Septate perfect mould are Oomycetes and Zygomycetes, the Septate perfect moulds are Ascomycetes and Basidiomycetes.

Cultural Characteristics

Some moulds look velvety on the upper surface, some look dry and powdery, and some wet or gelatinous. Some moulds are loose and fluffy and some are compact. The appearance of the moulds indicates its genus.

Physiological Characteristics

Temperature requirement: Most moulds grow well at ordinary temperature. A number of moulds grow well at refrigeration temperatures. A few can grow at a high temperature.

Moisture requirement: Moulds require less moisture to grow than yeast and bacteria. If dried food has a moisture content below 14 to 15 per cent, it will prevent or delay mould growth.

Oxygen requirement: Moulds are aerobic, so they require oxygen for their growth.

Mycelium

Mycelium (plural mycelia) is the vegetative part of a fungus, consisting of a mass of branching, thread-like hyphae. The mass of hyphae is sometimes called *shiro*, especially within the fairy ring fungi.

Fungal colonies composed of mycelia are found in soil and on or within many other substrates. A typical single spore germinates into a homokaryotic mycelium, which cannot reproduce sexually; when two compatible homokaryotic mycelia join and form a dikaryotic mycelium, that mycelium may form fruiting bodies such as mushrooms. A mycelium may be minute, forming a colony that is too small to see, or it may be extensive (Fig. 2.1).

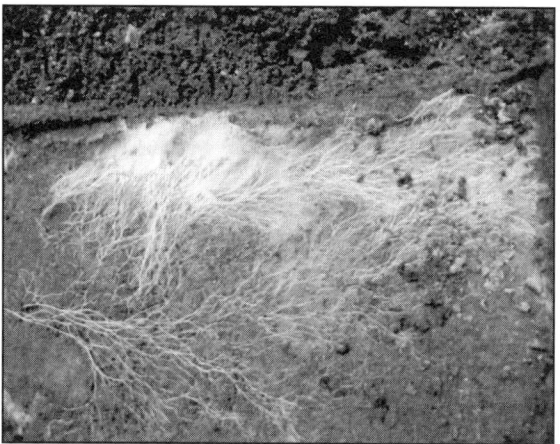

Fig. 2.1. Fungal mycelia.

It is through the mycelium that a fungus absorbs nutrients from its environment. It does this in a two-stage process. First, the hyphae secrete enzymes onto or into the food source, which break down biological polymers into smaller units such as monomers. These monomers are then absorbed into the mycelium by facilitated diffusion and active transport. Mycelium is vital in terrestrial and aquatic ecosystems for its role in the decomposition of plant material. It contributes to the organic fraction of soil, and its growth releases carbon dioxide back into the atmosphere. The mycelium of mycorrhizal fungi increases the efficiency of water and nutrient absorption of most plants and confers resistance to some plant pathogens. Mycelium is an important food source for many soil invertebrates. Sclerotia are compact or hard masses of mycelium (Fig. 2.2).

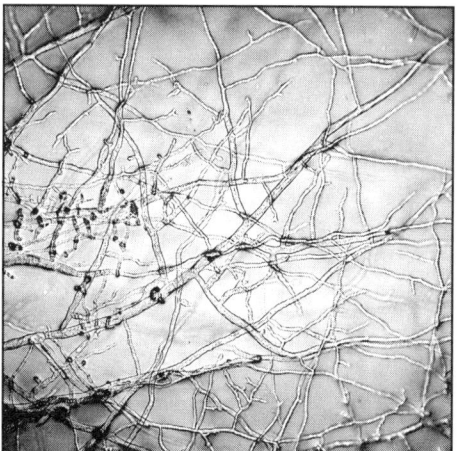

Fig. 2.2. Microscopic view of a mycelium. This image covers a one-millimetre square.

Hypha

A hypha (plural hyphae) is a long, branching filamentous structure of a fungus, and also of unrelated Actinobacteria. In most fungi, hyphae are the main mode of vegetative growth, and are collectively called a mycelium; yeasts are unicellular fungi that do not grow as hyphae (Fig. 2.3).

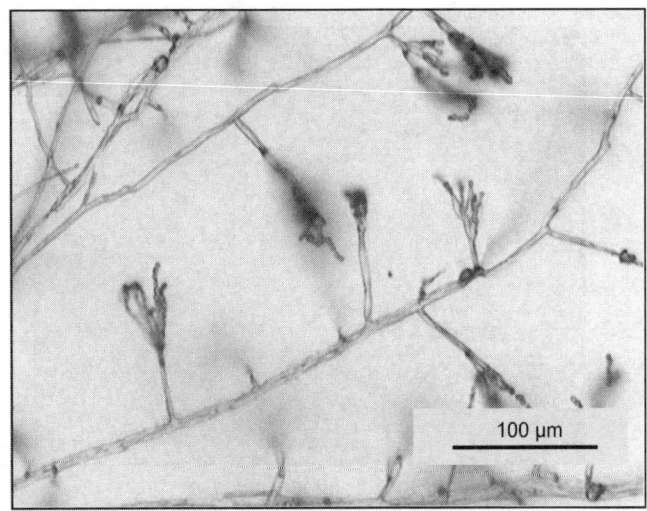

Fig. 2.3. Hyphae of *Penicillium*.

A hypha consists of one or more cells surrounded by a tubular cell wall. In most fungi, hyphae are divided into cells by internal cross-walls called 'septa' (singular septum). Septa are usually perforated by pores large enough for ribosomes, mitochondria and sometimes nuclei to flow between cells. The major structural polymer in fungal cell walls is typically chitin, in contrast to plants that have cellulosic cell walls. Some fungi have aseptate hyphae, meaning their hyphae are not partitioned by septa (Fig. 2.4).

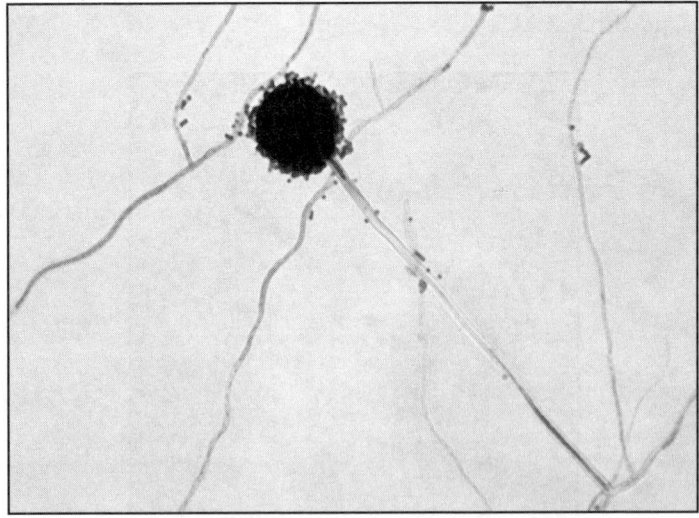

Fig. 2.4. *Aspergillus niger*.

Hyphae grow at their tips. During tip growth, cell walls are extended by the external assembly and polymerisation of cell wall components, and the internal production of new cell membrane. The spitzenkörper is an intracellular organelle associated with tip growth. It is composed of an aggregation of membrane-bound vesicles containing cell wall components. The spitzenkörper is part of the endomembrane system of fungi, holding and releasing vesicles it receives from the Golgi apparatus. These vesicles travel to the cell membrane via the cytoskeleton and release their contents outside the cell by the process of exocytosis, where it can then be transported to where it is needed. Vesicle membranes contribute to growth of the cell membrane while their contents form new cell wall. The spitzenkörper moves along the apex of the hyphal strand and generates apical growth and branching; the apical growth rate of the hyphal strand parallels and is regulated by the movement of the spitzenkörper (Fig. 2.5).

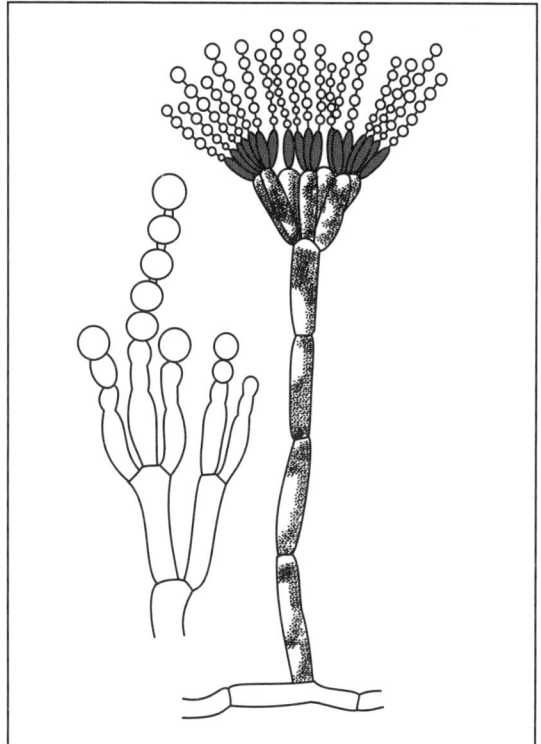

Fig. 2.5. Conidia on conidiophores.

As a hypha extends, septa may be formed behind the growing tip to partition each hypha into individual cells. Hyphae can branch through the bifurcation of a growing tip or by the emergence of a new tip from an established hypha.

Hyphae may be modified in many different ways to serve specific functions. Some parasitic fungi form haustoria that function in absorption within the host cells. The arbuscules of mutualistic mycorrhizal fungi serve a similar function in nutrient exchange, so are important in assisting nutrient and water absorption by plants. Hyphae are found enveloping the gonidia in lichens, making up a large part of their structure. In nematode-trapping fungi, hyphae may be modified into trapping structures such as constricting rings and adhesive nets. Mycelial cords can be formed to transfer nutrients over larger distances.

Types of hypha

Classification based on cell division

1. Septate (with septa).
   (a) *Aspergillus* and many other species have septate hyphae.
2. Aseptate or coenocytic (without septa).
   (a) Non-septate hyphae are associated with Mucor, some zygomycetes, and other fungi.
3. 'Pseudohyphae' are distinguished from true hyphae by their method of growth, relative frailty and lack of cytoplasmic connection between the cells.
   (a) Yeast can form pseudohyphae. They are the result of a sort of incomplete budding where the cells remain attached after division.

Classification based on cell wall and overall form

Characteristics of hyphae can be important in fungal classification. In basidiomycete taxonomy, hyphae that comprise the fruiting body can be identified as generative, skeletal or binding hyphae.

1. Generative hyphae are relatively undifferentiated and can develop reproductive structures. They are typically thin-walled, occasionally developing slightly thickened walls, usually have frequent septa, and may or may not have clamp connections. They may be embedded in mucilage or gelatinised materials.
2. Skeletal hyphae are of two basic types. The classical form is thick-walled and very long in comparison to the frequently septate generative hyphae, which are unbranched or rarely branched, with little cell content. They have few septa and lack clamp connections. Fusiform skeletal hyphae are the second form of skeletal hyphae. Unlike typical skeletal hyphae these are swollen centrally and often exceedingly broad, hence giving the hypha a fusiform shape.
3. Binding hyphae are thick-walled and frequent branched. Often they resemble deer antlers or defoliated trees because of the many tapering branches.

Based on the generative, skeletal and binding hyphal types, in 1932 E. J. H. Corner applied the terms monomitic, dimitic, and trimitic to hyphal systems, in order to improve the classification of polypores.

1. Every fungus must contain generative hyphae. A fungus which only contains this type, as do fleshy mushrooms such as agarics, is referred to as monomitic.
2. Skeletal and binding hyphae give leathery and woody fungi such as polypores their tough consistency. If a fungus contains all three types (example: *Trametes*), it is called trimitic.
3. If a fungus contains generative hyphae and just one of the other two types, it is called dimitic. In fact dimitic fungi almost always contain generative and skeletal hyphae; there is one exceptional genus, *Laetiporus* that includes only generative and binding hyphae.

Fungi that form fusiform skeletal hyphae bound by generative hyphae are said to have sarcodimitic hyphal systems. A few fungi form fusiform skeletal hyphae, generative hyphae, and binding hyphae, and these are said to have sarcotrimitic hyphal systems.

Classification based on refractive appearance

Hyphae are described as gloeoplerous (gloeohyphae) if their high refractive index gives them an oily or granular appearance under the microscope. These cells may be yellowish or clear (hyaline). They can sometimes selectively be coloured by sulphovanillin or other reagents. The specialised cells termed cystidia can also be gloeoplerous.

Asexual Reproduction

Asexual reproduction is a mode of reproduction by which offspring arise from a single parent, and inherit the genes of that parent only, it is reproduction which does not involve meiosis, ploidy reduction, or fertilisation. A more stringent definition is agamogenesis which is reproduction without the fusion of gametes. Asexual reproduction is the primary form of reproduction for single-celled organisms such as the archaea, bacteria, and protists. Many plants and fungi reproduce asexually as well. While all prokaryotes reproduce asexually (without the formation and fusion of gametes), mechanisms for lateral gene transfer such as conjugation, transformation and transduction are sometimes likened to sexual reproduction. A complete lack of sexual reproduction is relatively rare among multicellular organisms, particularly animals. It is not entirely understood why the ability to reproduce sexually is so common among them. Current hypotheses suggest that asexual reproduction may have short-term benefits when rapid population growth is important or in stable environments, while sexual reproduction offers a net advantage by allowing more rapid generation of genetic diversity, allowing adaptation to changing environments. Developmental constraints may underlie why few animals have relinquished sexual reproduction completely in their life-cycles.

Types of Asexual Reproduction

Binary fission

In binary fission the parent organism is replaced by two daughter organisms, because it literally divides in two. Many single-celled organisms, both prokaryotes (the archaea and the bacteria), and eukaryotes (such as protists and unicellular fungi), reproduce asexually through binary fission; most of these are also capable of sexual reproduction. Some single-celled organisms rely on one or more host organisms in order to reproduce.

Budding

Some cells split via budding (for example baker's yeast), resulting in a 'mother' and 'daughter' cell. The offspring organism is smaller than the parent. Budding is also known on a multicellular level; an animal example is the hydra, which reproduces by budding. The buds grow into fully matured individuals which eventually break away from the parent organism.

Vegetative reproduction

Vegetative reproduction is a type of asexual reproduction found in plants where new individuals are formed without the production of seeds or spores by meiosis or syngamy. Examples of vegetative reproduction include the formation of miniaturised plants called plantlets on specialised leaves (for example in kalanchoe) and some produce new plants out of rhizomes or stolon (for example in strawberry). Other plants reproduce by forming bulbs or tubers (for example tulip bulbs and dahlia tubers). Some plants produce adventitious shoots and suckers that form along their lateral roots. Plants that reproduce vegetatively may form a clonal colony, where all the individuals are clones, and the clones may cover a large area.

Spore formation

Many multicellular organisms form spores during their biological life cycle in a process called *sporogenesis*. Exceptions are animals and some protists, who undergo *gametic meiosis* immediately followed by fertilisation. Plants and many algae on the other hand undergo *sporic meiosis* where meiosis leads to the formation of haploid spores rather than gametes. These spores grow into multicellular individuals (called gametophytes in the case of plants) without a fertilisation event. These haploid individuals give rise to gametes through mitosis. Meiosis and gamete formation therefore occur in separate generations or 'phases' of the life cycle, referred to as alternation of generations. Since sexual reproduction is often more narrowly defined as the fusion of gametes (fertilisation), spore formation in plant sporophytes and algae might be considered a form of asexual reproduction (agamogenesis) despite being the result of meiosis and undergoing a reduction in ploidy. However, both events (spore formation and fertilisation) are necessary to complete sexual reproduction in the plant life cycle.

Fungi and some algae can also utilise true asexual spore formation, which involves mitosis giving rise to reproductive cells called mitospores that develop into a new organism after dispersal. This method of reproduction is found for example in conidial fungi and the red alga *Polysiphonia*, and involves sporogenesis without meiosis. Thus the chromosome number of the spore cell is the same as that of the parent producing the spores. However, mitotic sporogenesis is an exception and most spores, such as those of plants, most Basidiomycota, and many algae, are produced by meiosis.

Fragmentation

Fragmentation is a form of asexual reproduction where a new organism grows from a fragment of the parent. Each fragment develops into a mature, fully grown individual. Fragmentation is seen in many organisms such as animals (some annelid worms and sea stars), fungi, and plants. Some plants have specialised structures for reproduction via fragmentation, such as *gemmae* in liverworts. Most lichens, which are a symbiotic union of a fungus and photosynthetic algae or bacteria, reproduce through fragmentation to ensure that new individuals contain both symbionts. These fragments can take the form of *soredia*, dust-like particles consisting of fungal hyphae wrapped around photobiont cells.

Parthenogenesis

Parthenogenesis is a form of agamogenesis in which an unfertilised egg develops into a new individual. Parthenogenesis occurs naturally in many plants, invertebrates (e.g. water fleas, aphids, stick insects, some ants, bees and parasitic wasps), and vertebrates (e.g. some reptiles, amphibians, fish, very rarely birds). In plants, apomixis may or may not involve parthenogenesis.

Agamogenesis

Agamogenesis is any form of reproduction that does not involve a male gamete. Examples are parthenogenesis and apomixis.

Apomixis and nucellar embryony

Apomixis in plants is the formation of a new sporophyte without fertilisation. It is important in ferns and in flowering plants, but is very rare in other seed plants. In flowering plants, the term 'apomixis' is now most often used for agamospermy, the formation of seeds without fertilisation, but was once used to include vegetative reproduction. An example of an apomictic plant would be the triploid European dandelion. Apomixis mainly occurs in two forms. In gametophytic apomixis, the embryo arises from an unfertilised egg within a diploid embryo sac that was formed without completing meiosis. In nucellar embryony, the embryo is formed from the diploid nucellus tissue surrounding the embryo sac. Nucellar embryony occurs in some citrus seeds. Male apomixis can occur in rare cases, such as the Saharan Cypress where the genetic material of the embryo are derived entirely from pollen. The term 'apomixis' is also used for asexual reproduction in some animals, notably water-fleas, *Daphnia*.

Alternation between sexual and asexual reproduction

Some species alternate between the sexual and asexual strategies, an ability known as heterogamy, depending on conditions. For example, the freshwater crustacean *Daphnia* reproduces by parthenogenesis in the spring to rapidly populate ponds, then switches to sexual reproduction as the intensity of competition and predation increases. Many protists and fungi alternate between sexual and asexual reproduction.

For example, the slime mould *Dictyostelium* undergoes binary fission (mitosis) as single-celled amoebae under favourable conditions. However, when conditions turn unfavourable, the cells aggregate and follow one of two different developmental pathways, depending on conditions. In the social pathway, they form a multicellular slug which then forms a fruiting body with asexually generated spores. In the sexual pathway, two cells fuse to form a giant cell that develops into a large cyst. When this macrocyst germinates, it releases hundreds of amoebic cells that are the product of meiotic recombination between the original two cells.

The hyphae of the common mould (*Rhizopus*) are capable of producing both mitotic as well as meiotic spores. Many algae similarly switch between sexual and asexual reproduction. A number of plants use both sexual and asexual means to produce new plants, some species alter their primary modes of reproduction from sexual to asexual under varying environmental conditions.

CLASSIFICATION AND IDENTIFICATION OF MOULDS

Moulds are plants of the kingdom myceteae. They have no roots, stems, or leaves and are devoid of chlorophyll. They belong to the *Eumycetes* or true fungi, and are subdivided further to subdivisions, classes, orders, families, and genera.

The following criteria are used chiefly for differentiation and identification of moulds:

1. Hyphae septate or non-septate.
2. Mycelium clear or dark (smoky).
3. Mycelium coloured of colourless.
4. Whether sexual spores are produced and the type: oospores, zygospores, or ascospores.
5. Type of asexual spores: sporangiospores, conidia or arthrospores (oidia).
6. Characteristics of the spore head.
   (a) Sporangia: size, colour, shape, and location.
   (b) Spore heads bearing conidia: single conidia, chains, budding conidia, or masses; shape and arrangement of sterigmata or phialides; gumming together of conidia.
7. Appearance of sporangiophores or conidiophores: simple or branched, and if branched the type of branching; size and shape of columella at tip of sporangiophore; whether conidiophores are single or in bundles.
8. Microscopic appearance of the asexual spores, especially of conidia: shape, size, colour; smooth or rough; one-, or many-celled.
9. Presence of special structures (or spores): stolons, rhizoids, food cells, apophysis, chlamydospores, sclerotia, etc.

Moulds of Industrial Importance

Mucor

Mucor is a genus of about 3000 species of moulds commonly found in soil, digestive systems, plant surfaces, and rotten vegetable matter (Figs 2.6 and 2.7).

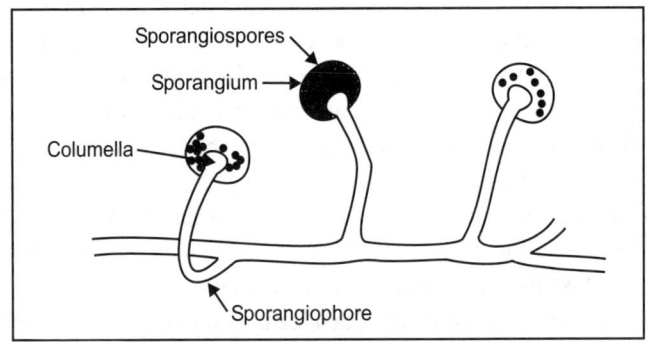

Fig. 2.6. *Mucor.*

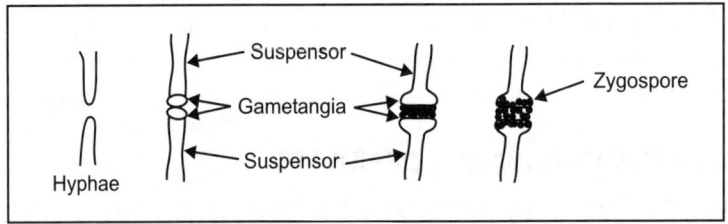

Fig. 2.7. Zygospore formation in *Mucor.*

Colonies of this fungal genus are typically white to beige or grey and fast-growing. Colonies on culture medium may grow to several centimeters in height. Older colonies become grey to brown in colour due to the development of spores.

Mucor sporangiophores can be simple or branched and form apical, globular sporangia that are supported and elevated by a column-shaped columella. *Mucor* species can be differentiated from moulds of the genera *Absidia*, *Rhizomucor*, and *Rhizopus* by the shape and insertion of the columella, and the lack of rhizoids. Some *Mucor* species produce chlamydospores.

Zygorrhynchus

These soil moulds are similar to Mucor except that the zygospore suspensors are markedly unequal in size (Fig. 2.8).

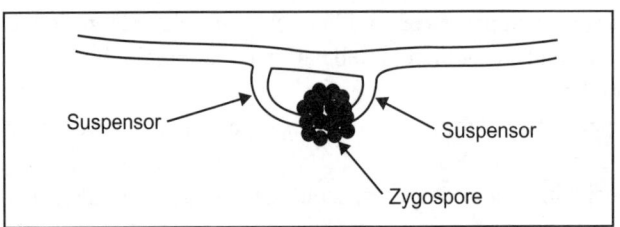

Fig. 2.8. Zygospore formation in *Zygorrhynchus*.

Rhizopus

Rhizopus is a genus of common saprobic fungi on plants and specialised parasites on animals. They are found on a wide variety of organic substrates, including 'mature fruits and vegetables', faeces, jellies, syrups, leather, bread, peanuts and tobacco. Some *Rhizopus* species are opportunistic agents of human zygomycosis (fungal infection) and can be fatal. *Rhizopus* infections are also an associated complication of diabetic ketoacidosis. The widespread genus contains about nine species (Fig. 2.9).

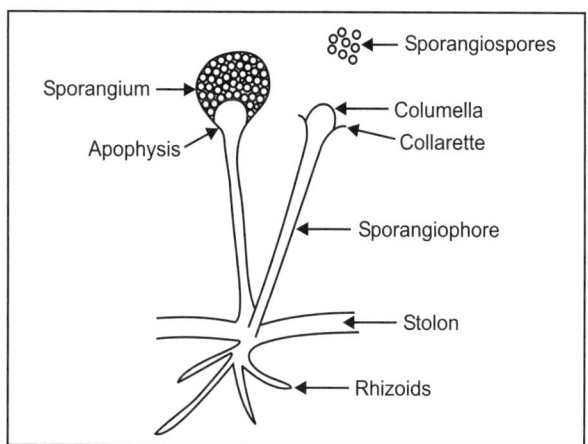

Fig. 2.9. Schematic diagram of *Rhizopus* spp.

Absidia

Absidia is a genus of fungi in the family Mucoraceae. The best known species is the pathogenic *Absidia corymbifera*, which causes zygomycosis, especially in the form of mycotic spontaneous abortion in cows. It can also cause mucormycosis in humans. It is an allergenic that could cause mucorosis in individuals with low immunity. It usually infects the lungs, nose, brain, eyesight and skin. *Absidia* spp. are ubiquitous in most environments. They are often associated with warm decaying plant matter, such as in compost heaps (Fig. 2.10).

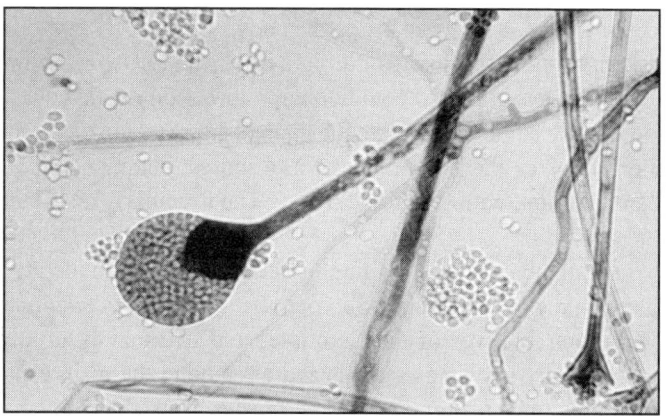

Fig. 2.10. Mature sporangium of a *Absidia* mould.

Thamnidium

Thamnidium elegans is found on meat in chilling storage, causing 'whiskers' on the meat (Fig. 2.11).

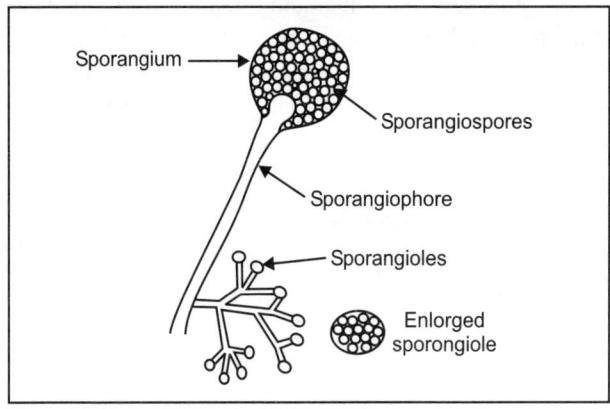

Fig. 2.11. *Thamnidium.*

Aspergillus

Aspergillus is a genus consisting of several hundred mould species found in various climates worldwide. *Aspergillus* was first catalogued in 1729 by the Italian priest and biologist Pier Antonio Micheli. Viewing the fungi under a microscope, Micheli was reminded of the shape of an aspergillum (holy water sprinkler), from Latin *spargere* (to sprinkle), and named the genus accordingly. Today 'aspergillum' is also the name of an asexual spore-forming structure common to all Aspergilli; around one-third of species are also known to have a sexual stage.

Aspergillus species are common contaminants of starchy foods (such as bread and potatoes), and grow in or on many plants and trees.

Penicillium

Penicillium is a genus of ascomycetous fungi of major importance in the natural environment as well as food and drug production. It produces penicillin, a molecule that is used as an antibiotic, which kills or stops the growth of certain kinds of bacteria inside the body.

The thallus (mycelium) typically consists of a highly branched network of multinucleate, septate, usually colourless hyphae. Many-branched conidiophores sprout on the mycelia, bearing individually constricted conidiospores. The conidiospores are the main dispersal route of the fungi, and often green.

Sexual reproduction involves the production of ascospores, commencing with the fusion of an archegonium and an antheridium, with sharing of nuclei. The irregularly distributed asci contain eight unicellular ascospores each.

Species of *Penicillium* are ubiquitous soil fungi preferring cool and moderate climates, commonly present wherever organic material is available. Saprophytic species of *Penicillium* and *Aspergillus* are among the best-known representatives of the Eurotiales and live mainly on organic biodegradable substances. They are commonly known as moulds and are among the main causes of food spoilage. Many species produce highly toxic mycotoxins. Some species have a blue colour, commonly growing on old bread and giving it a blue fuzzy texture.

Several species of the genus *Penicillium* play a central role in the production of cheese and of various meat products. To be specific, *Penicillium* moulds are found in Blue cheese. *Penicillium camemberti* and *Penicillium roqueforti* are the moulds on Camembert, Brie, Roquefort, and many other cheeses.

Trichothecium

The common species, *T. roseum* (Fig. 2.12), is a pink mould which grows on wood, paper, fruits such as apples and peaches, and vegetables such as cucumbers and cantaloupes. This mould is easily recognised by the clusters of two-celled conidia at the ends of short, erect conidiophores. Conidia have a nipplelike projection at the point of attachment, and the smaller of the two cells of each conidium is at this end.

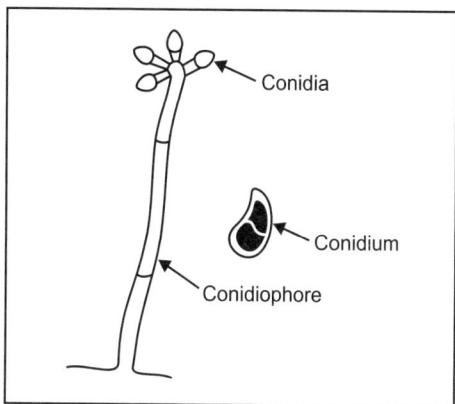

Fig. 2.12. *Trichothecium.*

Geotrichum

Geotrichum is a genus of fungi found worldwide in soil, water, air, and sewage, as well as in plants, cereals, and dairy products; it is also commonly found in normal human flora and is isolated from sputum and feces.

The genus *Geotrichum* includes several species. The most common species is *Geotrichum candidum*. *Geotrichum clavatum* and *Geotrichum fici* are among other *Geotrichum* species. *Geotrichum fici* has an intense smell resembling that of pineapple.

Neurospora

Neurospora is a genus of Ascomycete fungi. The genus name, meaning 'nerve spore' refers to the characteristic striations on the spores that resemble axons (Fig. 2.13).

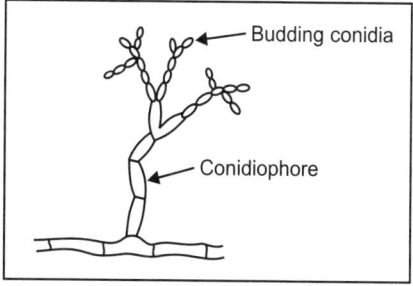

Fig. 2.13. *Neurospora (Monilia).*

The best known species in this genus is *Neurospora crassa*, a common model organism in biology. *Neurospora intermedia* var. *oncomensis* is believed to be the only mould belonging to *Neurospora* which is used in food production (to make oncom).

Sporotrichum

Among the saprophytic species is *S. carnis* (Fig. 2.14), found growing on chilled meats, where it causes 'white spot'.

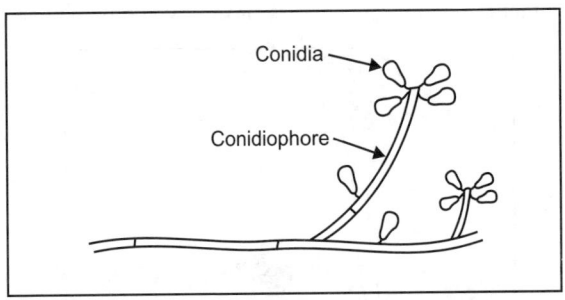

Fig. 2.14. Sporotrichum.

Botrytis

Botrytis may refer to:
1. *Botrytis*, the anamorphs of fungi of the genus *Botryotinia*.
   (a) *Botrytis cinerea*, a mould important in wine making.
2. *Botrytis*, the cauliflower cultivar group of *Brassica oleracea*.

Cephalosporium gramineum

Cephalosporium gramineum or *Hymenula cerealis* is a plant pathogen that causes Cephalosporium Stripe of wheat and other grasses. The disease can cause yield losses of up to 50 per cent by causing death of tillers and reducing seed production and seed size. The disease causes broad yellow or brown stripes along the length of the leaf and discolouration of the leaf veins.

There is very little natural resistance to the disease in wheat, control measures include crop rotation for 2–3 years in areas where the disease has become a particular problem. Currently there are no options for controlling the disease through the use of fungicides.

Trichoderma

Trichoderma is a genus of fungi that is present in all soils, where they are the most prevalent culturable fungi. Many species in this genus can be characterised as opportunistic avirulent plant symbionts.

There are 89 species in the *Trichoderma* genus. *Hypocrea* are teleomorphs of *Trichoderma* which themselves have *Hypocrea* as anamorphs.

Scopulariopsis

Scopulariopsis is a genus of anamorphic fungi that are saprobic and pathogenic to animals. The widespread genus contains 22 species.

Pullularia

Pullularia (Fig. 2.15) Ovate, hyaline conidia (blastospores of buds from preexisting cells) borne as lateral buds on all parts of the mycelium. Colonies are pale and slimy and yeastlike when young, becoming mycelial and dark and leathery in age. *P. pullulans* is a common species.

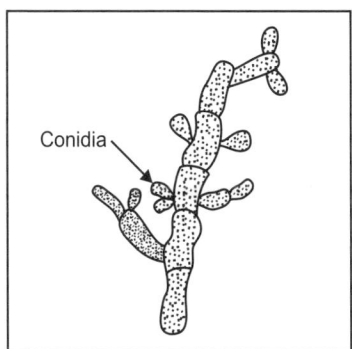

Fig. 2.15. *Pullularia.*

Cladosporium

Cladosporium is a genus of fungi including some of the most common indoor and outdoor moulds. Species produce olive-green to brown or black colonies, and have dark-pigmented conidia that are formed in simple or branching chains.

The many species of *Cladosporium* are commonly found on living and dead plant material. Some species are plant pathogens, others parasitise other fungi. *Cladosporium* spores are wind-dispersed and they are often extremely abundant in outdoor air. Indoors *Cladosporium* species may grow on surfaces when moisture is present.

Cladosporium fulvum, cause of tomato leaf mould, has been an important genetic model, in that the genetics of host resistance are understood.

Cladosporium species are rarely pathogenic to humans, but have been reported to cause infections of the skin and toenails, as well as sinusitis and pulmonary infections. If left untreated, these infections could turn into respiratory infections like pneumonia.

The airborne spores of *Cladosporium* species are significant allergens, and in large amounts they can severely affect asthmatics and people with respiratory diseases. Prolonged exposure may weaken the immune system. *Cladosporium* species produce no major mycotoxins of concern, but do produce volatile organic compounds (VOCs) associated with odours.

Helminthosporium

Helminthosporium (Fig. 2.16) Species of this genus are for the most part plant pathogens but may grow saprophytically on vegetable materials.

Alternaria

Alternaria is a genus of ascomycete fungi. *Alternaria* species are known as major plant pathogens. They are also common allergens in humans, growing indoors and causing hay fever or hypersensitivity reactions that sometimes lead to asthma. They readily cause opportunistic infections in immuno-compromised people such as AIDS patients.

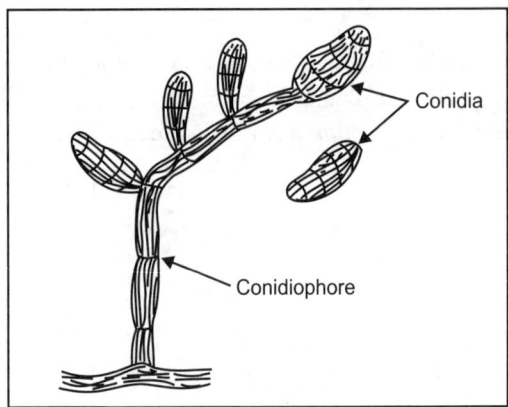

Fig. 2.16. *Helminthosporium.*

There are 299 species in the genus; they are ubiquitous in the environment and are a natural part of fungal flora almost everywhere. They are normal agents of decay and decomposition. The spores are airborne and found in the soil and water, as well as indoors and on objects. The club-shaped spores are single or form long chains. They can grow thick colonies which are usually black or gray.

At least 20 per cent of agricultural spoilage is caused by *Alternaria* species. Many human health disorders can be caused by these fungi, which grow on skin and mucous membranes, including on the eyeballs and within the respiratory tract. Allergies are common, but serious infections are rare, except in people with compromised immune systems. However, species of this fungal genus are often prolific producers of a variety of toxic compounds. The effects most of these compounds have on animal and plant health are not well known. The terms *alternariosis* and *alternariatoxicosis* are used for disorders in humans and animals caused by a fungus in this genus.

Not all *Alternaria* species are pests and pathogens; some have shown promise as biocontrol agents against invasive plant species.

Stemphylium

This, too, is a common genus. The conidia are dark and multicellular but have fewer cross walls than those a *Alternaria* and are rounded at both ends.

Fusarium

Fusarium is a large genus of filamentous fungi widely distributed in soil and in association with plants. Most species are harmless saprobes, and are relatively abundant members of the soil microbial community. Some species produce mycotoxins in cereal crops that can affect human and animal health if they enter the food chain. The main toxins produced by these *Fusarium* species are fumonisins and trichothecenes.

Fusarium contamination in barley can result in head blight, and in extreme contaminations, the barley can appear pink.

Monascus

Monascus is a genus of mould. Among the 24 known species of this genus, the red-pigmented *Monascus purpureus* is among the most important because of its use in the production of certain fermented foods in East Asia, particularly China and Japan.

Sclerotinia

Sclerotinia is a genus of fungi in the family Sclerotiniaceae. The widely distributed species contains 14 species.

YEASTS AND YEAST-LIKE FUNGI

Yeasts are eukaryotic micro-organisms classified in the kingdom Fungi, with the 1500 species currently described estimated to be only 1 per cent of all yeast species. Most reproduce asexually by budding, although a few do so by mitosis. Yeasts are unicellular, although some species with yeast forms may become multicellular through the formation of a string of connected budding cells known as pseudohyphae, or false hyphae, as seen in most moulds. Yeast size can vary greatly depending on the species, typically measuring 3–4 µm in diameter, although some yeasts can reach over 40 µm.

The yeast species *Saccharomyces cerevisiae* has been used in baking and in fermenting alcoholic beverages for thousands of years.

YEAST CULTURES

The benefit of the yeast culture comes from the metabolites produced during the fermentation process. It is suggested that the metabolites stimulate the bacteria in the hind gut of the horse, increasing their activity which results in an increase in digestion of feeds by the bacteria. The increase in activity is a result of changes in the bacteria population found in the hind gut. Moore found that the bacteria which digest fibre in the hind gut of the horse increased in numbers when the horses were supplemented with yeast culture. This increase in numbers can result in more nutrients from the feed being available to the horse. Research has shown that horses fed diets supplemented with yeast culture digested more of the dry matter and fibre than did unsupplemented horses. The digestion of fibre in the horse results in the production of volatile fatty acids which the horse uses as a source of energy.

Physiological Characteristics

Although species of yeasts may differ considerably in their physiology, those of industrial importance have enough physiological characteristics in common to permit generalisations, provided that it is kept in mind that there will be exceptions to every statement made.

In general, sugars are the best source of energy for yeasts, although oxidative yeast, e.g. the film yeasts, oxidise organic acids and alcohol. Carbon dioxide produced by bread yeasts accomplishes the leavening of bread, and alcohol made by the fermentative yeasts is the man product in the manufacture of wines, beer, industrial alcohol, and other products. They yeasts also aid in the production of flavours or 'bouquet' in wines.

Nitrogenous foods utilised vary from simple compounds such as ammonia and urea to amino acids and polypeptides. In addition, yeasts require accessory growth factors.

Yeasts may change in their physiological characteristics, especially the true, or ascospore-forming, yeasts which have a sexual method of reproduction. These yeasts can be bred for certain characteristics or may mutate to new forms. Most yeasts can be adapted to conditions which previously would not support good growth. Illustrative of different characteristics within a species in the large number of strains of *Saccharomyces cerevisiae* suited to different uses, e.g. bread strains, beer strains, wine strains, and high-alcohol-producing strains or varieties.

CLASSIFICATION AND IDENTIFICATION OF YEASTS

The true yeasts are in the subdivision *Ascomcotina*, and the false or asporogenous, yeasts are in the subdivision *Fungi imperfecti* or *Deuteromycotina*.

The principal bases for the identification and classification of genera of yeast are as follows:

1. Whether ascospores are formed.
2. If they are spore-forming:
   (a) The method of production of ascospores:
      (i) Produced without conjugation of yeast cells (parthenogenetically). Spore formation may be followed by: (a) conjugation of ascospores, and (b) conjugation of small daughter cells.
      (ii) Produced after isogamic conjugation (conjugating cells appear similar).
      (iii) Produced by heterogamic conjugation (conjugating cells differ in appearance).
   (b) Appearance of ascospores: shape, size, and colour. Most spores are spheroidal or ovoid, but some have odd shapes, e.g. most species of *Hansenula*, which look like derby hats.
   (c) the usual number of ascospores per ascus: one, two, four, or eight.
3. Appearance of vegetative cells: shape, size, colour, inclusions.
4. Method of asexual reproduction:
   (a) Budding.
   (b) Fission.
   (c) Combined budding and fission.
   (d) Arthrospores (oidia).
5. Production of a mycelium, pseudomycelium or no mycelium.
6. Growth as a film over surface of a liquid (film yeasts) or growth throughout medium.
7. Colour of macroscopic growth.
8. Physiological characteristics (used primarily to differentiate species or strains within a species):
   (a) Nitrogen and carbon sources.
   (b) Vitamin requirements.
   (c) Oxidative or fermentative: film yeasts are oxidative; other yeasts may be fermentative of fermentative and oxidative.
   (d) Lipolysis, urease activity, acid production or formation of starchlike compounds.

Yeasts of Industrial Importance

Schizosaccharomyces

Schizosaccharomyces is a genus of fission yeasts. The most well-studied species is *S. pombe*. Like the distantly related *Saccharomyces cerevisiae*, *S. pombe* is a significant model organism in the study of eukaryotic cell biology. It is particularly useful in evolutionary studies because it is thought to have diverged from the *Saccharomyces cerevisiae* lineage between 300 million and 1 billion years ago, and thus provides an evolutionarily distant comparison (Fig. 2.17).

Saccharomyces

Saccharomyces is a genus in the kingdom of fungi that includes many species of yeast. *Saccharomyces* is from Greek (sugar) and (mushroom) and means *sugar fungus*. Many members of this genus are considered very important in food production. One example is *Saccharomyces cerevisiae*, which is used in making wine, bread, and beer. Other members of this genus include *Saccharomyces bayanus*, used in making wine, and *Saccharomyces boulardii*, used in medicine.

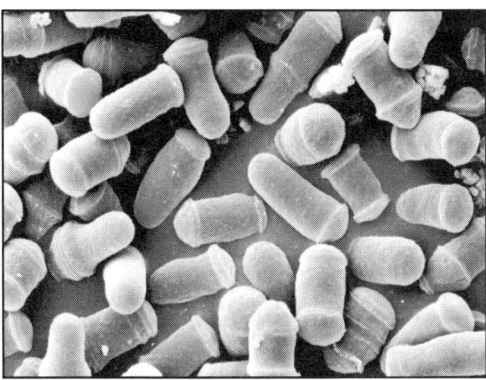

Fig. 2.17. *Schizosaccharomyces pombe.*

Colonies of *Saccharomyces* grow rapidly and mature in three days. They are flat, smooth, moist, glistening or dull, and cream to tannish cream in colour. The inability to use nitrate and ability to ferment various carbohydrates are typical characteristics of *Saccharomyces*.

Kluyveromyces

Kluyveromyces is a genus of ascomycetous yeasts in the family Saccharomycetaceae. Some of the species, such as *K. marxianus*, are the teleomorphs of *Candida species*.

Zygosaccharomyces

Zygosaccharomyces is a genus of yeast in the family Saccharomycetaceae. The yeast has a long history as a spoilage yeast within the food industry. This is mainly because it is tolerant to many of the common food preservation methods. The biochemical properties it possesses to achieve this includes high sugar tolerance (50–60 per cent), high ethanol tolerance (up to 18 per cent), high acetic acid tolerance (2.0–2.5 per cent), very high sorbic and benzoic acid tolerance (up to 800–1000 mg/l), very high molecular SO_2 tolerance (greater than 3 mg/l) and high xerotolerance.

Pichia

Pichia (*Hansenula* and *Hyphopichia* are obsolete synonyms) is a genus of yeasts in the family Saccharomycetaceae with real spherical, elliptical or oblong acuminate cells. *Pichia* is a teleomorph, and forms during sexual reproduction hat-shaped, hemispherical or round ascospores. The anamorphs of some *Pichia* species are *Candida* species. The asexual reproduction is by multilateral budding.

Today more than 100 species of this genus are known. Some of them interfere with the fermentation process for alcohol production. Most are found in decaying plants, some live in close symbiosis with insects, which live on decaying plants.

Some *Pichia* representatives can be found in raw milk and cheese, such as *P. anomola* (formerly named *Hansenula anomala*). *P. anomala* has been shown to combat the undesirable mould *Aspergillus flavus*, which contaminates food sources such as tree nuts and corn, and produces aflatoxins.

Hansenula polymorpha

Hansenula polymorpha (*Pichia angusta*) is a methylotrophic yeast with unusual characteristics. It is used as a protein factory for pharmaceuticals.

Hansenula polymorpha (*Pichia angusta*) belongs to a limited number of methylotrophic yeast species (yeasts that can grow on methanol). The range of methylotrophic yeasts includes *Candida boidinii*, *Pichia methanolica*, *Pichia pastoris* and *Hansenula polymorpha*. *H. polymorpha* is taxonomically a species of the Saccharomycetaceae family. The leading taxonomy monographs follow a recent proposal to merge the genera Pichia and Hansenula and to re-name *H. polymorpha* as *Pichia angusta*. However, many scientists desire to maintain the popular name *H. polymorpha*.

Debaryomyces

Debaryomyces is a genus of yeasts in the family Saccharomycetaceae.

Hanseniaspora

These lemon-shaped (apiculate) yeasts grow in fruit juices. *Nadsonia* yeasts are large and lemon-shaped.

Fungi Imperfecti

The Fungi imperfecti or imperfect fungi, also known as Deuteromycota, are fungi which do not fit into the commonly established taxonomic classifications of fungi that are based on biological species concepts or morphological characteristics of sexual structures because their sexual form of reproduction has never been observed; hence the name 'imperfect fungi'. Only their asexual form of reproduction is known, meaning that this group of fungus produces their spores asexually.

Fungi producing the antibiotic penicillin and those that cause athlete's foot and yeast infections are imperfect fungi. In addition, there are a number of edible imperfect fungi, including the ones that provide the distinctive characteristics of Roquefort and Camembert cheese.

Candida (fungus)

Candida is a genus of yeasts. Many species of this genus are endosymbionts of animal hosts including humans. While usually living as commensals, some *Candida* species have the potential to cause disease. Clinically, the most significant member of the genus is *Candida albicans*, which can cause infections (called candidiasis or thrush) in humans and other animals, especially in immunocompromised patients. Many *Candida* species are members of gut flora in animals, including *C. albicans* in mammalian hosts, whereas others live as endosymbionts in insect hosts.

Brettanomyces

Brettanomyces is a non-spore forming genus of yeast in the family Saccharomycetaceae, and is often colloquially referred to as '*Brett*'. The genus name *Dekkera* is used interchangeably with *Brettanomyces*, as it describes the teleomorph or spore forming form of the yeast. The cellular morphology of the yeast can vary from ovoid to long 'sausage' shaped cells. The yeast is acidogenic and when grown on glucose rich media produce large amounts of acetic acid. *Brettanomyces* is important to both the brewing and wine industries due to the sensory compounds it produces. In the wild, *Brettanomyces* lives on the skins of fruit.

Kloeckera

These are imperfect apiculate or lemon-shaped yeasts. *K. apiculata* is common on fruits and flowers and in the soil.

Trichosporon

Trichosporon is a genus of anamorphic fungi in the family Trichosporonaceae. All species of *Trichosporon* are yeasts with no known teleomorphs (sexual states). Most are typically isolated from soil, but several species occur as a natural part of the skin microbiota of humans and other animals. Proliferation of *Trichosporon* yeasts in the hair can lead to an unpleasant but non-serious condition known as white piedra. *Trichosporon* species can also cause severe opportunistic infections (trichosporonosis) in immunocompromised individuals.

Rhodotorula

Rhodotorula is a pigmented yeast, part of the Basidiomycota phylum, quite easily identifiable by distinctive orange/red colonies when grown on SDA (Sabouraud's Dextrose Agar). This distinctive colour is the result of pigments that the yeast creates to block out certain wavelengths of light that would otherwise be damaging to the cell. Colony colour can vary from being cream coloured to orange/red/pink or yellow.

Rhodotorula is a common environmental inhabitant. It can be cultured from soil, water, and air samples. It is able to scavenge nitrogenous compounds from its environment remarkably well, growing even in air which has been carefully cleaned of any fixed nitrogen contaminants. In such conditions, the nitrogen content of the dry weight of *Rhodotorula* can drop as low as 1 per cent, compared to around 14 per cent for most bacteria growing in normal conditions.

Groups of Yeasts

Film yeasts, in the general *Pichia, Hansenula, Debaryomyces, Candida*, and *Trichosporon*, grow on the surface of acid products such as sauerkraut and pickles, oxidise the organic acids, and enable less acid-tolerant organisms to continue the spoilage. *Hansenula* and *Pichia* tolerate high levels of alcohol and may oxidise it in alcoholic beverages. *Pichia* species are encouraged to grow on Jerez and Arbois wine, to which they are supposed to impart distinctive flavour and esters. *Debaryomyces* is very salt tolerant and can grow on cheese brines with as much as 24 per cent salt. The film yeasts produce little or no alcohol from sugars.

Apiculate or *lemon-shaped* yeasts, in *Saccharomycodes, hanseniaspora, nadsonia*, and *Kloeckera*, are considered objectionable in wine fermentations because they give off-flavours, low yields of alcohol, and highly volatile acid.

Osmophilic yeasts (*Saccharomyces rouxii* and *S. mellis*) grow well in an environment of high osmotic pressure, i.e. in high concentrations of sugars, salts or other solutes, causing spoilage of dry fruits, concentrated fruit juices, honey, maple sirup, and other high-sugar solutions.

Salt-tolerant yeasts grow in curing brines, salted meats and fish, soya sauce, miso paste, and tamari sauce. The most salt-tolerant of the film yeasts are species of *Debaryomyces*, which grow on curing brines and on meats and cucumbers in them, as does *Saccharomyces rouxii*, which can grow as a film on brine. Yeasts in various other genera (*Torulopsis, Brettanomyces*, and others) also grow in brines. Yeasts grow in soya sauce with its high content of salt (about 18 per cent). *Saccharomyces rouxii* is considered of great importance in the production of alcohol and flavour, but species of *Torulopsis, Pichia, Candida*, and *Trichosporon* also may grow. Film-forming *S. rouxii* and *Pichia* are sometimes involved in the spoilage of soy sauce. Similar yeasts are involved in miso production, but kinds will vary as the salt concentration is varied between 7 and 20 per cent.

BACTERIA

Bacteria are microscopic organisms whose single cells have neither a membrane-enclosed nucleus nor other membrane-enclosed organelles like mitochondria and chloroplasts. Another group of microbes, the archaea, meet these criteria but are so different from the bacteria in other ways that they must have had a long, independent evolutionary history since close to the dawn of life. In fact, there is considerable evidence that you are more closely related to the archaea than they are to the bacteria.

Morphological Characteristics Important in Food Bacteriology

One of the first steps in the identification of bacteria in food is microscopic examination to ascertain the shape, size, aggregation, structure, and staining reactions of the bacteria present. The following characteristics may be of special significance.

Encapsulation

The presence of capsules or slime may account for sliminess or ropiness of a food. In addition, capsules serve to increase the resistance of bacteria to adverse conditions, such as heat or chemicals. To the organism they may serve as a source of reserved nutrients. Most capsules are polysaccharides of dextrin, dextran or levan.

Endospore

An endospore is a dormant, tough, and temporarily non-reproductive structure produced by certain bacteria from the Firmicute phylum. The name 'endospore' is suggestive of a spore or seedlike form (*endo* means within), but it is not a true spore (i.e. not an offspring). It is a stripped-down, dormant form to which the bacterium can reduce itself. The endospore becomes important when the bacterium is experiencing an environment that is deleterious to the usual vegetative state of the bacterium, such as in desiccating conditions. Endospores enable bacteria to survive periods of environmental stress lasting at least several thousand years, and revival of spores many millions of years old has been claimed. When the environment becomes more favourable, the endospore can reactivate itself to the vegetative state. Most types of bacteria cannot change to the endospore form, but examples include *Bacillus* and *Clostridium*.

Endospores can survive without nutrients. They are resistant to ultraviolet radiation, desiccation, high temperature, extreme freezing and chemical disinfectants. Common antibacterial agents that work by destroying vegetative cell walls don't work on endospores. Endospores are commonly found in soil and water, where they may survive for long periods of time. Visualising endospores under the light microscope can be difficult due to the impermeability of the endospore wall to dyes and stains.

While the rest of a bacterial cell may stain, the endospore is left colourless. To combat this, a special stain technique called a Moeller stain is used. That allows the endospore to show up as red, while the rest of the cell stains blue.

Cultural Characteristics Important in Food Bacteriology

Bacterial growth in and on foods often is extensive enough to make the food unattractive in appearance or otherwise objectionable. Pigmented bacteria cause discolourations on the surfaces of foods; films may cover the surfaces of liquids; growth may make surfaces slimy; or growth throughout the liquids may result in undesirable cloudiness or sediment.

Physiological Characteristics Important in Food Bacteriology

The bacteriologist is concerned with the growth and activity of bacteria (and other micro-organisms) in foods and with the accompanying chemical changes. These changes include hydrolysis of complex carbohydrates to simple ones; hydrolysis of proteins to polypeptides, amino acids, and ammonia or amines; and hydrolysis of fats to glycerol and fatty acids. O–R reactions, which are utilised by the bacteria to obtain energy from foods (carbohydrates, other carbon compounds, simple nitrogen-carbon compounds, etc.), yield such products as organic acids, alcohols, aldehydes, ketones, and gases. A knowledge of the factors that favour or inhibit the growth and activity of bacteria is essential to an understanding of the principles of food preservation and spoilage.

Genera of Bacteria Important in Food Bacteriology

The following discussion emphasises the characteristics of genera of bacteria that make them important in foods and pays less attention to the characteristics used in their classification and identification.

Acetobacter

Acetobacter is a genus of acetic acid bacteria characterised by the ability to convert ethanol to acetic acid in the presence of oxygen. There are several species within this genus, and there are other bacteria capable of forming acetic acid under various conditions; but all of the *Acetobacter* are known by this characteristic ability.

Acetobacter are of particular importance commercially, because:
1. They are used in the production of vinegar (intentionally converting the ethanol in the wine to acetic acid).
2. They can destroy wine which they infect by producing excessive amounts of acetic acid or ethyl acetate, both of which can render the wine unpalatable.
3. They are used to intentionally acidify beer during long maturation periods in the production of traditional Flemish Sour Ales.
4. *A. xylinus* is the main source of microbial cellulose.

The growth of *Acetobacter* in wine can be suppressed through effective sanitation, by complete exclusion of air from wine in storage, and by the use of moderate amounts of sulphur dioxide in the wine as a preservative.

Aeromonas

Aeromonas is a Gram-negative, facultative anaerobic rod that morphologically resembles members of the family Enterobacteriaceae. Fourteen species of *Aeromonas* have been described, most of which have been associated with human diseases. The most important pathogens are *A. hydrophila*, *A. caviae*, and *A. veronii* biovar sobria. The organisms are ubiquitous in fresh and brackish water.

Although some potential virulence factors (e.g. endotoxins, hemolysins, enterotoxins, adherence factors) have been identified, their precise role is unknown. *Aeromonas* species cause:
1. Opportunistic systemic disease in immunocompromised patients.
2. Diarrheal disease in otherwise healthy individuals.
3. Wound infections.

Alcaligenes

Alcaligenes is a genus of Gram-negative, aerobic, rod-shaped bacteria. The species are motile with one or more peritrichous flagella.

Alcaligenes species have been used for the industrial production of non-standard amino acids; *A. eutrophus* also produces the biopolymer polyhydroxybutyrate (PHB).

Alteromonas

Alteromonas is a genus of Proteobacteria found in sea water, either in the open ocean or in the coast. It is Gram-negative. Its organelles consist of curved rods and a single polar flagellum.

Arthrobacter

Arthrobacter is a genus of bacteria that is commonly found in soil. All species in this genus are Gram-positive obligate aerobes that are rods during exponential growth and cocci in their stationary phase.

Colonies of *Arthrobacter* have a greenish metallic centre on mineral salts pyridone broth incubated at 20°C. This genus is distinctive because of its unusual habit of 'snapping division' in which the outer bacterial cell wall ruptures at a joint. One species, *A. crystallopoieties*, has been shown to reduce hexavalent chromium levels in contaminated soil, suggesting that it may be useful in bioremediation.

Bacillus

Bacillus is a genus of Gram-positive rod-shaped bacteria and a member of the division Firmicutes. *Bacillus* species can be obligate aerobes or facultative anaerobes, and test positive for the enzyme catalase. Ubiquitous in nature, *Bacillus* includes both free-living and pathogenic species. Under stressful environmental conditions, the cells produce oval endospores that can stay dormant for extended periods. These characteristics originally defined the genus, but not all such species are closely related, and many have been moved to other genera. Many *Bacillus* species are able to secrete large quantities of enzymes. *Bacillus amyloliquefaciens* is a species of *Bacillus* that is the source of a natural antibiotic protein barnase (a ribonuclease), alpha amylase used in starch hydrolysis, the protease subtilisin used with detergents, and the BamH1 restriction enzyme used in DNA research.

Brevibacterium

Brevibacterium is a genus of bacteria of the order Actinomycetales. They are Gram-positive soil organisms. It is the sole genus in the family Brevibacteriaceae. *Brevibacterium linens* is ubiquitously present on the human skin, where it causes foot odour. The same bacterium is also employed to ferment several cheeses such as Limburger, Port-du-Salut and Nasal. Its smell also attracts mosquitoes.

Brochotrix

These are Gram-positive rods which can form long filamentouslike chains that may fold into knotted masses. The optimum temperature for growth is 20° to 25°C, but growth can occur over a temperature range of 0° to 45°C depending on the strain. Growth can occur between pH 5.0 and 9.0 (optimum pH, 7.0) and in the presence of 6.5 to 10.0 per cent NaCl. The organisms will not survive heating at 63°C for 5 min. D values at 63°C have been calculated to be 0.1 min. They can spoil a wide variety of meats and meat products when they are stored aerobically or vacuum packed and held refrigerated. *B. thermosphacta* is the only species listed.

Campylobacter

Campylobacter is a genus of bacteria that are Gram-negative, spiral, and microaerophilic. Motile, with either uni- or bi-polar flagella, the organisms have a characteristic spiral/corkscrew appearance and are oxidase-positive. *Campylobacter jejuni* is now recognised as one of the main causes of bacterial foodborne disease in many developed countries. At least a dozen species of *Campylobacter* have been implicated in human disease, with *C. jejuni* and *C. coli* the most common. *C. fetus* is a cause of spontaneous abortions in cattle and sheep, as well as an opportunistic pathogen in humans.

Clostridium

Clostridium is a genus of Gram-positive bacteria, belonging to the Firmicutes. They are obligate anaerobes capable of producing endospores. Individual cells are rod-shaped, which gives them their name, from the Greek *kloster* or spindle. These characteristics traditionally defined the genus, however many species originally classified as *Clostridium* have been reclassified in other genera.

Corynebacterium

Corynebacterium is a genus of Gram-positive rod-shaped bacteria. They are widely distributed in nature and are mostly innocuous. Some are useful in industrial settings such as *C. glutamicum*. Others can cause human disease. *C. diphtheriae*, for example, is the pathogen responsible for diphtheria.

Desulfotomaculum

Desulfotomaculum is a genus of Gram-positive, obligately anaerobic soil bacteria. A type of sulphate-reducing bacteria, *Desulfotomaculum* can cause food spoilage in poorly processed canned foods. Their presence can be identified by the release of hydrogen sulphide gas with its rotten egg smell when the can is first opened. They are endospore-forming bacteria.

Enterobacter

Enterobacter is a genus of common Gram-negative, facultatively-anaerobic, rod-shaped bacteria of the family Enterobacteriaceae. Several strains of these bacteria are pathogenic and cause opportunistic infections in immunocompromised (usually hospitalised) hosts and in those who are on mechanical ventilation. The urinary and respiratory tract are the most common sites of infection. It is also a fecal coliform, along with *Escherichia*. Two clinically-important species from this genus are *E. aerogenes* and *E. cloacae*.

Erwinia

Erwinia is a genus of Enterobacteriaceae bacteria containing mostly plant pathogenic species. It is a Gram-negative bacterium related to *E. coli*, *Shigella*, *Salmonella* and *Yersinia*. It is primarily a rod-shaped bacteria. A well-known member of this genus is the species *E. amylovora*, which causes fireblight on apple, pear, and other Rosaceous crops. *Erwinia carotovora* (also known as *Pectobacterium carotovorum*) is another species, which causes diseases in many plants. These species produce pectolytic enzymes that hydrolyse pectin between individual plant cells. This causes the cells to separate, a disease plant pathologists term bacterial soft rot.

Escherichia

Escherichia is a genus of Gram-negative, non-spore forming, facultatively anaerobic, rod-shaped bacteria from the family Enterobacteriaceae. In those species which are inhabitants of the gastrointestinal tracts of warm-blooded animals, *Escherichia* species provide a portion of the microbially-derived vitamin K for their host. A number of the species of *Escherichia* are pathogenic. While *Escherichia coli* is responsible for the vast majority of *Escherichia*-related pathogenesis, other members of the genus have also been implicated in human disease.

Flavobacterium

Flavobacterium is a genus of Gram-negative, non-motile and motile, rod-shaped bacteria that consists of ten recognised species, as well as three newly proposed species (*F. gondwanense*, *F. salegens*, and *F. scophthalmum*). Flavobacteria are found in soil and freshwater in a variety of environments. Several species are known to cause disease in freshwater fish.

Gluconobacter

Species can oxidise ethanol to acetic acid. *G. oxydans* causes ropiness in beer following viscous growth in beer or wort.

Halobacterium

In taxonomy, *Halobacterium* is a genus of the Halobacteriaceae. The genus *Halobacterium* ('Salt' or 'Ocean Bacterium') consists of several species of archaea with an aerobic metabolism which require an environment with a high concentration of salt; many of their proteins will not function in low-salt environments. They grow on amino acids in their aerobic conditions. Their cell walls are also quite different from those of bacteria, as ordinary lipoprotein membranes fail in high salt concentrations. In shape, they may be either rods or cocci, and in colour, either red or purple. They reproduce using binary fission (by constriction), and are motile. *Halobacterium* grows best in a 42°C environment.

Klebsiella

Klebsiella is a genus of non-motile, Gram-negative, oxidase-negative, rod-shaped bacteria with a prominent polysaccharide-based capsule. Frequent human pathogens, *Klebsiella* organisms can lead to a wide range of disease states, notably pneumonia, urinary tract infections, septicemia, ankylosing spondylitis, and soft tissue infections. *Klebsiella* species are ubiquitous in nature.

Family Lactobacillaceae

Lactobacillus

Lactobacillus is a genus of Gram-positive facultative anaerobic or microaerophilic bacteria. They are a major part of the lactic acid bacteria group, named as such because most of its members convert lactose and other sugars to lactic acid. They are common and usually benign. In humans they are present in the vagina and the gastrointestinal tract, where they are symbiotic and make up a small portion of the gut flora. Many species are prominent in decaying plant material. The production of lactic acid makes its environment acidic, which inhibits the growth of some harmful bacteria. Several members of the genus have had their genome sequenced. Some *Lactobacillus* species are used for the production of yogurt, cheese, sauerkraut, pickles, beer, wine, cider, kimchi, chocolate, and other fermented foods, as well as animal feeds, such as silage. Sourdough bread is made using a 'starter culture,' which is a symbiotic culture of yeast and lactic acid bacteria growing in a water and flour medium. Lactobacilli, especially *L. casei* and *L. brevis*, are some of the most common beer spoilage organisms. The species operate by lowering the pH of the fermenting substance by creating the lactic acid, neutralising it to the desired extent.

Leuconostoc

Leuconostoc is a genus of Gram-positive bacteria, placed within the family of Leuconostocaceae. They are generally ovoid cocci often forming chains. *Leuconostoc* sp. are intrinsically resistant to vancomycin and are catalase-negative (which distinguishes them from staphylococci). All species within this genus are heterofermentative and are able to produce dextran from sucrose. They are generally slime-forming.

Blamed for causing the 'stink' when creating a sourdough starter, some species are also capable of causing human infection. Because they are an uncommon cause of disease in humans, standard commercial identification kits are often unable to identify the organism.

Leuconostoc is, along with other lactic acid bacteria such as *Pediococcus* and *Lactobacillus* responsible for the fermentation of cabbage, making it Sauerkraut. In this process the sugars in fresh cabbage are transformed to lactic acids which give it a sour flavour and good keeping qualities.

Listeria

Listeria is a bacterial genus containing six species. *Listeria* species are Gram-positive bacilli and are typified by *L. monocytogenes*, the causative agent of listeriosis. *Listeria ivanovii* is a pathogen of ruminants, and can infect mice in the laboratory, although it is only rarely the cause of human disease.

Listeria monocytogenes is a bacterium commonly found in soil, stream water, sewage, plants, and food. Each bacterium is Gram-positive and rod-shaped. *Listeria* are known to be the bacteria responsible for listeriosis, a rare but potentially lethal foodborne infection. Listeria has been found in uncooked meats, uncooked vegetables, unpasteurised milk, foods made from unpasteurised milk, and processed foods. Pasteurisation and sufficient cooking kill listeria; however, contamination may occur after cooking and before packaging. For example, meat-processing plants producing ready-to-eat foods, such as hot dogs and deli meats, must follow extensive sanitation policies and procedures to prevent listeria contamination.

Micrococcus

Micrococcus is a genus of bacteria in the Micrococcaceae family. *Micrococcus* occurs in a wide range of environments, including water, dust, and soil. Micrococci have Gram-positive spherical cells ranging from about 0.5 to 3 micrometres in diameter and typically appear in tetrads. *Micrococcus* has a substantial cell wall, which may comprise as much as 50 per cent of the cell mass. The genome of *Micrococcus* is rich in guanine and cytosine (GC), typically exhibiting 65 to 75 per cent GC-content. Micrococci often carry plasmids (ranging from 1 to 100 MDa in size) that provide the organism with useful traits.

Mycobacterium

Mycobacterium is a genus of Actinobacteria, given its own family, the Mycobacteriaceae. The genus includes pathogens known to cause serious diseases in mammals, including tuberculosis (*Mycobacterium tuberculosis*) and leprosy (*Mycobacterium leprae*). The Latin prefix '*myco*—' means both *fungus* and *wax*; its use here reflects the 'waxy' compounds that compose parts of the cell wall.

Pediococcus

Pediococcus is a genus of Gram-positive lactic acid bacteria, placed within the family of Lactobacillaceae. They usually occur in pairs or tetrads, and divide along two planes of symmetry, as do the other lactic acid cocci genera Aerococci and Tetragenococcus. They are purely homofermentative. *Pediococcus dextrinicus* has recently been reassigned to the genus *Lactobacillus*.

Pediococcus is, along with other lactic acid bacteria such as *Leuconostoc* and *Lactobacillus* responsible for the fermentation of cabbage, making it Sauerkraut. In this process the sugars in fresh cabbage are transformed to lactic acids which give it a sour flavour and good keeping qualities. *Pediococcus* bacteria are usually considered contaminants of beer and wine although their presence is sometimes desired in beer styles such as Lambic.

Photobacterium

Photobacterium is a genus of Gram-negative bacteria in the family *Vibrionaceae*. Members of the genus are bioluminescent, that is they have the ability to emit light.

Many species, including *Photobacterium leiognathi* and *Photobacterium phosphoreum*, live in symbiosis with marine organisms.

Species such as *Photobacterium profundum* are adapted for optimal growth in the deep cold seas making it both a psychrophile (an organism capable of growth and reproduction in cold temperatures) and a piezophile (an organism which thrives at high pressures).

Propionibacterium

Propionibacterium is a genus of bacteria named for their unique metabolism. They are able to synthesise propionic acid by using unusual transcarboxylase enzymes.

Its members are primarily facultative parasites and commensals of humans and other animals, living in and around the sweat glands, sebaceous glands, and other areas of the skin. They are virtually ubiquitous and do not cause problems for most people, but propionobacteria have been implicated in acne and other skin conditions.

The strain *Propionibacterium freudenreichii* subsp. *shermanii* is used in cheesemaking to create CO_2 bubbles that become 'eyes', round holes in the cheese.

Proteus

Bacteria of this genus have been involved in the spoilage of meats, seafood, and eggs. The presence of these bacteria in large numbers in unrefrigerated foods has made them suspect as a cause of food poisoning.

Pseudomonas

Pseudomonas is a genus of gamma proteobacteria, belonging to the larger family of pseudomonads. Recently, 16S rRNA sequence analysis has redefined the taxonomy of many bacterial species. As a result, the genus *Pseudomonas* includes strains formerly classified in the genera *Chryseomonas* and *Flavimonas*. Other strains previously classified in the genus *Pseudomonas* are now classified in the genera *Burkholderia* and *Ralstonia*.

Salmonella

Salmonella is a genus of rod-shaped, Gram-negative, non-spore-forming, predominantly motile enterobacteria with diameters around 0.7 to 1.5 µm, lengths from 2 to 5 µm, and flagella which grade in all directions (i.e. peritrichous). They are chemoorganotrophs, obtaining their energy from oxidation and reduction reactions using organic sources, and are facultative anaerobes.

Salmonella is closely related to the *Escherichia* genus and are found worldwide in cold- and warm-blooded animals (including humans), and in the environment. They cause illnesses like typhoid fever, paratyphoid fever, and the foodborne illness.

Serratia

Serratia is a genus of Gram-negative, facultatively anaerobic, rod-shaped bacteria of the Enterobacteriaceae family. The most common species in the genus, *S. marcescens*, is normally the only pathogen and usually causes nosocomial infections. However, rare strains of *S. plymuthica*, *S. liquefaciens*, *S. rubidaea*, and *S. odoriferae* have caused diseases through infection. Members of this genus produce characteristic red pigment, prodigiosin, and can be distinguished from other members of the family Enterobacteriaceae by its unique production of three enzymes: DNase, lipase, and gelatinase. *Serratia* infection has caused endocarditis and osteomyelitis in people addicted to heroin.

Shigella

Shigella is a genus of Gram-negative, non-spore forming rod-shaped bacteria closely related to *Escherichia coli* and *Salmonella*. The causative agent of human shigellosis, *Shigella* causes disease in primates, but not in other mammals. It is only naturally found in humans and apes. During infection, it typically causes dysentery.

Shigella infection is typically via ingestion (fecal–oral contamination); depending on age and condition of the host as few as 100 bacterial cells can be enough to cause an infection. *Shigella* causes dysentery that results in the destruction of the epithelial cells of the intestinal mucosa in the cecum and rectum. Some strains produce enterotoxin and Shiga toxin, similar to the verotoxin of *E. coli* O157:H7.

Sporolactobacillus

Sporolactobacillus is a genus of anaerobic endospore-forming Gram-positive motile rod-shaped lactic acid bacteria.

Members of this genus are catalase-negative, do not reduce nitrates to nitrites, and do not form indole. Lactic acid is produced actively without liberation of gas from glucose, fructose, mannose, sucrose, maltose, trehalose, raffinose, inulin, mannitol, sorbitol and alpha-methyl glucoside.

Sporolactobacillus grows readily at temperatures between 25°–40°C. The optimal temperature for growth lies around 35°C.

Sporosarcina

A Gram-positive coccus that forms endospores. *S. ureae* and *S. halophila* are the two species listed.

Staphylococcus

Staphylococcus is a genus of Gram-positive bacteria. Under the microscope they appear round (cocci), and form in grape-like clusters.

The *Staphylococcus* genus includes at least forty species. Of these, nine have two subspecies and one has three subspecies. Most are harmless and reside normally on the skin and mucous membranes of humans and other organisms. Found worldwide, they are a small component of soil microbial flora.

Streptococcus

Streptococcus is a genus of spherical Gram-positive bacteria belonging to the phylum Firmicutes and the lactic acid bacteria group. Cellular division occurs along a single axis in these bacteria, and thus they grow in chains or pairs, *streptos*, meaning easily bent or twisted, like a chain (twisted chain). Contrast this with staphylococci, which divide along multiple axes and generate grape-like clusters of cells. *Streptococci* are oxidase- and catalase-negative, and many are facultative anaerobes.

Streptomyces

Streptomyces is the largest genus of *Actinobacteria* and the type genus of the family Streptomycetaceae. Over 500 species of *Streptomyces* bacteria have been described. As with the other *Actinobacteria*, streptomycetes are Gram-positive, and have genomes with high GC-content. Found predominantly in soil and decaying vegetation, most streptomycetes produce spores, and are noted for their distinct 'earthy' odour which results from production of a volatile metabolite, geosmin.

Streptomycetes are characterised by a complex secondary metabolism. They produce over two-thirds of the clinically useful antibiotics of natural origin (e.g. neomycin, chloramphenicol). The now uncommonly-used streptomycin takes its name directly from *Streptomyces*. Streptomycetes are infrequent pathogens, though infections in human such as mycetoma can be caused by *S. somaliensis* and *S. sudanensis* and in plants can be caused by *S. caviscabies* and *S. scabies*.

Vibrio

Vibrio is a genus of Gram-negative bacteria possessing a curved rod shape, several species of which can cause foodborne infection, usually associated with eating undercooked seafood. Typically found in saltwater, *Vibrio* are facultative anaerobes that test positive for oxidase and do not form spores. All members of the genus are motile and have polar flagella with sheaths. Recent phylogenies have been constructed based on a suite of genes (multi-locus sequence analysis).

Several species of *Vibrio* are pathogens. Most disease causing strains are associated with gastroenteritis but can also infect open wounds and cause septicemia.

Yersinia

Yersinia is a genus of bacteria in the family Enterobacteriaceae. *Yersinia* are Gram-negative rod shaped bacteria, a few micrometres long and fractions of a micrometre in diameter, and are facultative anaerobes. Some members of *Yersinia* are pathogenic in humans; in particular, *Y. pestis* is the causative agent of the plague.

GROUPS OF BACTERIA IMPORTANT IN FOOD BACTERIOLOGY

Bacteria important in foods often are grouped on the basis of one common characteristic without regard for their systematic classification. It is obvious that some bacterial species might be included in two or more of these artificial groups.

Lactic Acid-Forming Bacteria, or Lactics

The most important characteristic of the lactic acid bacteria is their ability to ferment sugars to lactic acid. This may be desirable in making products such as sauerkraut and cheese but undesirable in terms of spoilage of wines. Because they form acid rapidly and commonly in considerable amounts, they usually eliminate for the time being much of the competition from other micro-organisms.

The major genera include *Leuconostoc, Lactobacillus, Streptococcus,* and *Pediococcus*.

Acetic Acid-Forming Bacteria, or Acetics

Most of acetic acid bacteria now belong to one of two genera, *Acetobacter* and *Gluconobacter*. Both oxidise ethyl alcohol to acetic acid, but *Acetobacter* is capable of oxidising acetic acid further to carbon dioxide. Characteristics that make the acetic acid bacteria important are (i) their ability to oxidise ethanol to acetic acid, making them useful in vinegar manufacture and harmful in alcoholic beverages, (ii) their strong oxidising power, which may result in the oxidation of the desired product, acetic acid, by undesirable species or by desirable species under unfavourable conditions; this oxidising power may be useful, as in the oxidation of D-sorbitol to L-sorbose in the preparation of ascorbic acid by synthetic methods, and (iii) excessive sliminess of some species, e.g. *Acetobacter aceti* subsp. *suboxydans*, that clog vinegar generators.

Butyric Acid-Forming Bacteria, or Butyrics

Most bacteria of this group are spore-forming anaerobes of the genus *Clostridium.*

Propionic Acid-Forming Bacteria, or Propionics

Most bacteria of this group are in the genus *Propionibacterium,* although propionic cocci have been reported.

Proteolytic Bacteria

This is a heterogeneous group of actively proteolytic bacteria which produce extracellular proteinases, so termed because the enzymes diffuse outside the cells. All bacteria have proteinases inside the cell, but only a limited number of kinds have extracellular proteinases. The proteolytic bacteria may be divided into those which are aerobic or facultative and may be spore-forming or not and those which are anaerobic and spore-forming. *Bacillus cereus* is an aerobic, spore-forming, proteolytic bacterium, *Pseudomonas fluorescens* is nonspore-forming and aerobic to facultative, and *Clostridium sporogenes* is spore forming and anaerobic. Many of the species of *Clostridium, Bacillus, Pseudomonas*, and *Proteus* are proteolytic. Some bacteria, termed 'acid-proteolytic', carry on an acid fermentation and proteolysis simultaneously. *Streptococcus faecalis* var. *liquefaciens* and *Micrococcus caseolyticus* are acid-proteolytic. Some bacteria are putrefactive, i.e. they decompose proteins anaerobically to produce foul-smelling compounds such as hydrogen sulphide, mercaptans, amines, indole, and fatty acids. Most proteolytic species of *Clostridium* are putrefactive, as are some species of *Proteus, Pseudomonas,* and other genera of nonsporeformers. Putrefaction of split products of proteins also can take place. Some *Pseudomonas* species are known to produce proteinase that can survive ultrahigh heat treatments.

Lipolytic Bacteria

This is a heterogeneous group of bacteria which produce lipases enzymes which catalyse the hydrolysis of fats to fatty acids and glycerol. Many of the aerobic, actively proteolytic bacteria also are lipolytic. *Pseudomonas fluorescens,* for example, is strongly lipolytic. *Pseudomonas, Alcaligenes, Staphylococcus, Serratia,* and *Micrococcus* are genera that contain lipolytic species. Many of the microbial lipases are resistant to processing techniques. The absence of viable lipolytic bacteria from a spoiled food should not be considered as proof that the product is free of microbial lipases.

Saccharolytic Bacteria

These bacteria hydrolyse disaccharides or polysaccharides to simpler sugars. A limited number of kinds of bacteria are amylolytic, i.e. possess amylase to bring about the hydrolysis of starch outside the cell. *Bacillus subtilis* and *Clostridium butyricum* are amylolytic. Few kinds of bacteria can hydrolyse cellulose. Species of *Clostridium* sometimes are classified as proteolytic ones that may or may not attack sugars or saccharolytic ones that attack sugars but not proteins. *C. lentoputrescens* is proteolytic but ordinarily does not ferment carbohydrates, whereas *C. butyricum* is nonproteolytic but ferments sugars.

Pectinolytic Bacteria

Pectins are complex carbohydrates that are responsible for cell-wall rigidity in vegetables and fruits. Pectic substances derived from citrus fruits can be used in commercial products as gelling agents. A variety of pectolytic enzymes called pectinase may be responsible for softening of plant tissues or loss of gelling power or body in various foods. Species of *Erwinia*, *Bacillus*, *Clostridium*, *Achromobacter*, *Aeromonas*, *Arthrobacter*, and *Flavobacterium* as well as species of moulds may be pectinolytic.

Thermophilic Bacteria or Thermophiles

These bacteria, with an optimal temperature at least above 45°C but usually 55°C be or above, are important in foods held at high temperatures. Thermophilic flat sour spoilage of low-acid canned foods is caused by *B. stearothermophilus*. Gaseous thermophilic spoilage of canned foods is a result of growth by *C. thermosaccharolyticum*.

Thermoduric Bacteria

Thermoduric bacteria are usually defined as those which can survive a heat treatment such as pasteurisation. *Bacillus* species, *micrococci*, and *enterococci* can survive pasteurisation of liquid eggs. Bacteria in the genera *Clostridium*, *Bacillus*, *Micrococcus*, *Streptococcus*, *Lactobacillus*, and *Microbacterium* are frequently encountered in foods. Occasionally moulds such as *Byssochlamys fulva* and even *Aspergillus* and *Penicillium* are thermoduric. Some thermoduric bacteria, such as *Bacillus* and enteroccocci, can also be psychrotrophic. In milk, where higher pasteurisation and longer refrigeration times are significant, these heat-resistant, or thermoduric, psychrotrophs often can be found.

Psychrotrophic Bacteria or Psychrotrophs

These bacteria are able to grow at commercial refrigeration temperatures. Unlike psychrophiles, psychrotrophs do not have their optimal temperature for growth at refrigeration temperatures; rather, their optimum is usually between 25°C and 30°C. Most of the bacteria responsible for the loss of quality in nonsterile refrigerated foods, excluding seafoods, are psychrotrophs. Psychrotrophic bacteria are found chiefly in the genera *Pseudomonas*, *Flavobacterium*, *Achromobacter*, and *Alcaligenes*, although *Micrococcus*, *Lactobacillus*, *Enterobacter*, *Arthrobacter*, and other genera may contain psychrotrophic species. Additionally, various yeasts and moulds are able to grow at refrigeration temperatures.

Halophilic Bacteria or Halophiles

Truly halophilic bacteria require certain minimal concentrations of dissolved sodium chloride for growth. Those bacteria, including *Pseudomonas*, *Moraxella*, *Flavobacterium*, *Acinetobacter*, and *Vibrio* species, which grow best in media with 0.5 to 3.0 per cent salt, are considered slightly halophilic. These micro-organisms are isolated from many species of fish and shellfish. Bacteria which are isolated from foods such as salted fish, brined meats, and some salted vegetables and which grow best in media with 3.0 to 15 per cent salt are referred to as moderate halophiles. Such bacteria are found in the genera *Bacillus*, *Micrococcus*, *Vibrio*, *Acinetobacter*, and *Moraxella*. Occasionally in heavily brined foods, 15 to 30 per cent salt, extreme halophiles such as *Halobacterium* and *Halococcus* species can be isolated. Frequently, they are also pigmented pink or red. Other bacteria are salt-tolerant, i.e. halotolerant bacteria can grow with or without salt. Usually they are capable of growing in foods containing 5.0 per cent salt or more;

they include some *Bacillus, Micrococcus, Corynebacterium, Streptococcus,* and *Clostridium* species. Other halophilic or halotolerant bacteria important in foods are found in the genera *Sarcina, Pseudomonas, Pediococcus,* and *Alcaligenes.*

Osmophilic or Saccharophilic Bacteria

The most frequently encountered osmophilic micro-organisms in foods are various species of yeasts. Osmophilic bacteria are those which grow in high concentrations of sugar; however, most bacteria called osmophiles are merely sugartolerant, e.g. species of *Leuconostoc.*

Pigmented Bacteria

Colours produced by pigmented bacteria growing on or in foods range through the visible spectrum and also include black and white. Examples will be numerous in a subsequent discussion of spoilage of foods. All species in some genera are pigmented, as in *Flavobacterium* (yellow to orange) and *Serratia* (red). Pigmented species are found in many genera; many species of *Micrococcus* are pigmented, for example. Also, pigmented varieties occur within some species, e.g. the rust-coloured *Lactobacillus plantarum* that discolours cheese. *Halobacterium* species are pigmented pink, red or red to orange. *Halococcus* species are pigmented red or red to orange.

Slime- or Rope-Forming Bacteria

Examples of these bacteria already have been given: *Alcaligenes viscolactis, Enterobacter aerogenes,* and *Klebsiella oxytoca,* causing ropiness of milk, and *Leuconostoc* spp., producing slime in sucrose solutions and slimy surface growth of various bacteria occurring on foods. Some of the species of *Streptococcus* and *Lactobacillus* have varieties that make milk slimy or ropy. A micrococcus makes curing solutions for meats ropy. Strains of *Lactobacillus plantarum* and other lactobacilli may cause ropiness in various fruit, vegetable, and grain products, e.g. in cider, sauerkraut, and beer. Some *Bacillus* species are responsible for ropiness in bread.

Gas-Forming Bacteria

Many kinds of bacteria produce such small amounts of gas and yield it so slowly that it ordinarily is not detected. This sometimes is true of the heterofermentative lactics, although under other conditions gas evolution is evident. Among the genera that contain gas-forming bacteria are *Leuconostoc, Lactobacillus* (heterofermentative), *Propionibacterium, Escherichia, Enterobacter, Proteus, Bacillus* (the aerobacilli), and *Clostridium.* Bacteria of the first three genera produce only carbon dioxide, and those of the other genera yield both carbon dioxide and hydrogen.

Coliform and Fecal Coliform Group

Coliforms are short rods that are defined as aerobic and facultative anaerobic, Gram-negative, non-spore-forming bacteria which ferment lactose with gas formation. The leading species of coliform bacteria are *Escherichia coli* and *Enterobacter aerogenes*; however, as many as twenty species may conform to these criteria, including species of other Enterobacteriaceae and even *Aeromonas* species. The fecal coliform group includes coliforms capable of growth at an elevated temperature (44.5° or 45°C). The original purpose of the elevated incubation tests was to differentiate coliforms of fecal origin from those of nonfecal origin. The designation 'fecal coliform' or 'coliform' is not taxonomically valid; rather, the terms refer to groups of bacteria that can grow under specific test conditions.

Procedures for coliform counts, fecal coliform counts, and even *E. coli* counts on foods are widely used and accepted as indicators. The use of 'indicator' micro-organisms began with the use of *E. coli* testing in water as a substitute for the testing of *Salmonella typhi*. The concept is based on Shardingen's suggestion in 1892 that members of the species we now call *E. coli* be used as an index or indicator of fecal pollution since they can be recovered with less difficulty than *Salmonella* species. Other indicator groups or tests suggested or used include the fecal streptococci or enterococci, the Enterobacteriaceae, *staphylococci* (suggesting the possible presence of *S. aureus* enterotoxin or handling abuse), and the presence of *Geotrichum candidum*, the machinery mould, as an indicator of plant sanitation and contaminated equipment.

Some of the characteristics that make the coliform bacteria important in food spoilage are: (i) their ability to grow well in a variety of substrates and to utilise a number of carbohydrates and some other organic compounds as food for energy and a number of fairly simple nitrogenous compounds as a source of nitrogen, (ii) their ability to synthesise most of the necessary vitamins, (iii) the ability of the group to grow well over a fairly wide range of temperatures, from below 10° to about 46°C, (iv) their ability to produce considerable amounts of acid and gas from sugars, (v) their ability to cause off-flavours, often described as 'unclean' or 'barny', and (vi) the ability of *E. aerogenes* to cause sliminess or ropiness of foods.

Chapter 3

Contamination of Foods

INTRODUCTION

Food contamination can come in the form of bacteria, viruses or parasitic organisms. People who become ill as a result of eating contaminated food may experience a variety of symptoms, including fever, abdominal pain, bloating, diarrhea, vomiting and dehydration. Most of these illnesses are short-lived and can be treated with fluids and electrolytes. Because of the extensive nature of the food industry when harvesting, preparing and handling food, contamination has a number of potential sources.

AGRICULTURAL CONTAMINATION

All cultivated or farmed food, whether fruits and vegetables or livestock and seafood, has a high potential for contamination by both biological organisms and chemicals. The sources of these contaminants can be air, dust, water, insects, rodents, equipment, sewage or employees who work hands-on with any of the foods during any stage of the cultivation or processing. Chemical contamination may occur from pesticide or herbicide use. Improper storage of food items also encourages the growth of microbial pathogens. Sanitation techniques, including cleanliness and proper disposal of sewage and waste products, may effectively minimise or eliminate the potential for contamination.

The natural surface flora of plants varies with the plant but usually includes species of *Pseudomonas*, *Alcaligenes*, *Flavobacterium*, and *Micrococcus* and coliforms and lactic acid bacteria. Lactic acid bacterial include *Lactobacillus brevis* and *plantarum*, *Leuconostoc mesenteroides* and *dextranicum*, and *Streptococcus faecium* and *faecalis*. *Bacillus* species, yeasts, and moulds also may be present. The numbers of bacteria will depend on the plant and its environment and may range from a few hundred or thousand per square centimetre of surface to millions. The surface of a well-washed tomato, for example, may show 400 to 700 micro-organisms per square centimetre, while an unwashed tomato would have several thousand. Outer tissue of unwashed cabbage might contain 1 million to 2 million micro-organisms per gram, but washed and trimmed cabbage might contain 2,00,000 to 5,00,000. The inner tissue of the cabbage, where the surface of the leaves would harbour primarily the natural flora, contains fewer kinds of lower numbers, ranging from a few hundred to 1,50,000 per gram. Exposed surfaces of plants become contaminated from soil, water, sewage, air, and animals, so that micro-organisms from these sources are added to the natural flora. Whenever conditions for growth of natural flora and contaminants are present, increases in number of special kinds of micro-organisms take place, especially following harvesting, as will be discussed subsequently. Some fruits have been found to contain viable micro-organisms in their interior. Normal, healthy tomatoes have been shown to contain *Pseudomonas*, coliforms, *Achromobacter*, *Micrococcus*, and *Corynebacterium*, and yeasts have been found inside undamaged fruits. Organisms also have been found in healthy root and tuber vegetables.

FROM ANIMALS

According to the Centres for Disease Control and Prevention, raw animal products are the most contaminated food sources. This category includes all meats and poultry, dairy products, eggs and shellfish. The actual source of the contamination may come from diseased animals, contaminated feed, water, storage or food processing. For example, hamburger may consist of meat from several different animals, but just one animal could be the source of contamination. Unsanitary conditions in processing plants are also a major cause of the spread of bacteria and viruses.

Sources of micro-organisms from animals include the surface flora, the flora of the respiratory tract, and the flora of the gastrointestinal tract. The natural surface flora of meat animals usually is not as important as the contaminating micro-organisms from their intestinal or respiratory tracts. However, hides, hooves, and hair contain not only large numbers of micro-organisms from soil, manure, feed, and water but also important kinds of spoilage organisms. Feathers and feet of poultry carry heavy contamination from similar sources. The skin of many meat animals may contain micrococci, staphylococci and beta-hemolytic streptococci. Staphylococci on the skin or from the respiratory tract may find their way onto the carcass and then to the final raw product. The feces and fecal-contaminated products of animals can contain many enteric organisms, including *Salmonella*. Salmonellosis in animals can result in contamination of animal products or by-products and thus contaminate foods derived from them with *Salmonella*.

Pig or beef carcasses may be contaminated with salmonellae. Because of further processing and handling, very few of these organisms result in human salmonellosis. Actually, meat from slaughtered animals is not frequently associated with human salmonellosis. Statistics in recent years have incriminated eggs and egg products much more frequently. Salmonellosis associated with eggs has been reduced because of the pasteurisation of egg products.

Many infectious disease agents of animals can be transmitted to people via foods, but this represents only one of several transmission routes. Many of these diseases have been reduced or eliminated by improvement in animal husbandry, but a listing of agents of animal disease causing infections from foods would include *Brucella*, *Mycobacterium tuberculosis*, *Coxiella*, *Listeria*, *Campylobacter*, beta-hemolytic streptococci, *Salmonella*, enteropathogenic *Escherichia coli*, parasites, and viruses.

Animals, from the lowest to the highest forms, contribute their wastes and finally their bodies to the soil and water and to plants growing there. Little attention has been paid to the direct contamination of food plants from this source, except insofar as coliform bacteria or enterococci may be added. Insects and birds cause mechanical damage to fruits and vegetables, introduce micro-organisms, and open the way for microbial spoilage.

Animal Feed Industry

There is considerable evidence that animal feed is frequently contaminated with foodborne bacterial pathogens. Non-Typhi serotypes of *S. enterica* were reported in US poultry feed. Studies from around the world have documented the presence of *S. enterica* in a wide variety of animal feeds. Outlines of the steps in animal feed manufacture are given in Fig. 3.1.

Surveys done by the rendering industry although limited in their scope, also show that animal protein-based animal feed is frequently contaminated with *S. enterica*.

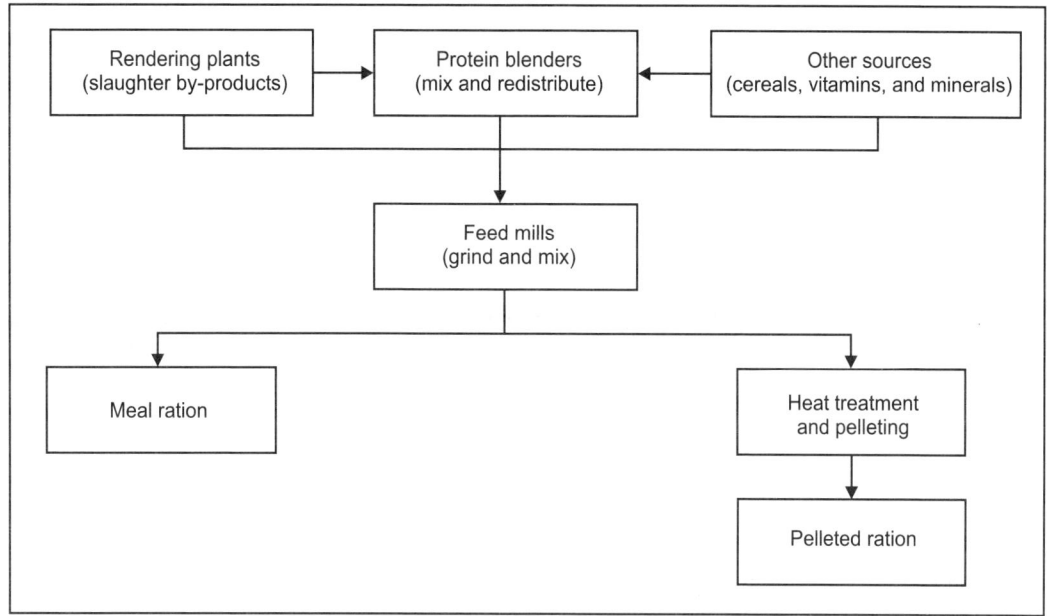

Fig. 3.1. Outlines of the steps in animal feed manufacture.

Evidence that Contaminated Animal Feed Results in Infection or Colonisation of Food Animals

It has long been known that infectious agents can be transmitted to animals through contaminated feed. For example, in 1948, workers in the United Kingdom demonstrated that non-Typhi serotypes of *S. enterica* could be transmitted to chicks through feed contaminated by the feces of infected rodents.

Experimental studies confirm that animals given feeds artificially contaminated with non-Typhi serotypes of *S. enterica* develop colonisation or infection with that organism. Furthermore, there are numerous examples of outbreaks of *Salmonella* infections in animals that were traced to contaminated feeds. These include cattle, pigs, chickens, turkeys, and mice. Although it is less well documented, bacteria that can cause human infections but may not cause illness in animals can also be readily transmitted to food animals via contaminated feed and appear on animal carcasses destined for human consumption.

Evidence that Consumption of Infected or Colonised Food Animals and Their Products Results in Human Illness

It has been well established that bacteria from colonised food animals can be transmitted to humans through the food supply. Humans become infected when they ingest contaminated meat or poultry products, raw produce contaminated with animal feces (e.g. from contaminated streams used for irrigation) or other foods, particularly uncooked foods, that have been cross-contaminated by contact with uncooked meat or poultry products. For example, *E. coli* O157:H7 is shed in the manure of cattle and contaminates beef during slaughter. Eating undercooked hamburger, a widespread practice, can lead to *E. coli* O157:H7 infection. *Campylobacter jejuni*, carried by poultry, can be spread to many poultry carcasses during the water-bath dressing process. Human infections occur when undercooked chicken or cross-contaminated food is consumed. Cattle, poultry, pigs, and other food animals are colonised with non-Typhi serotypes of *S. enterica*, which have multiple routes into the food supply. Consumption of meat or poultry products contaminated during slaughter leads to human salmonellosis. Consumption of produce grown adjacent to herds of animals colonised with bacterial pathogens may result in human infections if the crop is contaminated with animal feces.

In addition to causing outbreaks of illness, meat and poultry products also contribute to a large proportion of sporadic illness.

FROM UNTREATED SEWAGE

When untreated domestic sewage is used to fertilise plant crops, there is a likelihood that raw plant foods will be contaminated with human pathogens, especially those causing gastrointestinal diseases. The use of 'night soil' as a fertiliser still persists in some parts of the world. In addition to the pathogens, coliform bacteria, anaerobes, enterococci, other intestinal bacteria, and viruses can contaminate the foods from this source. Natural waters contaminated with sewage contribute their micro-organisms to shellfish, fish, and other seafood.

Treated sewage going onto soil or into water also contributes micro-organisms, although it should contain smaller numbers and fewer pathogens than does raw sewage.

FROM SOIL

The soil contains the greatest variety of micro-organisms of any source of contamination. Whenever microbiologists search for new kinds of micro-organisms or new strains for special purposes, they usually turn first to the soil. Not only numerous kinds of micro-organisms but also large total numbers are present in fertile soils, ready to contaminate the surfaces of plants growing on or in them and the surfaces of animals roaming over the land. Soil dust is whipped up by air currents, and soil particles are carried by running water to get into or onto foods. The soil is an important source of heat-resistant spore-forming bacteria.

No attempt will be made to list the micro-organisms important in food microbiology that could come from the soil, but it can be stated with certainty that nearly every important micro-organism can come from soil. Especially important are various moulds and yeasts and species of the bacterial genera *Bacillus*, *Clostridium*, *Enterobacter*, *Escherichia*, *Micrococcus*, *Alcaligenes*, *Flavobacterium*, *Chromobacterium*, *Pseudomonas*, *Proteus*, *Streptococcus*, *Leuconostoc*, and *Acetobacter* as well as some of the higher bacteria such as the actinomycetes and the iron bacteria.

Modern methods of food handling usually involve washing the surfaces of foods and hence the removal of much of the soil from those surfaces, and care is taken to avoid contamination by soil dust.

FROM WATER

Natural waters contain not only their natural flora but also micro-organisms from soil and possibly from animals or sewage. Surface waters in streams or pools and stored waters in lakes and large ponds vary considerably in their microbial content, from many thousands per millilitre after a rainstorm to the comparatively low numbers that result from self-purification of quiet lakes and ponds or of running water. Groundwaters from springs or wells have passed through layers of rock and soil to a definite level; hence most of the bacteria, as well as the greater part of other suspended material, have been removed. Bacterial numbers in these waters may range from a few to several hundred bacteria per millilitre.

The kinds of bacteria in natural waters are chiefly species of *Pseudomonas*, *Chromobacterium*, *Proteus*, *Micrococcus*, *Bacillus*, *Streptococcus* (enterococci), *Enterobacter*, and *Escherichia*. Bacteria of the last three genera probably are contaminants rather than part of the natural flora. These bacteria in the water surrounding fish and other sea life establish themselves on the surfaces and in the intestinal tracts of the sea fauna.

The food microbiologist is interested in two aspects of water bacteriology: (i) public health aspects, and (ii) economic aspects. From the public health point of view the water used about foods should be absolutely safe to drink, i.e. free from pathogens. Many nonfermenting bacteria such as Pseudomonas species actually grow in water lines and are not detected by traditional coliform analysis; therefore, total plate counts are important. Chlorination of drinking water is practiced when there is any doubt about the sanitary quality of the water, the amount of chlorine finally present ranging from 0.025 to 2 or more parts of available chlorine per million parts of water, depending on the composition of the water and the amount of contamination.

From the economic point of view, a water with agreeable chemical and bacteriological characteristics is desired for use in connection with the food being handled or processed. The water should have an acceptable taste, odour, colour, clarity, chemical composition, and bacterial content and should be available in sufficient volume at a desired temperature; it also should be uniform in composition. Desirable chemical composition is affected by hardness and alkalinity as well as by the content of organic matter, iron, manganese, and fluorine.

As has been stated, the water used about foods should meet the bacteriological standards for drinking water and should be acceptable from the sanitary viewpoint as well as the economic viewpoint. Usually, however, water is more important from the standpoint of the kinds of micro-organisms it may introduce into or onto foods than from the standpoint of the total numbers. Contamination may come from water used as an ingredient, for washing foods for cooling heated foods, and for manufactured ice for preserving foods. For each food product there will be certain micro-organisms to be feared especially. The gasforming coliform bacteria may enter milk from cooling-tank water and cause trouble in cheese made from the milk. Anaerobic gasformers may enter foods from soil-laden water. Cannery cooling water often contains coliform and other spoilage bacteria that enter canned foods during cooling through minute defects in the seams or seals of the cans.

This water commonly is chlorinated, but there have been reports that a chlorine-resistant flora can build up in time. Bacteria causing ropiness of milk, e.g. *Alcaligenes viscolactis* and *Enterobacter aerogenes*, usually come from water, as do slime-forming species of *Achromobacter*, *Alcaligenes*, and *Pseudomonas*, which cause trouble in cottage cheese. The bacterium causing the surface taint of butter, *Pseudomonas putrefaciens*, comes primarily from water. The iron bacteria, whose sheaths contain ferric hydroxide, may gum up an entire water supply and are difficult to eliminate. The bacterial flora of crushed ice to be applied to fish or other food consists mostly of *Corynebacterium*, *Alcaligenes*, *Flavobacterium*, *Pseudomonas*, and *cocci*.

FROM AIR

Contamination of foods from the air may be important for sanitary as well as economic reasons. Disease organisms, especially those causing respiratory infections, may be spread among employees by air, or the food product may become contaminated. Total numbers of micro-organisms in a food may be increased from the air, especially if the air is being used for aeration of the product, as in growing bread yeast, although the numbers of organisms introduced by sedimentation from air usually are negligible. Spoilage organisms may come from air, as may those interfering with food fermentations. Mould spores from air may give trouble in cheese, meat, sweetened condensed milk, and sliced bread and bacon.

Sources of Micro-organisms in Air

Air does not contain a natural flora of micro-organisms, for all that are present have come there by accident and usually are on suspended solid materials or in moisture droplets. Micro-organisms get into air on dust or lint; dry soil; spray from streams, lakes, or oceans; droplets of moisture from coughing, sneezing, or talking; and growths of sporulating moulds on walls, ceilings, floors, foods, and ingredients. Thus the air around a plant manufacturing yeast usually is high in yeasts, and the air of a dairy plant may contain bacteriophages or at least the starter bacteria being used there.

Kinds of Micro-organisms in Air

The micro-organisms in air have no opportunity for growth but merely persist there, and the kinds that are most resistant to desiccation will live the longest. Mould spores, because of their small size, resistance to drying, and large numbers per mould plant, are usually present in air. Many mould spores do not water-wet readily and therefore are less likely to sediment from humid air than are particles that wet readily. It is possible for any kind of bacterium to be suspended in air, especially on dust particles or in moisture droplets, but some kinds are more commonly found than others in undisturbed air. Cocci usually are more numerous than rod-shaped bacteria, and bacterial spores are relatively uncommon in dust-free air. Yeasts, especially asporogenous chromogenic ones, are found in most samples of air. Of course, whenever dusts or sprays of various materials are carried up into the air, the micro-organisms characteristic of those suspended materials will be present: soil organisms from soil and dust, water organisms from water spray, plant organisms from feed or fodder dust, etc.

Numbers of Micro-organisms in Air

The numbers of micro-organisms in air at any given time depend on such factors as the amount of movement, sunshine, humidity, location, and the amount of suspended dust or spray. Numbers vary from less than one per cubic foot at a mountaintop to thousands in very dusty air. Individual micro-organisms and those on suspended dust or in droplets settle out in quiet air; conversely, moving air brings organisms up into it. Therefore, numbers of micro-organisms in air are increased by air currents caused by movements of people, by ventilation, and by breezes. Direct rays from the sun kill micro-organisms suspended in air and hence reduce numbers. Dry air usually contains more organisms than does similar air in a moist condition. Rain or snow removes organisms from the air, so that a hard, steady rainfall may practically free the air of organisms.

According to a review of airborne contamination of foods by Heldman, various surveys have indicated that: (i) the microbial populations of different processing plants are similar, (ii) populations vary tremendously in numbers from one part of a given plant to another, (iii) populations in a plant are related to air quality outside the plant, and (iv) population levels are related to the level of activity of workers.

Treatment of Air

It has been pointed out that numbers of micro-organisms in air may be reduced under natural conditions by sedimentation, sunshine, and washing by rain or snow. Removal of micro-organisms from air by artificial means may involve these principles or those of filtration, chemical treatment, heat or electrostatic precipitation. The most frequently used of these methods is filtration through fibres of various sorts, e.g. cotton, fibre glass, etc. or activated carbon. The fibres are replaced periodically or sterilised with heat or a gas. Washing by means of a water spray or by bubbling air through water is not efficient and seldom is used by itself. Chemical treatments of air are finding increasing use. Passage of air through tunnels lined with ultraviolet lamps or installation of these lamps in a room or over an area where contamination from air is feared is used in some places. Electrostatic precipitation of dust particles and micro-organisms from air also has been accomplished successfully. Heat treatment of air at very high temperatures has been successful but expensive.

After the micro-organisms have been removed from air, precautions must be taken to prevent their re-entrance. Positive pressure in rooms keeps outside air away. Filters in ventilating or air-conditioning systems prevent the spread of organisms from one part of a plant to another, and ultraviolet-irradiated air locks at doors reduce the numbers of organisms carried in by workers.

DURING HANDLING AND PROCESSING

The contamination of foods from the natural sources just discussed may take place before the food is harvested or gathered or during handling and processing of the food. Additional contamination may come from equipment coming in contact with foods, from packaging materials, and from personnel. The processor attempts to clean and 'sanitise' equipment to reduce such contamination and to employ packaging materials that will minimise contamination. The term 'sanitise' is used here rather than 'sterilise' because although an attempt is made to sterilise the equipment, i.e. free it of all living organisms, sterility is seldom attained.

Personnel in food processing plants can contaminate foods during handling and processing. Various workers suggest that human beings shed from 10^3 to 10^4 viable organisms per minute. The numbers and types of organisms shed are closely related to the subjects working environment.

Chapter 4

Food Spoilage During Chemical Changes Caused by Micro-organisms

INTRODUCTION

The biochemical composition of a food, in particular, has a marked influence on the microbial population involved in the spoilage process and the microbial decomposition products associated with the spoilage of that food.

Effects of chemical properties on spoilage: The chemical properties of a food product influence the type of micro-organisms that can grow, and hence determine the changes in appearance, flavour, odour, and other qualities of food.

Composition: Proteins are degraded by proteolytic organisms. Many bacterial species, especially spore formers, gram negative rods such as *Pseudomonas* and *Proteus*, and a few cocci can attack proteins. Mould spoilage is also common. Carbohydrate foods are spoiled by carbohydrate fermenting, micro-organisms, particularly by yeast and moulds. Bacterial species of the genera *Streptococcus*, *Leuconostoc* and *Micrococcus* are saccharolytic and can also attack carbohydrates.

Fats are digested by relatively few micro-organisms, mainly moulds and few gram negative bacteria. Fats undergo hydrolytic decomposition and become rancid and malodorous fatty acids are set free.

Acidity: The reaction of nearly all foods is below pH 7.0. Foods are classified as acid or nonacid. The reaction of acid food is below pH 4.5, and that of nonacid food above pH 4.5. Most fruits are acid foods, while nearly all vegetables, fish, meats, and milk products are nonacid.

Acid foods have sufficiently low pH and, therefore, prevent the growth of almost bacterial species. They are spoiled mainly by yeast and moulds. Nonacid foods are particularly subject to bacterial spoilage, but will also support growth of moulds under proper conditions.

Moisture and osmotic pressure: Growth of micro-organisms require at least 13 per cent free water in foods. Moulds require the least free water and bacteria require the most. Foods of high sugar and salt concentration do not, support the growth of most micro-organism. Bacteria are generally inhibited by 5 to 11 per cent salt, whereas many moulds and some yeasts can tolerate salt concentrations greater than 15 per cent. Table 4.1 gives the influence of chemical properties of food on type of microbial growth. Chemical antimicrobials used in foods are given in Table 4.2.

CLASSIFICATION OF FOOD BASED ON PERISHABILITY

The techniques we need to adopt for preventing spoilage depend upon the quickness with which different foods undergo such spoilage as we have just discussed. Let us, therefore, classify food accordingly before we talk about storage.

Table 4.1. Influence of chemical properties of food on type of microbial growth.

Chemical properties	Predominant spoilage organisms
Composition	
Protein	Bacteria, moulds
Carbohydrate	Yeasts, moulds
Fat	Moulds, a few bacteria
Acidity	
Acid (pH < 4.5)	Moulds, yeasts
Nonacid (pH > 4.5)	Bacteria
Osmotic pressure	
Low	Moulds, bacteria, yeasts
High	Moulds

Table 4.2. Chemical antimicrobials used in foods.

Chemical	Max. permitted concentration
Benzoic acid	0.1 per cent
Methyl paraben	0.1 per cent
Propyl paraben	0.1 per cent
Sodium nitrite	500 ppm
Sodium nitrite	200 ppm
Sorbastes	0.1 per cent
Acetic acid	0.12–0.14 mg/ml in wines
Propylene oxide	300 ppm
Ethylene oxide	Residue not to exceed 50 ppm
Sulphites	Variable with foodstuff
Propionates	0.1 per cent
Potassium metabisulphite	0.05 per cent

Let us give a quick look at the purchasing habits of people. People generally buy milk, egg, fruits, etc. daily or once in two/three days or at most once a week. While other foodstuffs like atta, ghee, pulses, etc. are bought in bulk once in a week/fortnight/month. Can you give the reason for this? Some food items deteriorate/spoil easily as compared to others and need to be consumed in a day or two after the purchase. While others can be kept for a longer time without being spoilt. In fact, on the basis of the quickness with which a food item gets spoilt, we can place them into three categories:

1. Perishable foods.
2. Semi-perishable foods.
3. Non-perishable foods.

Perishable foods: These are foods which spoil easily unless special methods are used to prevent such spoilage. All animal foods like meat, fish, poultry, eggs, milk and milk products and most vegetables and fruits come in this category. The speed with which some of these spoil varies with the temperature, moisture and/or dryness of the environment; for example while in the cold season milk can remain at room temperature for a whole day without spoiling, in the hot season it would not last more than 3 to

4 hours. Fresh eggs, meats and fish spoil very fast in the hot weather unless refrigerated. As for vegetables and fruits, they spoil faster as the day progresses. Fresh coriander, lettuce and spinach plucked from the garden wilt within a matter of minutes unless stored adequately.

Semi-perishable foods: These are foods that can survive without any perceptible signs of spoilage for a couple of weeks or for a few months. Here again, the temperature and, humidity of the environment makes a big difference. Example of this category are all cereal and pulse products like wheat flour, refined wheat flour, semolina, vermicilli, broken wheat, bengal gram-flour, onions, potatoes, garlic, apples, citrus fruits, fats and oils. If properly handled and stored these will remain unspoiled for a fairly long period. In the cold climate like in most of the western countries these food items are considered non-perishable, but during the hot and humid seasons in our country they also perish unless we take special care.

Non-perishable foods: Cereals, pulses, sugar come in this category. They do not spoil unless handled and stored carelessly. Here again, we do need to take special care to make sure that they do not develop insects in storage. In the case of peanuts we have to worry about moulds in the monsoon season.

With the diverse environmental temperatures and levels of humidity prevailing in India, there can be no absolute classification of foods into these categories. With the exception of sugar and salt; there is nothing which would not spoil unless taken special care of. Even sugar and salt absorb moisture and become soggy during the rainy season unless we are careful. This makes the problem of storage even more significant for us, specially in the context of our population, what we produce, our transport facilities, and the low buying power of a large section of our population. Whatever we can produce needs to be looked after carefully till it is ready for use. As a nation and as a people we cannot afford to allow our food to get spoilt. We need to utilise every bit.

Factors Affecting Food Spoilage

Some factors like temperature, moisture affect the growth of micro-organisms, action of enzymes and hence effect food spoilage. Let us now study about these factors.

Temperature

Each micro-organism has an optimum growth temperature, i.e. the temperature at which it grows best and multiplies most rapidly. Similarly, enzymes are almost active at an optimum temperature. Microbial growth/enzyme action may be prevented by either decreasing or increasing the optimum temperature. Normally, freezing and chilling are adapted for storing foods at low temperature. Freezing process has a killing effect and bacteria continue to die during storage. Food can also be stored in refrigerator which has lower temperature, however not for a long time.

However, remember that excessive heat, as well as, cold can cause deterioration of food. Excessive heat can destroy proteins and vitamins and dry out food by removing moisture. Similarly excessive cold, if not controlled during freezing breaks the cell walls and membrane of food. Such a food during thawing allows micro-organisms to get in and spoil the food.

Moisture and dryness

Excessive moisture or dryness plays a very significant role in maintaining optimal quality in stored foods. Foods that are best when moist deteriorate on drying and those that should be kept in a dry state deteriorate when moist. Moisture is necessary for the growth of micro-organisms, as well as for enzyme action. Therefore, moisture on the surface of any food encourages multiplication of bacteria and growth of moulds. If temperature is also conducive to such multiplication and growth. Moisture need not be present in equal proportions throughout the food to have an effect on it. The surface moisture need not only come from the outside of atmosphere, the fruits and vegetables give off moisture from respiration and transpiration. When they are kept in a moistureproof package like a plastic bag, this moisture gets trapped inside and can support the growth of micro-organisms.

Hydrogen-ion Concentration (pH)

Every micro-organism has a minimal, a maximal, and an optimal pH for growth. Microbial cells are significantly affected by the pH of food because they apparently have no mechanism for adjusting their internal pH. In general, yeasts and moulds are more acid-tolerant than bacteria. The inherent pH of foods varies, although most foods are neutral or acidic. Foods with low pH values usually are not readily spoiled by bacteria and are more susceptible to spoilage by yeasts and moulds. A food with an inherently low pH would therefore tend to be more stable microbiologically than a neutral food. The excellent keeping quality of the following foods is related to their restrictive pH: fruits, soft drinks, fermented milks, sauerkraut, and pickles. Some foods have a low pH because of inherent acidity; others, e.g. the fermented products, have a low pH because of developed acidity from the accumulation of lactic acid during fermentation.

Moulds can grow over a wider range of pH values than can most yeasts and bacteria, and many moulds grow at acidities too great for yeasts and bacteria. Most fermentative yeasts are favoured by a pH of about 4.0 to 4.5, as in fruit juices, and film yeasts grow well on acid foods such as sauerkraut and pickles. On the other hand, most yeasts do not grow well in alkaline substrates and must be adapted to such media. Most bacteria are favoured by a pH near neutrality, although some, such as the acid formers, are favoured by moderate acidity, and others, e.g. the actively proteolytic bacteria, can grow in media with a high (alkaline) pH, as found in the white of a stored egg.

The buffers in a food, i.e. the compounds that resist changes in pH, are important not only for their buffering capacity but also for their ability to be especially effective within a certain pH range. Buffers permit an acid (or alkaline) fermentation to go on longer with a greater yield of products and organisms than would otherwise be possible. Vegetable juices have low buffering power, permitting an appreciable decrease in pH with the production of only small amounts of acid by the lactic acid bacteria during the early part of sauerkraut and pickle fermentations. This enables the lactics to suppress the undesirable pectin-hydrolyzing and proteolytic competing organisms. Low buffering power makes for a more rapidly appearing succession of micro-organisms during a fermentation than does high buffering power. Milk, on the other hand, is fairly high in protein (a good buffer) and therefore permits considerable growth and acid production by lactic acid bacteria in the manufacture of fermented milks before growth of the starter culture is finally suppressed.

The pH of a product can be readily determined with a pH meter, but this value alone may not be sufficient for predicting microbial responses. It is also desirable, for example, to know the acid responsible for a given pH, because some acids, particularly the organic acids, are more inhibitory than others. The inhibitory properties of many of the organic acids, including acetic, benzoic, citric, lactic, proprionic, and sorbic acids, make them widely used as acidulants or preservatives in foods. Also, changes in titratable acidity are not always evident from pH measurements.

Not only are the rates of growth of micro-organisms affected by pH, so are the rates of survival during storage, heating, drying, and other forms of processing. Also, the initial pH may be suitable, but because of competitive flora or growth of the organism itself, the pH may become unfavourable.

Conversely, the initial pH may be restrictive, but the growth of a limited number of micro-organisms may alter the pH to a range that is more favourable for the growth of many other micro-organisms.

NUTRIENT CONTENT

The kinds and proportions of nutrients in the food are all-important in determining what organism is most likely to grow. Consideration must be given to (i) foods for energy, (ii) foods for growth, and (iii) accessory food substances, or vitamins, which may be necessary for energy or growth.

Foods for Energy

The carbohydrates, especially the sugars, are most commonly used as an energy source, but other carbon compounds may serve, e.g. esters, alcohols, peptides, amino acids, and organic acids and their salts. Complex carbohydrates, e.g. cellulose, can be utilised by comparatively few organisms, and starch can be hydrolysed by only a limited number of organisms. Micro-organisms differ even in their ability to use some of the simpler soluble sugars. Many organisms cannot use the disaccharide lactose (milk sugar) and therefore do not grow well in milk. Maltose is not attacked by some yeasts. Bacteria often are identified and classified on the basis of their ability or inability to utilise various sugars and alcohols. Most organisms, if they utilise sugars at all, can use glucose.

The ability of micro-organisms to hydrolyse pectin, which is characteristic of some kinds of bacteria and many moulds, is important, of course, in the softening or rotting of fruits and vegetables or fermented products from them.

A limited number of kinds of micro-organisms can obtain their energy from fats but do so only if a more readily usable energy food, such as sugar, is absent. First, the fat must be hydrolysed with the aid of lipase to glycerol and fatty acids, which then can serve as an energy source for the hydrolysing organism or other organisms. In general, aerobic micro-organisms are more commonly involved in the decomposition of fats than are anaerobic ones, and the lipolytic organisms usually are also proteolytic. Direct oxidation of fats containing unsaturated fatty acids usually is chemical.

Hydrolysis products of proteins, peptides, and amino acids, for example, serve as an energy source for many proteolytic organisms when a better energy source is lacking and as foods for energy for other organisms that are not proteolytic. Meats, for example, may be low in carbohydrate and therefore decomposed by proteolytic species, e.g. *Pseudomonas* spp. with successive growth of weakly proteolytic or non proteolytic species that can utilise the products of protein hydrolysis. Organisms differ in their ability to use individual amino acids for energy. This is because it is the number of molecules (or moles) of sugar which affects a_w, and a percentage is usually expressed as weight per unit volume.

Not only is the kind of energy food important but also its concentration in solution and hence its osmotic effect and the amount of available moisture. For a given percentage of sugar in solution, the osmotic pressure will vary with the weight of the sugar molecule. Therefore, a 10 per cent solution of glucose has about twice the osmotic pressure of a 10 per cent solution of sucrose or maltose; i.e. it ties up twice as much moisture. In general, moulds can grow in the highest concentrations of sugars and yeasts in fairly high concentrations, but most bacteria grow best in fairly low concentrations. There are, of course, notable exceptions to this generalisation. Osmophilic yeasts grow in as high concentrations of sugar as moulds, and some bacteria can grow in fairly high concentrations of sugar.

Of course, an adequate supply of foods for growth will favour utilisation of the foods for energy. More carbohydrate will be used if a good nitrogen food is present in sufficient quantity than will be the case if the nitrogen is poor in kind or amount. Organisms requiring special accessory growth substances might be prevented from growing if one or more of these 'vitamins' were lacking, and thus the whole course of decomposition might be altered.

Foods for Growth

Micro-organisms differ in their ability to use various nitrogenous compounds as a source of nitrogen for growth. Many organisms are unable to hydrolyse proteins and hence cannot get nitrogen from them without help from a proteolytic organism. One protein may be a better source of nitrogenous food than another because of different products formed during hydrolysis, especially peptides and amino acids. Peptides, amino acids, urea, ammonia, and other simpler nitrogenous compounds may be available to some organisms but not to others or may be usable under some environmental conditions but not under others. Some of the lactic acid bacteria grow best with polypeptides as nitrogen foods, cannot attack casein, and do not grow well with only a limited number of kinds of amino acids present. The presence of fermentable carbohydrate in a substrate usually results in an acid fermentation and suppression of proteolytic bacteria and hence in what is called a 'sparing' action on the nitrogen compounds. Also, the production of obnoxious nitrogenous products is prevented or inhibited.

Many kinds of moulds are proteolytic, but comparatively few genera and species of bacteria and very few yeasts are actively proteolytic. In general, proteolytic bacteria grow best at pH values near neutrality and are inhibited by acidity, although there are exceptions, such as proteolysis by the acid-proteolytic bacteria that hydrolyse protein while producing acid.

Carbon for growth may come partly from carbon dioxide, but more often it comes from organic compounds. The minerals required by micro-organisms are neatly always present at the low levels required, but occasionally an essential mineral may be tied up so that it is unavailable, lacking, or present in insufficient amounts. An example is milk, which contains insufficient iron for pigmentation of the spores of Penicillium roqueforti. Bacteria causing septicemia usually have the ability to bind some of the iron in blood. Only strains which can compete for transferrin iron are able to grow well in human blood.

Accessory Food Substances, or Vitamins

Some micro-organisms are unable to manufacture some or all of the vitamins needed and must have them furnished. Most natural plant and animal foodstuffs contain an array of these vitamins, but some may be low in amount, or lacking. Thus meats are high in B vitamins and fruits are low, but fruits are high in ascorbic acid. Egg white contains biotin but also contains avidin,which ties up biotin, making it unavailable to micro-organisms and eliminating as possible spoilage organisms those which must have biotin supplied. The processing of foods often reduces the vitamin content. Thiamine, pantothenic acid, the folic acid group, and ascorbic acid (in air) are heat-labile, and drying causes a loss in vitamins such as thiamine and ascorbic acid. Even storage of foods for long periods, especially if the storage temperature is elevated, may result in a decrease in the level of some of the accessory growth factors.

Each kind of bacterium (or other micro-organism) has a definite range of food requirements. For some species the range is wide, and growth takes place in a variety of substrates, as is true for coliform bacteria; but for others, e.g. many of the pathogens, the range is narrow and the organisms can grow in only a limited number of kinds of substrates. Thus, bacteria differ in the foods that they can utilise for energy. Some can use a variety of carbohydrates, e.g. the coliform bacteria and *Clostridium* spp. and others only one or two, while some can use other carbon compounds such as organic acids and their salts, alcohols, and esters (*Pseudomonas* spp.). Some can hydrolyse complex carbohydrates, although others cannot. Likewise, the nitrogen requirements of bacteria such as *Pseudomonas* spp. may be satisfied by simple compounds such as ammonia or nitrates; or more complex compounds such as amino acids, peptides or proteins may be utilised or even required, as is true for the lactics. Bacteria also vary in their need for vitamins or accessory growth factors; some (*Staph. aureus*) synthesise part and others (*Pseudomonas* or *E. coli*) all of the factors needed, and still others must have them all furnished (the lactics and many pathogens). It should be emphasised that in general, the better the medium, for an organism, the wider the ranges of temperature, pH, and a_w over which growth can take place.

INHIBITORY SUBSTANCES AND BIOLOGICAL STRUCTURE

Inhibitory substances, originally present in the food, added purposely or accidentally, or developed there by growth of micro-organisms or by processing methods, may prevent growth of all micro-organisms or, more often, may deter certain specific kinds. Examples of inhibitors naturally present are the lactenins and anticoliform factor in freshly drawn milk, lysozyme in egg white, and benzoic acid in cranberries. A micro-organism growing in a food may produce one or more substances inhibitory to other organisms, products such as acids, alcohols, peroxides, and even antibiotics. Propionic acid produced by the propionibacteria in Swiss cheese is inhibitory to moulds; alcohol formed in quantity by wine yeasts inhibits competitors; and nisin produced by certain strains of *Streptococcus lactis* may be useful in inhibiting lactate-fermenting, gasforming clostridia in curing cheese and undesirable in slowing down some of the essential lactic acid streptococci during the manufacturing process. There also is the possibility of the destruction of inhibitory compounds in foods by micro-organisms. Certain moulds and bacteria are able to destroy some of the phenol compounds that are added to meat or fish by smoking or benzoic acid added to foods; sulphur dioxide is destroyed by yeasts resistant to it; and lactobacilli can inactivate nisin. Heating foods may result in the formation of inhibitory substances: Heating lipids may hasten autoxidation and make them inhibitory, and browning concentrated sugar sirups may result in the production of furfural and hydroxymethyl furfural, which are inhibitory to fermenting organisms. Long storage at warm temperatures may produce similar results.

The effect of the biological structure of food on the protection of foods against spoilage has been noted. The inner parts of whole, healthy tissues of living plants and animals are either sterile or low in microbial content. Therefore, unless opportunity has been given for their penetration, spoilage organisms within may be few or lacking. Often there is a protective covering about the food, e.g. the shell on eggs, the skin on poultry, the shell on nuts, and the rind or skin on fruits and vegetables, or we may have surrounded the food with an artificial coating, e.g. plastic or wax. This physical protection of the food not only may help its preservation but also may determine the kind, rate, and course of spoilage. Layers of fat over meat may protect that part of the flesh or scales may protect the outer part of the fish. On the other hand, an increase in exposed surface brought about by peeling, skinning, chopping; or comminution may serve not only to distribute spoilage organisms but also to release juices containing food materials for the invaders. The disintegration of tissues by freezing may accomplish a similar result.

In meat the growth of spoilage bacteria takes place mostly in the fluid between the small meat fibres, and it is only after rigour mortis that much of this food material is released from the fibres to become available to spoilage organisms.

Air and oxygen: Vitamins, particularly A and C as well as food colours and flavours get destroyed when exposed to air and oxygen. Oxygen also helps growth of moulds. In packaged foods effort is made to remove oxygen by vaccum or by flushing the food containers with nitrogen or carbon dioxide, in order to prevent such deterioration. Air also dries up food items and dryness in turn can cause deterioration in some foods as mentioned.

Light: Some vitamins, particularly riboflavin, vitamin A and vitamin C, and many food colours are destroyed by light. Sensitive foods are often protected from light by using containers that keep light out, for example dark coloured bottles and glazed pottery jars used for keeping pickles.

Time: Any food is at its peak quality for a certain time after it is harvested, slaughtered or manufactured, and this period is very short, from just a few hours after harvest as in the case of fresh peas and fresh corn, to may be a day or two. It generally depends on the time spent in the field itself after harvesting in view of the inadequate transport facilities in our country. All deteriorating factors like growth of micro-organisms, destruction by insects, action of food enzymes, loss of flavour, effects of heat, cold, oxygen, light and moisture progress with time.

The longer the time the greater the destructive influences. It is, however, also true that some food items improve with time, for example certain cheeses, wines and pickles, but the majority of foods decrease in quality with time.

CHEMICAL CHANGES CAUSED BY MICRO-ORGANISMS

Because of the great variety of organic compounds in foods and the numerous kinds of micro-organisms that can decompose them, many different chemical changes are possible and many kinds of products can result. The following discussion is concerned only with the important types of decomposition of main constituents of foods and the chief products produced.

Changes in Nitrogenous Organic Compounds

Most of the nitrogen in foods is in the form of proteins which must be hydrolysed by enzymes of the micro-organisms or of the food to polypeptides, simpler peptides, or amino acids before they can serve as nitrogenous food for most organisms. Proteinases catalyse the hydrolysis of proteins to peptides, which may give a bitter taste to foods. Peptidases catalyse the hydrolysis of polypeptides to simpler peptides and finally to amino acids. The latter give flavours, desirable or undesirable, to some foods; e.g. amino acids contribute to the flavour of ripened cheeses.

For the most part these hydrolyses do not result in particularly objectionable products. Anaerobic decomposition of proteins, peptides or amino acids, however, may result in the production of obnoxious odours and is then called putrefaction. It results in foul-smelling, sulphur-containing products, such as hydrogen, methyl, and ethyl sulphides and mercaptans, plus ammonia, amines (e.g. histamine, tyramine, piperidine, putrescine, and cadaverine), indole, skatole, and fatty acids.

When micro-organisms act on amino acids, they may deaminate them, decarboxylate them, or both, resulting in the products listed in *Escherichia coli*, for example, produces glyoxylic acid, acetic acid, and ammonia from glycine; *Pseudomonas* also produces methylamine and carbon dioxide; and clostridia give acetic acid, ammonia, and methane. From alanine these three organisms produce (i) an α-keto acid, ammonia, and carbon dioxide, (ii) acetic acid, ammonia, and carbon dioxide, and (iii) propionic acid, acetic acid, ammonia, and carbon dioxide, respectively. From serine, *E. coli* produces pyruvic acid for ammonia, and species of *Clostridium* give propionic acid, formic acid, and ammonia. As stated previously, the sulphur in sulphur-bearing amino acids may be reduced to foul-smelling sulphides or mercaptans. *Desulfotomaculum nigrificans* (formerly *C. nigrificans*), an obligate anaerobe, can reduce sulphate to sulphide and produces hydrogen sulphide from cystine.

Other nitrogenous compounds decomposed include (i) amides, imides, and urea, from which ammonia is the principal product, (ii) guanidine and creatine, which yield urea and ammonia, and (iii) amines, purines, and pyrimidines, which may yield ammonia, carbon dioxide, and organic acids (chiefly lactic or acetic).

Changes in Non-nitrogenous Organic Compounds

The main non-nitrogenous foods for micro-organisms, mostly used to obtain energy but possibly serving as sources of carbon, include carbohydrates, organic acids, aldehydes and ketones, alcohols, glycosides, cyclic compounds, and lipids. Food rich in carbohydrates are degraded by carbohydrate fermenting micro-organisms, particularly yeasts and moulds. Bacteria like *Micrococcus*, *Leuconostoc*, and *Streptococcus* can also degrade carbohydrates.

Carbohydrate foods + Carbohydrate fermenting micro-organisms → Acids + Alcohols + Gases.

Food rich in fats are attacked by relatively few micro-organisms such as moulds and some gram negative bacteria. These micro-organisms are, therefore, lipolytic in nature. Fatty food + Lipolytic micro-organisms → Fatty acids + Glycerol.

Carbohydrates

Carbohydrates, if available, usually are preferred by micro-organisms to other energy-yielding foods. Complex di-, tri- or polysaccharides usually are hydrolysed to simple sugars before utilisation. A monosaccharide, such as glucose, aerobically would be oxidised to carbon dioxide and water and anaerobically would undergo decomposition involving any of six main types of fermentation: (i) an alcoholic fermentation, as by yeasts, with ethanol and carbon dioxide as the principal products, (ii) a simple lactic fermentation, as by homofermentative lactic acid bacteria, with lactic acid as the main product, (iii) a mixed lactic fermentation, as by heterofermentative lactic acid bacteria, with lactic and acetic acids, ethanol, glycerol, and carbon dioxide as the chief products, (iv) the coliform type of fermentation, as by coliform bacteria, with lactic, acetic, and formic acids, ethanol, carbon dioxide, hydrogen, and perhaps acetoin and butanediol as likely products, (v) the propionic fermentation, by propionibacteria, producing propionic, acetic, and succinic acids and carbon dioxide, and (vi) the butyric-butyl-isopropyl fermentations, by anaerobic bacteria, yielding butyric and acetic acids, carbon dioxide, hydrogen, and in some instances acetone, butylene glycol, butanol, and 2-propanol. A variety of other products are possible from sugars when different micro-organisms are active, including higher fatty acids, other organic acids, aldehydes, and ketones.

Acidity

Generally the fruits are acid foods (pH below 4.5) while nearly all vegetables, fish, meats, and milk-products are non-acid (pH above 4.5). Since the pH of the acid foods (fruits) is sufficiently low, they do not allow bacterial growth and subsequent spoilage. They are spoiled mainly by yeasts and moulds, contrary to this, non-acid foods have sufficiently high pH and are spoiled mainly by bacteria.

Organic acids

Many of the organic acids usually occurring in foods as salts are oxidised by organisms to carbonates, causing the medium to become more alkaline. Aerobically the organic acids may be oxidised completely to carbon dioxide and water, as is done by film yeasts. Acids may be oxidised to other, simpler acids or to other products similar to those from sugars. Saturated fatty acids or lower ketonic derivatives are degraded to acetic acid, two carbons at a time, aided by coenzyme A. Unsaturated or hydroxy fatty acids may be degraded partially in a similar manner but must be converted to a saturated acid (or ketonic derivative) for complete beta oxidation.

Other compounds

Alcohols usually are oxidised to the corresponding organic acid, e.g. ethanol to acetic acid. Glycerol may be dissimilated to products similar to those from glucose. Glycosides, after hydrolysis to release the sugar, will have the sugar dissimilated characteristically. Acetaldehyde may be oxidised to acetic acid or reduced to ethanol. Cyclic compounds are not readily attacked.

Lipids

Fats are hydrolysed by microbial lipase to glycerol and fatty acids, which are then dissimilated as outlined previously. Micro-organisms may be involved in the oxidation of fats, but auto-oxidation is more common. Phospholipids may be degraded to their constituent phosphate, glycerol, fatty acids, and nitrogenous base, e.g. choline. Lipoproteins are made up of proteins, cholesterol esters, and phospholipids.

Pectic substances

Protopectin, the water-insoluble parent pectic substance in plants, is converted to pectin, a water-soluble polymer of galacturonic acid which contains methyl ester linkages and varying degrees of neutralisation by various cations. It gels with sugar and acid. Pectinesterase causes hydrolysis of the methyl ester linkage of pectin to yield pectic acid and methanol. Polygalacturonases destroy the linkage between galacturonic acid units of pectin or pectic acid to yield smaller chains and ultimately free D-galacturonic acid, which may be degraded to simple sugars. Moisture and osmotic concentration average 13 per cent free water is required in food for usual microbial growth. This is the reason why the foods of high sugar salt concentrations do not allow most of the micro-organisms to grow. But, specific microbial growths cannot be over ruled 65–70 per cent sugar concentration is required to prevent mould-growth and 50 per cent to prevent bacterial and yeast growth.

SECTION II

Principles of Food Preservation

Chapter 5

General Principles of Food Preservation

INTRODUCTION

The term food preservation refers to any one of a number of techniques used to prevent food from spoiling. It includes methods such as canning, pickling, drying and freeze-drying, irradiation, pasteurisation, smoking, and the addition of chemical additives. Food preservation has become an increasingly important component of the food industry as fewer people eat foods produced on their own lands, and as consumers expect to be able to purchase and consume foods that are out of season.

The vast majority of instances of food spoilage can be attributed to one of two major causes: (i) the attack by pathogens (disease-causing micro-organisms) such as bacteria and moulds, and (ii) oxidation that causes the destruction of essential biochemical compounds and/or the destruction of plant and animal cells. The various methods that have been devised for preserving foods are all designed to reduce or eliminate one or the other (or both) of these causative agents.

For example, a simple and common method of preserving food is by heating it to some minimum temperature. This process prevents or retards spoilage because high temperatures kill or inactivate most kinds of pathogens. The addition of compounds known as BHA and BHT to foods also prevents spoilage in another different way. These compounds are known to act as antioxidants, preventing chemical reactions that cause the oxidation of food that results in its spoilage. Almost all techniques of preservation are designed to extend the life of food by acting in one of these two ways.

The search for methods of food preservation probably can be traced to the dawn of human civilisation. People who lived through harsh winters found it necessary to find some means of insuring a food supply during seasons when no fresh fruits and vegetables were available. Evidence for the use of dehydration (drying) as a method of food preservation, for example, goes back at least 5000 years. Among the most primitive forms of food preservation that are still in use today are such methods as smoking, drying, salting, freezing, and fermenting.

Early humans probably discovered by accident that certain foods exposed to smoke seem to last longer than those that are not. Meats, fish, fowl, and cheese were among such foods. It appears that compounds present in wood smoke have antimicrobial actions that prevent the growth of organisms that cause spoilage. Today, the process of smoking has become a sophisticated method of food preservation with both hot and cold forms in use. Hot smoking is used primarily with fresh or frozen foods, while cold smoking is used most often with salted products. The most advantageous conditions for each kind of smoking—air velocity, relative humidity, length of exposure, and salt content, for example—are now generally understood and applied during the smoking process. For example, electrostatic precipitators can be employed to attract smoke.

PRESERVATION PROCESSES

Types of Preservation Processes

Preservation processes include:

1. Heating to kill or denature micro-organisms (e.g. boiling).
2. Oxidation (e.g. use of sulphur dioxide).
3. Toxic inhibition (e.g. smoking, use of carbon dioxide, vinegar, alcohol, etc.).
4. Dehydration (drying).
5. Osmotic inhibition (e.g. use of syrups).
6. Low temperature inactivation (e.g. freezing).
7. Ultra high water pressure (e.g. fresherised, a kind of 'cold' pasteurisation, the pressure kills naturally occurring pathogens, which cause food deterioration and affect food safety.).
8. Combinations of these methods.

Drying

One of the oldest methods of food preservation is by drying, which reduces water activity sufficiently to prevent or delay bacterial growth.

Refrigeration

Refrigeration preserves food by slowing down the growth and reproduction of micro-organisms and the action of enzymes which cause food to rot.

Freezing

Freezing is also one of the most commonly used processes commercially and domestically for preserving a very wide range of food including prepared food stuffs which would not have required freezing in their unprepared state. For example, potato waffles are stored in the freezer, but potatoes themselves require only a cool dark place to ensure many months' storage. Cold stores provide large volume, long-term storage for strategic food stocks held in case of national emergency in many countries.

Vacuum packing

Vacuum-packing stores food in a vacuum environment, usually in an air-tight bag or bottle. The vacuum environment strips bacteria of oxygen needed for survival, slowing spoiling. Vacuum-packing is commonly used for storing nuts to reduce loss of flavour from oxidation.

Salt

Salting or curing draws moisture from the meat through a process of osmosis. Meat is cured with salt or sugar or a combination of the two. Nitrates and nitrites are also often used to cure meat and contribute the characteristic pink colour, as well as inhibition of *Clostridium botulinum*.

Sugar

Sugar is used to preserve fruits, either in syrup with fruit such as apples, pears, peaches, apricots, plums or in crystallised form where the preserved material is cooked in sugar to the point of crystallisation and the resultant product is then stored dry. This method is used for the skins of citrus fruit (candied peel), angelica and ginger.

Artificial food additives

Preservative food additives can be antimicrobial; which inhibit the growth of bacteria or fungi, including mould or antioxidant; such as oxygen absorbers, which inhibit the oxidation of food constituents.

Pickling

Pickling is a method of preserving food in an edible anti-microbial liquid. Pickling can be broadly categorised as chemical pickling for example. In chemical pickling, the food is placed in an edible liquid that inhibits or kills bacteria and other micro-organisms. In fermentation pickling, the food itself produces the preservation agent, typically by a process that produces lactic acid. Fermented pickles include sauerkraut, nukazuke, kimchi, surströmming, and curtido. Some pickled cucumbers are also fermented. In commercial pickles, a preservative like sodium benzoate or EDTA may also be added to enhance shelf life.

Lye

Sodium hydroxide (lye) makes food too alkaline for bacterial growth. Lye will saponify fats in the food, which will change its flavour and texture. Lutefisk uses lye in its preparation, as do some olive recipes. Modern recipes for century eggs also call for lye. Masa harina and hominy use agricultural lime in their preparation and this is often misheard as 'lye'.

Canning and bottling

Canning involves cooking food, sealing it in sterile cans or jars, and boiling the containers to kill or weaken any remaining bacteria as a form of sterilisation.

Jellying

Food may be preserved by cooking in a material that solidifies to form a gel. Such materials include gelatine, agar, maize flour and arrowroot flour.

Potting

A traditional British way of preserving meat (particularly shrimp) is by setting it in a pot and sealing it with a layer of fat.

Jugging

Meat can be preserved by jugging, the process of stewing the meat (commonly game or fish) in a covered earthenware jug or casserole. The animal to be jugged is usually cut into pieces, placed into a tightly-sealed jug with brine or gravy, and stewed. Red wine and/or the animal's own blood is sometimes added to the cooking liquid.

Irradiation

Irradiation of food is the exposure of food to ionising radiation; either high-energy electrons or X-rays from accelerators or by gamma rays (emitted from radioactive sources as Cobalt-60 or Caesium-137). The treatment has a range of effects, including killing bacteria, moulds and insect pests, reducing the ripening and spoiling of fruits, and at higher doses inducing sterility.

Pulsed electric field processing

Pulsed electric field (PEF) processing is a method for processing cells by means of brief pulses of a strong electric field. PEF holds potential as a type of low temperature alternative pasteurisation process for sterilising food products.

Modified atmosphere

Modifying atmosphere is a way to preserve food by operating on the atmosphere around it. Salad crops which are notoriously difficult to preserve are now being packaged in sealed bags with an atmosphere modified to reduce the oxygen (O_2) concentration and increase the carbon dioxide (CO_2) concentration.

Burial in the ground

Burial of food can preserve it due to a variety of factors: lack of light, lack of oxygen, cool temperatures, pH level, or desiccants in the soil. Burial may be combined with other methods such as salting or fermentation.

Controlled use of micro-organism

Some foods, such as many cheeses, wines, and beers will keep for a long time because their production uses specific micro-organisms that combat spoilage from other less benign organisms. These micro-organisms keep pathogens in check by creating an environment toxic for themselves and other micro-organisms by producing acid or alcohol.

High pressure food preservation

High pressure food preservation refers to high pressure used for food preservation.

PRINCIPLES OF FOOD PRESERVATION

Food preservation operates according to three principles, namely:
1. Prevention or delay of microbial decomposition.
    (a) Asepsis: Process of keeping micro-organisms out of food and its surroundings.
        (i) Proper packaging of the product.
        (ii) Maintenance of sanitary conditions.
    (b) Removal of micro-organisms.
        (i) Washing.
        (ii) Trimming ingredients.
        (iii) Discarding dirt.
        (iv) Filtering clear liquid.
    (c) Hindering the growth and activity of micro-organisms.
        (i) Low temperature-freezing.
        (ii) Drying-reduces moisture.
        (iii) Maintenance of anaerobic conditions—removal of air, e.g. hotdogs, bacon
        (iv) Use of chemicals—preservatives.
    (d) Killing micro-organisms by heat or irradiation.
        (i) micro-organisms are killed by heat.
2. Prevention or delay of self-decomposition of foods.
    (a) Destroying or inactivating food enzymes.
        (i) Blanching is an example of this kind of prevention.

(ii) Low temperature.

(iii) Chemical preservatives.

(iv) Drying.

(b) Preventing oxidation with the use of antioxidants.

(i) Oxygen speeds up decomposition of food antioxidants deprives food from oxygen.

(ii) Butter, margarine and other fatty foods.

3. Prevention of damage because of external factors such as insects, rodents, dust, odour, fumes, and mechanical, fire, heat or water damage.

(a) Styrofoam boxes, cartons, and shock absorbing materials.

(b) Sealed tight, vacuum-packed.

GROWTH CURVE

Growth of micro-organisms refers to an increase in the number of unicellular organisms. Under favourable conditions of nutrition, oxygen, pH, moisture, and temperature, some kinds of bacteria may double in number about every 20 minutes. This time interval is called generation time. Simple arithmetic shows the magnitude of the result if this rate of increase were to continue for only a few days. Fortunately, there are several factors that help control the situation. In some cases, the food supply may become depleted or the accumulation of waste products may slow the process. However, when these conditions are controlled by the continuous addition of nutrients and removal of waste products, the bacterial population always reaches a maximum before the medium in which it is growing becomes a solid mass of cells.

Four Phases

Different species of bacteria show various shapes of growth curves depending on the generation time and the maximum population attainable under the prevailing growth conditions. The growth curve is determined by plotting the numbers of bacteria per millilitre of culture against incubation time. The counts are plotted with logarithms of numbers. The growth curve of micro-organisms is composed of four phases (Fig. 5.1).

1. The initial lag phase (A to B), during which there is no growth or even a decline in numbers.
2. The phase of positive acceleration (B to C), during which the rate of growth is continuously increasing.
3. The logarithmic or exponential phase of growth (C to D), during which the rate of multiplication is most rapid and is constant.
4. The phase of negative acceleration (D to E), during which the rate of multiplication is decreasing.
5. The maximal stationary phase (E to F), where numbers remain constant.
6. The accelerated death phase (F to G).
7. The death phase or phase of decline (G to H), during which numbers decrease at a faster rate than new cells are formed.
8. The survival phase (H to I), during which no cell division occurs but remaining cells survive on endogenous nutrients. With many bacteria (or other micro-organisms) the numbers do not decrease at a fixed rate to zero, as indicated by the unbroken line in the figure, but taper off very gradually as low numbers are approached, as shown by the broken line, and a few viable cells remain for some time.

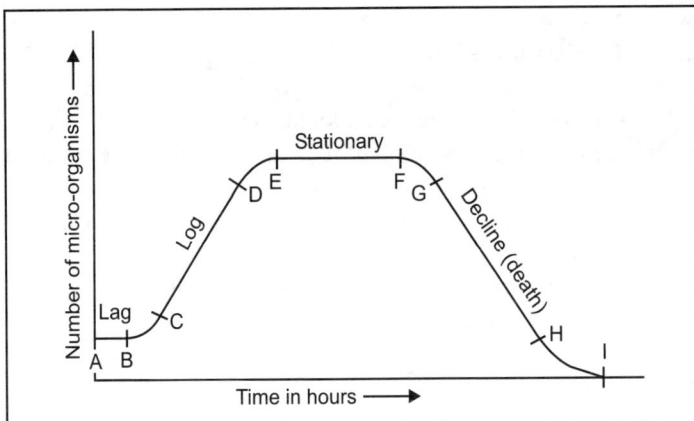

Fig. 5.1. Growth curve. *A* to *B*, lag phase; *B* to *C*, phase of positive acceleration; *C* to *D*, logarithmic or exponential phase; *D* to *E*, phase of negative acceleration; *E* to *F*, maximal stationary phase; *F* to *G*, accelerated death phase; *G* to *H*, death phase; and *H* to *I*, survival phase.

Prevention of Microbial Decomposition

Microbial decomposition of foods will be prevented if all spoilage organisms are killed or removed and recontamination is prevented. Merely stopping the multiplication of micro-organisms, however, does not necessarily prevent decomposition, for viable organisms or their enzymes may continue to be active. As will be pointed out in later chapters, killing micro-organisms by most agencies is easier when smaller initial numbers are present than with larger number; this re-emphasises the importance of contamination. Especially important is the introduction of building up of micro-organisms resistant to the lethal agent being employed, for example, heat-resistant bacterial spores when foods are to be heat-processed. Vegetative cells of organisms in their logarithmic phase of growth are least resistant to lethal agencies, and they are more resistant in their late lag maximal stationary phase of growth.

ASEPSIS

Asepsis is the state of being free from disease-causing contaminants (such as bacteria, viruses, fungi, and parasites) or preventing contact with micro-organisms. The term asepsis often refers to those practices used to promote or induce asepsis in an operative field in surgery or medicine to prevent infection. Ideally, a surgical field is 'sterile'—free of all biological contaminants, not just those that can cause disease, putrefaction or fermentation—but that is a situation that is difficult to attain, especially given the patient is often a source of infectious agents. There is no current method to safely eliminate all of the patients bacterial flora without causing significant tissue damage. However, elimination of infection is the goal of asepsis, not sterility.

Today's techniques include a series of steps that complement each other. Foremost remains good hygienic practice. The procedure room is laid out according to specific guidelines, subject to regulations concerning filtering and airflow, and kept clean between surgical cases. A patient who is brought for the procedure is washed and wears a clean gown. The surgical site is washed, possibly shaved, and skin is exposed to a germicide (i.e. an iodine solution such as betadine). In turn, members of the surgical team wash hands and arms with germicidal solution. Operating surgeons and nurses wear sterile gowns and gloves. Hair is covered and a surgical mask is worn. Instruments are sterilised through autoclaving or if disposable, are used once. Irrigation is used in the surgical site. Suture material or xenografts have been sterilised beforehand. Dressing material is sterile. Antibiotics are often not necessary in a 'clean' case, that is, a surgical procedure where no infection is apparent; however, when a case is considered 'contaminated', they are usually indicated. Dirty and biologically contaminated material is subject to regulated disposal.

REMOVAL OF MICRO-ORGANISMS

Removal may be accomplished by means of filtration, centrifugation (sedimentation of clarification), washing, or trimming.

Filtration is the only successful method for the complete removal of organisms, and its use is limited to clear liquids. The liquid is filtered through a previously sterilised 'bacteriaproof' filter made of sintered glass, diatomaceous earth, unglassed porcelain, membrane pads, or similar material, and the liquid is forced through by positive or negative pressure. This method has been used successfully with fruit juices, beer, soft drinks, wine, and water.

Centrifugation or sedimentation, generally is not very effective, in that some but not all of the micro-organisms are removed. Sedimentation is used in the treatment of drinking water but is insufficient by itself. When centrifugation (clarification) is applied to milk, the main purpose is not to remove bacteria but to take out other suspended materials, although centrifugation at high speeds removes most of the spores.

Washing raw foods can be helpful in their preservation but may be harmful under some conditions. Washing cabbage heads or cucumbers before their fermentation into sauerkraut and pickles, respectively, removes most of the soil micro-organisms on the surface and in this way increases the proportion of desirable lactic acid bacteria in the total flora. Washing fresh fruits and vegetables removes soil organisms that may be resistant to the heat process during the canning of these foods. Obviously the removal of organisms and of food for them from equipment coming into contact with foods, followed by a germicidal treatment of the apparatus, is an essential and effective procedure during the handling of all kinds of foods. Washing foods may be dangerous if the water adds spoilage organisms or increases the moisture so that growth of spoilage organisms is encouraged.

Trimming away spoiled portions of a food or discarding spoiled samples is important from the standpoint of food laws and may be helpful in food preservation. Although large numbers of spoilage organisms are removed in this way, heavy contamination of the remaining food may take place. Trimming the outer leaves of cabbage heads is recommended for the manufacture of sauerkraut.

MAINTENANCE OF ANAEROBIC CONDITIONS

A preservative factor in sealed, packaged foods may be the anaerobic conditions in the container. A complete fill, evacuation of the unfilled space (the head space in a can) or replacement of the air by carbon dioxide or by an inert gas such as nitrogen will bring about anaerobic conditions. Spores of some of the aerobic spore-formers are especially resistant to heat and may survive in canned food but are unable to germinate or grow in the absence of oxygen. Production of carbon dioxide during fermentation and accumulation at the surface will serve to make conditions anaerobic there and prevent the growth of aerobes.

Chapter 6

Preservation by Use of Low Temperature

INTRODUCTION

Low temperatures are used to retard chemical reactions and action of food enzymes and to slow down or stop the growth and activity of micro-organisms in food. The lower the temperature, the slower will be chemical reactions, enzyme action, and microbial growth; a low enough temperature will prevent the growth of any micro-organism.

Any raw plant or animal food may be assumed to contain a variety of bacteria, yeasts, and moulds which need only conditions for growth to bring about undesirable changes in the food. Each micro-organisms present has an optimal or best, temperature for growth and minimal temperature below which it cannot multiply. As the temperature drops from this optimal temperature toward the minimal, the rate of growth of the organisms decreases and is slowest at the minimal temperature. Cooler temperatures will prevent growth, but slow metabolic activity may continue. Therefore, the cooling of the food from ordinary temperatures has a different effect on the various organisms present.

Freezing and cold storage are among the oldest methods of preservation. Low temperature retards chemical reactions as well as the activity of food enzymes and slows down or stops the growth and activity of micro-organisms in food. The benefits of low temperature processing or preservation include: (i) preservation of food without any adverse effects on the nutritional values and flavour, colour and textural characteristics of the food, (ii) control of the rate of chemical/enzymes as in ageing of beef, (iii) control of the growth and metabolic activity of starter cultures of desirable food micro-organisms as practised in cheese ripening, and ageing of wines, (iv) enhanced ease and efficiency of unit operations such as peeling and depitting of vegetables and fruits for canning, as also cutting and slicing of bread, (v) reduced loss in flavour and associated changes during extraction of juice from citrus fruits, (vi) ease of precipitation of waxes from edible oils, and (vii) increased solubility of carbon dioxide in water used for aerated drinks.

LOW TEMPERATURE TREATMENT

Temperature approaching 0°C and lower retard the growth and metabolic activities of micro-organisms. Modern refrigeration and freezing equipment has made it possible to transport and store perishable foods for long periods of time. Refrigerated trucks and railway cars, ship's storage vaults, and the home refrigerator and freezer have improved the quality of the human diet and increased the variety of food available. Any food that needs to be preserved must be freed as best as possible from micro-organisms before subjecting it to this method because low temperature do not kill them but only inhibit their activity. Low temperature preservation includes two different methods, viz. chilling and freezing. The effect of low temperatures on micro-organisms depends on the particular microbe and the intensity of application. For example, at temperatures of ordinary refrigerators (0°C), the metabolic rate of some microbes is so reduced that they cannot reproduce or synthesise toxins. In other words, ordinary refrigeration has a bacteriostatic effect, but does not kill many microbes. Heat is much more effective than cold at killing micro-organism.

Yet psychrotrophs do grow slowly at refrigerator temperatures and will alter the appearance and taste of foods after a time. For example, a single microbe reproducing only three times a day would reach a population of more than 2 million within a week. Advantage by medical point of view: Pathogenic bacteria generally will not grow at refrigerator temperature. Uses of cold temperature: Refrigeration is used to prevent food spoilage. Freezing, drying, and freeze-drying are used to preserve both foods and micro-organism, but these methods do not achieve sterilisation.

Optimum conditions: Surprisingly, some bacteria can grow at temperatures several degrees below freezing. Most foods remain unfrozen until –2°C or lower. Rapidly attained subfreezing temperatures tend to render microbes dormant but do not necessarily kill them. Slow freezing is more harmful to bacteria; the ice crystals that form and grow disrupt the cellular and molecular structure of the bacteria. Thawing, being inherently slower is actually the more damaging part of a freeze-thaw cycle. Once frozen, one third of the population of some vegetative bacteria might survive a year, whereas other species might have very few survivors after this time.

Results of low temperature treatment: Many eukaryotic parasites, such as the roundworms that cause trichinosis, are killed by several days of freezing temperatures.

Conditions: Many fresh foods can be prevented from spoiling by keeping them at 5°C (ordinary refrigerator temperature).

Limitations: However, storage should be limited to a few days because some bacteria and moulds continue to grow at this temperature. To convince yourself of this, recall some of the strange things you have found growing on left over of the back of your refrigerator. In rare instances strains of *Clostridium botulinum* have been found growing and producing lethal toxins in a refrigerator when the organism were deep within a container of food, where anaerobic conditions exist.

COOLING, CHILLING AND COLD STABILISATION

Cooling can be defined as a processing technique that is used to reduce the temperature of the food from one processing temperature to another or to a required storage temperature. Chilling is a processing technique in which the temperature of a food is reduced and kept at a temperature between –1°C and 8°C. The objective of cooling and chilling is to reduce the rate of biochemical and microbiological changes in foods, in order to extend the shelf-life of fresh and processed foods or to maintain a certain temperature in a food process, e.g. in the fermentation and treatment of beer. Cooling is also used to promote a change of state of aggregation, e.g. crystallisation. In the wine industry, cooling (chilling) is applied to clarify the must before fermentation. The objective of cold stabilisation is to obtain the precipitation of tartrates (in wines) or fatty acids (in spirits) before bottling.

Field of Application

Cooling is a process step in many food production processes. Chilling for food preservation is widely applied for a lot of perishable foods. The main application of cold stabilisation in the food industry is in the wine and spirit sector.

The supply of chilled foods to consumers requires a sophisticated distribution system, involving chilled stores, refrigerated transport and chilled retail display cabinets. Chilled foods can be grouped into four categories according to the storage temperature:

1. $-1°$ to $+1°C$ (fresh fish, meats, sausages and ground meats, smoked meats and fish).
2. $0°$ to $+5°C$ (pasteurised canned meat, milk and milk products, prepared salads, baked goods, pizzas, unbaked dough and pastry).
3. $0°$ to $+8°C$ (fully cooked meats and fish pies, cooked or uncooked cured meats, butter, margarine, cheese and soft fruits).
4. $8°$ to $12°C$ in the wine industry. The must is kept at this temperature between 6 and 24 hours.

Description of Techniques, Methods and Equipment

Cooling of liquid foods is commonly carried out by passing the product through a heat exchanger (cooler) or by cooling the vessels. The cooling medium in the cooler can be groundwater, water recirculating over a cooling tower, or water (eventually mixed with agents like glycol) which is recirculated via a mechanical refrigeration system (ice-water). Cooling and chilling of solid foods is carried out by contacting the food with cold air, or directly with a refrigerant like liquid carbon dioxide or liquid nitrogen. The equipment used for freezing can also be used for cooling and chilling.

Typical applications

1. Cooling of sugar: Sugar to be stored in silos must be dedusted and cooled to the storage temperature. This is done in a sugar cooler, which is a device in which warm and dried sugar is intensively aerated by cold filtered external air to cool the sugar to the storage temperature, approximately $20°–30°C$. The most common systems in use are coolers (typically drum or fluidised-bed coolers) with chilling systems with countercurrent or cross-current phase flow.
2. Cryogenic cooling: In cryogenic cooling the food is in direct contact with the refrigerant, which may be solid or liquid carbon dioxide or liquid nitrogen. As the refrigerant evaporates or sublimates it removes heat from the food, thereby causing rapid cooling. Both liquid nitrogen and carbon dioxide refrigerants are colourless, odourless and inert.
3. Cold stabilisation: Cold stabilisation is a technique of chilling wines before bottling to cause the precipitation of harmless tartrate crystals. For spirits, this technique consists of bringing the spirit to a temperature of between $-1°$ and $-7°C$, depending on the operators, and possibly performing a stabulation (storing at low temperature) in a tank at constant temperature for between 24 and 48 hours. A cold filtration (around $-1°C$) allows the fatty acid esters to be retained.

For wines, three techniques can be employed: Stabilisation by batch and stabulation. This is the oldest technique and consists of bringing the wine to a temperature below zero close to the freezing point, then stabulating in an isothermal tank during a period of 5 to 8 days.

But currently the most widely-used techniques are: Continuous stabilisation, where the stabulation tank is replaced by a cylindro-conical crystalliser and an agitator, in which the wine will remain for only between 30 and 90 minutes, stabilisation by crystal seeding consisting of refrigerating at between $-1°$ and $-2°C$, and seeding at 4 g/l of tartaric crystals with agitation over 2 to 4 hours, and later storage in tank, and decantation after 12 to 48 hours. There can be many variations on these basic schemes.

MICROBIAL ACTIVITY AT LOW-TEMPERATURES

Most food spoilage micro-organisms grow rapidly at temperatures above $10°C$ while some food poisoning organisms grow slowly even at about $3°C$. Psychrotropic micro-organisms grow slowly between $4.4°C$

and –9.4°C (15°F) provided the food is not solidly frozen. These organisms will not produce food poisoning or disease but even below –3.9°C cause the deterioration of the food quality. Below –9.4°C there is no significant growth of micro-organisms in the food and there is a gradual reduction in their numbers due to slow death. But complete death of all the micro-organisms does not occur merely due to low temperatures and when the food is thawed there can be a rapid multiplication of micro-organisms.

REFRIGERATION AND COOL STORAGE

This is most common method of food preservation as it has no adverse effects on taste, texture and nutritive value. Ideally, refrigeration of perishables should start immediately after harvest or slaughter and should be maintained throughout transportation, warehousing and storage prior to ultimate use. This is particularly true of certain metabolically active fruits and vegetables. These foods give off heat from respiration and convert initially formed metabolites into other compounds. For example, sweet corn metabolises its own sugar even at 0°C resulting in the loss of sweetness to the extent of 8 per cent in a day and 22 per cent in 4 days whereas at 20°C the loss is as high as 25 per cent in one day. Hence a hydrocooler, where jets of cold water are sprayed on the corn soon after harvest to lower the temperature and also to inactivate surface micro-organisms and wash off any pesticide residues, is used. The corn is then transported by trucks to warehouses.

Refrigeration influences agricultural and marketing practices and sets the economic climate of the food industry. Storage and shipment of refrigerated foods helps in maintaining the food supply uniformly throughout the year and to areas of deficiency. Control of prices during different seasons is also possible.

Cooling does not simply mean the placement of bulk foods into a refrigerated container. It means the removal of heat out of a body. Hence cold nitrogen gas volatilising off liquid nitrogen is allowed to pass over the food products to bring about quick cooling. The changes that occur in foods during cool storage are many and are influenced by factors such as growing conditions and varieties of plants, feeding practices of animals, harvest and slaughter, sanitation, damage to tissues and mixture of foods in the storage. Thus apples store well at 2.2° to 4.4°C and grapefruits at 11°C. Pigs fed on peanuts and soyabeans (high unsaturated fat foods) produce soft pork and lard than animals fed on cereal grains. However, flesh of the latter keeps better in cold storage. Animals permitted to rest before slaughter build up glycogen reserves in their muscles which is converted to lactic acid after slaughter. Lactic acid is a mild preservative and enhances the keeping quality of meat in cold storage. Too low temperatures cause cold damage to fruits and vegetables. In the case of bananas and tomatoes, storage below 13°C slows down natural ripening and results in poor ripened colours. Loss of nutrients also occur even during cool storage, e.g. loss of sweetness of sweet corn and vitamins from vegetables. Loss crispness and firmness of vegetables and fruits, loss of flavour and lumping or caking of granular foods are some of the problems associated with cool storage.

Some foods should not be refrigerated at all. Bread is an example. The rate of staling of bread is greater at refrigeration temperatures than at room temperature. However, freezing at –22°C or below can arrest staling and frozen bread retains its freshness for many months. Cakes, cookies, waffles and pancakes are also frozen and marketed.

Factors of Importance in Refrigerated Storage

Factors to be considered in connection with refrigeration include: (i) control of low temperatures, (ii) relative humidity and air circulation, (iii) composition of atmosphere in the storage chamber and (iv) food variability (types of food).

Control of low temperature is achieved by the use of properly designed refrigerators and refrigerated store rooms to maintain temperatures at ±1°C of the selected temperature. The quantity of heat to be removed from food depends on the specific heat of the particular food. Fruits and vegetables produce heat due to respiration. Hence information of the specific heat and respiration rates is necessary to calculate the refrigeration load, which is the quantity of heat that must be removed from the food and the storage area to go from an initial temperature to a selected cold temperature and maintain this temperature for a specified time. Fruits and vegetables, for example, produce heat due to respiration. The amount of heat expressed in terms of British thermal units Btu at 0°C varies with the type of fruit or vegetable (1 Btu = 52 cal. = 1055 joules). For example, the heat given off by apples is of about 300 to 880; cabbage, 1200; carrots, 2130; onions, 600 to 1100; oranges, 420 to 1030; potatoes, 440 to 880; green tomatoes, 580 and ripe tomatoes, 1020 Btu.

Air circulation is of importance because proper air circulation helps in removing the heat away from the vicinity of the food surface to the refrigerator coils/plates. The air circulated within a cold storage room must not be too dry or too moist. Air of high humidity can condense moisture on the surface of cold food allowing the growth of moulds. On the other hand, if air is too dry it will cause excessive drying out of foods.

The optimum humidity to be maintained in cool storage rooms for most foods has been determined. Most foods store best at refrigerated temperatures when air humidity is in the range of 80–95 per cent. The optimum relative humidity is 90–95 per cent for crisp vegetables, about 70 per cent for nuts and 50 per cent for dry and granular products such as milk powder and eggs.

In case refrigerated storage is required for prolonged periods, precautions are to be adopted to maintain food quality. Packaging can protect foods that tend to lose moisture. Thus plastic sacks sprayed with moisture-resistant coatings are used to cover large cuts of meat. Cheeses, which are ripened for many months in cold warehouses, are protected with a wax dip. This minimises the moisture loss and also protects against contamination and growth of surface moulds. Eggs tend to lose moisture and carbon dioxide. Dipping the eggs in thin mineral oil to seal the pores of the eggshell retards these losses. Conventionally, ageing of beef is done at about 2°C (35°F) for a period of several weeks. If the humidity of the storage room is much below 90 per cent the beef dries out, and if it is above 90 per cent mould growth occurs. Precise control of relative humidity is difficult. Hence in the accelerated ageing process (Tenderay process) beef is aged in 2 or 3 days by combining high humidity with a temperature of 18°C (65°F). The accelerated ageing also speeds-up microbial growth which is kept in check by irradiating the beef with ultraviolet light. However, UV irradiation dosage must be regulated because excessive exposure to UV light can cause surface fat to become rancid.

Controlled 'atmospheric storage is practised in cool storage. Fruits in cold storage, respire, ripen and then become overripe. Respiration depends on the availability of oxygen and carbon dioxide content in the surrounding atmosphere. Slow down in respiration and the accompanying undesirable physiological changes in such foods are achieved by the use of (i) low temperature, (ii) depletion of oxygen in the atmosphere and (iii) increase in the level of carbon dioxide. The optimum temperature, relative humidity and gas composition of the cold room atmosphere differs for different fruits and vegetables. Apples can be stored without any deterioration in quality for about six months by maintaining the temperature at 2.8°C, relative humidity at 87 per cent, oxygen concentration at 3 per cent (depletion from the 21 per cent) and increase of carbon dioxide level from the normal 0.03 per cent in air to 3 per cent and the remaining percentage being nitrogen.

Other examples of modified gas atmospheres include the use of diphenyl vapours to inhibit mould growth on citrus fruits and the use of ethylene gas to speed up ripening and colour development of citrus fruits and bananas. The term hypobaric storage refers to storage of food in refrigerated conditions at reduced pressure (to decrease the amount of air) with high humidity (to prevent drying of food).

Food variability or types of foods that can be stored in a cold room is of relevance. Refrigerated storage permits exchange of flavours between types of foods stored near one another. For example, butter and milk absorb odour from fish, and fruits and eggs absorb odour from onions. Hence odourous foods should be stored separately or packaged properly.

Freezing

This process is used for preserving perishable plant and animal products for long periods, from weeks to months. Before freezing the foods are stored, trimmed, washed and blanched. Blanching consists of immersing the food in boiling water or exposing it to live steam for a few minutes. Blanching destroys most of the micro-organisms and inactivates enzymes that would alter the product even at low temperatures. The food is then immediately packaged and frozen. Quick freezing, which is preferred to slow freezing, implies a freezing time of 30 minutes or less and the temperature between $-180°C$ to $-340°C$. Quick freezing produces smaller ice crystals and less damage to the food tissues. Slow freezing products large crystals of ice which rupture cell structures and cause extensive drip or loss of fluid upon thawing.

Frozen fruits may be stored between $-10°C$ and $-180°C$ with little further change. It should be emphasised that freezing cannot be relied upon to kill all micro-organisms no matter what the temperature. The number and types of viable and non-viable micro-organisms present in frozen foods reflect the degree of contamination of the raw product, the sanitation in the processing plant, and the speed and care with which the product was processed. The microbial count of most frozen foods decrease during storage; but many organisms, including pathogens, e.g. species of salmonella survive for long periods of time at $-9°$ and $-170°C$. However, frozen food should be immediately used after thawing because the surviving micro-organisms begin to multiply as soon as they are warmed. Frozen foods are not expected to lose their nutritional value but, the flavour and aroma of fresh food is lost with the length of storage period.

Uses of Freezing: Freezing at $-20°C$ is used to preserve foods in homes and in the food industry. Although freezing does not sterilise foods, it does significantly slow the rate of chemical reactions so that micro-organism does not cause food to spoil. Frozen foods should not be thawed and refrozen. Repeated freezing and thawing of foods causes large ice crystals to form in the foods during slow freezing. Cell membranes in the foods are ruptured, and nutrients leak out. The texture of foods is thus altered, and they become less palatable. It also allows bacteria to multiply while food is thawed, making the food more susceptible to bacterial degradation.

Freezing can be used to preserve micro-organisms, but this requires a much lower temperature than that used for food preservation. Micro-organism are usually suspended in glycerol or protein to prevent the formation of large ice crystal (which could puncture cells), cooled with solid carbon dioxide (dry ice) to a temperature of $-78°C$, and then held there. Alternatively, they can be placed in liquid nitrogen and cooled to $-180°C$.

FACTORS AFFECTING FROZEN FOOD QUALITY

If foods have only partially thawed, and still have ice crystals in the package, they can be safely refrozen, though their quality will be lower.

Frozen foods should be stored at zero degrees Fahrenheit or less. Refrigerator-freezer combinations can be used for storing frozen food; if the freezer is a true freezer. A true freezer compartment will maintain a temperature of zero degrees Fahrenheit or below. If the freezer compartment is not a true freezer, store food for only one to two weeks for best quality. Food may not spoil if the compartment temperature is above zero degrees Fahrenheit. However, the quality will decline. The overall quality of frozen foods will decline if the food is held much longer than the recommended storage time, although it will still be safe to eat. Freezing does not improve the quality of the food product. Frozen food is only as good as the quality of the fresh food, so select only high quality products at optimum maturity and freshness.

Freezing does not Kill Germs Present in Food

It does prevent the growth and multiplication of germs, if food is held at zero degree Fahrenheit or less. When thawed, the surviving organisms can grow again. Meat, fish, poultry, prepared foods, vegetables, and fruit can be refrozen if the freezer temperature is 40°F or below and if the colour and odour are good. A freezer thermometer is the surest way to check and maintain the freezer's temperature.

Adding large amounts of room temperature food to a freezer at one time can also bring the freezer temperature up. It can also cause slight thawing of some frozen foods, as well as, slow freezing of the newly added food. Add only the amount of food that will freeze within 24 hours. The general rule is to allow two to three pounds of food per cubic foot or storage space. Turning the freezer temperature down below zero degree at least 12 hours before new food is added will also help the freezer maintain a zero degree Fahrenheit or below temperature.

Packaging at Zero Degrees

When foods are held at zero degree Fahrenheit, their packaging becomes very important. Freezer burn is dehydration or drying that occurs on the surface of a product if it is improperly wrapped. The food is safe to eat but poorer in quality. To prevent freezer burn, the package must be free of air and tightly sealed.

Packaging materials must be moisture-vapour resistant, durable and leak proof and resistant to oil, grease of water. Good freezing materials include rigid containers made of aluminum, glass, plastic, tin, or heavily waxed cardboard; bags and sheets of moisture-vapour resistant wraps and laminated papers made especially for freezing. Heavy duty aluminum can be used as a freezer wrap, but because it can be torn or punctured easily, it is wise to use an over wrap. Light weight or household aluminum foil is not satisfactory for home freezing.

FOOD PRESERVATION AND SHELF-LIFE EXTENSION

The more common industrial gases typically employed in the production of safe food include nitrogen, CO_2, oxygen, SO_2, ozone and hydrogen. These gases are used to provide improved functionality of food ingredients like cryogenically crystallised fats which can increase the shortening power by 30 per cent due to its unique crystal morphology. Rapid freezing and chilling can also improve the product quality by reducing dehydration losses and reducing the risk of 'freezer burn'.

By reducing temperatures of fresh products like poultry from 10° to –1°C deep chilling can be achieved in less than 2 hours hence substantially reducing the risk of microbiological spoilage and increase the shelf-life. Yield improvements of up to 4 per cent can also be realised by for instance crust freezing small goods prior to slicing in high-speed slicers. During mixing and grinding a significant amount of heat is generated, and CO_2 chilling processes can offset this added heat load and also further reduce temperatures for optimum forming or further processing. Equipment has been developed to meet all the processing and quality requirements, whether batch or continuous processes.

These include batch freezers and continuous belt freezers like tunnel, spiral and fluid bed freezers to deliver individually quick frozen value added products. Automated CO_2 based chilling equipment has been specially adapted to suit in-process requirements and conditions. CO_2 chilling systems fitted to blenders have the capability to control the temperature to 0.1°C. All this equipment has been designed to allow for easy internal access for the purpose of sanitation. Gas mixing systems have been specially designed to consistently supply the required gas mixes and flow rate required for modified atmosphere packaging. In the wine industry, the control of wild yeast can be maintained by an accurate SO_2 dosing system, critical where tight limitations exist for the presence of residual SO_2 in food stuff. Process audits assess the efficiency of gas related applications and provide recommendations of how to improve yields, reduce costs and improve food safety.

In the first stage, or in the case of minimally processed food, the predominant needs are to rapidly reduce temperatures and/or control the atmosphere to prevent microbial spoilage or senescence. Products like oil are prone to oxidation of the fatty acids, and hence need to be blanketed in a nitrogen atmosphere.

The presence of oxygen in MAP gases can reduce the risk of botulism in seafood and hence severe food poisoning. CO_2 when dissolved in aqueous solutions forms a weak acid inhibiting microbial spoilage and also anaerobic conditions which in turn inhibit aerobic micro-organisms. During sparging applications nitrogen is used to sparge liquids like wine and oils to remove dissolved oxygen which can potentially degrade product.

In modified atmosphere packaging, gas mixtures are specifically tailor made to target the predominant spoilage mechanisms and hence enhance shelf life and provide another hurdle for reducing microbial spoilage. Temperature control is as critical to extend shelf-life and inhibit spoilage mechanisms in the case of produce as well as primary meat production facilities. Dry ice or CO_2 snow may be applied to grapes during harvesting for rapid chilling or applied into combo bins or trays to chill poultry prior to distribution to secondary processing facilities.

Particularly poultry is prone to microbial spoilage if insufficient heat is removed from the carcass by the spin chillers, and hence dry ice or CO_2 snow can rapidly reduce the temperature below 4°C, to inhibit the onset of spoilage and enhance shelf-life.

A very diverse range of innovative solutions has evolved over recent years covering atmosphere, microbe and temperature control. In conjunction with local and overseas research organisations new technologies continue to emerge. In wine processing, levels of dissolved oxygen are continually monitored and both gases CO_2 and N_2 are used in varying ratios to control dissolved levels of CO_2 and oxygen, depending on the type of wine that is being produced. This results in a wine with an extended shelf life and the desired flavour profile and functionality.

Hydrogen is used in the hydrogenation process to change liquid into hard fats by changing the molecular structure whilst the high solubility of CO_2 in aqueous solutions (1 volume to 1 volume at 1 atm) provides soft drinks with the effervescence and slightly acidic taste. Sulphur Dioxide and Ozone, a strong oxidising agent, have strong anti-microbial properties and are used in food preservation, preventing cross contamination and sanitising processing equipment. Temperature control during processing is also very important and can impact on quality, yield and food safety.

Temperatures in blenders for beef patties manufacturing have to be controlled within 0.1°C, at a maximum temperature of −1.2°C in order to achieve a coined edge Pattie during the forming process. Bottom injection of liquid CO_2 via injection nozzles at the bottom of the blender delivers CO_2 snow at a very high rate achieving rapid and uniform temperature throughout the mix. Viscosity control allows for the control of the CO_2 to be injected at the exact amount to achieve the target temperature.

The temperature of some dough like cookie dough is critical, and fluctuations especially due to ambient conditions can result in increased rejects, production losses and quality issues. By reducing the temperature of the flour, the main ingredient in pneumatic conveying systems, the dough temperature can be maintained at the target temperature irrespective of seasonal fluctuations in temperatures. Optimising the temperatures so that the product or product surface is more rigid for a cleaner cut can attain improved slicing and dicing yields.

A cryogenic spiral freezer can ensure that the product temperature is brought down to near 0°C to ensure a clean cut and reduce yield losses by as much as 4 per cent. The final product is packaged and sold as either a 'fresh' or frozen commodity. Fresh products stored at either refrigerated or ambient temperatures, can benefit from modified atmospheres, and hence extending shelf life. The drivers for increasing shelf life may be financially driven or improved market penetration, or simply another hurdle to improved food safety.

For example, red meat for retail display is commonly being packaged centrally rather than in retail stores. Centralised packaging is growing in popularity, as it requires less labour, equipment and also a reduced risk of microbial contamination. Consumers associate the bright red colour in red meat with freshness and this can be attained with high oxygen MAP gas mix, containing also CO_2.

The carbon dioxide inhibits bacterial spoilage whilst the oxygen is needed to give the bloom that appeals to customers. A wide range of equipment exists for temperature control covering both chilling and freezing. Cryogenic freezing involves a rapid temperature reduction using specialised equipment to a final temperature of −18°C or colder, and in the case of chilling to below 4°C.

Due to the cold operating temperatures within the freezers, dehydration is substantially less than in conventional freezing equipment, and there is a reduced risk of spoilage of food due to the rapid temperature reduction. For individually quick frozen products like pizza topping or diced cooked poultry, fluid bed freezers have been developed which have superior performance over other equipment.

The product is initially immersed in liquid nitrogen, to be crust frozen, to prevent product from clumping followed by further heat removal in a fluidised bed. Cryogenic freezers are typically a quarter of the capital cost, and with a much smaller foot print than conventional system, the added flexibility allows customers to trial new products, and adapt to changing market conditions.

The final product may be transferred into tankers or into storage silos or tanks. Wine or fruit juice transported in bulk must be protected from oxidation and is blanketed in a nitrogen or CO_2-atmosphere. Atmosphere control in cool rooms is commonly employed to extend the shelf life of apples and other fruit, and hence extend the availability of these perishable products. Oxygen is used in the aquaculture industry to transport live fish.

In transit refrigeration in trucks using CO_2 or N_2 provides increased flexibility and more rapid temperature pull-down, and can provide back up if the mechanical refrigeration system fails. In transit refrigeration with CO_2 snow is commonly utilised where products require chilling from loading through to delivery to the customer.

Thaw Recorder Indicator

The thaw indicators (labels) are irreversible and can record thaw temperature exceeded. They enable the receiver of the goods to check out whether a certain temperature has been exceeded during transport or not. The thaw indicators have some kinds of active mechanism, before used, they stay in not activated state (not ready to change colour). When the thaw indicators get ready to record temperature changing in transport or other situation (the indicator need to be activated).

Instructions

1. Leave food in the refrigerator to thaw all day or overnight.
2. Place food in a watertight container or bag and submerge it in cold water. Change the water every 30 minutes until thawing is complete.
3. Use the defrost setting on a microwave oven for the quickest results. Leave a 2 inch space between the food and the side of the microwave for better heat circulation.
4. Cut food into smaller pieces (if you can, or when it defrosts enough to allow you to) to allow it to thaw more evenly. Turn the food over several times as it defrosts.

The best way to thaw food is in the refrigerator at 41°F or lower. Another way is under cool running water with the water running over the covered product which thaws the ice crystals. After thawing food in the microwave, you must always continue the cooking process, never refrigerate and cook later as you will give harmful organisms the time, temperature, moisture that they need to reproduce. Put your food in a ziplock and then put in a microwave safe bowl with enough water to cover the defrost setting from cooking the thinner parts of your food. For meat this is also a good time to marinate.

Chapter 7

Preservation by Use of High Temperature

INTRODUCTION

Exposure to heat denatures proteins leading to inactivation of enzymes required for metabolism. The heat treatment necessary to kill micro-organisms or their spores varies with the kind of organism, its physiological state and the environment during heating. The heat treatment selected depends on kind of organisms to be killed, other preservative methods to be employed and the effect of heat on food. Certain factors affect the heat resistance of cells or spores like:

1. Initial concentration of cells/spores in food to be heated.
2. Previous history of cells/spores, that is the conditions under which they have been grown like culture medium, temperature, growth phage, desiccation, etc.

Culture medium components influence heat resistance of micro-organisms. Glucose increases heat resistance, phosphate and magnesium ions reduce heat resistance in bacteria. Temperature of incubation influences heat resistance of micro-organisms. Resistance increases if the cells are incubated at optimum temperature of growth. Growth phase of bacteria has influence on their sensitivity to heat. Bacterial cells are resistant to heat during late log and stationary phases. They are most susceptible during log phase. Water content in cells influences their sensitivity to heat. Desiccation makes them to resist high temperatures. Therefore spores are more resistant to heat than their vegetative cells. Composition of substrate in which cells/spores are heated influences response of micro-organisms to high temperature. Moisture of substrate increases effectiveness of heat as moist heat is more effective in killing micro-organisms than dry heat. Substrate at neutral pH is less susceptible to heat than that at acidic or alkaline pH. Solutes containing salt and sugar reduce susceptibility of cells or spores to heat. For efficient application of high temperature used for food preservation, heat resistance of micro-organisms in terms of thermal death time and thermal death point have to be taken into consideration.

FACTORS AFFECTING HEAT RESISTANCE OF MICRO-ORGANISMS

Cells and spores differ widely in their ability to resist high temperatures. Even within a population of cells and spores the heat resistance varies as indicated by the thermal death time or frequency distribution. In general, a small number of cells have low resistance, most of the cells have a medium resistance and a small number have a high resistance. The various factors influencing the thermal death time (heat resistance) of micro-organisms include the following:

1. Temperature time relationship: The time required for killing cells or spores under a given set of conditions decreases as temperature is increased. For example, the time required to kill the

spores of *C. botulinum* at an initial population of 6×10^{10} in buffered medium at pH 7 has been estimated to be 260 minutes at 100°C, 120 minutes at 105°C, 36 minutes at 110°C and 5 minutes at 120°C.

2. Initial concentration of spores or cells: The more the number of spores or cells present, greater is the heat treatment required to kill them. For instance, the time required to kill spores of a thermophilic organism in spoiled canned corn juice with a pH of 6.0 at a temperature of 120°C has been found to be 14 minutes for an initial concentration of 50,000/ml, 10 minutes for 5000/ml and 9 minutes for 500/ml. Similarly, the thermal death time of the spores of *C. botulinum* (in a buffer of pH 7) at 100°C was found to be 110 minutes for an initial population of 3.2×10^7 and 50 minutes for an initial population of 1.64×10^4.

3. Previous history of the vegetative cells or spores: The conditions under which the cells have been grown and spores have been produced and their treatment thereafter will influence their resistance to heat.

   (a) Culture medium: The medium in which growth takes place is especially important. The effect of the nutrients in the medium, their kind, and the amount vary with the organism, but in general the better the medium for growth, the more resistant the cells or spores. The presence of an adequate supply of accessory growth factors usually favours the production of heat-resistant cells or spores. This probably is why vegetable infusions and liver extract increase heat resistance. According to Curran, spores formed and aged in soil or oats are more resistant than those in broth or agar. Carbohydrates, amino acids, and organic acid radicals have an effect, but it is difficult to predict. A small amount of glucose in a medium may lead to increased heat resistance, but more sugar may result in the formation of enough acid to cause decreased heat resistance. Some salts seem to have an effect; phosphate and magnesium ions, for instance, are said to decrease the heat resistance of bacterial spores produced in a medium containing them. Prolonged exposure to metabolic products reduces the heat resistance of cells and spores.

   (b) Temperature of incubation: The temperature of growth of cells and the temperature of sporulation influences their heat resistance. In general, resistance increases as the incubation temperature is raised toward the optimum for the organism and for many organisms increases further as the temperature approaches the maximum for growth. *Escherichia coli*, for example, is considerably more heat-resistant when grown at 38.5°C, which is near its optimal temperature, than at 28°C. Spores of *Bacillus subtilis*, grown at different temperatures in 1 per cent peptone water, were heated with the results.

   (c) Phase of growth or age: The heat resistance of vegetative cells varies with the stage of growth and of spores with their age. Bacterial cells show their greatest resistance during the late lag phase but almost as great resistance during their maximum stationary phase, followed by a decline in resistance. The cells are least resistant during their phase of logarithmic growth. Very young (immature) spores are less resistant than are mature ones. Some spores increase in resistance during the first weeks of storage but later begin to decrease in resistance.

   (d) Desiccation: Dried spores of some bacteria are harder to kill by heat than are those kept moist, but this apparently does not hold for all bacterial spores.

4. Composition of the substrate in which cells or spores are heated: The material in which the spores or cells are heated is so important that it must be stated if a thermal death time is to have meaning.

(a) Moisture: Moist heat is a much more effective killing agent than dry heat, and as a corollary dry materials require more heat for sterilisation than moist ones. In the bacteriological laboratory about 15 to 30 min at 121°C in the moist heat of an autoclave will effect sterilisation of ordinary materials, but 3 to 4 hr at 160° to 180°C is necessary when the dry heat of an oven is employed. Spores of *Bacillus subtilis* are killed in less than 10 min in steam at 120°C, but in anhydrous glycerol 170°C for 30 min is required.

(b) Hydrogen-ion concentration (pH): In general, cells or spores are most heatresistant in a substrate that is at or near neutrality. An increase in acidity or alkalinity hastens killing by heat, but a change toward the acid side is more effective than a corresponding increase in alkalinity. Spores of *B. subtilis* heated at 100°C in 1:15 m phosphate solutions, adjusted to various pH values, gave the results. Other examples will be given in the discussion of the heat processing of canned foods. Cameron divided canned foods into the acid food, the pH values of which are below 4.5, and the low-acid foods, with a pH above 4.5. Acid foods include the common fruits and certain vegetable products, and the low-acid foods are those such as meat, seafood, milk, and most of the common vegetables. A further subdivision was suggested by Cameron.

Low-acid foods: With a pH above 5.3, including such foods as peas, corn, lima beans, meats, fish, poultry, and milk (although Cameron included only vegetables and fruits in his original grouping).

Medium-acid foods: With a pH between 5.3 and 4.5, including such foods as spinach, asparagus, beets, and pumpkin.

Acid foods: With a pH between 4.5 and 3.7, including such foods as tomatoes, pears, and pineapple.

High-acid foods: With a pH of 3.7 and below, including such foods as berries and sauerkraut. The effect of the pH of the substrate is complicated by the fact that heating at high temperature causes a decrease in the pH of low- or medium-acid foods; and the higher the original pH, the greater the drop in pH caused by heating. Foods with an original pH of less than 5.5 to 5.8 change little in acidity as a result of heating.

(c) Other constituents of the substrate: The only salt present in appreciable amounts in most foods is sodium chloride, which in low concentrations has a protective effect on some spores. Sugar seems to protect some organisms or spores but not others. The optimal concentration for protection varies with the organism: it is high for some osmophilic organisms and low for others, high for spores and low for non osmophilic cells. The protective effect of sugar may be related to a resulting decrease in a_w. A reduced a_w does result in an increase in observed heat resistance.

Solutes differ in their effect on bacteria. Glucose, for example, protects *Escherichia coli* and *Pseudomonas fluorescens* against heat better than sodium chloride at a_w levels near the minimum for growth. On the other hand, glucose affords practically no protection or is even harmful to *Staphylococcus aureus*, whereas sodium chloride is very protective.

Since the concentration of solutes may affect the heat process necessary for sterilisation, canners sometimes further classify foods as high-soluble-solids foods, such as sirups and concentrates, and low-soluble-solids foods, such as fruits, vegetables, and meats.

Colloidal materials, especially proteins and fats, are protective against heat. This is well illustrated in Table 7.1 by the data of Brown and Peiser who used thermal death points.

Table 7.1. Effect of protective substance on heat resistance of bacteria.

Substance	Temperature, °C		
	S. lactis	*E. coli*	*L. bulgaricus*
Cream	69–71	73	95
Whole milk	65	69	91
Skim milk	59–63	65	89
Whey	57–61	63	83
Broth	55–57	61	

It will be observed that as the content of protective substances (proteins and fat) decreased in the media, the temperature needed to kill the organism in 10 minutes decreased.

Antiseptic or germicidal substances in the substrate aid heat in the destruction of organisms. Thus hydrogen peroxide plus heat is used to reduce the bacterial content of sugar and is the basis of a process for milk.

THERMAL DEATH TIME

Thermal death time is a concept used to determine how long it takes to kill a specific bacteria at a specific temperature. It was developed for food canning and has found applications in cosmetics and pharmaceuticals.

Thermal death time: It is defined as the time taken at a given temperature to kill specified number of micro-organisms under defined conditions.

Thermal death point: It is the temperature necessary to kill all micro-organisms present in a given substance in defined time (minutes).

For efficient application of high temperature for preservation of food, the rate of heat penetration into food should be efficient and this is influenced by material of the container, consistency, size and shape of contents, initial temperature of food, prior treatments if any, etc. Material of container make like glass has slower rate of penetration than metal. Consistency of can contents and size and shape of food item, like larger one takes longer time, smaller one takes shorter time. Food items could retain their identity, lose their form and become viscous or layer out. Initial temperature of food, like lower the initial temperature, longer time of exposure and higher the initial temperature, shorter the time of exposure required for treatment. Prior treatments like asepsis, removal of micro-organisms, etc. affect by reducing the bioburden of food items.

Mathematical Formulas

Thermal death time can be determined one of two ways: (i) by using graphs, and (ii) by using mathematical formulas.

Graphical method

This is usually expressed in minutes at the temperature of 250°F or 121°C. This is designated as F_0. Each 18°F or 10°C change results in a time change by a factor of 10. This would be shown either as F_{121}^{10} = 10 minutes (SI) or F_{250}^{18} = 10 minutes (American English).

A lethal ratio (L) is also a sterilising effect at 1 minute at other temperatures with (T).

$$L = 10^{(T - T_{Ref})/z}$$

where, T_{Ref} is the reference temperature, usually 250°F or 121°C; z is the z-value, and T is the slowest heat point of the product temperature.

Formula method

Prior to the advent of computers, this was plotted on semilogarithmic paper though it can also be done on spreadsheet programs. The time would be shown on the x-axis while the temperature would be shown on the y-axis. This simple heating curve can also determine the lag factor (j) and the slope (f_h). It also measures the product temperature rather than the can temperature.

$$j = \frac{jI}{I}$$

where, I = RT (Retort temperature) – IT (Initial temperature) and where j is constant for a given product. It is also determined in the equation shown below:

$$\text{Log } g = \log jI - \frac{B_B}{f_h}$$

where, g is the number of degrees below the retort temperature on a simple heating curve at the end of the heating period, B_B is the time in minutes from the beginning of the process to the end of the heating period, and f_h is the time in minutes required for the straight-line portion of the heating curve plotted semilogarithmically on paper or a computer spreadsheet to pass through a log cycle.

A broken heating curve is also used in this method when dealing with different products in the same process such as chicken noodle soup in having to dealing with the meat and the noodles having different cooking times as an example. It is more complex than the simple heating curve for processing.

Applications

In the food industry, it is important to reduce the amount of microbes in products to ensure proper food safety. This is usually done by thermal processing and finding ways to reduce the number of bacteria in the product. Time-temperature measurements of bacterial reduction is determined by a D-value, meaning how long it would take to reduce the bacterial population by 90 per cent or one $\log_{10}$ at a given temperature. This D-value reference (D_R) point is 250°F or 121°C. z is used to determine the time values with different D-values at different temperatures with its equation shown below:

$$z = \frac{T_2 - T_1}{\log D_1 - \log D_2}$$

where, T is temperature in °F or °C.

This D-value is affected by pH of the product where low pH has faster D-values on various foods.

The target of reduction in canning is the 12-D reduction of *C. botulinum*, which means that processing time will reduce the amount of this bacteria by 10^{12} bacteria per gram or millilitre. The D_R for *C. botulinum* is 0.21 minute (12.6 seconds). A 12-D reduction will take 2.52 minutes (151 seconds).

THERMAL DESTRUCTION OF MICRO-ORGANISMS

Heat is lethal to micro-organisms, but each species has its own particular heat tolerance. During a thermal destruction process, such as pasteurisation, the rate of destruction is logarithmic, as is their rate of growth. Thus bacteria subjected to heat are killed at a rate that is porportional to the number of organisms present. The process is dependent both on the temperature of exposure and the time required at this temperature to accomplish to desired rate of destruction. Thermal calculations thus involve the need for knowledge of the concentration of micro-organisms to be destroyed, the acceptable concentration of micro-organisms that can remain behind (spoilage organisms, for example, but not pathogens), the thermal resistance of the target micro-organisms (the most heat tolerant ones), and the temperature time relationship required for destruction of the target organisms.

The extent of the pasteurisation treatment required is determined by the heat resistance of the most heat-resistant enzyme or micro-organism in the food. For example, milk pasteurisation historically was based on *Mycobacterium tuberculosis* and *Coxiella burnetti*, but with the recognition of each new pathogen, the required time temperature relationships are continuously being examined.

A thermal death curve for this process is shown in Fig. 7.1. It is a logarithmic process, meaning that in a given time interval and at a given temperature, the same percentage of the bacterial population will be destroyed regardless of the population present. For example, if the time required to destroy one log cycle or 90 per cent is known, and the desired thermal reduction has been decided (for example, 12 log cycles), then the time required can be calculated. If the number of micro-organisms in the food increases, the heating time required to process the product will also be increased to bring the population down to an acceptable level. The heat process for pasteurisation is usually based on a 12-*D* concept or a 12 log cycle reduction in the numbers of this organism (Fig. 7.1).

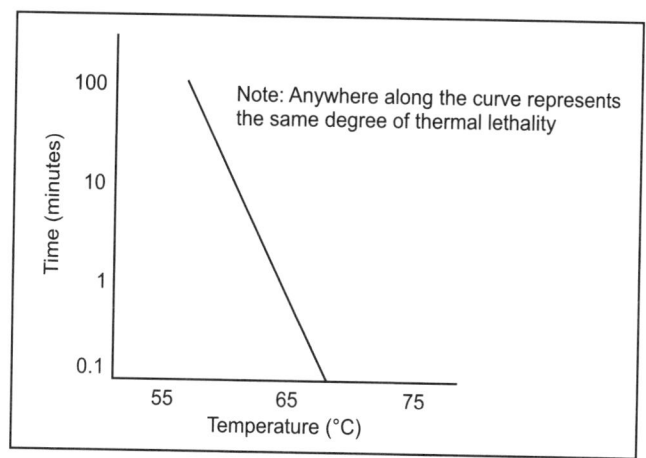

Fig. 7.1. Thermal death time curve for *Coxiella burnetti*, $z = 4°C$.

Several parameters help us to do thermal calculations and define the rate of thermal lethality. The *D* value is a measure of the heat resistance of a micro-organism. It is the time in minutes at a given temperature required to destroy 1 log cycle (90 per cent) of the target micro-organism. (Of course, in an actual process, all others that are less heat tolerant are destroyed to a greater extent.) For example, a *D*-value at 72°C of 1 minute means that for each minute of processing at 72°C the bacteria population of the target micro-organism will be reduced by 90 per cent. In the illustration (Fig. 7.2) the *D* value is 14 minutes (40–26) and would be representative of a process at 72°C. The *Z*-value reflects the temperature dependence of the reaction. It is defined as the temperature change required to change the *D*-value by a factor of 10. In the illustration (Fig. 7.3) the *Z*-value is 10°C.

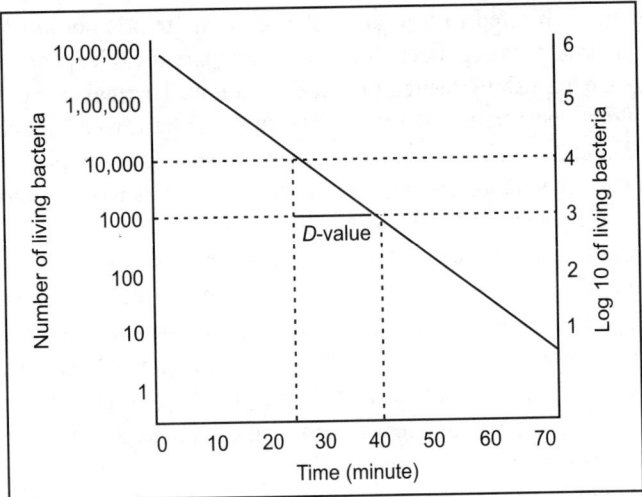

Fig. 7.2. Illustration showing *D*-value.

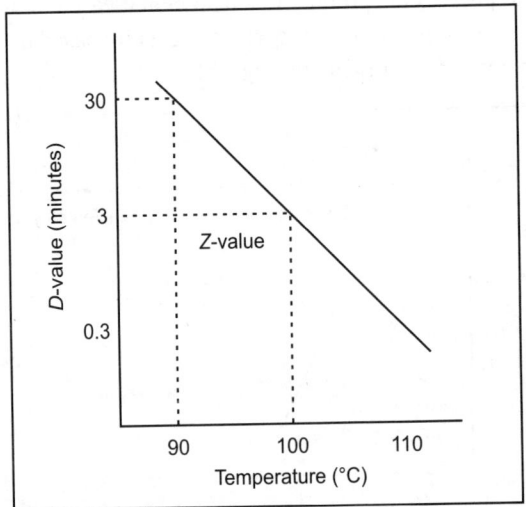

Fig. 7.3. Illustration showing *Z*-value.

Reactions that have small *Z*-values are highly temperature dependent, whereas those with large *Z*-values require larger changes in temperature to reduce the time. *A Z*-value of 10°C is typical for a spore forming bacterium. Heat induced chemical changes have much larger *Z*-values that micro-organisms, as shown in Table 7.2.

Table 7.2. Heat induced chemical changes.

	Z (°C)	*D121 (min)*
Bacteria	5–10	1–5
Enzymes	30–40	1–5
Vitamins	20–25	150–200
Pigments	40–70	15–50

The Fig. 7.4 illustrates the relative changes in time temperature profiles for the destruction of micro-organisms. Above and to the right of each line the micro-organisms or quality factors would be destroyed, whereas below and to the left of each line, the micro-organisms or quality factors would not be destroyed. Due to the differences in Z-values, it is apparent that at higher temperatures for shorter times, a region exists (shaded area) where pathogens can be destroyed while vitamins can be maintained. The same holds true for other quality factors such as colour and flavour components. Thus in milk processing the higher temperature, shorter time (HTST) process (72°C/16 sec) is favoured compared to a lower temperature longer time (batch or vat) process since it results in a slightly lower loss of vitamins and better sensory quality.

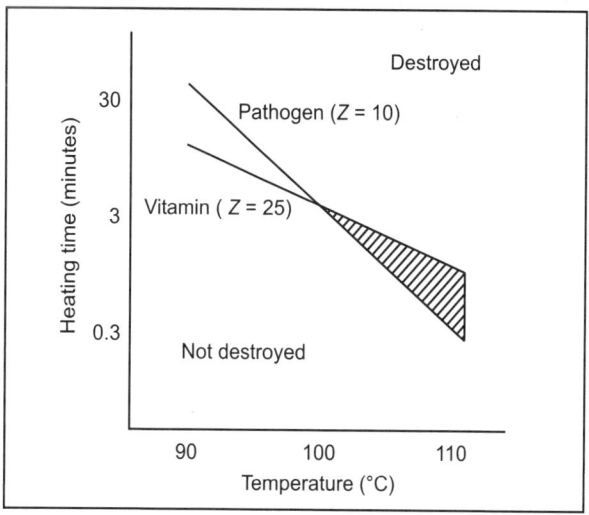

Fig. 7.4. Relative changes in time temperature profiles for the destruction of micro-organisms.

Alkaline phosphatase is a naturally-occurring enzyme in raw milk which has a similar Z-value to heat-resistant pathogens. Since the direct estimation of pathogen numbers by microbial methods is expensive and time consuming, a simple test for phosphatase activity is routinely used. If activity is found, it is assumed that either the heat treatment was inadequate or that unpasteurised milk has contaminated the pasteurised product.

HEAT PENETRATION

The rate of penetration of heat into a food must be known in order to calculate the thermal process necessary for its preservation. Since every part of the food in a can or other container must receive an adequate heat treatment to prevent spoilage, that part which heats the most slowly is the critical one, and rates of change in the temperature of that part—usually near the center of containers of foods heating by conduction and farther down when heating is by convection are measured.

Heat penetration from an external source to the center of the can may take place by conduction, where heat passes from molecule to molecule; by convection, where heat is transferred by movement of liquids or gases; or, as is usually the case, by a combination of conduction and convection. Conduction is slow in foods and rapid in metals. The rate of heat transfer by convection depends on the opportunity for currents in the liquid and the rate of flow of these currents.

When both conduction and convection are involved in the heating of foods, they may function simultaneously or successively. When solid particles of food are suspended in a liquid, the particles heat by conduction and the liquid heats by convection. Some foods change in consistency during heating, and a broken heating curve results. This is true of sugar sirups, brine-packed whole-grain corn, and certain thick soups and tomato juices.

STERILISATION

The aim is complete destruction of micro-organisms. Because of the resistance of certain bacterial spores to heat, a treatment at 121°C (250°F) of wet heat for 15 minutes or its equivalent is necessary for sterilisation. Every particle of the food must receive this heat treatment. If a can of food is to be sterilised, immersing it into a pressure cooker or retort at 121°C for 15 minutes will not be sufficient because of the low rate of heat transfer through the food. Depending upon the size of the can and the type of food, sterilisation may require several hours. During this time, many changes can occur to depreciate the quality of the food. Fortunately, many of the foods need not be sterilised completely. Most of the canned and bottled products are commercially sterile. It means a degree of sterilisation at which all pathogenic and toxin forming organisms as well as all other types of food spoilage organisms have been destroyed. Commercially sterilised food may still contain a very small number of resistant bacterial spores, but these will not normally multiply in food. However, if they are isolated from the food and given suitable environmental conditions they will multiply. Commercially sterile canned foods have a shelf life of 2 years or more. Even after longer periods, deterioration in the quality of such foods is generally due to texture or flavour changes rather than to growth of micro-organisms.

Canning: A variety of foods are canned. These include whole fruits and vegetables, sliced or diced fruits and vegetables, meat and meat products, fish and fish products and soups. Two general methods of sterilisation are commonly used in industry: (i) in-pack sterilisation (sterilisation inside containers), and (ii) sterilisation of the food before placing in the containers.

The in-pack sterilisation involves several steps. These include: (i) cleaning and grading of food raw materials, (ii) blanching to inactivate native enzymes (particularly in vegetables and fruits), (iii) filling or placing the cleaned raw food in a sealable container, with added brine in the case of vegetables, meat and fish or sugar syrup in the case of fruits, (iv) deaeration (to prevent bulging or bursting of can during heating) followed by closing and sealing the container, (v) heating the container in a retort at specified temperature for a specific holding time, (vi) cooling partially under pressure in the retort followed by cooling in a cooling tank, and (vii) labelling, storing and/or marketing. The sterilisation process may be operated in batch or continuous mode involving vertical or horizontal retorts, pressure cooker, rotary or reel cooker or hydrostat cooker or non-pressurised methods. All these procedures use temperatures above 100°C and hence the pressure developed is greater than atmospheric pressure. The containers may be cans, necked-in flange type (to control postcanning infection) or tin-free steel type cans, glass jars, film pouches or sterilisable plastic containers of rigid, semi-rigid or flexible forms. Heat penetration in these packs is controlled by the geometry of the pack and by the thermal properties of the food, the container and the heating medium. Hence sterilisation of food placed within the containers is a slow process.

Asceptic canning involves: (i) sterilising the food separately outside the containers, (ii) placing the food in previously sterilised cans under asceptic conditions, and (iii) sealing the containers. The advantages in this method include:

1. High temperature processing at temperatures up to 150°C using high speed heat exchangers cutting down the processing time appreciably.

2. A better product quality as deterioration due to over heating is prevented. The food is passed continuously through a plate or tubular heat exchanger where it is brought to sterilising temperature almost instantaneously. The holding period is about 1–2 seconds at this temperature and the technique is known as *Ultra-high temperature* (UHT) *sterilisation*. The sterilised food is then quickly cooled by another heat exchanger and enters the asceptic canning line, which consists of a tunnel maintained under sterile conditions through which sterilised cans are conveyed, filled and sealed.

Hot packing or hot filling technique involves the filling of previously sterilised food, while still hot, into clean but not necessarily sterile containers under clean but not necessarily asceptic conditions. The heat of the food and the holding time before cooling ensures commercial sterility of the filled product. Hot packing or hot filling is suitable for acid foods because most of the micro-organisms include *C. botulinum* which do not survive at pH less than 4.5. Most fruit juices such as orange, grape, grapefruit, tomato and acid fruits and vegetables and pickled vegetables such as sauerkraut are hot packed or hot filled. For example, fruit juices are heated in the range of 77°–100°C for 30–60 seconds, hot filled at about 90°C and held at this temperature for about 3 minutes with an inversion of the can before cooling.

Hot packing of low acid foods requires the presence of other preservative measures such as high concentration of sugar as in the case of fruit jams. An alternative technique 'Flash 18' process or pressure canning is used for low acid foods. Low acid foods need to be heated to temperatures above 100°C under pressure for sterilisation. If the food at this temperature is filled into containers for sealing at atmospheric pressure, there will be violent boiling. In flash 18 process, the entire canning line is placed inside a pressure chamber at about 1.1 to 1.4 atmospheric pressure and at this pressure water will not boil at temperatures below 124°–127°C. Hence low acid foods sterilised at higher than 100°C are conveyed to the pressure chamber and filled into previously sterilised cans and sealed. A filling temperature of 124°C held over several minutes at this pressure gives commercial sterility to the product.

ASEPTIC PROCESSING

Aseptic processing is the process by which a sterile (aseptic) product (typically food or pharmaceutical) is packaged in a sterile container in a way that maintains sterility.

Sterility is achieved with a flash-heating process (temperature between 195° and 295°F (91° to 146°C), which retains more nutrients and uses less energy than conventional sterilisation techniques such as retort or hot-fill canning. Aseptic food preservation methods allow processed food to keep for long periods of time without preservatives, as long as they are not opened. The aseptic packages are typically a mix of paper (70 per cent), polyethylene (LDPE) (24 per cent), and aluminum (6 per cent), with a tight polyethylene inside layer. Together the materials form a tight seal against microbiological organisms, contaminants, and degradation, eliminating the need for refrigeration.

Aseptic processing is commonly used for the packaging of milks, fruit juices, liquid whole eggs, gravies, and tomatoes. Fresh tomatoes are aseptically processed and packaged for year-round remanufacture into various food products.

ASEPTIC PACKAGING SYSTEM

Aseptic packaging can be defined as the filling of a commercially sterile product into a sterile container under aseptic conditions and hermetically sealing the containers so that reinfection is prevented. This results in a product, which is shelf-stable at ambient conditions. The term 'aseptic' is derived from the Greek word 'septicos' which means the absence of putrefactive micro-organisms.

In practice, generally there are two specific fields of application of aseptic packaging technology:

1. Packaging of presterilised and sterile products. Examples are milk and dairy products, puddings, desserts, fruit and vegetable juices, soups, sauces, and products with particulates.

2. Packaging of nonsterile product to avoid infection by micro-organisms. Examples of this application include fermented dairy products like yoghurt.

Aseptic packaging technology is fundamentally different from that of conventional food processing by canning. In canning, the process begins with treating the food prior to filling. Initial operations inactivate enzymes so that these will not degrade the product during processing. The package is cleaned, and the product is introduced into the package, usually hot. Generally, air that can cause oxidative damage is removed from the interior. The package is hermetically sealed and then subjected to heating. The package must be able to withstand heat up to about 100°C for high acid products and up to 127°C for low acid products, which must receive added heat to destroy heat-resistant microbial spores. Packages containing low-acid (above pH 4.5) food must withstand pressure as well.

Although conventional canning renders food products commercially sterile, the nutritional contents and the organoleptic properties of the food generally suffer in the processing. Moreover, tinplate containers are heavy in weight, prone to rusting and are of high cost.

Figure 7.5 is a simple illustration comparing the basic difference between conventional canning and aseptic packaging processes for the production of shelf-stable food products.

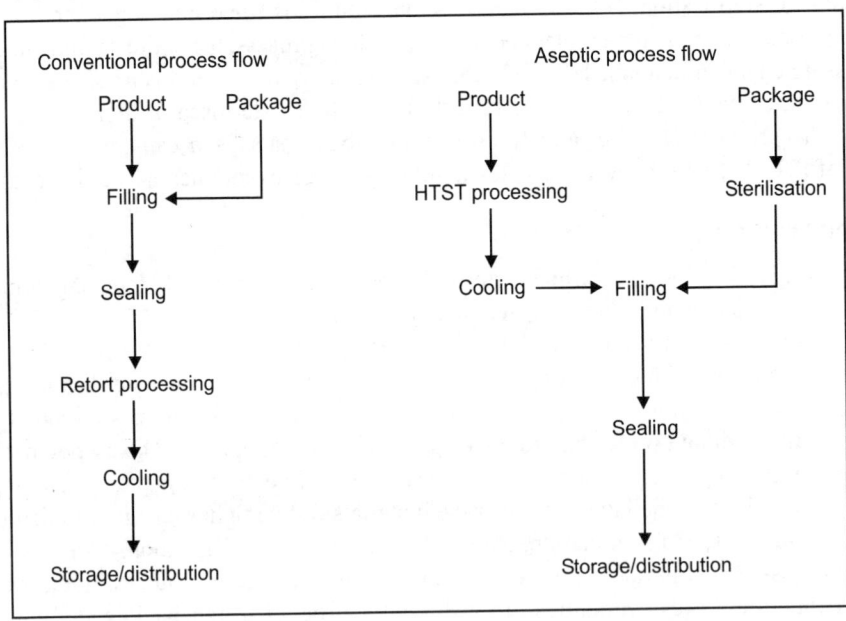

Fig. 7.5. Conventional canning v/s aseptic packaging.

Advantages of Aseptic Packaging Technology

The three main advantages of using aseptic packaging technology are:

1. Packaging materials, which are unsuitable for in-package sterilisation can be used. Therefore, light weight materials consuming less space offering convenient features and with low cost such as paper and flexible and semi-rigid plastic materials can be used gainfully.

2. Sterilisation process of high-temperature-short time (HTST) for aseptic packaging is thermally efficient and generally gives rise to products of high quality and nutritive value compared to those processed at lower temperatures for longer time.

3. Extension of shelf-life of products at normal temperatures by packing them aseptically.

Besides the features mentioned above, additional advantages are that the HTST process utilises less energy, as part of the process-heat is recovered through the heat exchangers and the aseptic process is a modern continuous flow process needing fewer operators.

Aseptic Processing Methodology

Aseptic processing comprises the following:
1. Sterilisation of the products before filling.
2. Sterilisation of packaging materials or containers and closures before filling.
3. Sterilisation of aseptic installations before operation (UHT unit, lines for products, sterile air and gases, filler and relevant machine zones).
4. Maintaining sterility in this total system during operation; sterilisation of all media entering the system, like air, gases, sterile water.
5. Production of hermetic packages.

Sterilisation of Products

In aseptic processing, the design to achieve commercial stability is based on the well-founded principles of thermal bacteriology and integrated effect of time/temperature treatment on spores of micro-organisms.

Presterilisation of a product usually consists of heating the product to the desired UHT temperature, maintaining this temperature for a given period in order to achieve the desired degree of sterility, with subsequent cooling, usually to ambient temperature and sometimes to an elevated temperature to achieve right viscosity for filling. Heating and cooling should be performed as rapidly as possible to achieve the best quality, depending upon the nature of the product. A fast heat exchange rate is desired for cost reasons.

Various heat transfer methods are used, but essentially the systems can be divided into direct and indirect heat exchange methods. Table 7.3 summarises the characteristics of the heat exchange systems used for aseptic processing of liquids.

Table 7.3. Characteristics of the heat exchange systems used for aseptic processing of liquids.

Equipment type	Product quality	Aroma retention	Energy saving	Capital cost	Space	Pulp capability	Fouling length of run	Turn-down*
Steam injection/ infusion	Excellent	No	Poor	High	Fair	Fair-good	Excellent	Fair
Plate heat Exchanger	Good	Yes	Excellent	Low	Excellent	Limited	Limited	Good
Tubular:								
Small tubes	Medium	Yes	Fair	Medium	Good	Good	Limited	Good
Large tubes	Poor	Yes	Fair	Low	Fair	Good	Good	Good
Swept surface	Good	Yes	Very poor	Very high	High	Fair-good	Good	Good

(*Turndown is the capability of the system to process at different rates to accommodate different number of fillers or different package sizes.)

Some of the latest methods of sterilisation of products include:
1. Microwaves.
2. Electrical resistance heating.
3. High voltage discharge.
4. Ultra high pressure.

Sterilisation of Aseptic Packaging Materials and Equipment

Sterilisation agents

Heat, chemicals and radiation have been used, alone or in combination, for sterilisation of aseptic equipment and packaging materials. Practical considerations and regulatory requirements have limited the number of sterilants, which are used for aseptic systems.

Heat

Initially, heat was used as the sterilant for aseptic systems as a natural extension of thermal processing. Product supply lines and fillers are commonly sterilised by 'moist' heat in the form of hot water or saturated steam under pressure. 'Dry' heat, in the form of superheated steam or hot air, may also be used to sterilise equipment. However, due to the relatively high dry heat resistance of bacterial endospores, the time-temperature requirements for dry heat sterilisation are considerably higher than those for moist heat sterilisation.

Since, relatively large masses of metal are often present in aseptic filling and packaging systems, high temperatures and relatively long holding periods are necessary to assure that appropriate sterilisation has occurred. Systems employing moist heat are frequently sterilised at temperatures ranging from 121° to 129°C, while 176° to 232°C is used for sterilisation by dry heat. In addition, sterilisation of air by incineration usually is conducted at temperatures ranging from 260° to 315°C.

Chemicals

Hydrogen peroxide is the overwhelming choice for use as a chemical sterilant. Other chemicals which have been used as sterilants, primarily for use in systems for acid food, include various acids, ethanol, ethylene oxide and peracetic acid. Hydrogen peroxide is not an efficient sporicide when used at room temperature. However, the sporicidal activity increases substantially with increasing temperatures. Therefore, most aseptic packaging systems use hydrogen peroxide (at concentrations of 30 to 35 per cent) as a sterilant for packaging materials followed by hot air (60° to 125°C) to dissipate residual hydrogen peroxide.

Radiation

Gamma-radiation has been used for decades to decontaminate packaging materials for use in aseptic systems for packing acid and acidified food. Due to the penetrating powers of gamma-radiation, packages are treated in bulk at commercial irradiators. A dose of approximately 1.5 Megaradians (Mrad) is commonly used to decontaminate containers for acid and acidified food. Recently, processes for low acid food aseptic filling and packaging systems are also being accepted. Doses required to sterilise containers for use with low acid food are considerably higher than those required for acid and acidified food.

Other types of radiation are not widely used in aseptic systems. Ultraviolet (UV-C) light has been used to decontaminate food contact surfaces. The low penetration and problems associated with 'shadowing', limit the use of UV-C for aseptic systems packaging of low acid food. While equipment size, speed and costs have precluded use of electron beam irradiators until now; it is only a matter of time before such a system is developed.

Filling

1. Once the product has been brought to the sterilisation temperature, it flows into a holding tube. The tube provides the required residence time at the sterilisation temperature. The process is designed to ensure that the fastest moving particle through the holding tube will receive a time/temperature process sufficient for sterilisation. Since there is some loss of temperature as product passes through the holding tube, the product temperature must be sufficiently high on entering, so that even with some temperature drop, it will still at least be at the prescribed minimum temperature at the exit of the holding tube. No external heating of the holding tube should take place.

2. A deaerator is used to remove air, as most products, which are aseptically processed, must be deaerated prior to packaging. The air is removed to prevent undesirable oxidative reactions, which occur as the product temperature is increased during the process. The deaerator generally consists of a vessel in which the product is exposed to a vacuum on a continuous flow.

3. The sterilised product is accumulated in an aseptic surge tank prior to packaging. The valve system that connects the surge tank between the end of the cooling section and the packaging system, allows the processor to carry out the processing and packaging functions more or less independently. The product is pumped into the surge tank and is removed by maintaining a positive pressure in the tank with sterile air or other sterile gas. The positive pressure must be monitored and controlled to protect the tank from contamination.

Seals and Closures

Any aseptic system must be capable of closing and/or sealing the package hermetically to maintain sterility during handling and distribution. The integrity of the closure and seal is therefore of paramount importance. The integrity of the heat-seals used in most aseptic systems is principally influenced by the efficiency of the sealing system used and by contamination of the heat seal area by the product. To avoid recontamination, the production units, which are tight are required. Two systems are manufactured in the Tetrapak system—the longitudinal and the transverse seam.

In the longitudinal system, a flat web of packaging material is used, supplied in reels. This flat material web is formed into a tube, which is sealed longitudinally resulting in a cylinder shaped structure. The strength of this longitudinal seam is determined partly by an 'overlap seal' and partly by a plastic longitudinal strip. This strip is first sealed to one edge of the packaging material web and once the packaging material tube has been formed—sealed to the inner surface of the packaging material. Both these operations, the strip application and the actual longitudinal sealing are done by using sterile, hot air and pressure.

Transversal sealing is done below the level of the product in the packaging material tube. By constantly moving sealing and pressure jaws, pressure is applied from the outside of the packaging material tube squeezing the product from the sealing area. An electrical impulse is passed through the sealing jaw and heat is transferred from the outside to the inside plastic layer of the packaging material. The polyethylene layer is heated, melted and pressed together between a pair of jaws. While pressure is maintained, the melted plastic layer cools down and a bonding is effectuated between the two opposite packaging material surfaces: they are sealed transversally.

Maintenance and preventive maintenance is needed to ensure satisfactory seam quality as well as to prevent damage of the packaging material in general, which may interfere with the tightness of the container. Thus, units are produced which are sufficiently tight to prevent re-infection of the product.

Types of Aseptic Packs

Consumer packages

A great variety of packages may be aseptically filled now as listed.

1. Carton boxes: Some of the existing aseptic carton boxes may now be filled with particulates, also aseptically.
2. Bags and pouches: Pillow pouches are usually used for packaging of milk; three-sided sealed pouch, however, is suitable also for aseptic packaging of particulates up to particle sizes of 12μ and bag sizes from 1–5 litres. For standing pouches a Japanese machine uses closed pouches from a reel with sterile interior surfaces, the exterior of which is sterilised in a hydrogen peroxide bath when the web with pouches enters the aseptic cabinet. The bags are then cut from the web, filled and sealed.
3. Cups and trays: These are either used pre-made or formed, filled and sealed in thermoform/fill/seal machines. Both types of machines exist for filling particulates and also in packs suitable for microwave heating. Usually polypropylene-based multilayer materials with EVOH barrier are applied for this purpose.
4. Bottles and jars: Glass bottles may be aseptically filled with food containing small particles, for instance for baby food. Jars may be filled with larger particles 12 mm cube size or larger—if one dimension is smaller. In a recent development, returnable bottles are filled aseptically, which up to now were applied only for UHT–treated milk.

    Basically, the same products can be filled into plastic bottles and jars as into glass containers. Closing is usually done by heat-sealing aluminium lids. For this reason, much attention has to be paid to avoid contamination of heat-sealing rims.
5. Metal cans: As mentioned earlier, only the Dole system is able to apply to cans from steel and aluminium for aseptic filling. The existing slit filler, however, limits applications to liquids with very small particles, such as rice.
6. Plastic cans: An aseptic machine for filling and closing of two-piece plastic cans, 'gourmet cans', was recently developed. They are sterilised with hydrogen peroxide, UV radiation and heat-sealed inductively. The can is presently offered for liquids only—for example coffee.
7. Composite Cans: These may, at present, not be filled with particulate food, but only with fruit juice with long fibres.

Aseptic Packaging Materials

Packaging materials must meet following factors:

1. The packaging material must be compatible with the product intended to be packed and must comply with applicable material migration requirements.
2. Physical integrity of the package is necessary to assume containment of the product and maintenance of sterility.
3. The package material must be able to withstand sterilisation and be compatible with the methods of sterilisation.
4. The package must protect the product from oxygen, also package must retain the aroma of the product.

Special Need of Plastics in Aseptic Packaging

Packaging for aseptics was particularly demanding of the long shelf-life, high seal integrity and consumer appeal. However, because plastic material is so important to aseptic packaging, it is useful to discuss some special properties demanded of plastics by aseptic process itself. They are as follows:

1. Chemical resistance and wettability.
2. Thermal stability.
3. Low levels of contaminating micro-organisms.
4. Resistance to ionising radiations.

Package Structure and Composition

Aseptic package has not only to protect the product but also to maintain the quality of the product. Hence the structure as well as composition of aseptic packaging are more complex and vary depending on product application, package size and package type. Factors such as seal strength and integrity, package shape, stiffness and durability, as well as barrier properties determine the choice and/or combination of materials required. Generally to achieve all required properties, aseptic packages incorporate more than one material in the structure that is assembled by lamination or co-extrusion process.

Advantages of bulk aseptic packaging: It offers the following advantages:

1. Safety.
2. Reliability.
3. Extended shelf-life.
4. Product quality.

Safety due to:

1. Steam sterilisation of spout, and sterilisation effect can be controlled and recorded.
2. No chemical sprays used to sterilise the chamber.
3. Spout is tamper proof.
4. Safer sterilisation and easier to monitor.
5. No risk of adding chemicals to the product.
6. No risk of laminate material relating with chemicals.

Reliability, because:

1. The filling machine is uncomplicated as there is no sterile chamber.
2. Filling is controlled by weight. This ensures accuracy as no adjustments for specific gravity need to be made.
3. Customer will have one partner with worldwide service organisations and long experience in processing and packaging technology.

Extended shelf-life due to:

1. High oxygen barrier of the laminate. Laminate is less susceptible to flex cracking.
2. Secure spout with limited possibility of oxygen permeation. Spout is made of HDPE, which has three times less oxygen transmission rate compared to LDPE.
3. There is no head space in the bag.

Product quality because:

1. Chemical browning is minimised due to high oxygen barrier properties of pouch material.

PASTEURISATION

Pasteurisation destroys most disease producing organisms and limits fermentation in milk, beer, and other liquids by partial or complete sterilisation. The pasteurisation process heats milk to 161°F (63°C) for 15 seconds, inactivating or killing organisms that grow rapidly in milk. Pasteurisation does not destroy organisms that grow slowly or produce spores.

While pasteurisation destroys many micro-organisms in milk, improper handling after pasteurisation can recontaminate milk. Many dairy farms use a home-pasteurising machine to pasteurise small amounts of milk for personal use. Raw milk can also be pasteurised on the stovetop. Microwaving raw milk is not an effective means of pasteurisation because of uneven heat distribution.

Ultra-high temperature (UHT) processing destroys organisms more effectively and the milk is essentially sterilised and can be stored at room temperature for up to 8 weeks without any change in flavour.

Requirements for Safe Handling of Milk

The requirements for proper pasteurisation and handling of milk are:
1. A potable water supply and proper dispensing system must be available to avoid contamination: A pure hot and cold water supply for the animals' health, and for proper cleaning of the animals, milk handlers and utensils. Regular inspection and maintenance of the system is necessary.
2. Clean and healthy animals, clean hands, and clean utensils are essential: The animals' hair should be clipped regularly around the flanks and udder to keep it from collecting dirt. Milkers should wash their hands and the udder with clean water or use an approved germicidal solution before milking. Milk from diseased animals or those under antibiotic treatment may not be used. All equipment and utensils should be cleaned immediately after use. Stainless steel utensils are preferred since they are durable and easy to clean.
3. Rapid cooling, cold storage, proper pasteurisation, and clean cold storage of pasteurised are necessary for the prevention of foodborne illness. Milk must be promptly cooled to 40°F (4°C) or less and stored in a closed container before and after pasteurisation to maintain the quality and flavour of the milk.

Care should be taken not to transfer barnyard dirt from the bottom or sides of the storage container to the countertop or to utensils in the pasteurisation and storage areas.

Do not mix fresh milk with previously cooked milk unless you plan to pasteurise the entire batch immediately.

Pasteurisation of Milk

Milk must be heated, with agitation, in such a way that every particle of the milk, including the foam, receives a minimum heat treatment of 150°F (66°C) continuously for 30 minutes or 161°F (72°C) for 15 seconds. The temperature should be monitored with an accurate metal or protected glass thermometer. Commercial operations commonly use a high-temperature, short-time process in which the milk is heated to 170°F (77°C) for 15 seconds and then cooled immediately to below 40°F (4°C) to increase storage life without any noticeable flavour change in the milk.

Pasteurisation of fluid milk has very specific requirements for time and temperature as listed in the Table 7.4.

Table 7.4. Temperature–time pasteurisation requirements for fluid milk.

Temperature	Time
150°F (66°C) (vat pasteurisation)	30 minutes
161°F (72°C) (high temperature, short-time pasteurisation)	15 seconds
191°F (89°C)	1 second
212°F (100°C)	0.01 second

Appertisation

The term for the heat-processing of foods at temperatures above 120°C, in particular, retorting and high temperature short-time (HTST) processing. This process does not guarantee complete sterility but any spores present should be non-pathogenic and unable to grow in the processed food environment.

Chapter 8

Preservation by Drying

INTRODUCTION

Drying is a method of food preservation that works by removing water from the food, which inhibits the growth of micro-organisms and hinders quality decay. Drying food using sun and wind to prevent spoilage has been practised since ancient times. Water is usually removed by evaporation (air drying, sun drying, smoking or wind drying) but, in the case of freeze-drying, food is first frozen and then the water is removed by sublimation. Bacteria yeasts and moulds need the water in the food to grow. Drying effectively prevents them from surviving in the food.

FOOD TYPES

Many different foods are prepared by dehydration. Dried and salted reindeer meat is a traditional Sami food. First the meat is soaked/pickled in saltwater for a couple of days to guarantee the conservation of the meat. Then the meat is dried in the sun in spring when the air temperature is below zero. The dried meat can be further processed to make soup. Fruits change character completely when dried: the plum becomes a prune, the grape a raisin; figs and dates are also transformed in new, different products, that can be eaten as they are or else after rehydration.

Home drying of vegetables, fruit and even meat (to produce jerky) may be carried out by a do-it-yourself practice, employing electrical dehydrators (household appliance). If the user does not like to use additives as potassium metabisulphite or BHA, BHT for meats, dried products may be hermetically shelf stored if it is to be consumed soon or else in the refrigerator or even freezer if a long storage is to be expected. Freeze dried vegetables are often found in backpackers food, hunters, military, etc. The exception to this rule are bulbs, such as garlic and onion, which are often dried. Also chilis are frequently dried. Edible and psilocybin mushrooms, as well as other fungi, are also sometimes dried for preservation purposes, to affect the potency of chemical components or so they can be used as seasonings.

For centuries, much of the European diet depended on dried cod, known as salt cod or bacalhau (with salt) or stockfish (without). It formed the main protein source for the slaves on the West Indian plantations, and was a major economic force within the triangular trade. Dried shark meat, known as Hákarl, is a delicacy in Iceland.

GRAIN DRYING

Hundreds of millions of tonnes of wheat, corn, soyabean, rice and other grains as sorghum, sunflower seeds, rapeseed/canola, barley, oats, etc. are dried in grain dryers. In the main agricultural countries, drying comprises the reduction of moisture from about 17–30 per cent w/w to values between 8 and 15 per cent w/w, depending on the grain. The final moisture content for drying must be adequate for storage. The more oil the grain has, the lower its storage moisture content will be (though its initial moisture for drying will also be lower). Cereals are often dried to 14 per cent w/w, while oilseeds, to 12.5 per cent (soyabeans), 8 per cent (sunflower) and 9 per cent (peanuts). Drying is carried out as a requisite for safe storage, in order to inhibit microbial growth. However, low temperatures in storage are also highly recommended to avoid degradative reactions and, especially, the growth of insects and mites. A good maximum storage temperature is about 18°C. The largest dryers are normally used 'Off-farm', in elevators, and are of the continuous type: Mixed-flow dryers are preferred in Europe, while Cross-flow dryers in the USA.

Grain drying is an active area of manufacturing and research. Now it is possible to simulate the performance of a dryer with computer programs based on equations (mathematical models) that represent the phenomena involved in drying: physics, physical chemistry, thermodynamics and heat and mass transfer. Most recently the evolution of quality indices is beginning to be predicted with some confidence, in order to add an essential performance parameter with which to establish a compromise of reasonably fast drying rate, limited energy consumption, and satisfactory grain quality. A typical quality parameter in wheat drying is the breadmaking quality and germination percentage whose reductions in drying are somewhat related.

Methods of Drying

There are many different methods for drying, each with their own advantages for particular applications. Some of the important methods of drying are given below:

1. Bed dryers.
2. Drum drying.
3. Freeze drying.
4. Shelf dryers.
5. Spray drying.
6. Sunlight.
7. Commercial food dehydrators.
8. Household oven.

Drum drying

Drum drying is a method used for drying out liquids; for example, milk is applied as a thin film to the surface of a heated drum, and the dried milk solids are then scraped off with a knife. Powdered milk made by drum drying tends to have a cooked flavour, due to caramelisation caused by greater heat exposure. Compared to spray drying, drum drying is a more intense heat treatment which results in more denatured proteins. The powder is less soluble as a result. The temperature uniformity of the heated roller/drum is poor so spray drying results in better quality milk powder.

Other products were drum drying can be used are for example starches, breakfast cereals, baby food, instant mashed potatoes to make them cold water soluble.

Freeze-drying

Freeze-drying (also known as lyophilisation or cryodesiccation) is a dehydration process typically used to preserve a perishable material or make the material more convenient for transport. Freeze-drying works by freezing the material and then reducing the surrounding pressure and adding enough heat to allow the frozen water in the material to sublime directly from the solid phase to the gas phase.

Freeze-drying process

There are four stages in the complete drying process: pretreatment, freezing, primary drying, and secondary drying.

Pretreatment

Pretreatment includes any method of treating the product prior to freezing. This may include concentrating the product, formulation revision (i.e. addition of components to increase stability and/or improve processing), decreasing a high vapour pressure solvent or increasing the surface area. In many instances the decision to pretreat a product is based on theoretical knowledge of freeze-drying and its requirements, or is demanded by cycle time or product quality considerations. Methods of pretreatment include: Freeze concentration, solution phase concentration, formulation to preserve product appearance, formulation to stabilise reactive products, formulation to increase the surface area, and decreasing high vapour pressure solvents.

Freezing

In a lab, this is often done by placing the material in a freeze-drying flask and rotating the flask in a bath, called a shell freezer, which is cooled by mechanical refrigeration, dry ice and methanol or liquid nitrogen. On a larger scale, freezing is usually done using a freeze-drying machine. In this step, it is important to cool the material below its triple point, the lowest temperature at which the solid and liquid phases of the material can coexist. This ensures that sublimation rather than melting will occur in the following steps. Larger crystals are easier to freeze-dry. To produce larger crystals, the product should be frozen slowly or can be cycled up and down in temperature. This cycling process is called annealing. However, in the case of food or objects with formerly-living cells, large ice crystals will break the cell walls (a problem discovered, and solved, by Clarence Birdseye), resulting in the destruction of more cells, which can result in increasingly poor texture and nutritive content. In this case, the freezing is done rapidly, in order to lower the material to below its eutectic point quickly, thus avoiding the formation of ice crystals. Usually, the freezing temperatures are between $-50°$ and $-80°C$. The freezing phase is the most critical in the whole freeze-drying process, because the product can be spoiled if badly done.

Amorphous materials do not have a eutectic point, but they do have a critical point, below which the product must be maintained to prevent melt-back or collapse during primary and secondary drying.

Primary drying

During the primary drying phase, the pressure is lowered (to the range of a few millibars), and enough heat is supplied to the material for the water to sublime. The amount of heat necessary can be calculated using the sublimating molecules latent heat of sublimation. In this initial drying phase, about 95 per cent of the water in the material is sublimated. This phase may be slow (can be several days in the industry), because, if too much heat is added, the material's structure could be altered.

In this phase, pressure is controlled through the application of partial vacuum. The vacuum speeds sublimation, making it useful as a deliberate drying process. Furthermore, a cold condenser chamber and/or condenser plates provide a surface(s) for the water vapour to re-solidify on. This condenser plays no role in keeping the material frozen; rather, it prevents water vapour from reaching the vacuum pump, which could degrade the pump's performance. Condenser temperatures are typically below $-50°C$ ($-60°F$).

It is important to note that, in this range of pressure, the heat is brought mainly by conduction or radiation; the convection effect is considered to be inefficient.

Secondary drying

The secondary drying phase aims to remove unfrozen water molecules, since the ice was removed in the primary drying phase. This part of the freeze-drying process is governed by the material's adsorption isotherms. In this phase, the temperature is raised higher than in the primary drying phase, and can even be above $0°C$, to break any physico-chemical interactions that have formed between the water molecules and the frozen material. Usually the pressure is also lowered in this stage to encourage desorption (typically in the range of microbars or fractions of a pascal). However, there are products that benefit from increased pressure as well.

After the freeze-drying process is complete, the vacuum is usually broken with an inert gas, such as nitrogen, before the material is sealed.

At the end of the operation, the final residual water content in the product is extremely low, around 1 to 4 per cent.

Properties of freeze-dried products

If a freeze-dried substance is sealed to prevent the reabsorption of moisture, the substance may be stored at room temperature without refrigeration, and be protected against spoilage for many years. Preservation is possible because the greatly reduced water content inhibits the action of micro-organisms and enzymes that would normally spoil or degrade the substance.

Freeze-drying also causes less damage to the substance than other dehydration methods using higher temperatures. Freeze-drying does not usually cause shrinkage or toughening of the material being dried. In addition, flavours, smells and nutritional content generally remain unchanged, making the process popular for preserving food. However, water is not the only chemical capable of sublimation, and the loss of other volatile compounds such as acetic acid (vinegar) and alcohols can yield undesirable results.

Freeze-dried products can be rehydrated (reconstituted) much more quickly and easily because the process leaves microscopic pores. The pores are created by the ice crystals that sublimate, leaving gaps or pores in their place. This is especially important when it comes to pharmaceutical uses. Freeze-drying can also be used to increase the shelf-life of some pharmaceuticals for many years.

Applications of freeze-drying

Food industry

Freeze-drying is used to preserve food, the resulting product being very lightweight. The process has been popularised in the forms of freeze-dried ice cream, an example of astronaut food. It is also widely used to produce essences or flavourings to add to food. Because of its light weight per volume of reconstituted food, freeze dried product is also popular and convenient for hikers. More dried food can be carried per the same weight of wet food, and has the benefit of 'long-life' compared to wet food that will go off. The hikers then reconstituted the food with water available at point of use. Instant coffee is sometimes freeze-dried, despite the high costs of the freeze-driers used. The coffee is often dried by vapourisation in a hot air flow, or by projection on hot metallic plates. Freeze-dried fruit is used in some breakfast cereal. Culinary herbs are also freeze-dried, although air-dried herbs are far more common and less expensive.

Freeze-drying equipment

There are essentially three categories of freeze-driers: The rotary evaporator freeze-drier, the manifold freeze-drier, and the tray freeze-drier. Rotary freeze-driers are usually used with liquid products, such as pharmaceutical solutions and tissue extracts.

Manifold freeze-driers are usually used when drying a large amount of small containers and the product will be used in a short period of time. A manifold drier will dry the product to less than 5 per cent moisture content. Without heat, only primary drying (removal of the unbound water) can be achieved. A heater must be added for secondary drying, which will remove the bound water and will produce a lower moisture content.

Tray freeze-driers are more sophisticated and are used to dry a variety of materials. A tray freeze-drier is used to produce the driest product for long-term storage. A tray freeze-drier allows the product to be frozen in place and performs both primary (unbound water removal) and secondary (bound water removal) freeze-drying, thus producing the driest possible end-product. Tray freeze-driers can dry products in bulk or in vials. When drying in vials, the freeze-drier is supplied with a stoppering mechanism that allows a stopper to be pressed into place, sealing the vial before it is exposed to the atmosphere. This is used for long-term storage, such as vaccines.

Improved freeze drying techniques are being developed to extend the range of products that can be freeze dried, to improve the quality of the product, and to produce the product faster with less labour.

Spray drying

Spray drying is a method of producing a dry powder from a liquid or slurry by rapidly drying with a hot gas. This is the preferred method of drying of many thermally-sensitive materials such as foods and pharmaceuticals. A consistent particle size distribution is a reason for spray drying some industrial products such as catalysts. Air is the heated drying media; however, if the liquid is a flammable solvent such as ethanol or the product is oxygen-sensitive then nitrogen is used (Fig. 8.1).

All spray dryers use some type of atomiser or spray nozzle to disperse the liquid or slurry into a controlled drop size spray. The most common of these are rotary nozzles and single-fluid pressure swirl nozzles. Alternatively, for some applications two-fluid or ultrasonic nozzles are used. Depending on the process needs drop sizes from 10 to 500 micrometres can be achieved with the appropriate choices. The most common applications are in the 100 to 200 micrometre diameter range. The dry powder is often free-flowing.

The hot drying gas can be passed as a co-current or counter-current flow to the atomiser direction. The co-current flow enables the particles to have a lower residence time within the system and the particle separator (typically a cyclone device) operates more efficiently. The counter-current flow method enables a greater residence time of the particles in the chamber and usually is paired with a fluidised bed system.

Alternatives to spray dryers are:

1. Freeze dryer: A more-expensive batch process for products that degrade in spray drying. Dry product is not free-flowing.
2. Drum dryer: A less-expensive continuous process for low-value products; creates flakes instead of free-flowing powder.
3. Pulse combustion dryer: A less-expensive continuous process that can handle higher viscosities and solids loading than a spray dryer, and that sometimes gives a freeze-dry quality powder that is free-flowing.

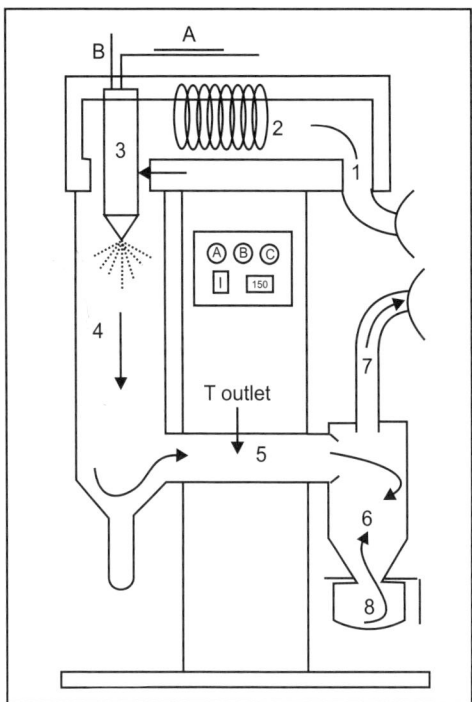

Fig. 8.1. Laboratory-scale spray dryer. A = Solution or suspension to be dried in, B = Atomisation gas in, 1 = Drying gas in, 2 = Heating of drying gas, 3 = Spraying of solution or suspension, 4 = Drying chamber, 5 = Part between drying chamber and cyclone, 6 = Cyclone, 7 = Drying gas is taken away, 8 = Collection vessel of product, arrows mean that this is co-current lab-spraydryer.

Spray dryer

A spray dryer is a device used in spray drying. It takes a liquid stream and separates the solute or suspension as a solid and the solvent into a vapour. The solid is usually collected in a drum or cyclone. The liquid input stream is sprayed through a nozzle into a hot vapour stream and vapourised. Solids form as moisture quickly leaves the droplets. A nozzle is usually used to make the droplets as small as possible, maximising heat transfer and the rate of water vapourisation. Droplet sizes can range from 20 to 180 μm depending on the nozzle.

Spray dryers can dry a product very quickly compared to other methods of drying. They also turn a solution, or slurry into a dried powder in a single step, which can be advantageous for profit maximisation and process simplification.

Micro-encapsulation

Spray drying often is used as an encapsulation technique by the food and other industries. A substance to be encapsulated (the load) and an amphipathic carrier (usually some sort of modified starch) are homogenised as a suspension in water (the slurry). The slurry is then fed into a spray drier, usually a tower heated to temperatures well over the boiling point of water.

As the slurry enters the tower, it is atomised. Partly because of the high surface tension of water and partly because of the hydrophobic/hydrophilic interactions between the amphipathic carrier, the water, and the load, the atomised slurry forms micelles. The small size of the drops (averaging 100 micrometres in diameter) results in a relatively large surface area which dries quickly. As the water dries, the carrier forms a hardened shell around the load.

Load loss is usually a function of molecular weight. That is, lighter molecules tend to boil off in larger quantities at the processing temperatures. Loss is minimised industrially by spraying into taller towers. A larger volume of air has a lower average humidity as the process proceeds. By the osmosis principle, water will be encouraged by its difference in fugacities in the vapour and liquid phases to leave the micelles and enter the air. Therefore, the same percentage of water can be dried out of the particles at lower temperatures if larger towers are used. Alternatively, the slurry can be sprayed into a partial vacuum. Since the boiling point of a solvent is the temperature at which the vapour pressure of the solvent is equal to the ambient pressure, reducing pressure in the tower has the effect of lowering the boiling point of the solvent.

The application of the spray drying encapsulation technique is to prepare 'dehydrated' powders of substances which do not have any water to dehydrate. For example, instant drink mixes are spray dries of the various chemicals which make up the beverage. The technique was once used to remove water from food products; for instance, in the preparation of dehydrated milk. Because the milk was not being encapsulated and because spray drying causes thermal degradation, milk dehydration and similar processes have been replaced by other dehydration techniques. Skim milk powders are still widely produced using spray drying technology around the world, typically at high solids concentration for maximum drying efficiency. Thermal degradation of products can be overcome by using lower operating temperatures and larger chamber sizes for increased residence times.

Spray drying applications
1. Food: Milk powder, coffee, tea, eggs, cereal, spices, flavourings.
2. Pharmaceutical: Antibiotics, medical ingredients, additives.
3. Industrial: Paint pigments, ceramic materials, catalyst supports.

Solar Drying Technology for Food Preservation

Preserving fruits, vegetables, grains, and meat has been practiced in many parts of the world for thousands of years. Methods of preservation include: canning, freezing, pickling, curing (smoking or salting), and drying. Food spoilage is caused by the action of moulds, yeasts, bacteria, and enzymes. The drying process removes enough moisture from food to greatly decrease these destructive effects.

Moisture content: The moisture content of fresh foods ranges from 20 to 90 per cent. Foods require different levels of dryness for safe storage, as shown in Table 8.1. For example: the moisture content of rice must be reduced from 24 to 14 per cent of the total weight. Therefore, drying 1000 kg of rice requires the removal of 100 kg of water. Safe storage generally requires reducing the moisture content to below 20 per cent for fruits, 10 per cent for vegetables, and 10–15 per cent for grains. If food is properly dried, no moisture will be visible when it is cut.

Moisture absorption: The length of time required to dry food depends upon how quickly air absorbs moisture out of the food. Fast drying primarily depends upon three factors: the air should be warm, dry, and moving. The dryness of air is measured in terms of relative humidity (RH). If air is at 100 per cent relative humidity, it has absorbed 100 per cent of the water it can hold at that temperature. If air has a RH near 100 per cent, it must be heated before it will be able to absorb moisture out of food.

Table 8.1. Moisture contents.

Food	Moisture content (wet basis)	
	Initial	Desired
Rice	24%	14%
Maize	35%	15%
Potatoes	75%	13%
Apricots	85%	18%
Coffee	50%	11%

Energy requirements: The amount of energy that must be added in order to dry produce depends on the local climate. Air drops in temperature as it absorbs moisture from food, and thus supplies some energy for drying. Therefore, if the air is warm and dry enough, food will dry slowly without additional heating from fuel or the sun. However, additional heat shortens the drying process and yields a higher quality product. Under typical conditions 100 kg of maize might be dried with roughly 3 kg of kerosene, or with 10 kg of biomass such as wood or rice husks. Alternatively, a 6 m² solar collector will dry the maize over three sunny days, if the relative humidity is low. The size of solar collector required for a certain size of drier depends on the ambient temperature, amount of sun, and humidity.

Solar drying essentials

Solar drier components: Solar driers may be viewed as three main components—a drying chamber in which food is dried, a solar collector that heats the air, and some type of airflow system. Figure 8.2 shows one type of solar drier with each of these three components labelled. The drying chamber protects the food from animals, insects, dust, and rain. It is often insulated (with sawdust, for example) to increase efficiency. The trays should be safe for food contact; a plastic coating is best to avoid harmful residues in food. A general rule of thumb is that one m² of tray area is needed to lay out 10 kg of fresh produce. The solar collector (or absorber) is often a dark coloured box with a transparent cover. It raises the air temperature between 10° and 30°C above ambient. This may be separate from the drier chamber, or combined (as with direct driers). Often the bottom surface of the absorber is dark to promote solar absorption, and occasionally charred rice chaff serves this purpose. Glass is recommended for the absorber cover, although it is expensive and difficult to use. Plastic is acceptable if it is firm or supported by a rib such that it does not sag and collect water.

Solar driers use one of two types of airflow systems; natural convection utilises the natural principle that hot air rises, and forced convection driers force air through the drying chamber with fans. The effects of natural convection may be enhanced by the addition of a chimney in which exiting air is heated even more. Additionally, prevailing winds may be taken advantage of. Natural convection driers require careful use; stacking the product too high or a lack of sun can cause air to stagnate in the drier and halt the drying process. The use of forced convection can reduce drying time by three times and decrease the required collector area by 50 per cent. Consequently, a drier using fans may achieve the same throughput as a natural convection drier with a collector six times as large. Fans may be powered with utility electricity if it is available, or with a solar photovoltaic cell. For comparison, one study showed that the installation of three small fans and a photovoltaic cell was equivalent to the effect of a 12 m chimney.

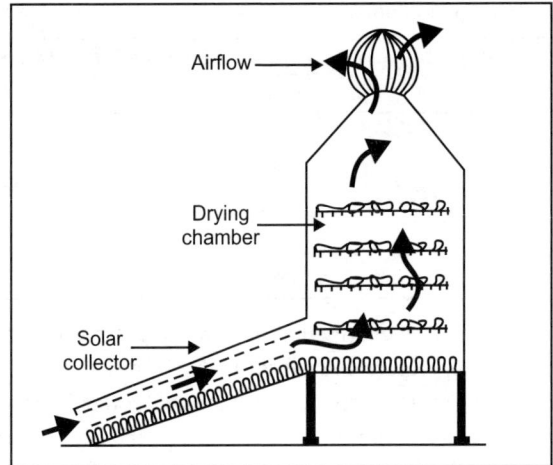

Fig. 8.2. Solar drier components.

The drying process: Producing safe, highquality dried produce requires careful procedures throughout the entire preservation process. Foods suffer only a slight reduction in nutrition and aesthetics if dried properly; however, incorrect drying can dramatically degrade food and brings the risk of food poisoning. A process similar to the following seven steps is usually used when drying fruits and vegetables (and fish, with some modifications):

1. Selection (fresh, undamaged produce).
2. Cleaning (washing and disinfection).
3. Preparation (peeling, slicing, etc.).
4. Pre-treatment (e.g. sulphurising, blanching, salting).
5. Drying.
6. Packaging.
7. Storage or export.

Only fresh, undamaged food should be selected for drying to reduce the chances of spoilage and help insure a quality product. After selection, it is important to clean the produce. This is because drying does not always destroy micro-organisms, but only inhibits their growth. Fruits, vegetables, and meats generally require a pretreatment before drying.

The quality of dried fruits and vegetables is generally improved with one or more of the following pretreatments: anti-discolouration by coating with vitamin C, de-waxing by briefly boiling and quenching, and sulphurising by soaking or fumigating. Fish is often salted. A small amount of chemical will treat a large amount of produce, and thus the cost for these supplies is usually small. However, potential problems with availability and the complexity of the process should be considered. The best pretreatment procedure may be determined through a combination of experimentation and consulting literature on the subject.

After selection, cleaning, and pretreatment, produce is ready to place in the drier trays. Solar driers are usually designed to dry a batch every three to five days. Fast drying minimises the chances of food spoilage. However, excessively fast drying can result in the formation of a hard, dry skin — a problem known as case hardening. Case hardened foods appear dry outside, but inside remain moist and susceptible to spoiling. It is also important not to exceed the maximum temperature recommended, which ranges from 35° to 45°C depending upon the produce. Learning to properly solar dry foods in a specific location usually requires experimentation. For strict quality control, the drying rate may be monitored and correlated to the food moisture content to help determine the proper drying parameters.

After drying is complete, the dried produce often requires packaging to prevent insect losses and to avoid re-gaining moisture. It should cool first, and then be packaged in sanitary conditions. Sufficient drying and airtight storage will keep produce fresh for six to twelve months. If possible, the packaged product should be stored in a dry, dark location until use or export. If produce is to be exported, it must meet the quality standards of the target country. In some cases this will require a chemical and microbiological analysis of dried samples in a laboratory.

Food drying requires significant labour for pretreatment (except for grains), and minimal involvement during the drying process such as shifting food to insure even drying. Solar drying equipment generally requires little maintenance.

Capabilities of solar driers: Solar drying can preserve a variety of fruits, vegetables, grains, and some meat. It can also be used for cash crops such as coffee, herbs, cashew, and macadamia. Solar driers exist for treating timber, although they are not discussed here. Fruits are ideal for preservation by drying since they are high in sugar and acid, which act to preserve the dried fruit. Vegetables are more challenging to preserve since they are low in sugar and acid. Drying meat requires extreme caution since it is high in protein, which invites microbial growth. Fish drying, for example, requires thorough cleaning of the drier after each batch.

Lists are available explaining which foods are suited to drying. For example, apples, apricots, coconuts, dates, figs, guavas, and plums are fruits that dry quite easily, while avocados, bananas, breadfruit, and grapes are more difficult to dry. Most legumes are easily dried, as well as chilies, corn, potatoes, cassava root, onion flakes, and the leaves of various herbs and spices. On the other hand, asparagus, beets, broccoli, carrots, celery, various greens, pumpkin, squash, and tomatoes are more difficult to dry successfully.

Classification and selection of driers

Classification of food driers: Drying techniques may be divided into six general categories based on the way the food is heated (summarised in Table 8.2). Open-air or unimproved, solar drying takes place when food is exposed to the sun and wind by placing it in trays, on racks or on the ground. Although the food is rarely protected from predators and weather, in some cases screens are used to keep out insects, or a clear roof is used to shed rain. Direct sun driers enclose food in a container with a clear lid, such that sun shines directly on the food. In addition to the direct heating of the solar radiation, the greenhouse effect traps heat in the enclosure and raises the temperature of the air. Vent holes allow for air exchange. Indirect sun driers heat fresh air in a solar collector separate from the food chamber, so the food is not exposed to direct sunlight.

This is of particular importance for foods which loose nutritional value when exposed to direct sunlight. Mixed mode driers combine the aspects of direct and indirect types; a separate collector pre-heats air and then direct sunlight adds heat to the food and air. Hybrid driers combine solar energy with a fossil fuel or biomass fuel such as rice husks. (It is interesting to note that a harvest of 1000 kg of rice yields 200 kg of husks, and requires burning only 25 kg of husks to be dried.) Fueled driers use conventional fuels or utility supplied electricity for heat and ventilation.

Table 8.2. Classification of food driers.

Classification	Description
Open-air	Food is exposed to the sun and wind by placing in trays, on racks or on the ground. Food is rarely protected from predators and the weather
Direct sun	Food is enclosed in a container with a clear lid allowing sun to shine directly on the food. Vent holes allow for air circulation
Indirect sun	Fresh air is heated in a solar heat collector and then passed through food in the drier chamber. In this way the food is not exposed to direct sunlight
Mixed mode	Combines the direct and indirect types; a separate collector preheats air and direct sunlight adds heat to the food and air
Hybrid	Combines solar heat with another source such as fossil fuel or biomass
Fueled	Uses electricity or fossil fuel as a source of heat and ventilation

Comparing solar drying with other options: A first step when considering solar drying is to compare it with other options available. In some situations open-air drying or fuelled driers may be preferable to solar. If either of these is already used in a certain location, solar drying will only be successful if it has a clear advantage over the current practice (Table 8.3).

Table 8.3. Solar driers compared with open-air and fuel drying.

Type of drying	Benefits (+) and disadvantages (–) of solar driers
Solar vs. open-air	+ Can lead to better quality dried products, and better market prices
	+ Reduces losses and contamination from insects, dust, and animals
	+ Reduces land required (by roughly 1/3)
	+ Some driers protect food from sunlight, better preserving nutrition and colour
	+ May reduce labour required
	+ Faster drying time reduces chances of spoilage
	+ More complete drying allows longer storage
	+ Allows more control (sheltered from rain, for example)
	– More expensive, may require importing some materials
	– In some cases, food quality is not significantly improved
	– In some cases, market value of food will not be increased
Solar vs. fueled	+ Prevents fuel dependence
	+ Often less expensive
	+ Reduced environmental impact (consumption of non-renewables)
	– Requires adequate solar radiation
	– Hot and dry climates preferred (usually RH below 60% needed)
	– Requires more time
	– Greater difficulty controlling process, may result in lower quality product

The above comparison will assist in deciding among solar, open-air, and fueled driers. The local site conditions will also play an important role in this decision. Some indications that solar driers may be useful in a specific location include:
1. Conventional energy is unavailable or unreliable (making fuel driers unattractive).
2. Plenty of sunshine.

3. Dry climate (relative humidity below 60 per cent).
4. Quality of open-air dried products needs improvement.
5. Land is extremely scarce (making open-air drying unattractive).
6. Introducing solar drying technology will not have harmful socio-economic effects.

In addition to local conditions, the type of product to be dried plays a role in the decision process. For example, in some locations traditional open-air drying may be suitable for coffee, whereas fruit would largely be lost to predators. High-value cash crops often require consistent high quality without risking lost produce, and thus the use of fuel driers may be best.

The uses of solar dried products might include: self-consumption, local sale, large markets, and export. Therefore, the potential market for solar dried foods is often another important consideration. Preservation always slightly reduces nutrition and aesthetics, and therefore dried foods are only desirable if fresh is not available. Even where fresh is not available, consumer acceptance may be problematic if dried foods are not already on the market.

Existing infrastructure may be available to facilitate marketing dried produce. The expected market price will influence how much can be invested in a drier. Unfortunately, higher quality from solar driers doesn't always bring higher market prices than open-air drying. In some cases local markets are not willing to pay extra for higher quality solar dried products.

In some cases a centralised operation is more economical than numerous small driers, due to economies of scale. The appropriate amount of centralisation is different for simple natural convection driers than for more sophisticated forced convection driers.

Natural convection may be more effective with multiple small driers rather than one large unit. This is because the construction of small driers is simpler, and independent operation allows more flexibility. However, for forced convection driers, economies of scale favour centralisation to maximise use of the ventilation equipment.

Some useful criteria for selecting a solar drier: If the use of solar driers appears favourable, the next step is to consider which type of solar drier to use. Table 8.4 presents four general categories of solar driers along with advantages and disadvantages of each.

Table 8.4. Advantages and disadvantages of the four types of solar food driers.

Classification	Advantages	Disadvantages
Direct sun	+ Least expensive + Simple	– UV radiation can damage food
Indirect sun	+ Products protected from UV + Less damage from temperature extremes	– More complex and expensive than direct sun
Mixed mode	+ Less damage from temperature extremes	– UV radiation can damage food – More complex and expensive than direct sun
Hybrid	+ Ability to operate without sun reduces chance of food loss + Allows better control of drying + Fuel mode may be up to 40x faster than solar (Drying, ITDG)	– Expensive – May cause fuel dependence

Choosing a solar drier is a subjective decision, and is heavily dependent upon local conditions and the product to be dried. The following aspects should be considered when selecting a drier:

1. Can the drier be made from locally available materials and skills?
2. What are the purchase and maintenance costs?
3. What is the drying capacity?
4. What range of foods can be dried?
5. What is the drying time required?
6. What is the quality of the dried product?
7. Is the drier adaptable to local conditions?

Solar drying has the potential to improve the quality of life in some areas. The decision of whether solar, open-air or fueled driers are best may be made according to the criteria in Table 8.3. If solar drying is the best option, Table 8.4 and the selection criteria given may be used to choose a drier. Once a particular drier has been chosen, it may be purchased (if available) or constructed. Experience shows that the best configuration of a solar drier is different for each location, and therefore successful food drying usually requires a period of experimentation and adjustments at the local site.

Chapter 9

Preservation by Radiation

INTRODUCTION

Food irradiation is the process of exposing food to ionising radiation to destroy micro-organisms, bacteria, viruses or insects that might be present in the food. Further applications include sprout inhibition, delay of ripening, increase of juice yield, and improvement of rehydration. Irradiated food does not become radioactive, but in some cases there may be subtle chemical changes.

Irradiation is a more general term of the exposure of materials to radiation to achieve a technical goal (in this context 'ionising radiation' is implied). As such it is also used on non-food items, such as medical hardware, plastics, tubes for gas pipelines, hoses for floor heating, shrink-foils for food packaging, automobile parts, wires and cables (isolation), tyres, and even gemstones.

Food irradiation acts by damaging the target organism's DNA beyond its ability to repair. Micro-organisms can no longer proliferate and continue their malignant or pathogenic activities. Spoilage-causing micro-organisms cannot continue their activities. Insects do not survive or become incapable of reproduction. Plants cannot continue their natural ripening processes.

The energy density per atomic transition of ionising radiation is very high; it can break apart molecules and induce ionisation, which is not achieved by mere heating. This is the reason for both new effects and new concerns. The treatment of solid food by ionising radiation can provide an effect similar to heat pasteurisation of liquids, such as milk. However, the use of the term 'cold pasteurisation' to describe irradiated foods is controversial, since pasteurisation and irradiation are fundamentally different processes.

PROCESSING OF FOOD BY IONISING RADIATION

By irradiating food, depending on the dose, some or all of the harmful bacteria and other pathogens present are killed. This prolongs the shelf-life of the food in cases where microbial spoilage is the limiting factor. Some foods, e.g. herbs and spices, are irradiated at sufficient doses (five kilograys or more) to reduce the microbial counts by several orders of magnitude; such ingredients do not carry over spoilage or pathogen micro-organisms into the final product. It has also been shown that irradiation can delay the ripening of fruits or the sprouting of vegetables.

Furthermore, insect pests can be sterilised (be made incapable of proliferation) using irradiation at relatively low doses. In consequence, the United States department of agriculture (USDA) has approved the use of low-level irradiation as an alternative treatment to pesticides for fruits and vegetables that are considered hosts to a number of insect pests, including fruit flies and seed weevils; the US food and drug administration (FDA) has cleared among a number of other applications the treatment of hamburger patties to eliminate the residual risk of a contamination by a virulent *E. coli*. The United Nations food and agricultural organisation (FAO) has passed a motion to commit member states to implement irradiation technology for their national phytosanitary programs; the general assembly of the International atomic energy agency (IAEA) has urged to make wider use of the irradiation technology. Additionally, the USDA has made a number of bilateral agreements with developing countries to facilitate the imports of exotic fruits and to simplify the quarantine procedures.

The European Union has regulated processing of food by ionising radiation in specific directives since 1999; the relevant documents and reports are accessible online. The 'implementing' directive contains a 'positive list' permitting irradiation of only dried aromatic herbs, spices, and vegetable seasonings.

Other countries, including New Zealand, Australia, Thailand, India, and Mexico, have permitted the irradiation of fresh fruits for fruit fly quarantine purposes, amongst others. Such countries as Pakistan and Brazil have adopted the Codex Alimentarius Standard on Irradiated Food without any reservation or restriction, i.e. any food may be irradiated to any dose.

Radiation Absorbed Dose

Dose is the physical quantity governing the radiation processing of food, relating to the beneficial effects to be achieved.

Unit of measure for irradiation dose

The dose of radiation is measured in the SI unit known as the gray (Gy). One gray of radiation is equal to 1 joule of energy absorbed per kilogram of food material. In radiation processing of foods, the doses are generally measured in kilograys (kGy, 1000 Gy).

Dosimetry

The measurement of radiation dose is referred to as dosimetry and involves exposing dosimeters jointly with the treated food item. Dosimeters are small components attached to the irradiated product made of materials that, when exposed to ionising radiation, change specific, measurable physical attributes to a degree that can be correlated to the dose received. Modern dosimeters are made of a range of materials, such as alanine pellets, perspex (PMMA) blocks, and radiochromic films, as well as special solutions and other materials. These dosimeters are used in combination with specialised read out devices. Standards that describe calibration and operation for radiation dosimetry, as well as procedures to relate the measured dose to the effects achieved and to report and document such results, are maintained by the American Society for Testing and Materials (ASTM international) and are also available as ISO/ASTM standards.

Applications

On the basis of the dose of radiation the application is generally divided into three main categories as detailed under:

Low dose applications (up to 1 kGy)

1. Sprout inhibition in bulbs and tubers 0.03–0.15 kGy.
2. Delay in fruit ripening 0.25–0.75 kGy.
3. Insect disinfestation including quarantine treatment and elimination of food borne parasites 0.07–1.00 kGy.

Medium dose applications (1 kGy to 10 kGy)

1. Reduction of spoilage microbes to prolong shelf-life of meat, poultry and seafoods under refrigeration 1.50–3.00 kGy.
2. Reduction of pathogenic microbes in fresh and frozen meat, poultry and seafoods 3.00–7.00 kGy.
3. Reducing the number of micro-organisms in spices to improve hygienic quality 10.00 kGy.

High dose applications (above 10 kGy)

1. Sterilisation of packaged meat, poultry, and their products that are shelf stable without refrigeration 25.00–70.00 kGy.
2. Sterilisation of hospital diets 25.00–70.00 kGy.
3. Product improvement as increased juice yield or improved rehydration.

Irradiation treatments are also sometimes classified as radappertisation, radicidation and radurisation.

Technologies

Electron irradiation

Electron irradiation uses electrons accelerated in an electric field to a velocity close to the speed of light. Electrons are particulate radiation and, hence, have cross section many times larger than photons, so that they do not penetrate the product beyond a few inches, depending on product density. Electron facilities rely on substantial concrete shields to protect workers and the environment from radiation exposure.

Gamma irradiation

Gamma radiation is radiation of photons in the gamma part of the electromagnetic spectrum. The radiation is obtained through the use of radioisotopes, generally cobalt-60 or, in theory, caesium-137. Cobalt-60 is bred from cobalt-59 using neutron irradiation in specifically designed nuclear reactors. Caesium-137 is recovered during the processing of spent nuclear fuel. Because this technology — except for military applications — is not commercially available, insufficient quantities of it are available on the global isotope markets for use in large scale, commercial irradiators. Presently, caesium-137 is used only in small hospital units to treat blood before transfusion to prevent Graft-versus-host disease.

Food irradiation using cobalt-60 is the preferred method by most processors, because the deeper penetration enables administering treatment to entire industrial pallets or totes, reducing the need for material handling. A pallet or tote is typically exposed for several minutes to hours depending on dose. Radioactive material must be monitored and carefully stored to shield workers and the environment from its gamma rays.

During operation this is achieved by substantial concrete shields. With most designs the radioisotope can be lowered into a water-filled source storage pool to allow maintenance personnel to enter the radiation shield. In this mode the water in the pool absorbs the radiation. Other uncommonly used designs feature dry storage by providing movable shields that reduce radiation levels in areas of the irradiation chamber.

One variant of gamma irradiators keeps the Cobalt-60 under water at all times and lowers the product to be irradiated under water in hermetic bells. No further shielding is required for such designs.

X-ray irradiation

Similar to gamma radiation, X-rays are photon radiation of a wide energy spectrum and an alternative to isotope based irradiation systems. X-rays are generated by colliding accelerated electrons with a dense material (target) such as tantalum or tungsten in a process known as bremsstrahlung-conversion. X-ray irradiators are scalable and have deep penetration comparable to Co-60, with the added effect of using an electronic source that stops radiating when switched off. They also permit dose uniformity. However, these systems generally have low energetic efficiency during the conversion of electron energy to photon radiation requiring much more electrical energy than other systems. Like most other types of facilities, X-ray systems rely on concrete shields to protect the environment and workers from radiation.

Nominal X-ray energy is usually limited to 5 MeV; however, USA has provisions for up to 7.5 MeV, which increases conversion efficiency. Another development is the availability of electron accelerators with extremely high power output, up to 1000 kW beam. At a conversion efficiency of up to 12 per cent, the X-ray power may reach (including filtering and other losses) 100 kW. This power would be equivalent to a gamma facility with Co-60 of about 6.5 MCi.

Food irradiation is sometimes referred to as 'cold pasteurisation' or 'electronic pasteurisation' because ionising the food does not heat the food to high temperatures during the process, as in heat-pasteurisation (at a typical dose of 10 kGy, food that is physically equivalent to water would warm by about 2.5°C). The treatment of solid food by ionising radiation can provide an effect similar to heat pasteurisation of liquids, such as milk. However, the use of the term, cold pasteurisation, to describe irradiated foods is controversial, because pasteurisation and irradiation are fundamentally different processes, although the intended end results can in some cases be similar.

Alternatives

Other methods to reduce several pathogens in food include heat-pasteurisation, ultra-high temperature processing, UV radiation, ozone or fumigation with ethylene oxide.

For quarantine purposes, insect pests can also be eliminated by fumigation with methyl bromide or aluminum phosphine, vapour heat, forced hot air, hot water dipping, or cold treatment.

Other methods to extend shelf-life of food items include modified atmosphere packaging, carbon monoxide, dehydration, vacuum packaging, freezing and flash freezing as well as chemical additives.

MICROWAVE RADIATION

Microwave heating refers to the use of electromagnetic waves of certain frequencies to generate heat in a material. In microwave heating, continuous electromagnetic waves are produced in the magnetron and transmitted through a hollow metallic tube into a resonant cavity where the food is processed. Foods are heated because of molecular friction caused by alternating polarisation of molecules. Foods absorb microwave energy in the form of orientational and ionic polarisation. Orientational polarisation results from dipolar molecules, such as water, which tend to align according to the applied electric field. The electric field oscillates at 2450 or 915 million times per second (MHz), making the dipolar molecules rotate, thus promoting molecular friction, which in turn results in heat dissipation. Ionic polarisation occurs when dissolved salts are present.

Positive and negative ions tend to migrate to opposite-charged regions, colliding with other ions and converting kinetic energy into heat. Dipole rotation is more important than ionic polarisation as a microwave heating mechanism.

Effects of Microwaves on Microbial Inactivation

Heat sensitive nutrients such as vitamins and flavour constituents can be retained better through rapid heating than by conventional heat treatments. However, little conclusive evidence exists for any real flavour differences between many conventionally and microwave-heated foods microwave energy inactivates microbes via conventional thermal mechanisms, including thermal irreversible denaturation of enzymes, proteins, and nucleic acids.

Applications of microwave heating are found for most of the heat treatment operations in the food-processing industries. Microwave heating offers the opportunity of shortening the time required in conventional heat treatments to achieve the desired food-processing temperature. Microwave pasteurisation and sterilisation promise fast heat processing.

Are Microwave Ovens Safe

Microwave ovens offer a fast way to prepare and reheat food, which is perfect for today's fast paced world. In fact, microwaves have become commonplace in American homes and have even replaced the conventional oven and stove-top for preparing meals. However, there has long been concern about the safety of microwave ovens.

Dangers of microwave radiation

Obviously, the dangers of microwave radiation are very real. These devices can cause a variety of health problems in humans. Here are just a few of the possible health effects related to microwave ovens:
1. Microwave ovens turn some minerals into cancerous agents.
2. Foods from a microwave may cause tumours in the stomach or intestine. This may be an explanation for the increased rate of colon cancer in America.
3. Regularly eating microwaved foods may cause an increase in cancerous cells in human blood.
4. The radiation dangers involved with microwaved food may cause decreased immune system function in humans.
5. There is even a mental danger to eating foods from a microwave. Regularly doing so may cause memory loss, emotional problems, and a decrease in intelligence.
6. A steady diet of microwave-cooked food may cause your body to shut down its hormones production.

Microwave radiation is a very serious concern that many people will overlook in order to maintain their toxic paces. Many people have not even heard of the threat of microwave cooking and heating. That doesn't make it any less harmful. In fact, that makes it all the more insidious because there are people in key positions who could bring these dangers to the forefront. As it happens, they don't. So, once again, we must look to ourselves to seek out the answers to make the best decisions that we can. We have the indicators that we need when you consider these: if it's not safe for infants and hospitals, the rest of us should steer clear of it too.

Health Effects of Microwave Radiation—Microwave Ovens

Because the body is electrochemical in nature, any force which disrupts or changes human electrochemical phenomena will affect the physiology of the body.

Microwave ovens emit two types of radiation: the microwaves or high frequency radio waves, and the 60 hz magnetic fields common to other home appliances. This comes from the transformers in the back. The oven door is the most dangerous place for microwave leakage, but magnetic field can occur all around the oven. This is not good news for children, who love to watch the foods bubbling inside.

In addition to oven leakage, microwaving causes adverse effects in food. They include: formation of cancer-causing substances, leakage of toxic chemicals from the packaging into the foods, and destruction of nutrients.

What happens to people who ingest microwaved foods or who are exposed to external sources of microwave radiation.

Carcinogenic substances in microwaved food

Carcinogens were formed in virtually all foods tested. No test food was subjected to more microwaving than necessary to accomplish the purpose, e.g. cooking or thawing or heating to insure sanitary ingestion. Here's a summary of some of the results:

1. Microwaving prepared meats sufficiently to insure sanitary ingestion caused formation of *d*-Nitrosodienthanolamines, a well known carcinogen.
2. Microwaving milk and cereal grains converted certain of their amino acids into carcinogens.
3. Thawing frozen fruits converted their glucoside and galactoside containing fractions into carcinogenic substances.
4. Extremely short exposure of raw, cooked or frozen vegetables converted their plant alkaloids into carcinogens.
5. Carcinogenic free radicals were formed in microwaved plants, especially root vegetables.

Decrease in nutritive value of microwaved foods

Russian researchers reported a marked acceleration of structural degradation leading to a decreased food value of 60 to 90 per cent in all foods tested. Among the changes observed were:

1. Deceased bioavailability of vitamin B complex, vitamin C, vitamin E, essential minerals and lipotropics factors in all food tested.
2. Various kinds of damaged to many plant substances, such as alkaloids, glucosides, galactosides and nitrilosides.
3. The degradation of mucleoproteins in meats.

Leakage of chemicals from the package into food

Microwave ovens cannot make foods brown and crisp or crunchy. No problem! Heat susceptors are visible thin, gray strips or disks of metallised plastic that absorb microwave energy and turn the surface of the package into a very hot little frying pan which does the trick!

There are many chemicals that can be used in heat-susceptor packages, all approved of by the FDA. What was not recognised, however, was that susceptors can reach temperatures of 300° to 500°F in the microwave. When they do, the chemicals in the plastic migrate from the susceptors into your food, the FDA tested susceptors packages in 1988. Every package tested released chemicals into the food. Among these were PET (polyethylene terpthalate, a petroleum derived product), and other known or suspected carcinogens, such as benzene, toluene and xylene.

Pathogenic changes observed in consumers of microwaved food

Changes are observed in the blood chemistries and the rates of certain diseases among consumers of microwaved foods. The following is a sample of these changes:

1. Lymphatic disorders were observed, leading to decreased ability to prevent certain types of cancers.
2. An increased rate of cancer cell formation was observed in the blood.

3. Increased rates of stomach and intestinal cancers were observed.

4. Higher rates of digestive disorders and a grandual breakdown of the systems of elimination were observed.

According to US researcher William Kopp, Russian forensic teams observed the following key effects:

1. People who ingested microwaved foods showed a statistically higher incidence of stomach and intestinal cancers, plus a general degeneration of peripheral cellular tissues and a gradual breakdown of the function of the digestive and excretory systems.

2. Due to chemical alterations within food substances, malfunctions occurred within the lymphatic system, causing a degeneration in the immune system's ability to protect the body against neoplastic (cancerous) growth.

3. Microwave exposure caused significant decreases in the nutritional value of all foods studied, most significantly in the bioavailability of B-complex vitamins, vitamin C, vitamin E, essential minerals and lipotropics (substances that prevent abnormal accumulation of fat).

4. Heating prepared meats in a microwave sufficiently for human consumption creates the cancer-causing agent *d*-nitrosodiethanolamine.

5. Cancer-causing free radicals were formed within certain trace-mineral, molecular formations in plant substances—particularly in raw root vegetables.

6. Ingestion of microwaved foods caused a higher percentage of cancerous cells within the blood serum.

7. Microwaving foods alters their elemental food substances, leading to disorders in the digestive system.

PASCALISATION

Pascalisation or high pressure processing (HPP), is a method of preserving and sterilising food, in which a product is processed under very high pressure, leading to the inactivation of certain micro-organisms and enzymes in the food.

Pascalisation stops chemical activity caused by micro-organisms that play a role in the deterioration of foods. The treatment occurs at low temperatures and does not include the use of food additives. From 1990, some juices, jellies, and jams have been preserved using pascalisation in Japan. The technique is now used there to preserve fish and meats, salad dressing, rice cakes, and yogurts. An early use of pascalisation in the United States was to treat guacamole.

It did not change the guacamole's taste, texture or colour, but the shelf-life of the product increased to thirty days, from three days without the treatment. However, some treated foods still require cold storage because pascalisation does not stop all enzyme activity caused by proteins, some of which affects shelf-life.

In pascalisation, food products are sealed and placed into a steel compartment containing a liquid, often water, and pumps are used to create pressure. The pumps may apply pressure constantly or intermittently. The application of high hydrostatic pressures (HHP) on a food product will kill many micro-organisms, but the spores of some bacteria may need to be separately treated with acid to prevent their reproduction. Pascalisation works especially well on acidic foods, such as yogurts and fruits, because pressure-tolerant spores are not able to live in environments with low pH levels. The treatment works equally well for both solid and liquid products.

During pascalisation, the food's proteins are denatured, hydrogen bonds are fortified, and noncovalent bonds in the food are disrupted, while the product's main structure remains intact. Because pascalisation is not heat-based, covalent bonds are not affected, causing no change in the food's taste. High hydrostatic pressure can affect muscle tissues by increasing the rate of lipid oxidation, which in turn leads to poor flavour and decreased health benefits.

Because hydrostatic pressure is able to act quickly and evenly on food, neither the size of a product's container nor its thickness play a role in the effectiveness of pascalisation. There are several side effects of the process, including a slight increase in a product's sweetness, but pascalisation does not greatly affect the nutritional value, taste, texture, and appearance. As a result, high pressure treatment of foods is regarded as a 'natural' preservation method, as it does not use chemical preservatives.

Chapter 10

Preservation by Food Additives

INTRODUCTION

A food additive is a substance or mixture of substances, other than the basic food stuff, which is present in food as a result of any aspect of production processing, storage or packaging. Those food additives which are specifically added to prevent the deterioration or decomposition of food have been referred to as chemical preservatives. Preservatives may inhibit micro-organisms by interfering with their cell membranes, their enzyme activity or their genetic mechanisms. Other preservatives may be used as antioxidants to hinder the oxidation of unsaturated fats, as neutralisers of acidity, as stabilisers to prevent physical changes, as firming agents, and as coatings or wrappers to keep out micro-organisms, prevent loss of water or hinder undesirable microbial enzymatic and chemical reactions. An ideal antimicrobial preservative should have wide range of microbial activity, should be non-toxic to consumers, should be economical, should not affect organoleptic properties of food, should not be inactivated by food, should not promote the growth of resistant strains, and should kill rather than inhibit microbes. Factors that influence the effectiveness of chemical preservatives in killing micro-organisms or inhibiting their growth and activity are: (i) concentration of the chemical, (ii) kind, number, age, and previous history of the organism, (iii) temperature, (iv) time, and (v) the chemical and physical characteristics of the substrate in which the organism is found (moisture content, pH, kinds and amounts of solutes, surface tension, and colloids and other protective substances). A chemical agent may be bactericidal at a certain concentration, only inhibitory at a lower level, and ineffective at still greater dilutions.

ANTIOXIDANTS AND ANTIMICROBIAL PRESERVATIVES

Antioxidants and antimicrobial preservatives are substances which are used to extend the shelf-life of medicines by respectively retarding the oxidation of active ingredients and excipients, and by reducing microbial proliferation.

The properties of these substances are due to certain chemical groups which are usually aggressive towards living cells and which lead to certain risks when used in man (and animals).

For each antioxidant and antimicrobial preservative the application should contain:
1. Reason for inclusion.
2. Proof of efficacy.
3. The method of control in the finished product.
4. Details of the labelling of the finished product.
5. Safety information.

Antioxidants

Antioxidants are used to reduce the oxidation of active substances and excipients in the finished product. Antioxidants should not be used to disguise poorly formulated products or inadequate packaging. The need to include an antioxidant should be explained and fully justified. Oxidative degradation can be accelerated by light and by the presence of mineral impurities, due to the formation of free radicals. There are three types of antioxidants (Table 10.1).

Table 10.1. There are three types of antioxidants.

Type	Definition	Example
True antioxidants	These are thought to block chain reactions by reacting with free radicals	Butylated hydroxytoluene
Reducing agents	These have a lower redox potential than the drug or excipient they are protecting	Ascorbic acid
Antioxidant synergists	These enhance the effects of antioxidants	Sodium edetate

The efficacy obtained for an antioxidant depends on its nature, its concentration, the stage at which it is incorporated into the finished product, the nature of the container and the formulation. The efficacy of antioxidants must be assessed in the finished product in conditions which simulate actual use by measuring the extent of degradation in the finished product, with and without the antioxidant. Antioxidants should only be included in a formulation if it has been proved that their use cannot be avoided. This applies to cases where the manufacturing process is optimised to minimise the potential for oxidation.

Antimicrobial Preservatives

Antimicrobial preservatives are used to prevent or inhibit the growth of micro-organisms which could present a risk of infection or degradation of the medicinal product. These micro-organism may proliferate during normal storage conditions or use of the product by the patient, particularly in multidose preparations. On no account should preservatives be used as an alternative to good manufacturing practice. Preparations at greatest risk of contamination are those which contain water such as solutions, suspensions and emulsions to be taken orally, solution for external use, creams, and sterile preparations used repeatedly (e.g. injectable multidose preparations and eyedrops).

The level of efficacy obtained will vary according to the chemical structure of the preservative, its concentration, the physical and chemical characteristics of the medicinal product (especially pH) and the type and level of initial microbial contamination. The design of the pack and the temperature at which the product is stored will also affect the level of activity of any antimicrobial preservatives present. The antimicrobial efficacy of the preservative in the finished product should be assessed during product development using the European Pharmacopoeia test.

If products do not contain a preservative and do not have adequate inherent preservative efficacy they must not be packaged in multidose presentations without a sound justification.

Grouping of antimicrobial preservatives

Antimicrobial preservatives added to food can be grouped as follows:
1. Those added preservatives not defined as such by law: Natural organic acids (lactic, malic, citric, etc.) and their salts, vinegars (acetic is a natural acid), sodium chloride, sugars, spices and their oils, woods smoke, carbon dioxide, and nitrogen.

2. Substances generally recognised as safe (GRAS) for addition to food: Propionic acid and sodium and calcium propionates, caprylic acid, sorbic acid and potassium, sodium, and calcium sorbates, benzoic acid and benzoates and derivatives of benzoic acid such as methylparaben and propylparaben, sodium diacetate, sulphur dioxide and sulphites, potassium and sodium bisulphite and metabisulphite, and sodium nitrite (Limitations on the use of some of these should be considered during usage).
3. Chemicals considered to be food additives: These include all not listed in the first two categories. They can be used only when proved safe for humans or animals, and they then fall into group 4.
4. Chemicals proved safe and approved by the food and drug administration. Preservatives added to inhibit or kill micro-organisms may be classified on various other criteria, such as their chemical composition, mode of action, specificity, effectiveness, and legality.

Formulation

Antimicrobial preservative and antioxidants should be chemically defined (reference to existing pharmacopoeia monographs may be used) and designated by the chemical abstract service (CAS) registry number if they are not referenced in the pharmacopoeia. The purpose for the inclusion of any antioxidant or antimicrobial preservative should be stated (antioxidant for the benefit of active ingredient or excipient or both, or antimicrobial preservative).

Development Pharmaceutics

During the pharmaceutical development of the product the applicant should demonstrate:
1. The necessity to add an antioxidant or a preservative to the finished product at the level chosen.
2. The physical and chemical compatibility of the antioxidant and of the preservative with other constituents of the finished product, the container and the closures.

The concentration used must be justified in terms of efficacy and safety, such that the minimum concentration of preservative is used which gives the required level of efficacy.

The appropriate test method for efficacy of antimicrobial preservation is that of the European Pharmacopoeia. This should be used to determine whether the required level of activity is achieved.

In the case of antioxidants, these should only be used once it has been shown that their use cannot be avoided, even if the manufacturing process is optimised to minimise the potential for oxidation, for example by manufacturing and filling products under an inert headspace gas.

The safety of the antioxidant or preservative should be supported by bibliographic and/or experimental data. Some antioxidants or antimicrobial preservatives may be undesirable under certain circumstances, e.g. mercury containing preservatives, benzyl alcohol (when used in parenteral products for children under the age of 2 years or in new-born animals or in cats), benzoic acid esters (when used in any medicinal products for injection), sulphites and metabisulphite.

Parenteral infusions do not contain any added antimicrobial preservatives and no antimicrobial preservatives are added when the medicinal product is intended for administration by routes where for medical reasons an antimicrobial preservative is unacceptable, such as intercisternally or by any other route of administration which gives access to the cerebrospinal fluid or retroocularly.

Control of the Finished Product

The finished product release specifications should include an identification test and limits for any antioxidants and antimicrobial preservatives present in the formulation. The finished product specification against which the product is tested throughout its shelf-life should also include limits for the antimicrobial preservatives present. Where antioxidants are used during the manufacture of the product, the release limits should be justified by batch data. The adequacy of specified limits should be justified on the basis of controlled conditions and in use stability testing to ensure that sufficient antioxidant remains to protect the product throughout its entire shelf life and during the proposed in use period.

The control of antioxidants and antimicrobial preservatives should comply with the requirements identified in the note for guidance specifications and control tests of the finished product.

Stability

The application should follow the current EU guidelines on the stability of new dosage forms and should ensure that antimicrobial preservative and antioxidants levels are quantified periodically throughout the shelf-life of the finished product. In addition the efficacy of preservatives should be established using the test for efficacy of antimicrobial preservation of the European Pharmacopoeia. This should be performed on the finished product at the end of the shelf life and at the lower preservative limit in the end of shelf-life specification.

The former is necessary, even if no evidence of degradation of the antimicrobial preservative and of the antioxidant is observed on storage, as other chemical and physical changes in the finished product may influence the efficacy of the antimicrobial preservative and of the antioxidant. In the case of products presented in multidose containers, the efficacy of the antimicrobial preservative under simulated in use conditions must be established.

The tests should be performed under the same condition as it is expected to be used by the user. It may also be appropriate to examine the efficacy of the antimicrobial preservative following storage of opened or used containers for the proposed in use shelf-life.

Labelling

Labelling must be in accordance with relevant community directives-council directive 92/27/EEC and 81/851/EEC. However, if a product is presented in a multidose container without a preservative because:

1. It is intended for single use only (e.g. cytotoxic).
2. The product is self-preserving.
3. The product is oil based.

The labelling and product literature should indicate the absence of a preservative. This would not only emphasise the increased risk associated with the use of such products, but also aid the physician to specifically identify a product without preservative.

Organic Acids and Their Salts

Lactic, acetic, propionic, and citric acids or their salts may be added to or developed in food. Citric acid is used in syrups, drinks, jams, and jellies as a substitute for fruit flavours and for preservation:

1. Acids, chiefly acetic and lactic, can be present in preserved foods as a result of acid addition to non-fermented foods, or as a result of microbial fermentation of tissue carbohydrates.
2. Acids have two anti-microbial effects: One is due to their effect in pH, and the other is the specific toxicity of the undissociated acid which carries for different acids.

Salt

1. Salt was used by man as one of the earliest methods of food preservation.

2. Smoking and drying is used extensively in combination with salt, particularly for meat and fish product.

3. Salt and acid are used extensively in the preservation of vegetable product of which cucumbers, cabbage, and onions are important examples.

Sugar

1. Sugar are involved in the preservation and manufacture of wide range of food products.

2. Some of the more common include: Jams, jellies, fruit juice concentrates, sweetened condensed milk.

3. When sugars are added to foods in high concentration (at least 40 per cent soluble solids), some of the water present becomes unavailable for microbial growth and the a_w of the food is reduced.

Chemical preservatives

To be in accord with good manufacturing practices, the use of preservatives:

1. Should not result in deception.

2. Should not adversely affect the nutritive value of the food.

3. Should not permit the growth of food-poisoning organisms while suppressing growth of the others that would make spoilage evident.

4. Chemical preservatives vegetables preservation are sulphur dioxide (SO_2), benzoates, and sorbates.

5. The efficiency of chemical preservatives depends primarily on the concentration of the preservative, the composition of the food, and the type of organisms to be inhibited.

6. The concentration of preservative permitted by food regulations.

7. It is essential that the microbiological population of the food to be preserved is kept to a minimum by handling and processing.

Anti-microbial properties of salt and acid

1. Salt produces a number of effects when added to fresh plant tissues.

2. Salt exerts a selective inhibitory action on certain contaminating micro-organisms.

3. Salt also affects the water activity (a_w) of the substrate, thus controlling microbial growth by a method independent of its toxic effects.

Propionates

Sodium or calcium propionate is used most extensively in the prevention of mould growth and rope development in baked goods and for mould inhibition in many cheese food and spreads. Propionic acid is a short-chain fatty acid (CH_3CH_2COOH) and, like some other fatty acids, perhaps affects the cell-membrane permeability, although its precise mode of fungistatic action is not known.

Experimentally or on a limited scale, they have been used in butter, jams, jellies, figs, apple slices, and malt extract. They are effective against moulds, with little or no inhibition of most yeast and bacteria. Their effectiveness decreases with an increase in pH, with an optimal upper limit of about pH 5 to 6, depending on the food item. They appear to be ideal preservatives for bread and baked goods. Although the heat of baking destroys most moulds, contamination of the loaves can occur during slicing and/or wrapping, hence the need for the propionates. Since they have little inhibitory effect on yeasts, they can be added to the dough of yeast-raised baked goods without interfering with leavening.

Benzoates

The sodium salt of benzoic acid has been used extensively as an antimicrobial agent in food. It has been incorporated into jams, jellies, margarine, carbonated beverage, fruit salads, pickles, relishes, fruit juices, etc. Sodium benzoate is relatively ineffective at pH values near neutrality, and the effectiveness increases with increase in acidity, an indication that the undissociated and is the effective agent. The pH at which sodium benzoate is most effective (2.5 to 4.0) is in itself enough to inhibit the growth of most bacteria, but some (not all) yeasts and moulds are inhibited at pH levels that would otherwise permit their growth. Two esters of *p*-hydroxybenzoic acid, methylparaben, and propylparaben, are also used extensively in foods, and to lesser extent the butyl and ethylesters. These compounds are similar to benzoic acid in their effectiveness.

Their distinct advantage is that they tend to be more effective at higher pH values than the other banzoates because the esterification of the carboxyl group means that the undissociated molecule is retained over a wider pH range; since it is the undissociated molecule that exerts inhibition, the esters are effective at higher pH values. The mechanism of action of the benzoates is not clear; it is known, however, that the effectiveness of the benzoic acid esters increases with an increase in the chain length of the ester group.

Sorbates

Sorbic acid, as the calcium, sodium, or potassium salt, is used as a direct antimicrobial additive in food and as a spray, dip or coating on packaging materials. It is widely used in cheeses, cheese products, baked goods, beverages, syrups, fruit juices, jellies, jams, fruit cocktails, dried fruits, pickles, and margaine. Sorbic acid and its salts are known to inhibit yeast and moulds but are less effective against bacteria. They are most effective at low pH values with a maximal level of use at about pH 6.5. These compounds are more effective than sodium benzoate at pH values above 4.0.

Acetates

Derivatives of acetic acid, e.g. monochloroacetic acid, peracetic acid, dehydroacetic acid, and sodium diacetate, have been recommended as preservatives. Dehydroacetic acid has been used to impregnate wrappers for cheese to inhibit the growth of moulds and as a temporary preservative for squash.

Acetic acid in the form of vinegar is used in mayonnaise, pickles, catsup, pickled sausages, and pigs' feet. Acetic acid is more effective against yeasts and bacteria than against moulds, and its effectiveness increases with a decrease in pH, which would favour the presence of the undissociated acid.

Sodium diacetate has been used in cheese spreads and malt sirups and as treatment for wrappers used on butter.

Nitrites and nitrates

Combinations of these various salts have been used in curing solutions and curing mixtures for meats. Nitrites decompose to nitric acid, which forms nitrosomyoglobin when it reacts with the pigments in meats and thereby forms a stable red colour. Nitrate probably only acts as a reservoir for nitrite. Nitrites can react with secondary and tertiary amines to form nitrosamines, which are known to be carcinogenic. They are currently added in the form of sodium nitrite, potassium nitrite, sodium nitrate, and potassium nitrate. Recent work has emphasised the inhibitory property of nitrites towards *Clostridium botulinum* in meat products, particularly in bacon and canned or processed hams. Nitrates have a limited effect on limited number of organisms and would not be considered a good chemical preservative.

Sulphur dioxide and sulphites

The Egyptians and Romans burned sulphur to form sulphur dioxide as a means of sanitising their wine-making equipment and storage vessels. Today sulphur dioxide and sulphites are used in the wine industry to sanitise equipment and to reduce the normal flora of the grape must. In aqueous solutions, sulphur dioxide and various sulphites, including sodium sulphite, potassium sulphite, sodium bisulphite, potassium bisulphite, sodium metabisulphite, and potassium metabisulphite, form sulphurous acid, the active antimicrobial compound. Many mechanisms for the action of sulphurous acid on microbial cells have been suggested, including the reduction of disulphide linkages, formation of carbonyl compounds, reaction with ketone groups, and inhibition of respiratory mechanisms.

The fumes of burning sulphur are used to treat most light-coloured dehydrated fruits, while dehydrated vegetables are exposed to spray of neutral bisulphite and sulphites before drying. Sulphur dioxide has also been used in sirups and fruit juices and, of course, wine making. Some countries permit the use of sulphites on meats and fish. In addition to the antimicrobial action of sulphites, they are also used to prevent enzymatic and nonenzymatic changes or discolouration in some foods.

Ethylene and propylene oxide

Ethylene oxide kills all micro-organisms, propylene oxide, although it kills many micro-organism, is not as effective as that of ethylene oxide. They are thought to act strong alkylating agents attacking labile hydrogen. They have also been used successfully in dried fruits, dries eggs, gelatine, cereals, dried yeast, and spices. The FDA restricts the use of ethylene oxide to spices and other processed natural seasonings except mixtures containing added salt. Propylene oxide is permitted only as a package fumigant for dried prunes or glace fruits and as a fumigant for cocoa, gums, spices, starch, and processed nutmeats (but not peanuts).

Alcohol

Ethanol, a coagulant and denaturiser of cell proteins, is most germicidal in concentrations between 70 and 95 per cent. Flavouring extracts, e.g. vanilla and lemon extracts, are preserved by their content of alcohol.

The alcoholic content of beer, ale, and unfortified wine is not great enough to prevent their spoilage by micro-organisms but limits the types able to grow. Liqueurs and distilled liquors usually contain enough alcohol to ensure freedom from microbial attack. Methanol is poisonous and should not be added to foods, the traces added to foods by smoking are not enough to be harmful. Glycerol is antiseptic in high concentrations because of its dehydrating effect but is unimportant in food preservation. Propylene glycol has been used as a mould inhibitor and as a spray to kill airborne micro-organisms.

Formaldehyde

The addition of formaldehyde to food is not permitted, except as a minor constituent of woods smoke, but this compound is effective against moulds, bacteria, and viruses and can be used where its poisonous nature and irritating properties are not objectionable.

Thus it is useful in the treatment of walls, shelves, floors, etc. to eliminate moulds and their spores. Paraformaldehyde can be used to control bacterial and fungal growth in tapholes of maple trees. Formaldehyde probably combines with free amino groups of the proteins of cell protoplasm, injures nuclei, and coagulates proteins.

Wood smoke

The smoking of food usually has main purposes like adding desired flavours and preserving. Woods smoke contains a large number of volatile compounds that may have bacteriostatic and bactericidal effect. Formaldehyde is considered the most effective of these compounds, with phenols and cresols next in importance. Other compounds in the smoke are aliphatic acids from formic through caproic; primary and secondary alcohols, ketones, and acetaldehyde and other aldehydes; waxes; resins; guaiacol and its methyl and propyl isomers; and catechol, methyl, catechol and pyrogallol and its methyl ester. Wood smoke is more effective against vegetative cells than against bacterial spores, and the temperature varies with the kind of wood employed.

The residual effect of the smoke in the food has been reported to be greater against bacteria than against moulds. The concentration of mycostatic materials from wood smoke necessary to prevent mould growth increases with a rise in the humidity of the atmosphere of storage.

The application of 'liquid smoke', a solution of chemicals similar to those in wood smoke, to the outside of foods has little or no preservative effect although it contributes to flavour.

Spices and other condiment

Spices and other condiments do not have any marked bacteriostatic effect in the concentrations customarily used but may help other agents in preventing the growth of organisms in food. The inhibitory effect of spices differs with the kind of spice and the micro-organism being tested. Mustard flour and the volatile oil of mustard, for example, are very effective against *Saccharomyces cerevisiae* but are not as potent as cinnamon and cloves against most bacteria. The essential oils of spices are more inhibitory than the corresponding ground spices. Cinnamon and clove, containing cinnamic aldehyde and eugenol, respectively, usually are more bacteriostatic than are other spices.

Cinnamon and cloves, containing cinnamic aldehyde and eugenol, respectively, usually are more bacteriostatic than are other spices. Ground peppercorn and allspice are less inhibitory, and mustard, mace, nutmeg, and ginger still less. Thyme, bay leaves, marjoram, savory, rosemary, black pepper, and others have only weak inhibitory power against most organisms and may even stimulate some, e.g. yeasts and moulds. Fairly heavy concentrations of the more effective spices permit mycelial growth of some of the moulds but inhibit the formation of asexual spores. Of the oils tested, the volatile oil of mustard is most effective against yeasts; oils of cinnamon and cloves are fairly effective, and oils of thyme and bay leaves are least effective.

Unless spices have been treated to reduce their microbial content, they may add high numbers and undesirable kinds of micro-organisms to foods of which they are ingredients.

Other plant materials used in seasoning foods, such as horseradish, garlic, and onion, may be bacteriostatic or germicidal. Extracts of these plants, as well as of cabbage and turnip, have been shown to be inhibitory to *Bacillus subtilis* and *Escherichia coli*. Acrolein is supposedly the active principle in onions and garlic, and butyl thiocyanate in horseradish. These volatile compounds are lost from the condiment on exposure to the air, with a corresponding loss in bacteriostatic properties.

Other food additives

Halogens are added to water for washing food or equipment, for cooling, and for addition to some products, i.e. washing butter; water for drinking may be chlorinated by the direct addition of chlorine, or hypochlorites or chloramines may be used. Iodine-impregnated wrappers have been employed to lengthen the keeping time of fruits. Iodophors, which are combinations of iodine with non-ionic wetting agents and acid, are being used in the sanitisation of dairy utensils. Halogens kill organisms by oxidation, injury to cell membranes or direct combination with cell proteins.

Hypochlorites, usually of calcium or sodium, yield hypochlorous acid, a powerful oxidising agent, and are effective germicidal agents; their effectiveness is reduced by the presence of organic matter in any considerable amount. The hypochlorites are used in the treatment of water used in food plants for drinking, processing, and cooling and on plant equipment. They have been incorporated in ice for icing fish in transit and in water for washing the exterior of fruits and vegetables. Micro-organisms are harmed by oxidation or by direct chlorination of cell proteins. Phosphoric is used in some soft drinks, e.g. the colas.

The oxidising agent hydrogen peroxide has been used as a preservative, usually in conjunction with heat. One method for the pasteurisation of milk for cheese involves the addition of H_2O_2 and the use of a comparatively low heating temperature. Excess peroxide is decomposed by catalase. Thermophiles are destroyed in the processing of sugar by a combination of heat and H_2O_2. Other peroxides are used in foods but not for the prevention of microbial growth.

Gas storage of foods was mentioned in connection with preservation by chilling on the preservation of specific foods. Most often used is carbon dioxide in combination with chilling. Oxygen or air under pressure is combined with chilling, as in the Hofius process for milk. Nitrogen is used as an inert gas over foods that should not be exposed to air.

Boric acid and borates still are used in some countries as preservatives for foods, but their use is forbidden in the United States. Powdered boric acid has been dusted onto foods, e.g., meats, but it is a very weak antiseptic and is not considered healthful. Borax (sodium tetraborate) has been used to wash vegetables and whole fruits, such as oranges.

Antibiotics

Most of the better-known antibiotics have been tested on raw food, chiefly proteinaceous ones like meats, fish, and poultry, in an endeavour to lengthen the storage time at chilling temperatures. Aureomycin (chlortetracycline) has been found superior to other antibiotics tested because of its broad spectrum of activity. Terramycin (oxytetracycline) is almost as good for lengthening the time of preservation of food.

Some success also has been claimed with chloromycetin (chloramphenicol). These three antibiotics inhibit protein synthesis in the cell. Streptomycin, neomycin, polymyxin, nisin, subtilin, bacitracin, and others are not as satisfactory, and penicillin is of little use. Nisin has been employed in Europe to suppress anaerobes in cheese and cheese products. Natamycin is effective against yeasts and moulds; it is used, or tested, in orange juice, fresh fruits, sausage, and cheese.

Experimentally, antibiotics have been combined with heat in attempts to reduce the thermal treatment necessary for the preservation of low and medium-acid canned foods. Most tests have been with the peptides, subtilin and nisin, and tylosin. It has been suggested that a botulinum cook, i.e. enough of a heat treatment to inactivate all spores of *Clostridium botulinum*, be given canned foods, combined with the addition of enough antibiotic to inhibit germination and outgrowth of surviving spores of the most heat-resistant thermophilic spoilage bacteria and putrefactive anaerobes. Subtilin supposedly has no effect on the heat resistance of bacterial spores but inhibits heat-damaged cells during outgrowth, whereas nisin apparently interferes with spore germination and with lysis of the spore coat. Tylosin may inhibit cell growth.

It has been recommended that antibiotics selected for use in food preservation be other than those being used in the treatment of human diseases. Canners feel that when used in the processing of canned foods, the antibiotic plus the heat treatment must destroy all spores of *Clostridium botulinum* and allow a margin of safety, and preferably the treatment should destroy all spoilage organisms and their spores. If spores survive, the antibiotic must remain in sufficient concentration in the food to prevent germination, outgrowth, or vegetative growth of cells. This means that the antibiotic must persist in bacteriostatic or sporostatic concentration throughout the storage life of the canned food.

The food and drug administration had approved the use of a chlortetracycline and oxytetracycline dip for preserving poultry, setting up a 7 ppm tolerance in the uncooked, dressed fowls. This quantity of antibiotic has been shown to double or triple the storage life of the poultry. Apparently approval had been granted because evidence was given to prove that: (i) use of the material affords added protection to the consumer, (ii) basic sanitation procedures are not replaced because of the method, and (iii) the antibiotic is destroyed during cooking of the poultry, leaving no harmful end products. This permission for use FDA has been revoked. Now it is permissible to use these tetracyclines at 5 ppm only on fresh fish, shucked scallops, and unpeeled shrimp. The antibiotic may be applied as a dip or an ice.

Developed preservatives

Preservatives could be produced in food by microbes like lactic acid, alcohol, bacterixin, etc. Their preservative effect is mostly supplemented by one or more additional preservative methods like low temperature, high temperature, anaerobic conditions, sodium chloride, sugar, etc. Developed acidity plays a part in preservation of sauerkraut, pickles, green olives, fermented milk and cheese, and certain sausages and in various fermented foods of plant origin. Development of the full amount of acidity from the sugar available may be permitted in the pickle and green-olive fermentations or the fermentation may be stopped by chilling or canning before the maximum acidity is attained in other fermentations, e.g. that for fermented, milks or sauerkraut. The approximate acidity developed in some of these products, expressed as lactic acid, is sauerkraut, 1.7 per cent; salt-stock or dill pickles and green olives, 0.9 per cent; and fermented milks, 0.6 to 0.85 per cent. The acidity of cheese usually is expressed in terms of hydrogen-ion concentration; most freshly made cheeses have a pH of about 5.0 to 5.2 and become more alkaline during curing.

The alcohol content of beer, ale, fermented fruit juices, and distilled liquors has a preservative effect but was not produced primarily for that purpose.

SECTION III

Contamination, Preservation and Spoilage of Various Foods

Chapter 11

Contamination, Preservation and Spoilage of Vegetables and Fruits

INTRODUCTION

All living creatures, including humans, depend on nature for their food. Humans are not only hunters and gatherers, but also farmers. We live from hunting and fishing, agriculture and animal husbandry. Most of our food consists of agricultural products, which are usually seasonal and spoil quickly. To make food available throughout the year, humans have developed methods to prolong the storage life of products to preserve them. The rotting process can be postponed by adding preservatives, optimising storage conditions or applying modern techniques.

Fruits and vegetables provide an abundant and inexpensive source of energy, body-building nutrients, vitamins and minerals. Their nutritional value is highest when they are fresh, but it is not always possible to consume them immediately. During the harvest season, fresh produce is available in abundance, but at other times it is scarce. Moreover, most fruits and vegetables are only edible for a very short time, unless they are promptly and properly preserved.

FOOD SPOILAGE: CAUSES, EFFECTS AND PREVENTION

Every change in food that causes it to lose its desired quality and eventually become inedible is called food spoilage or rotting. As noted earlier, this chapter focuses specifically on fruits and vegetables. As long as they are not harvested, their quality remains relatively stable—if they are not damaged by disease or eaten by insects or other animals. However, the harvest cannot be postponed indefinitely: when the time is right, it is time to act. As soon as the fruits and vegetables are cut off from their natural nutrient supply, their quality begins to diminish. This is due to a natural process that starts as soon as the biological cycle is broken by harvesting. Once it is harvested, the agricultural product is edible for only a limited time, which can vary from a few days to weeks. The product then begins to spoil or 'rot'. We distinguish between various types of spoilage:

1. Physical spoilage.
2. Physiological ageing.
3. Spoilage due to insects or rodents.
4. Mechanical damage.
5. Chemical and enzyme spoilage.
6. Microbial spoilage.

Physical spoilage is caused for example by dehydration. Physiological ageing occurs as soon as the biological cycle is broken through harvesting. Neither process can be prevented, but they can be delayed by storing the agricultural products in a dry and draft-free area at as low a temperature as possible.

Insects and rodents can cause a lot of damage. Not only by eating the products, but also by passing on micro-organisms through their hair and droppings. The affected parts of the plants are then especially susceptible to diseases.

Chemical and enzyme spoilage occurs especially when vegetables and fruit are damaged by falling or breaking. Such damage can release enzymes that trigger chemical reactions. Tomatoes become soft, for example, and apples and other types of fruit turn brown. The fruit can also become rancid. The same processes can also be triggered by insects: the fruit becomes damaged, which causes enzymes to be released. Enzymes can be deactivated by heating the fruit or vegetables. The same effect can be achieved by making the fruit or vegetables sour or by drying them, but the enzymes become active again as soon as the acidity is reduced or water is added.

The peel of a fruit or vegetable provides natural protection against micro-organisms. As soon as this shield is damaged by falling, crushing, cutting, peeling or cooking, the chance of spoilage increases considerably. Crushing occurs most often when fruits or vegetables are piled up too high.

To prevent harvested products from spoiling, they can be preserved: physiological ageing and enzyme changes are then stopped and micro-organisms are prevented from multiplying on the product. To retain the desired quality of a product longer than if it were simply stored after harvesting, it must be preserved. To preserve food it must first be treated, with the goal of stopping physiological ageing and enzyme changes and preventing the growth of micro-organisms.

Before discussing the specific treatment methods, we will first focus on the subject of micro-organisms. What are micro-organisms? Why are they dangerous? How can you prevent them from making you sick? The answers to these questions will help you understand the steps required to safely preserve food.

What are Micro-organisms and What Factors Affect their Growth?

Micro-organisms are very small, one-celled animals. There are three types: bacteria, moulds and yeasts. Bacteria and yeasts cannot be seen with the naked eye, but moulds are often visible because they form visible thin threads (filaments) or a solid cluster. Just like humans, micro-organisms require certain minimum living conditions. They cannot survive without:

1. Sufficient water.
2. Oxygen.
3. The right degree of acidity.
4. Nutrients.
5. The right temperature.

Water is necessary for maintaining many physical processes. Where there is a shortage or lack of water micro-organisms cannot grow, such as in dried legumes. Drying is therefore one way to prevent spoilage. Meat and fish do not have to be 100 per cent dry in order to preserve them. By adding salt, the remaining water becomes unsuitable for micro-organisms. The same effect can be achieved by adding sugar to fruit. Enzymatic spoilage is also inhibited by drying.

Most micro-organisms need oxygen. If there is a shortage of oxygen, it is difficult for bacteria to survive, let alone multiply. But there are always a few that manage to survive. As soon as the oxygen supply is increased, these remaining bacteria will again grow and multiply. Some types of micro-organisms even thrive in an oxygen-poor environment.

Bacteria grow best in an environment that is not too acidic. Less acidic products are therefore especially susceptible to bacterial spoilage. Examples of such products are meat, eggs, milk and various types of vegetables. Beer, yoghurt, wine, vinegar and fruit are less sensitive because they are more acidic. Adding acidity to products slows down the process of microbial spoilage. The degree of acidity is measured as a pH level. A neutral product like milk has a pH of 7; meat has a pH of about 6, carrots have a pH of 5 and oranges about 4. The more acidic a product is, the lower the pH value will be.

Just like humans, micro-organisms also need nutrients: sugars, proteins, fats, minerals and vitamins. These are rarely in short supply, because they can be found in all food products. To thrive, micro-organisms need a temperature of between 5° and 65°C. At temperatures above 65°C it becomes very difficult for them to survive; and they definitely die if boiled, as long as they are boiled for a certain length of time, such as 10 minutes.

When heated, the micro-organisms slowly die off, but not all at the same time. Heating at temperatures lower than 100°C thus has to be sustained for a longer period. The growth of micro-organisms is also slowed down significantly at temperatures between 0 and 5°C (as in a refrigerator), which makes it possible to store the food products for a few additional days. At temperatures below 0°C microbial growth is stopped completely, but the micro-organisms themselves remain alive. They will become active again as soon as the temperature rises above 0°C.

To preserve food, it is sometimes necessary to make drastic changes to the micro-organisms' living conditions. We can remove water (drying), increase the acidity, or first heat the products (to kill the bacteria) and then store them in air-tight containers to prevent oxygen from entering (preserving/canning).

Do Micro-organisms Grow Differently on Vegetables and Fruits?

Vegetables and fruit have a lot in common. But there are also important differences, which determine the type of spoilage they are most susceptible to. Damaged fruits, which are usually somewhat acidic, are very susceptible to the growth of yeasts and moulds. Vegetables are generally less acidic, and their spoilage is usually caused by bacteria. Though not visible to the naked eye, bacteria can still be present in large numbers.

What Types of Micro-organisms Grow on What Products?

1. Moulds can be found on almost all food products. They are often very visible and can significantly alter the taste of the products. They grow the best in low temperatures in an acidic environment and on dry products such as grains and bread. Some moulds produce poisonous substances, especially in moist seeds such as peanuts, corn and soyabeans.
2. Yeasts can also cause food to spoil. They prefer low temperatures and acidic products.
3. Bacteria can grow on almost all types of fresh food that is not too acidic: meat, fish, milk and vegetables. One type of bacteria carries a kind of seed, called a spore. Spores can survive at a temperature of 100°C, even though the bacteria themselves die. Once the temperature drops, new bacteria can grow out of the spores. To kill the spores, they must be exposed to a temperature of 121°C. This is called sterilisation.

WHAT DO MICRO-ORGANISMS DO TO FRUITS AND VEGETABLES?

Micro-organisms take from food products the various substances they need to survive and multiply. Their secreted waste products can have either a negative or positive effect on the affected food and the humans who eat it.

Positive Effects of Micro-organisms on Food

The waste products secreted by some micro-organisms can have a positive effect on food. Lactic acid bacteria, for example, are used to make cheese and yoghurt from milk, and sauerkraut from white cabbage. Moulds are used to make tempeh from soyabeans, and yeasts are used to make beer and bread. These substances influence the taste and structure of the food products and generally increase their shelf-life. The products can be kept longer because the desired micro-organisms decrease the food's pH level or because they are present in such huge numbers that other micro-organisms have no chance to grow. This use of micro-organisms for the preparation of food is called fermentation.

Negative Effects of Micro-organisms on Food

Sometimes the negative effects of bacteria are clearly apparent, such as when milk has turned sour and curdled, when meat is covered in slime, when moulds and gasses have formed, and when food has a distinctly putrid smell. However, food spoilage is not always this obvious. There are bacteria whose presence in food does not always cause a change in its taste or appearance. In any case, it is important to avoid eating rotten food, because it can make a person seriously ill.

Eating rotten food can cause contamination or poisoning. A food contamination occurs when a person consumes a large number of living micro-organisms in a meal. These can multiply rapidly in the person's gastrointestinal tract and severely disturb the digestive system. The result is often diarrhoea and sometimes also bleeding. The symptoms appear between 3 and 24 hours after eating the rotten food. A food contamination can be prevented by frying or boiling the food thoroughly, since sufficient heating will kill the micro-organisms.

Food poisoning occurs when a person consumes food containing the poisonous waste products secreted by the bacteria. Heating the food does not help in this case: the bacteria will be killed, but the poisonous waste will remain unharmed. Both food poisoning and food contaminations can be *lethal,* but usually they only make a person sick.

How do Micro-organisms Come in Contact with Fruits and Vegetables?

Spoilage caused by yeasts, moulds and bacteria develops slowly and is not always noticeable. The most important sources of microbial contaminations are sand, water, air, and pests such as insects and rodents. Food products can also be infected by people. Micro-organisms are everywhere around us. To prevent them from reaching our food in great numbers, it is important to work as hygienically as possible when handling fruits and vegetables, for example.

The following practices are therefore recommended:
1. Wash your hands thoroughly with hot water and soap before beginning to prepare food.
2. Make sure that kitchen utensils and appliances are well cleaned and disinfected.
3. Always store food in a clean place.
4. Use herbs and spices as little as possible, because they are an important source of contamination.
5. Use clean and pure salt only—if the salt is not pure, heat it on a dry, metal sheet above the fire.
6. Allow only clean drinking water to come in contact with fruits and vegetables.
7. Never allow anyone who is sick or has open wounds to come in contact with food that is to be preserved.

PREPARATION OF FRUITS AND VEGETABLES

Fruits and vegetables should be prepared for preservation as soon as possible after harvesting, in any case within 4 to 48 hours. The likelihood of spoilage increases rapidly as time passes.

Cleaning and Washing

First, the fruits or vegetables have to be thoroughly cleaned to remove any dirt or insecticide residues. The outer layers of onions also have to be removed. This cleaning process usually involves washing the products under a faucet with running drinking-water or in a bucket with clean water that is regularly refreshed. When cleaning leafy vegetables, it is best to first remove the stems. Some types of fruit, such as cherries, strawberries and mushrooms are not washed, because this would actually increase the spread of micro-organisms. It is also not advisable to wash cucumbers, because this shortens their shelf-life.

Dried beans and nuts are soaked in water for 16–20 hours before being processed further. To prevent the beans and nuts from turning black, a stainless steel pan or bowl, or other galvanised material, should be used. The temperature of the soaking water should remain constant.

Lye Dip

Some products, such as plums and grapes, are immersed for 5–15 seconds in a pan of hot, almost boiling, lye (NaOH; 10–20 g lye/litre water) to make the peel rough and to thereby speed up the general drying process. The peel then also separates more readily from the fruit, which makes it easier to remove. After such a treatment, the fruit has to be rinsed vigorously with cold water to remove the lye residues. Lemon juice can also be used to neutralise any remaining lye residues.

The preparation method described above is considered to be ecologically harmful because alkaline is transported by the waste-water into the environment. Other disadvantages of using lye are that the food can become discoloured and the metal pan could become corroded. The use of too-high concentrations of lye is also unhealthy for the people working with it.

Sorting

To achieve a uniformly sized product, fruits and vegetables are sorted immediately after cleaning according to their size, shape, weight or colour. Sorting by size is especially important if the products are to be dried or heated, because their size will determine how much time will be needed for these processes.

Peeling

Many types of fruits and vegetables have to be peeled in order to be preserved. This can easily be done with a stainless steel knife. It is extremely important that the knife be made of stainless steel because this will prevent the discolouration of the plant tissues. It is best to first submerge citrus fruits, tomatoes and peaches, whose peels are all securely connected to the fruit, in hot water for 1 ½ to 3 minutes. The softened peel can then be removed without too much effort.

Cutting

Cutting is important because you will need approximately uniform pieces for the heating, drying and packing stages. Fruits and vegetables are usually cut into cubes, thin slices, rings or shreds. The cutting utensils have to be sharp and clean to prevent micro-organisms from entering the food. From the moment they are cut, the quality of the products decreases due to the release of enzymes and nutrients for micro-organisms. A decrease in quality is also caused by the damage done to the plant tissues. For this reason, the interval between peeling/cutting and preserving has to be as short as possible.

BLANCHING

Blanching or precooking is done by immersing fruits or vegetables in water at a temperature of 90°–95°C. Exposing them to steam is also possible. The result is that fruits and vegetables become somewhat soft and the enzymes are inactivated. Leafy vegetables shrink in this process and some of the micro-organisms die. Blanching is done before a product is dried in order to prevent unwanted colour and odour changes and an excessive loss of vitamins. Fruit that does not change colour generally does not need to be blanched. Onions and leek are not at all suited for blanching.

Blanching is quite simple. The only thing you need is a large pan with a lid and a metal, or in any case heat-resistant, colander (Fig. 11.1). Place the fruit or vegetable in the colander (a linen cloth with a cord will also do) and immerse this in a pan with sufficient nearly boiling water to cover the food completely. Leave the colander in the pan for a few minutes and turn the food occasionally to make sure that it is heated evenly. Immediately after the colander is removed from the pan the food has to be rinsed with cold, clean running water. Make sure that the extra water can run off. If no faucet is available, a container with drinking-water can also be used, as long as the water is cold and clean. During the blanching process, it is important to monitor the time and the water temperature (Appendix 11.4 gives an overview of recommended blanching times per vegetable).

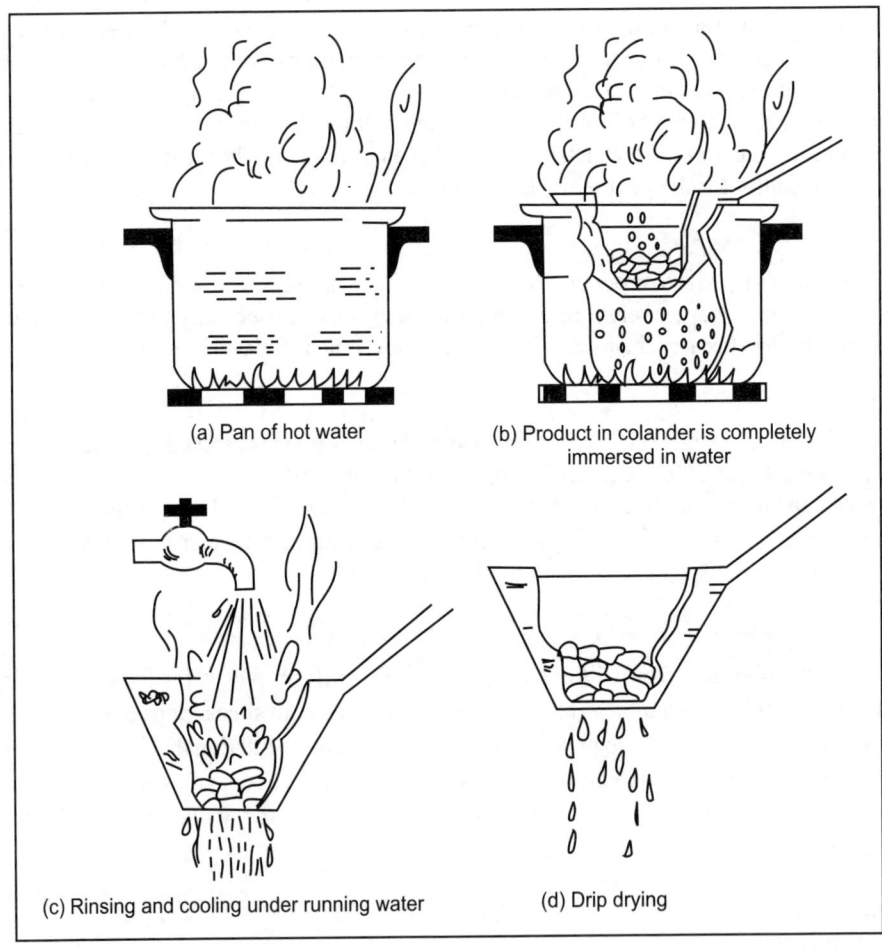

(a) Pan of hot water

(b) Product in colander is completely immersed in water

(c) Rinsing and cooling under running water

(d) Drip drying

Fig. 11.1. Blanching.

The disadvantage of this blanching method is that many vitamins are lost in the hot water. Steaming is therefore a better alternative. Only a small amount of water has to be added to the pan and brought to the boil. Make sure that the fruit or vegetable in the colander is touched by the steam but not by the water.

PRESERVING BY HEATING

One of the most common and effective ways to preserve fruits and vegetables is to prepare them and place them in air-tight containers, which are then heated. The high temperatures ensure that micro-organisms are killed and the enzymes are inactivated. Any remaining spores will not have the right conditions to grow into bacteria and microbial contamination from outside is prevented. However, it is important to remember that some micro-organisms are unfortunately less sensitive to heat: *Clostridium* and *Staphylococcus* can still multiply and spoil the food through the poisonous substances they produce. *Clostridium* can cause botulism and result in tragic deaths. This bacteria does not thrive as well in more acidic products such as fruit (pH < 4.5).

The heating method for fruit is different than for most vegetables. As noted above, fruit has a low pH level. It can be heated in boiling water (100°C), whereas most vegetables have to be heated at temperatures above 100°C, because they have a higher pH and are thus more susceptible to bacterial contamination.

This preservation method produces the best results, but only if fresh products are used and the instructions for heating are followed exactly. As with other methods, heating has advantages and disadvantages as outlined below.

Advantages

1. Most micro-organisms are destroyed so there is less chance of spoilage.
2. After being sterilised and stored, the food can be kept longer and more safely.

Disadvantages

1. Heating requires the following investments:
    (a) Heat-resistant storage containers (which can be difficult to obtain) such as cans or glass jars. The latter are preferred because they can be reused.
    (b) Cooking utensils, such as a steamer.
    (c) Fuel.
2. These investment costs will have to be represented in the final cost of the product.
3. This method is labour intensive.
4. It requires access to abundant clean water.
5. Preserved fruits and vegetables have a lower nutritional value and generally less taste than fresh products. However, fewer nutrients are lost using the heating method than any other preservation method.

Pasteurisation and sterilisation are two methods of heating food products to prevent them from rotting and to prepare them for storage in glass jars or tins. These methods will be explained later in this chapter, but first we will discuss the packing and preparation of vegetables.

PACKING

Even though increasing the container volume decreases the cost per kilogram of packing a product, there are two reasons to avoid using large containers. First, the entire content of the container has to be consumed within 24 hours after opening it; and second, it will take much longer before the food in the middle of the container is heated sufficiently to kill all the bacteria. Heating the product longer will increase the energy costs. If large volumes are desired, it is best to work with flat tin containers, since the distance from the nearest edge of the container to the centre is smaller and the product will therefore heat up quicker.

Of course the packing material must be clean. The more micro-organisms that come in contact with the food, the longer the heating process will have to take. The two types of containers used to preserve food with the heating method (tins and glass) are described below.

Tins

These are iron cans, which are covered with a thin layer of tin. They are especially used for sterilising, and are very suitable for sterilising larger amounts. Unfortunately, they can only be used once. There are many different types available with varying volumes and shapes (cylindrical tins are long, round and narrow, while flat tins are wide and shallow). A few common volumes are: 0.58 l/0.85 l/0.95 l/3.1 l.

Tins can also vary with respect to the presence or absence of a varnish layer on the inside. Unvarnished tins are often good enough. However, varnished tins must be used for special products, such as cherries, berries and plums, in order to maintain good colour and taste. In these and other products, tin triggers chemical reactions that change the product's colour and/or taste. Varnish thus avoids contact between the tin and the product.

Every tin comes with a lid, which can be hermetically sealed with the help of a tin sealer. Various types are available, ranging from simple hand-operated tools to new automatic machines. The seal must be properly adjusted to prevent leakage. This can be checked by closing the tin with a little water inside and immersing it in boiling water. If, after a few minutes, steam is seen to escape, the seal must be readjusted.

Tins delivered from the factory are fairly clean, and do not require extra washing. Store them upside down to keep out contaminants. If they are not clean, wash them in hot soda water (1.5 per cent), rinse with hot water and let them drip dry on a clean cloth. The lids must also be clean.

Glass

Glass bottles and jars can be used for sterilisation and pasteurisation and they are normally reusable. However, they are also breakable and they do not protect food from the negative effects of light. This problem can be alleviated by storing the filled bottles and jars in a dark place.

Glass bottles, those previously used for soft drinks or beer for example, are well suited for heating and storing fruit pulp, puree or juice. They have to be sealed with a metal screw cap. Their volume can vary from 0.2 to even 2 litres. These bottles and their screw caps can easily be reused.

It is important that the bottles or jars be completely hermetically sealed. This can be done by inserting a soft layer of rubber or other similar material between the bottle or jar and the cap or lid. Producers of glass bottles and jars often also sell accompanying rubber rings and lids or caps. The best results are achieved when the glass containers and sealing mechanisms (rings, caps and lids) are made by the same company.

The bottles or jars and their caps or lids must first be thoroughly cleaned with soda (15 gram/litre) and hot water. Allow them to soak in the hot water until the moment they are used.

PREPARATION

Before a product is heated in its storage container, it must be prepared as already explained. Specific information about the appropriate ways to prepare and preserve the various types of fruits and vegetables can be found in Appendixes 11.1, 11.2 and 11.3.

1. Pasteurisation (heating up to 100°C) for products that will be subsequently stored at temperatures below 20°C (Appendix 11.1).
2. Sterilisation at 100°C only for acidic products (Appendix 11.2).
3. Sterilisation (above 100°C) in a pressure cooker or an autoclave (large pressure cooker) (Appendix 11.3).

Each appendix consists of two tables. The first table lists the recommended preparation method for each product and the content of the fluid with which the fruit or vegetable is preserved. The second table lists the temperature at which the glass container or tin should be filled and the recommended duration of heating for various sizes of glass and tins. The food to be preserved is usually heated in a large pan and then packed while still hot, before the actual heating process even begins. This is the most efficient method, because it is faster to thoroughly heat a large amount of food in a large pan by continually stirring it than to heat smaller amounts of food in individual sealed bottles or tins. It takes much more time for the heat to penetrate to the centre of the food in the jars.

THREE TYPES OF HEATING

As mentioned above three types of heating (1, 2 and 3). Before discussing each of these in detail, we will give an example of how tins, jars and bottles should be filled. The products are first prepared as described in the appendixes. The following example demonstrates how these appendixes should be used:

> To preserve white beans in 0.85 litre tins: First peel and wash the beans and then blanch them for 3 minutes. Large beans should first be soaked in water overnight. After blanching and straining the beans, put them in the cans, which are then filled almost to the brim with boiling, salted (2 per cent) water (Appendix 11.3). Seal the cans while the content is at a temperature of at least 60°C. Place the cans in a pressure cooker and heat them for 85 minutes at a temperature of 115°C (see Appendix 11.3).

The tins or jars have to be filled up to 0.5 cm below the sealing edge. For leafy greens the fluid has to be poured into the tin or glass container first, followed by the vegetable. Make sure to eliminate as many air bubbles as possible. The sealing temperature is very important. It may never be lower than indicated in the appendix. If the temperature of the food is lower, the jars and tins must be quickly reheated in a shallow water bath until the temperature of the food in the middle of the tin is equal to or higher than the indicated temperature. Always measure the temperature in the middle of the tin. Seal quickly and apply the recommended heat treatment. Put the filled bottles or jars in the water before it boils to prevent the glass from breaking due to the sudden increase in temperature. Tins can be placed immediately in boiling water.

Important: If a sugar solution of 40 per cent has to be used, this is not 400 grams of sugar with 1000 ml (1 litre) water, but 400 grams of sugar in 600 ml water.

Pasteurisation

Pasteurisation is a mild heating treatment at temperatures up to 100°C (which is the boiling point of water at elevations up to 300 metres above sea level). This method causes only a slight decrease in taste and nutritional value. The enzymes are inactivated and most, but not all, bacteria are killed. Pasteurised products therefore spoil faster than sterilised products. To prevent the surviving spore-producing micro-organisms from multiplying, the products should be stored in temperatures below 20°C. To extend the shelf-life of fruit preserves, a lot of sugar is often added, which allows them to remain edible for months.

The more acid or sugar contained in a pasteurised product, the longer it will stay good because the remaining micro-organisms do not have a chance to develop.

A product is pasteurised by heating it for a time in a closed glass or tin container in a pan of hot water. It is important that the lid of a glass jar fit well, but it should not be twisted tightly closed, because some air should be allowed to escape while it is being heated. Close the lid tightly immediately after removing the jar from the pan. As the product cools, a vacuum will develop within the container. In this way the food has no chance of coming in contact with the air and becoming contaminated.

The water in the pan has to be warm and at least the same temperature as the filled bottles and tins. Start monitoring the heating time as soon as the water has reached the recommended temperature listed in the appendix. Remove the bottles or tins as soon as the recommended time has elapsed and allow them to cool.

Remember that the boiling point of water decreases as elevation increases. In areas up to 300 metres above sea level the boiling point is 100°C. At higher elevations the heating time will have to be increased as indicated in the following table in order to compensate for the lower boiling temperatures (Table 11.1).

Table 11.1. Heating time at different altitudes.

Altitude in metres	Heating time in minutes	Example
0–300	a	$a = 10$ minutes
300–600	$a + 1/5\ a$	Total 12 minutes
600–900	$a + 2/5\ a$	Total 14 minutes
900–1200	$a + 3/5\ a$	Total 16 minutes

Since pasteurisation sometimes requires heating at 100°C and the food can be kept for only a limited time, it is better not to pasteurise food (as described in Appendix 11.1) at elevations higher than 300 m, but rather to sterilise it (possibly under pressure) as explained in Appendix 11.3. Products that have to be heated at temperatures below 100°C can be made at higher elevations, as long as the required temperature can be achieved.

Fruit juices, which are not listed in the appendixes, have to be pasteurised at temperatures between 60° and 95°C. More information on fruit juices can be found. Always cook the preserved vegetables for 15 minutes before eating them. Never eat spoilt food and never eat from jars that have opened during storage.

Sterilisation in a Bath of Boiling Water

Sterilisation in a boiling water bath is performed at 100°C. This process will kill all the micro-organisms present, but not the spores they produced. Under the right conditions, these spores can grow into spoilage-causing bacteria. Since the spores do not grow well in acidic conditions, acid is often added to the preserved food. Sugar has the same preventative effect. Thus by adding sugar or acid, you can ensure that even after heating at just 100°C the preserved product can be considered to be sterilised: its shelf-life is much longer than a product heated at 100°C to which no extra acid or sugar has been added. Appendix 11.2 provides the information you will need to sufficiently sterilise various types of fruits and vegetables.

Sterilisation with a Pressure Cooker or Autoclave

Sterilisation carried out properly in an autoclave or pressure cooker will kill not only the micro-organisms but also the spores. In this way a long shelf-life can be achieved without adding extra acid or sugar. In an autoclave or pressure cooker the boiling point of water is at a temperature higher than 100°C. If the atmospheric pressure (at sea level) is increased by 0.7 bar, then the water in this pan will boil at 115°C; if the pressure is increased by 1 bar the boiling point becomes 121°C. Here too, the boiling temperature is lower the higher above sea level you are. This decrease can be compensated by increasing the pressure by 0.1 bar for every 1000 metres above sea level. To sterilise canned vegetables the temperature is allowed to reach 115°–121°C. In general, all foods with a high pH (which includes most vegetables) have to be preserved at a temperature above 100°C. We recommend that a pressure cooker be purchased for this purpose. Appendix 11.4 provides temperature and time combinations needed to sterilise foods in a pressure cooker or autoclave. The following instructions generally apply when sterilising foods:

1. Place a rack on the bottom of the pan to ensure that the jars/bottles/tins do not come in too close contact with the heat source.
2. Remember not to place the filled glass jars or bottles directly in boiling water, because they will most likely break. Heat the water in the pan up to about the same temperature as the filled jars or bottles, and then place them in the water.
3. Do not screw the lids on too tightly, to ensure that some air will be able to escape.
4. Do not pack the jars or bottles too tightly in the pan. Leave some space between them and between the jars/bottles and the sides of the pan.
5. The jars or bottles should be covered by at least 5 cm of water.
6. The sterilisation time begins at the moment the water reaches the desired temperature.
7. For optimal results use jars of the same size and volume.
8. Never try to open the autoclave or pressure cooker while the water is boiling. The high pressure in the pan and the high temperature of the water make this very dangerous.

Remember the following points when sterilising under high pressure using tins or glass.

Tins

After the processing, let the steam escape from the pan slowly. This can be done quicker with small tins than with bigger ones, but still should be done slowly and carefully, as the tins can deform or even burst. When the pressure is again normal the lid of the pan can be opened. Remove the tins and immerse them in cold water, which should be refreshed occasionally to keep it cold. When the tins are cool dry them.

Glass jars

Wait until the pressure cooker cools down and the pressure inside of it has gone down before opening the lid. Remove the jars and tighten the lids immediately. The disadvantage of glass jars is that they cannot be cooled quickly. The safest way to cool them is to set them in the open air until they are lukewarm, and then put them in cold water. The advantage of an autoclave over a pressure cooker is that it can be cooled down faster. On the other hand, an autoclave requires more water and thus more energy to heat.

STORAGE AND CONSUMPTION

Always store the preserved food in a cool place, at a temperature preferably below 20°C. Keep glass bottles and jars out of the light. Label the containers so that you know what they contain and the date they were preserved. Always consume the older products first. The storage area has to be dry and have a consistent temperature. Moisture will make tins rust. Pay close attention when opening preserved food. A bulging lid or tin indicates gas formation by bacteria and thus food spoilage. Look carefully at the food and smell it. Heat the food if necessary and never eat anything you suspect may be spoilt.

Remember that preserving vegetables and fruit is always a risky undertaking. Always follow the rules described in this booklet and keep in mind that the heating times given in the appendixes represent the minimum time that is required. Never heat products for a shorter time than indicated. Heating food for a longer time decreases the chance of spoilage, but it also decreases the food's taste and nutritional value.

DRYING

Drying is one of the oldest preservation methods. The moisture level of agricultural products is decreased to 10–15 per cent so that the micro-organisms present cannot thrive and the enzymes become inactive. Further dehydration is usually not desired, because the products then often become brittle. To ensure that the products do not spoil after being dried, they have to be stored in a moisture-free environment.

Drying is generally not difficult. Since the products lose water, they also become much lighter and thus easier to transport. Two disadvantages, however, are that the products also lose vitamins, and they change in appearance. The most common drying method is exposure to air. Air can absorb water; and the warmer the air is, the more it will absorb. For optimal results, the air should be hot, dry and in motion. In a closed environment, the air has to be refreshed regularly because it will otherwise become saturated with the moisture it absorbs from the products. Good ventilation is therefore essential. For drying, the relative humidity (RH) of the air should be less than 65 per cent. If the RH is higher than 65 per cent the fruits and vegetables will eventually dry out, but not in the right way. When the sun is shining, the RH is usually lower than 65 per cent, but when it is cloudy and definitely when it is raining the humidity is usually higher. Sunshine is therefore extremely important! For this reason, it is not possible to dry products in this way in every season of the year.

Before drying, the vegetables and fruits have to be thoroughly washed and cut into pieces if necessary. Sometimes extra preparation is needed to retain the product's colour and to minimise nutrient loss.

The various preparation methods are described already in this chapter, and a list of methods required for drying each agricultural product is given in Appendix 11.4. The final quality of the dried product is determined by a large number of factors, which can be divided into four groups:

1. Quality of the product to be dried.
2. The preparation of the product.
3. The drying method used.
4. The packing and storage conditions.

These four points are discussed in the following sections, followed by examples of drying potatoes, tomatoes and mango.

Quality of the Fresh Product

The fruits and vegetables to be dried should be of good quality. Fruit that is rotten or damaged in any way should be separated from the good fruit. To prevent the product from losing its quality, the time between harvesting and drying should be as short as possible. Of course it is possible to wait longer before drying hard fruits and root vegetables than before drying soft fruit and leafy vegetables. The time normally allowed between harvesting and consumption can also be seen as the maximum time allowable between harvesting and drying.

Preparation

Before describing the various preparation methods used specifically for drying, we would like to remind the reader that the hygiene rules described already in this chapter must also be followed when drying food.

Washing and cutting

Wash the fruits and vegetables thoroughly. Remove sand, rotten spots and seeds. Peeled and cut fruit dries quicker. It is important that all of the pieces are about the same size, so that they will dry at the same rate. Tubers and roots should be cut into slices that are 3–6 mm long or pieces that are 4–8 mm thick. Leafy vegetables such as cabbage should be cut into pieces that are 3–6 mm thick.

Lye dip and blanching

Already discussed in this chapter.

Osmotic drying

Some fruits can be prepared by immersing them for some time in a strong sugar solution. In fact this is not just a preparation, but already the start of the drying process because the sugar extracts water from the fruit. The fruit also adsorbs part of the sugar and is therefore allowed to retain more water at the end of drying process, which makes the product softer than if it were dried only in the air. Normally sugar solutions of 40–60 per cent are used. Good results are obtained by dipping the product for 18 hours in a 40 per cent sugar solution. To make such drying profitable it is necessary to have a good use for the diluted sugar solutions, such as the production of jams or syrups.

Preservatives

Fruit is sometimes treated with the smoke from burning sulphur or dipped in a sulphite or bisulphite-salt solution to prevent browning. Taste and vitamin C content are also better preserved with these treatments. The residual sulphite in the product can, however, be dangerous in high concentrations and can also affect the taste. As this method needs more specific information we cannot discuss it here in detail.

DRYING METHODS

Drying in the open air is called natural drying. We speak of artificial drying when the air is first heated to decrease the relative humidity to a desired level. Both methods are described below.

Natural Drying

Drying in the open air is a simple and inexpensive process. It does not require any costly energy, just sunlight and wind. The product to be dried is placed in thin layers on trays (Fig. 11.2) or black plastic and exposed to direct sunlight. The trays are usually made of wood, and lined with plastic or galvanised nets. The trays should be placed 1 metre above the ground on stands set on a flat surface. This way no dirt can come in contact with the food from below and the food can receive maximum sun exposure. If necessary, the trays can be covered to protect the food from rain, dust, birds, insects and other pests. Mosquito netting probably offers the best protection from pests. To ensure that the fruits or vegetables dry uniformly, it is best to turn them regularly or at least to shake the trays. This does not apply to tomatoes, peaches or apricots, which are cut in half and arranged in a single layer on the trays.

Fruit dries very well in the sun, but some products are damaged by exposure to direct sunlight and are therefore dried preferably in a hung up under some type of shelter. Of course, drying these products takes more time.

In areas with a high chance of rain, it is advisable to have an artificial dryer that can be used when it is raining or when the RH is too high. This will prevent interruption in the drying process and thus also a loss of food quality. In the event of rain, the (moveable) trays should be covered with plastic or placed under a shelter. Afterwards, they should be returned as soon as possible to the drying spot. It takes about two to four days to dry tropical vegetables.

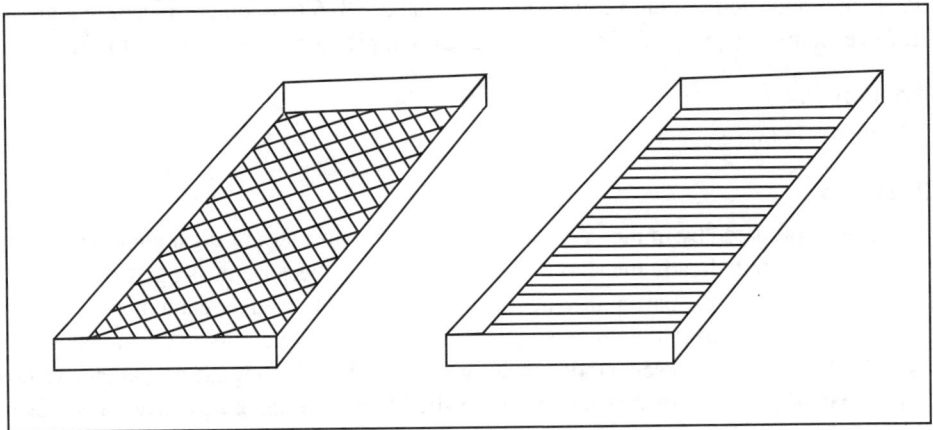

Fig. 11.2. Drying tray.

Artificial Drying

The temperature of outside air often needs to be increased only by a few degrees to make drying possible. For example, during a rain shower at 30°C the air must be heated to at least 37°C to be able to dry fruits or vegetables. Heating it further increases the speed at which the product will be dried because:

1. The air can absorb more water.
2. The product releases water faster at higher temperatures.

The air can be heated with solar energy or by burning natural or fossil fuels. Appendix 11.4 gives information about preparation, drying conditions and maximum temperatures for several types of vegetables and fruit.

The maximum drying temperature is important because above this temperature the quality of the dried product decreases quickly. Another reason for not drying at very high temperatures is that the product then dries quickly on the outside, but remains moist on the inside. Different types of artificial drying will be discussed below.

Improved sun drying

Products dry quicker when the trays are placed in a structure that allows the sunlight to enter through a glass cover, thereby trapping the warmth. This raises the temperature to 60°–75°C. Overheating can be avoided by regulating the ventilation (Fig. 11.3).

Without ventilation the temperature can reach 90°–100°C, especially towards the end of the drying process. The ventilation must be good enough to prevent condensation on the glass. This is a direct drying method.

It is also possible to heat the air in special boxes before leading it to the product (Fig. 11.4). This method is called indirect drying, because there is no direct solar radiation on the product. These techniques will speed up the sun drying in dry areas (beware of overheating), resulting in a better product.

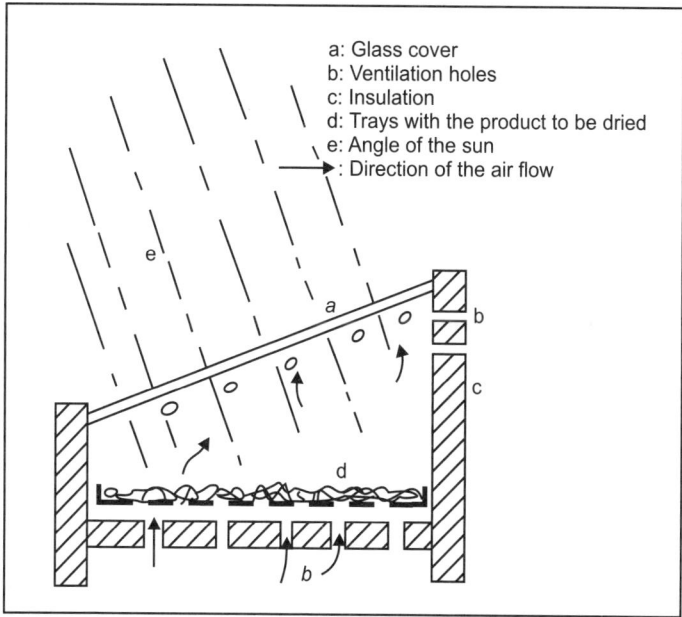

Fig. 11.3. Improved indirect sun dryer.

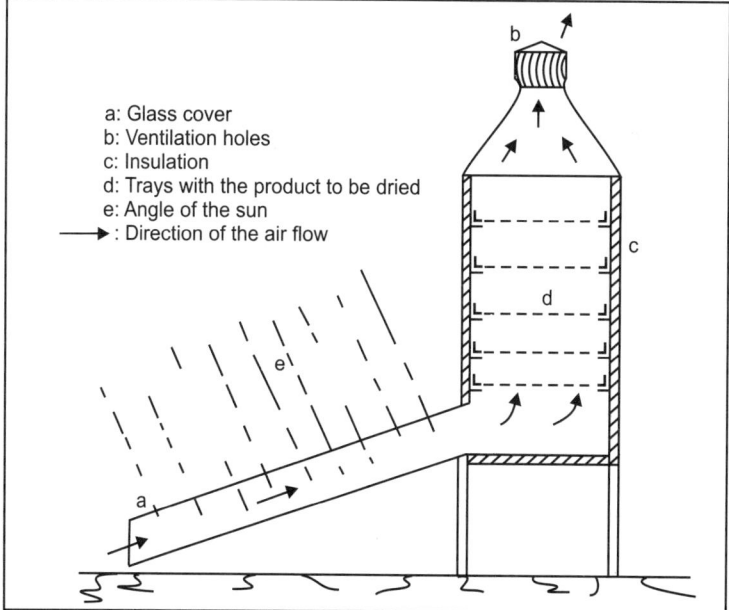

Fig. 11.4. Improved direct sun dryer.

These techniques also make drying possible in areas with high humidity, as the relative moisture decreases with a higher temperature, as explained earlier in this chapter. An extra advantage of this technique is that the product is protected from rain.

Heating with fuel

In wet climates, or when large quantities (over 100 kg/day) have to be processed, one should consider heating the air, if fuel is available. Vegetables dry better with this method than in the sun, and the colour, odour and taste of the end products are better. Two methods will be briefly described to give an idea of the technique.

Bush dryer

A fire in an oven made from oil drums heats the surrounding air. The heated air rises through a thin layer of the product that is to be dried on the racks. The fire must be watched at all times, and the product has to be shaken or stirred at regular intervals.

Specifications of the bush dryer:

Capacity	0.1 to 1 ton/day (24 hours).
Material	Oil drums, galvanised iron sheets, netting, wire, wood, nails, one sack portland cement, sand, stones.
Costs	Building costs, material costs, high fuel costs and attendance.
Construction	Accurate work is required.

Air dryers with artificial ventilation

A motor-powered ventilator can be used to blow warm air from the motor (or air warmed by a burner) through the product.

When is the Drying Process Finished?

To test whether a product is sufficiently dry, it first has to be cool. A warm product is softer and seems to contain more water. Fruit may contain 12–14 per cent water; vegetables should be dryer, containing 4-8 per cent water depending on the type, since vegetables contain less sugar. The moisture content is difficult to measure without a drying oven or moisture content meter. As rules of thumb use the following:

Fruit:
1. It should not be possible to squeeze juice out.
2. The fruit must not be so dry that it rattles when the drying trays are emptied.
3. It should be possible to knead a handful of fruit pieces, but they should not stick to each other.

Vegetables: Dried greens should be brittle and can be easily rubbed into a powder.

Packing and Storage

At the end of the drying period all foreign material (stems, etc.) should be removed, as well as pieces that are not yet dry enough. Dried vegetables can easily absorb water from the surrounding air because of their low water content, so packing has to take place in a dry room. It is a good idea to finish drying during the warmest part of the day when the relative humidity is at its lowest. The product can be cooled in the shade and if the work has been done hygienically, the cooled products can be packed immediately. The packing material must be waterproof, airtight and insect-proof.

The dried products will only remain good if stored in such a way that they are dry and protected from insects. Normal plastic bags (properly sealed) will do for some time, but are not entirely gas and waterproof. It is also possible to use polymer-coated cellophane bags, which are water and airtight. These can be closed with a hot iron or a sealing machine (where electricity is available). Unfortunately, this kind of plastic is not as easily obtained, and it is not too strong.

A plastic bag of a thicker quality (polyethylene, 0.05 mm thick) is the best. These can be closed tightly with a metal clip or with cellophane tape, although the quality of the closure also depends on the force with which the bag is closed and on the flexibility of the material. The plastic bags still have to be stored in a cool place and must be protected against rats and mice. It is, therefore, better to put a number of small bags in bigger jars or tins, which can be closed tightly as well. Small bags are useful, as the products will not absorb water despite regular opening of the tin. Each bag can best be filled with a quantity sufficient for one family meal.

Gourds can also serve as a packing/storage material. They must be closed well and smeared with linseed oil, varnish or other sealing material. Ground products absorb water quicker, so it is wise to grind them just before use, rather than storing the products in ground form. Properly dried and packed vegetables can be stored for about one year. After that, the quality can decrease quickly. Cool storage (e.g. in a cellar) makes longer storage possible.

Consuming Dried Products

Soak the product in a small amount of water in a pan. Fruit should be soaked for 8–12 hours; the ratio of dried fruit to water is 2:3. Vegetables need only be soaked for half an hour; the ration of dried vegetables to water is 2:2.5–4.5. Products in powder form do not need to be soaked before they are consumed. After soaking, the product should be cooked for 10 to 15 minutes. Some types of fruit have a shorter cooking time than this, while others require even more time.

Three Examples

Drying potatoes

Choose potatoes that are firm and undamaged. Peel the potatoes, wash them under the faucet or in a container with clean water, and cut them in slices about 3 mm thick. Immerse the slices in boiling water, let them cook for 3–5 minutes, rinse them off with clean water, dry them with a clean cloth and place them on a piece of black plastic or on trays to dry for 2 to 3 days in the sun. Turn them regularly, about 2 to 3 times per day. The drying process is finished when the potatoes are hard and crumble easily when squeezed in your hand. The dried potatoes have to be soaked in water before they can be consumed.

Drying tomatoes

Use firm, not too ripe, undamaged tomatoes. Wash and then cut them in half or in quarters (or in smaller pieces), and remove the seeds. Blanch the tomato pieces for one minute at 90°C and then allow them to cool off quickly under cold, running water. Once cooled, they have to be immersed for 10 minutes in water to which lemon juice has been added. Strain and then dry them with a clean cloth. Place the tomatoes on a piece of black plastic and let them dry in the sun. To make sure that they dry evenly, turn them 2 to 3 times per day. Place them under a shelter in the evenings. After 2 to 3 days they will feel brittle, and the drying process will have been completed.

Drying mangos

Use firm, harvest-ripe mangos. The varieties Ameli and Kent are particularly good for drying. Wash and peel the mangos and then cut them in pieces about 6–8 mm thick. You can then choose to either blanch them in water at 56°C with two tablespoons of lemon juice added per litre of water or immerse them in a 40 per cent sugar solution for 18 hours, with the same amount of lemon juice added. In both cases, add 3 grams of sodium bisulphate ($Na_2S_2O_3$) per litre of water to prevent the fruit from discolouring and to protect it from moulds and insects. After this preparation, the pieces of fruit should be briefly rinsed with hot water to keep them from sticking together. Finally, place the mango pieces to dry on trays, preferably made of plastic mesh (metal trays cause food products, especially fruit, to discolour quickly) and coated with glycerine to prevent sticking.

PRESERVING VEGETABLES WITH SALT AND/OR VINEGAR

Adding salt is one of the oldest ways to preserve food, except fruit, especially in areas that have easy access to inexpensive salt. Since salt absorbs much of the water in food, it makes it difficult for micro-organisms to survive. There are two salting methods. One uses a lot of salt, and the other only a small amount. The disadvantage of using a lot of salt is that it has a very negative impact on the taste of the food. To overcome this problem, the food can be rinsed or soaked in water before it is eaten, but this also decreases the nutritional value of the food. It is, therefore, advisable to use a lot of salt only when there is a surplus of fresh vegetables and no other preservation method is possible. The use of a small amount of salt is in itself not enough to prevent the growth of bacteria, but it does result in the development of a certain kind of acid-producing bacteria that limits the growth of other bacteria. One example of a product made in this way is sauerkraut, which has a high nutritional value. Another way to preserve vegetables is by adding vinegar.

Preserving with Salt

This section describes the two salting methods and the equipment that is needed. In both cases, the vegetables have to be hygienically prepared. Detailed information can be found in Appendix 11.5, which lists the method recommended and the amounts of salt needed per type of vegetable.

Preserving with a large amount of salt

Heavy salting means that approximately 1 part salt is used for 5 parts of vegetables. This gives the vegetables a very salty taste, which makes it necessary for the vegetables to be soaked in water a few times before they can be eaten. The salt can be added as dried granules or as brine (a salt-water solution in various concentrations).

Sometimes a little bit of vinegar also has to be added. Heavy salting is a simple preservation method, and much less labour intensive than preserving with a small amount of salt.

Heavy salting (20–25 per cent)

Mix the vegetables and the salt well, using 250 g of salt per kg of vegetables. Fill crocks with the mixture of vegetables and salt, cover with muslin cloth, a pressure plate and a weight. Add brine (250 g of salt per litre of water) until the pressure plate is just submerged.

After about two weeks the salted product must be repacked into smaller jars. These jars should only be big enough to contain enough for one meal, as contamination can occur quickly in an opened jar. Pour the remaining liquid from the crocks over the salted product in the smaller jars, until the vegetables are completely covered. Seal the jars tightly and then store them at as cool a temperature as possible.

Before using, the vegetables normally have to be soaked in freshwater for half a day (1 kg vegetables in 10 litres of water). However, the vegetables lose nutrients during soaking, and this should therefore be avoided where possible, for example, when the vegetables are to be used in soup. Always cook the vegetables before use.

Heavy brine (20 per cent)

Fill the crocks or jars with the prepared vegetables (to which no salt has yet been added). Pour the brine (in this case 200 g salt + 65 ml vinegar per litre water) over the vegetables until the pressure plate is just submerged. The required quantity of brine is about half of the volume of the vegetables. To maintain the proper salt concentration sprinkle 200 g of salt per kg of vegetables over the pressure plate. Store the crocks at 21°–25°C and make sure that the vegetables remain under the brine. Add fresh brine (200 g salt + 65 ml vinegar per litre water) when necessary. The vegetables have to be packed into smaller jars after about two weeks. Shell peas and brown beans if this has not been done yet. After repacking the vegetables add the old brine plus fresh brine where necessary so that the vegetables are submerged. Close the jars tightly. Before use, soak the vegetables as described above.

Use of small amounts of salt

Enough salt is added to the vegetables to create appropriate conditions for the growth of micro-organisms that form acids, which will in turn preserve the vegetables. The acid gives the product a special taste that is often appreciated. Add 1 part salt to 20 parts of vegetables as dry salt or as light brine. When vinegar is also added to this light brine less salt is needed. The brine method is easier than the dry salt method, as brine gives an even distribution of salt and vegetables. This even distribution is a necessary condition for success. With the dry salt method, the product will shrink as liquid leaves the product. However, the colour, odour and taste are better when preserved with salt than with brine.

The preparation for salted or pickled vegetables is the same as for fresh vegetables, although longer cooking times are sometimes necessary. A description of the equipment needed for salting and the special product data, followed by exact instructions, are given in this section.

Light salting (2.5–5 per cent)

One product made according to this method is sauerkraut. Mix the prepared vegetables with salt (25 g salt per kg vegetables; for green beans 50 g salt + 50 ml vinegar per kg). Fill the crocks with the vegetables and salt mixture, packing tightly. Cover the vegetables with several layers of muslin cloth, the pressure plate and the weight. The salt draws the liquid from the vegetables, which should gradually become covered with brine. If this does not happen within a few hours, add light brine (25 g salt per litre of water). Brine for green beans should be made from 50 g salt plus 50 ml vinegar per litre of water. Store the crocks at 20°–25°C. The vegetables will undergo an acid fermentation lasting 2–3 weeks. Skim the froth regularly from the surface of the vegetables, using the following method.

A white layer of froth will appear on the vegetables after a few days when fermenting with the light brine and light salting methods (sometimes with other methods as well). This is caused by the growth of undesirable micro-organisms. If this froth is left undisturbed it will use up the acid from the fermentation process and can cause an unpleasant smell and taste in the vegetables.

The froth is best removed by first removing the weight and pressure plate and carefully lifting the muslin cloth, keeping the froth on the cloth. Rinse this, together with the pressure plate and weight. This treatment should be carried out every other day, especially when the froth is produced in large quantities.

If the vegetables are to be kept longer than 2–3 weeks, they have to be repacked into smaller containers after fermentation. Vegetables fermented in small jars do not need repacking. The fermented product is packed tightly into glass jars of 0.5–1 litre with a screw cap. Pour brine over the product until it is covered, using the old brine plus, where necessary, fresh brine made from 25 g salt plus 50 ml vinegar per litre of water. Close the jars, but make sure that air can escape by twisting the lid closed and then giving it a quarter turn (back the turn back should be less than one quarter). Heat the jars in a boiling water bath for 25 minutes (for 0.5 litre jars) or 30 minutes (for 1 litre jars). The jars should be tightly closed immediately after heating. This process will pasteurise the contents and stop fermentation.

Light brine (5 per cent)

Fill jars or crocks with the prepared vegetables and cover with the muslin cloth, the pressure plate and the weight. Add brine (50 g salt + 50 ml vinegar per litre of water) until the pressure plate is just submerged. You will need about half of the volume of the vegetables in brine. Keep the jars or crocks in a cool place (+/–15°C). An acid fermentation will take place during the next 2–3 weeks. Remove the froth regularly (as described above). After the fermentation, it is best to repack the vegetables from the crocks into smaller jars with twist lids. Pack the glass jars tightly and add brine until the vegetables are submerged. Where necessary fresh brine can be made using 50 g salt + 50 ml vinegar per litre of water. Close the jars so that air can escape by closing the twist lid and giving it a quarter turn back. Pasteurise the contents by heating the jars in a boiling water bath (25 minutes for 0.5 l jars and 30 minutes for 1 litre jars). Close the jars tightly immediately after heating. The vegetables need only be drained and rinsed before use.

Requirements for Salting

1. Salt: This should be finely granulated and without a drying agent. Disinfect salt that is not pre-packed or that is locally extracted by sprinkling the salt on a metal sheet and heating this over a hot fire.
2. Vinegar: Use white or cider vinegar with a 4–5 per cent concentration.
3. Jars and crocks or other vessels: These can be made of wood, plastic, ceramic, glass or stainless steel. Barrels made from pinewood should be avoided as they can change the taste of the vegetables. The jars must be very clean. Wash them in hot soda water and rinse with clean hot water.
4. Muslin cloth: This is laid over the vegetables and under the pressure plate. The cloth is used to remove the froth from the surface of the vegetables.
5. Pressure plate: This is a plate or grid of wood, ceramic, glass, stainless steel or plastic. A weight is put on top of this to keep the vegetables under the surface of the liquid. The pressure plate should be slightly smaller than the diameter of the vessel. A pressure plate that catches under the neck can be used with certain jars, in which case a weight is not needed.
6. Weight: This is put on the pressure plate to keep the vegetables under the level of the liquid. The weight can be a clean stone or a waterfilled glass jar.
7. Scales and/or measuring cup: These are needed to weigh or measure correct amounts of vegetables, salt and vinegar.
8. Knives: Stainless steel knives are needed to cut the vegetables.

Warning

Peas, beans, sweet corn and greens preserved with salt always have to be cooked for at least 10 minutes before use. Do not eat (even for tasting) preserved vegetables that have not yet been cooked. It is important that the vegetables are always kept submerged below the level of the liquid.

Preserving in Vinegar

Pickling in vinegar or acetic acid can also preserve food. This method of preserving can be done with vegetables (cabbage, beets, onions, cucumber) and fruits (lemons, olives). To obtain a product that can be stored, the food first has to be salted and heated before being put into vinegar. An example of a vinegar-preserved food is Atjar Tjampoer.

When ordinary vinegar is used (5 per cent acetic acid in water), it has to be heated in a closed pan. The utensils should be made of enamel or stainless steel, because the high acid concentration of the vinegar corrodes other materials. The vinegar should have a minimum concentration of 4 per cent. (The pH has to be lower than 3.5; this can be checked with pH papers.) The following vinegars can be used: white or cider vinegar (5 per cent acetic acid) or pickling vinegar (concentrations vary up to 100 per cent acetic acid).

Vinegar can be homemade by fermenting fruit juice with water and sugar. A kind of wine is produced first, which subsequently turns into vinegar when it comes in contact with the oxygen in the air. Experiment to find the best way to make wine and vinegar using local ingredients.

The following method is generally used: The prepared fruits or vegetables are put into cold heavy brine (200 g of salt per litre of water) for several hours, depending upon the size and shape of the product. Next they are put into a boiling salt solution, boiled, and cooled to 70°–80°C. At this temperature the product (with herbs and spices if necessary, but without the brine) is transferred to jars. The jars are filled to 1.5 cm under the rim and the product is covered with warm vinegar so that all pieces are covered by at least 1 cm of the liquid. The jars are thus filled to 0.5 cm under the rim. The vinegar used must have a final concentration of about 5 per cent after dilution. Always use clean glass jars. Close the jars as quickly as possible and cool quickly in a cool, airy place. Store the products at as cool a temperature as possible.

Gherkins are sometimes fermented first (lactic acid fermentation) by storing them for some time in a salt-vinegar solution in crocks, after which they are packed into jars. If you have no previous experience with this process, caution is advised.

JAM AND JUICE MAKING, SYRUPS, JELLIES AND CANDIED FRUIT

There are several possible methods of preserving fruit. Canning, sterilising and drying have already been dealt with in the preceding chapters. This section discusses the possibilities of making juice, jams, jellies and candied fruit. This can be done with all kinds of fruit. A mixture of two or more kinds of fruit often gives a better, more rounded taste in the final product. Apricots and peaches combine very well with orange or grapefruit juice. Orange and grapefruit juices can also be mixed. Pineapple is often mixed with orange, grapefruit, or apricot juice. The juices are best mixed before preserving, not just before use. Choose the proportion of the fruit in the mixtures according to your individual taste. The proportions have no effect on the shelf-life of the product. The methods described in this section are based on preserving with sugar or heat or a combination of these two.

It is best to start with fresh, undamaged fruit that is not overripe. Mouldy fruit increases the chance of spoilage and of causing food poisoning. Overripe fruit results in a tasteless or sometimes slightly musty-tasting product. All materials with which the fruit comes into contact, such as knives, pots, kettles, cans, pans and bottles, should be made of stainless steel, glass, undamaged enamel or good-quality plastic. Avoid using aluminium or galvanised tools and kettles, as the acid in the fruit will attack these. The acid can dissolve the aluminium and the zinc layer of the galvanised materials, resulting in a metallic taste and possible zinc poisoning.

This section first describes drink preparation, followed by methods for the preparation of other fruit products such as jelly, candied fruit, jam and chutney.

Making Fruit Juices

This section gives an overview of fruit juice preparation, followed by a description of different types of packing, bottling methods and storage of the bottled product. Examples are also given of the preservation of tomato juice and the preparation of fruit juice concentrates.

Juice extraction

Preserved fruit juices keep their fresh taste and attractive colour as long as they are not heated for too long or at too high a temperature. Prolonged boiling or heating changes the taste, except with tomato and apricot juice.

Appendix 11.6 lists methods for the preparation and juice extraction of several types of fruit. Be sure not to heat the juice any longer than is indicated.

The extraction of fruit juice can be done in three ways. It is important to work as quickly as possible and to expose the juice as little as possible to the open air. Heating the fruit aids juice extraction and gives the juice a deeper colour. Heating also inactivates the enzymes and increases the shelf-life of the juice. The Table 11.2 shows which fruits should or should not be heated before extraction.

Table 11.2. Heating or not heating before extraction.

Heat before extraction		Do not heat before extraction
Apricots	Rhubarb	Apples
Berries	Tomatoes	Morello (sour) cherries
Red cherries	Plums	Green grapes
Peaches	Purple grapes	Citrus fruit
	Mango	

Method 1

Clean the fruit and cut it into pieces. Heat the fruit with very little water until sufficient liquid has been extracted. Turn the mass onto a wet muslin cloth, put this into a sieve, and let the juice drip without with squeezing, but this will make the juice cloudy.

Method 2

This extraction method requires a fruit press or a fruit mill. Figure 11.5 shows a popular basket press. This method gives cloudy juice. The juice can be cleared by heating it to 60°C and then straining it through a cloth (use a clean, washed, finely woven cloth such as muslin or several layers of cheese cloth). The advantage of this juice is that it retains the smell and nutritional value of the fresh fruit, because the juice is extracted without boiling.

Method 3

Steaming fruit is a labour-intensive method that produces a lot of clear juice. Wash and cut fruit into pieces (remove pits if necessary). Put the fruit into a juice steamer. Bring the water in the kettle to a boil and allow the steam to build up. The steam and the heat extract the juice from the fruit; the juice drips through the cloth and is collected in a small pan. For soft fruit this method takes about one hour, for hard fruit about 1½ hours.

The material needed for a juice steamer is:
1. A kettle or pan with a lid without holes.

2. A plate or grate which is laid on the bottom of the pan; a small enamelled pan or bowl or a dish of glazed pottery, which is put on the plate or grate to catch the juice (glazed pottery can sometimes contain a lead compound that can cause lead poisoning; be sure to inquire before using).
3. Two boiled white (preferably muslin) cloths, one of coarse weave and one of fine weave, that serve as juice filters and are pulled over the edge of the kettle or pan.
4. A piece of strong parchment paper (grease-proof paper) to be put over the fruit on the cloth to catch the condensation.

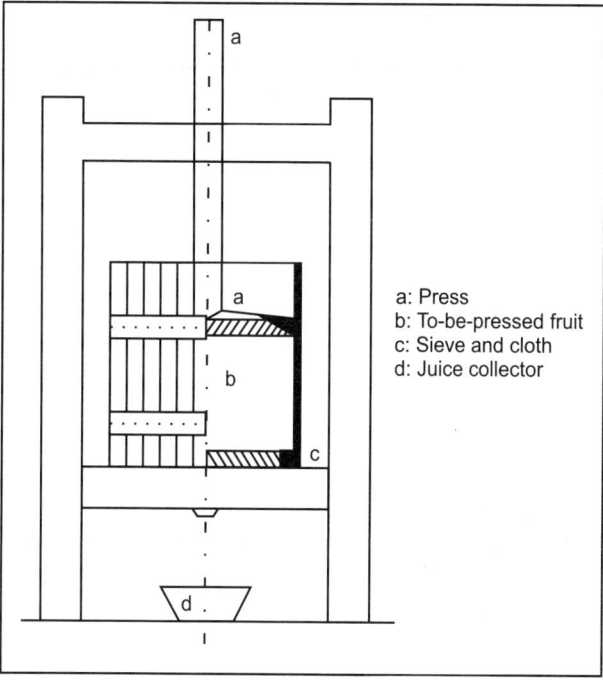

a: Press
b: To-be-pressed fruit
c: Sieve and cloth
d: Juice collector

Fig. 11.5. Fruit press.

Fruit can be processed using any of the three methods, but as mentioned above, apples, sour cherries (morellos), green grapes and citrus fruit are best squeezed without heating (method 2). The fruit pulp left over after extraction can be used as a spread on bread, with sugar added if necessary, or as a base for fruit yoghurt. Before bottling the extracted juices, one can add sugar and/or acid to them. Mixing sweet with sour juices is a good idea because it makes it unnecessary to add expensive sugar.

Materials

Jars and bottles of 0.5–1 litre are best. Bottles bigger than 1 litre are less suitable, as they need a longer heating time. One-litre bottles are of course cheaper and easier to use than 0.5 litre bottles, as they hold twice as much juice. Clean jars or bottles with soda, sterilise (boil), and keep in hot water (95°–100°C) until ready for filling.

Jars: Follow the manufacturer's instructions for heating the jars, lids and rubber sealing rings. If no instructions are available, heat the jars and lids in hot water just before use.

Bottles: Use bottles that can be closed with metal tops. Always use clean tops that have never been used. Tops with a plastic layer on the inside are the best. Bottle tops with a cork layer inside can infect the product, while those with metal foil on the inside can give a metallic taste and cause food poisoning.

Bottle top sealers are available. Make sure that the bottle sealer is properly adjusted, in accordance with the manufacturer's instructions.

Sulphured bottles: Bottling in sulphured bottles is a special preserving method. A burning piece of sulphur ribbon is put into the washed bottle and the cork is put into place. When the bottle is full of sulphur vapour the ribbon is removed and doused in a bowl of water. The bottle is closed with the top and is held upside down for 10 minutes to disinfect the cork. The vapour is let out of the bottle, which is then quickly filled.

Bottling fruit juices

Sour fruit juices can be kept in cleaned and sulphured or sterilised bottles. Other juices can also be kept this way, but the chance of spoilage is greater. It is better to always pasteurise or sterilise in those cases. The juice can be pasteurised or sterilised in two ways. Either the juice is pasteurised first and then poured into the bottles or the bottles are filled first and then pasteurised. Both methods are described below. The second method is preferable.

Method 1: Pasteurising before packing

The juice is heated in a pan and brought to boiling point, while being stirred constantly. Juice preserved in this way will have a mildly boiled taste. Better results can be achieved by placing the pan with the juice inside a larger pan containing boiling water. Stir gently but thoroughly and heat to 88°C. Remove the pan from the fire and fill the bottles or jars. Tomato juice cannot be treated in this way because of its low acid concentration. It must be boiled and sterilised. When the juice is ready for pouring, remove the bottles or jars from the hot water or reopen sulphured bottles. Fill all bottles or jars immediately to the brim with the hot juice. Remove any froth and add extra juice to fill the bottles again to the top. Keep the juice at the proper temperature (hold above a fire or in a hot water bath). If the temperature of the juice falls below 85°C, the juice must be reheated to 85°C. Put the tops on the bottles and invert them immediately for 5 minutes. Close the lids on the jars tightly and invert them for 3 minutes. Do not place the bottles or jars on a cold surface. Cool the vessels after turning.

Method 2: Packing before pasteurising

Remove the bottles from the hot water bath, drain quickly and fill immediately to 2 cm under the rim. When using jars the neck of the jar must be cleaned well, removing any spills, before the sealing ring and lid are placed on the jar. Ordinary bottles are sealed loosely with sterilised (boiled) corks, which are secured with string or with a damp piece of cellophane with a hole in the centre, again secured with string.

Fill a kettle or pan with water until it reaches the level of the juice in the bottle or jars. Bring the water to the boil (for sterilising) or to 75°C (for pasteurising) and heat the bottles for 20 minutes. After this, take the bottles out of the kettle, press the corks securely into the bottles or place a second piece of damp cellophane (without a hole) over the cellophane squares. Cover the bottles with a cloth and let cool to hand temperature (+/–60°C). Cooling of jars and bottles (for both methods 1 and 2). When the bottles or jars are still hot to the touch, they can be placed into a big crock or pail with lukewarm water. After a few minutes, drain 1/3 of the water from the crock or pail and replace it with cold water. Repeat this once or twice. To remove the last of the heat, put the jars or bottles into cold running water for 5 minutes. Take care not to aim the flow directly at the bottles.

Storage of the bottles and jars

Wipe the bottles dry and put them into a dark, cool and dry place. The lower the storage temperature is, the longer the shelf-life will be.

Hygienically prepared juices will not spoil quickly, even if they are stored in warmer places. However, they will slowly lose taste and vitamins, and their colour will change. At higher temperatures, for example 20°C and above, the loss will be faster than at lower temperatures. Check the bottles regularly for fungus and remove any bottles that show signs of spoilage. Never use the contents of these bottles.

Preservation of tomato juice

Tomato juice is preserved by sterilising it in a boiling water bath. Boil the pieces of tomato and press the pulp through a fine colander or sieve to remove the seeds and to soften the mass. Add, to taste, a teaspoon of salt per litre of juice or 3–5 g citric acid. The bottling is the same as with the other juices. Pour the boiling juice into the bottles and close the bottles. Place the bottles and jars into a boiling water bath and heat them for 15–20 minutes.

Preparation of fruit syrup

Where storage space is limited or bottles are hard to obtain, you can still make fruit syrups. For this method you need a lot of sugar. With most fruits, start with the juice obtained by extraction method 2. Boil the juice and add 1.5 kg of sugar per litre of juice. Dissolve the sugar while stirring. Skim the liquid (where necessary) and then allow it to cool. When using citric acid, first dissolve it in hot water and then let it cool. Mix the cooled lemon juice or citric acid with the syrup and then pour this into the bottles.

Fruits such as berries, cherries and plums should be ground down raw and forced through a sieve; oranges, grapefruit, etc. should be squeesed. Sieve the juice, and then while stirring add the lemon juice or citric acid solution to taste and 1.5 kg of sugar per litre of juice. Cover the liquid, but remember to stir it regularly until all the sugar is dissolved. This can take a day or even longer. When all the sugar is dissolved, pour the syrup into bottles and close these tightly.

Preparation of Other Fruit Products

The following sections describe the preparation of fruit jelly, candied fruit, jam and chutney.

Fruit jelly

Jelly is prepared from fruit juice and sugar. Extract the juice using method 3. Apple, grape, red currant, black currant and elderberry juice are especially good for making jelly. A general recipe is given below. Reduce the fruit juice to 2/3 of its original volume by boiling. While stirring, add 3/4 kg sugar per litre of reduced juice. Add, if desired, lemon juice or citric acid. Boil the jelly mass until a few drops, when sprinkled onto a plate and cooled, have the thickness of jelly. Skim off any froth. Fill well-cleaned jars with the jelly and seal these immediately with cellophane, a metal, glass or plastic lid or with grease proof paper. The jelly can also be covered with hot paraffin wax; after setting, this has to be covered with a second layer to completely seal all sides.

Another recipe for jelly, which uses less fuel but more sugar, is as follows: heat one litre of juice to boiling and add 1.5 kg of sugar. Boil for 5 minutes. Fill the jars and close as described above. Jelly can also be made with pectin (see directions on the pectin packet) or with albedo (the white of orange peel).

Candied fruit

With candying, the fruit is slowly impregnated with sugar until the sugar concentration is very high, approximately 65–70 per cent. Peel and cut the fruit into pieces of 1–2 cm thick. Boil these pieces in water until they can be easily pierced with a fork. Soak them overnight in a 30 per cent sugar solution. After this the sugar solution is increased by 10 per cent and the mass is momentarily brought to the boil again before being allowed to stand overnight. This process is repeated until the sugar solution contains +/–72 per cent sugar. The sugar concentration can be checked with a sugar refractometer, a small, handy and inexpensive instrument. Keep the fruits for several weeks in this saturated sugar solution of +/–72 per cent and then dry them. To prevent crystallisation, the sugar solution must consist of glucose as well as beet or cane sugar. If this is not available, 'inverted' sugar can be used. This can be prepared by boiling a concentrated solution of beet or cane sugar for 20 minutes with a generous dash of acid (vinegar, lemon juice, citric acid, hydrochloric acid, etc).

Jam

Two methods for jam making are given below.

Volume reduction method

Peel and cut the fruit into large pieces. Heat the fruit with a small amount of water in a covered pan until soft. Mash the fruit. Reduce the fruit to 2/3 of its original volume by cooking it in an uncovered pan. Stir the sugar (3/4 kg per 1 kg of fresh fruit) gradually into the fruit mass and boil for another few minutes. Lemon juice or citric acid can be added to increase acidity. Boil the jam until a few drops, scattered on a plate and cooled, have the thickness of jam. Skim the mass if necessary. Fill jars as described for fruit jelly. If you use a strong lid that can withstand heat, put the jars upside down so the hot jam will kill micro-organisms present on the lid.

Pectin method

Pectin is a jellying agent used to set the jam. Follow the directions for use enclosed in the package. Apple pulp (apple sauce) or ground albedo (the white of orange peel) can be used instead of pectin.

Preparation of chutney and marmalade

For 1 kg of fruit (tomato, rhubarb, etc.) use 1 dl vinegar (5 per cent), 125 g brown sugar, onions, Spanish peppers, ginger powder and mustard powder to taste. Mix all the ingredients and heat it until thick. Complete the preparations using the recipe for jam making. Marmalade is made from citrus fruit. The peel can also be used, in which case pectin is not needed. If the jam is to be kept for a long time, sodium benzoate can be added as a preservative. Use up to 250 mg per kg of jam.

APPENDIX 11.1: PASTEURISATION OF FRUITS AND VEGETABLES

Table 11.3 has given preparation methods and packing liquid.

Table 11.3. Preparation methods and packing liquid.

Product	Preparation	Add to product when packing into jar, bottle or tin
Apricots	Peel, split and remove pits	Cold 75% sugar solution
Applesauce	Make applesauce, reduce liquid, do not add any sugar	–
Broad beans	Shell, wash, boil in lightly salted water for 5 minutes	Boiling water

(Contd ...)

Product	Preparation	Add to product when packing into jar, bottle or tin
Carrots	Clean, wash, boil in lightly salted water for 5 minutes	Boiling water, plus salt to taste
Cauliflower	Cut, wash, boil 1–2 minutes	Boiling water
Cherries	Wash, remove stems	Cold water, sugar (sweet cherries need 25% sugar solution, sour cherries need 75% sugar)
Currant juice	Wash currents, remove stems, boil shortly, simmer 1 hour, strain if cloudy	–
Endive	Cut, wash, boil 10 minutes in 1% salt, pack tightly	Boiling water
Green beans	Wash, break, boil 10 minutes in lightly salted water	Boiling water
Mango	Steam 2 minutes, peel, slice, remove pit, pack into flat jars or tins	Boiling water, 40% sugar + 0.25% vinegar
Pears	Hard: peel, cook for 1/2 hour Soft: peel and cut	Cold water, 40% sugar
Peaches	Peel, halve and remove pits	Cold water, 40% sugar
Peas	Shell, wash, do not boil	Boiling water
Plums	Wash, peel if desired, halve, remove pits	Cold water, 40% sugar
Raspberries	Wash, sprinkle with 1/4 weight in sugar, let stand 2 hours before packing	–
Rhubarb	Clean, cut into pieces, sprinkle with 1/4 of the product weight in sugar. Pack with juices after 2 hours.	–
Snow peas	Remove ends, wash, boil in lightly salted water for 10 minutes	Boiling water
Spinach	Use fresh leaves only; wash, boil without water for 5 minutes with some salt, pack tightly	Boiling water
Strawberries	Wash, sprinkle with 1/4 of product weight in sugar, let stand 2 hours before packing	–
Tomatoes	Wash	Warm salted water (1% salt solution)
Tomato puree	Wash tomatoes, boil for short time, strain, reduce juice	–
Turnip tops	Wash, boil for 5 minutes	Boiling water

Table 11.4 has given pasteurisation times and temperatures.

Table 11.4. Pasteurisation times and temperatures.

Product	Pasteurisation time (jars of 1–2 litre)	Temperature
Apricots	30 min.	80°C
Applesauce	30 min.	80°C

(Contd ...)

Product	Pasteurisation time (jars of 1–2 litre)	Temperature
Broad beans	1½ hr	100°C
Carrots	1½ hr	100°C
Cauliflower	1½ hr, wash, boil 1-2 minutes	100°C
Cherries	30 min.	80°C
Currant juice	20 min.	75°C
Endive	1½ hours	100°C
Green beans	1 hr	100°C
Mango	10 min.	91°C
Pears	30 min.	80°C
Peaches	30 min.	80°C
Peas	1½ hr—repeat after 24 hr	100°C
Plums	30 min.	80°C
Raspberries	20 min.	75°C
Rhubarb	30 min.	80°C
Snow peas	1 hr	100°C
Spinach	1½ hr	100°C
Strawberries	30 min.	80°C
Tomato puree	30 min.	80°C
Tomatoes	20 min.	80°C
Turnip tops	1½ hr	100°C

APPENDIX 11.2: STERILISATION IN A BOILING WATER BATH

Unless otherwise stated, all products are blanched and sterilised in the boiling water bath. Table 11.5 has given preparation and packing liquid.

Table 11.5. Preparation and packing liquid.

Product	Preparation	Add to product when packing into jar, bottle or tin
Apples (whole)	Peel, blanch 3 minutes, pack tightly in jars or tins	Boiling water or 20% weight in sugar
Apples (slices)	Peel, remove core, slice, blanch 3 minutes in 1% salt	Boiling water or 20% sugar
Applesauce	Pulp apples, boil 10 minutes, pack at 82°C (minimum)	5% sugar
Apricots	Remove stalks, wash, halve, remove pits	Boiling water, 25% sugar
Banana	Peel, cut into slices, pack into jars or cans immediately	Boiling water, 3.5% sugar + 0.5% vinegar + 0.1% calcium chloride
Berries	Remove stalks and overripe fruit, wash carefully	Boiling water, 30% sugar
Cherries	Remove stalks, wash, remove pits.	Boiling water, 30% sugar. For sour cherries add extra sugar

(Contd ...)

Product	Preparation	Add to product when packing into jar, bottle or tin
Figs	Remove stalks, boil in 30% sugar until the syrup contains 65% sugar, fill at 100°C	Boiling water
Fruit puree	Prepare, pack into jars or cans at 70–80°C	–
Grapefruit	Peel, remove seeds, split segments, fill jars first with water	Boiling water, 40% sugar
Grapes	Remove stalks, wash	Boiling water, 15% sugar
Lychee	Peel, halve, remove pits	Boiling water, 50% sugar + 0.25% vinegar
Oranges	Peel, remove seeds, split segments	Boiling water, 15% sugar
Papaya	Peel, halve or slice	Boiling water, 50% sugar + 0.25% vinegar
Peaches	Boil 1 minute in water, peel, halve, remove pits	Boiling water, 25% sugar
Pears	Peel, halve, keep under water until packing	80°C water, 20% sugar
Pineapple	Peel, core, cut into rings	Boiling water, 30% sugar
Plums	Remove any overripe fruit, wash, remove stalks, halve, remove pits	Boiling water, 30% sugar
Sauerkraut	Boil 10 minutes and pack hot	–
Strawberries	Remove tops, wash	Boiling water, 20% sugar
Sweet pepper	Cut, (peel after boiling in 10% lye), blanch for 3 minutes, puree if desired	Boiling water, 1.5% salt
Tomatoes	Wash, steam 15 seconds, dip in cold water, remove skins	0.5% dry salt + 0.07% calcium chloride

Table 11.6 has given sterilisation times and sealing temperatures.

Table 11.6. Sterilisation times and sealing temperatures.

Product	Sealing temp. °C	Sterilisation times in boiling water bath (minutes)				
		Glass jars		Tins		
		½ l	1 l	0.58 l	0.85 l	3.1 l
Apples	60	20	20	15	15	20
Applesauce	82	5	5	5	5	10
Apricots	60	25	25	15	20	30
Banana	71	15	15	10	12	20
Berries	70	25	25	15	20	30
Cherries	70	25	25	15	20	30
Figs	95	15	15	15	20	30
Fruit puree	71	20	20	15	15	25
Grapefruit	60	10	10	15	18	20
Grapes	77	20	20	12	15	20

(Contd ...)

| Product | Sealing temp. °C | Sterilisation times in boiling water bath (minutes) | | | | |
| | | Glass jars | | Tins | | |
		½ l	1 l	0.58 l	0.85 l	3.1 l
Lychee	77	15	15	10	12	20
Oranges	77	10	10	15	18	20
Papaya	77	20	20	15	20	30
Peaches	71	20	20	20	25	40
Pears	71	35	35	30	30	30
Pineapple	75	20	20	20	30	40
Plums	82	20	20	15	22	35
Sauerkraut	71	10	10	15	18	20
Strawberries	77	10	10	15	18	20
Sweet pepper	60	20	20	20	25	–
Tomatoes	60	45	45	45	55	90

APPENDIX 11.3: STERILISATION IN A PRESSURE COOKER OR AUTOCLAVE

Unless otherwise stated, all products are blanched and sterilised in a pressure cooker or autoclave. Table 11.7 has given preparation and packing liquid.

Table 11.7. Preparation and packing liquid.

Product	Preparation	Add to product when packing into jar, bottle or tin
Beet root	Wash, blanch 20 minutes, peel (slice if desired)	Boiling salted (1%) water, sugar to taste
Broad beans	Shell, wash, blanch 3 minutes	Boiling salted (2%) water
Green beans	Wash, cut tips, break or cut, for young beans blanch 1½ minutes, for old beans blanch 3 minutes, fill, shaking tin to pack tightly	–
Cabbage	Use only solid cabbages; cut, wash, blanch until soft (±10 minutes)	Boiling salted (1.5%) water
Carrots	Remove tops and tips, blanch 5 minutes, peel and scrape, cut if desired	Boiling salted (2%) water
Celery (roots)	Cut, blanch 4 minutes in 2% citric acid	Boiling salted (1.5%) water
Cauliflower	Cut into small rosettes (soak a few hours in 1% salt), wash, blanch 4 minutes in 0.5% citric acid	Boiling salted (1.5%) water + 0.1 citric acid
Sweet corn	Remove kernels from cob, wash	Boiling salted (0.5%) water
Eggplant	Wash, cut into pieces ±2 cm long	Boiling salted (1%) water
Greens	Sort, wash well, blanch 3 minutes, add boiling liquid to the jars or cans first, then lower greens into the liquid	Boiling salted (3%) water

(Contd ...)

Product	Preparation	Add to product when packing into jar, bottle or tin
Mushrooms	Use fresh mushrooms, scrape caps, cut off base, soak in lemon juice 10 minutes, rinse with cold water, blanch 8 minutes	Boiling salted (2%) water + 0.1% citric acid
Okra (fermented)	Remove stems, soak in 2% salt for 18 hours, blanch 3 minutes, cut	Boiling salted (2%) water
Okra (fresh)	Blanch 2 minutes, rinse in cold water immediately	Boiling salted (2%) water
Olives	Soak in 1% sodium lye for 6–8 hours, oxidise in the open air, soak again in 1% lye for 6 hours, soak in water 4-6 days until all lye has been removed, then soak 1 day in 1% salt, 1 day in 2% salt and 1 day in 3% salt	Boiling salted (2%) water
Onions	Remove outer skins, blanch 5 minutes	Boiling salted (1.5%) water
Peas	Shell, wash, blanch 2 minutes, rinse with cold water immediately	Boiling salted (2.5%) water
Potatoes	Peel, wash, blanch 5 minutes	Boiling salted (1.5%) water
Pumpkin	Remove dirt, brush, halve, remove seeds, steam for 45 minutes	–
Salsify	Wash, scrape, blanch 5 minutes	Boiling salted (3%) water
Summer squash	Wash, halve, remove seeds, cut into pieces	–
Swedes	Wash, scrape, blanch 10 minutes, pack immediately	Boiling salted (2%) water
Sweet potato	Wash, cook, remove skin while hot, pack while hot	Boiling salted water or boiling sugar water to taste
Yams	Wash, cook, peel, pack while still hot	Boiling water
White beans (soya, kidney)	Peel, wash, blanch 3 minutes, big, dry beans need to be soaked overnight	Boiling salted (2%) water

Table 11.8 has given sterilising in a pressure cooker or autoclave.

Table 11.8. Sterilising in a pressure cooker or autoclave.

Product	Sealing temp. °C	Sterilisation times (minutes)							
		Glass jars, 115°C		Tins, 115°C			Tins, 121°C		
		½ l	1 l	0.58 l	0.85 l	3 l	0.58 l	0.85 l	3 l
Green beans	74	35	40	21	26	37	12	15	22
White beans	60	80	90	70	85	100	35	50	55
Broad beans	71	35	40	–	30	–	–	–	–
Beet root	71	35	40	35	35	50	23	23	35
Cabbage	66	–	–	40	40	60	25	25	35
Carrots	66	35	40	30	35	50	20	23	35

(Contd ...)

Product	Sealing temp. °C	Glass jars, 115°C		Tins, 115°C			Tins, 121°C		
		½ l	1 l	0.58 l	0.85 l	3 l	0.58 l	0.85 l	3 l
Cauliflower	75	–	–	30	–	–	20	20	–
Celery, roots	85	30	35	28	33	45	–	–	–
Sweet corn	85	60	70	55	65	85	30	35	45
Eggplant	71	–	–	–	–	–	35	40	60
Greens	77	60*	65*	–	–	–	55	55	85
Mushrooms	66	35	40	25	30	–	20	20	35
Okra, fresh	66	35	40	35	40	55	25	30	45
Okra, fermented	66	–	–	20	23	40	–	–	–
Olives	66	60	70	60	70	70	45	48	50
Onions	66	–	–	20	–	35	–	–	–
Peas	71	40	45	36	50	55	25	35	40
Potatoes	70	40	45	35	55	23	30	38	–
Pumpkin	85	60*	75*	85	115	235	75	85	185
Salsify	66	–	–	40	–	–	–	–	–
Summer squash	66	–	–	–	–	–	25	35	40
Swedes	66	–	–	30	30	40	–	–	–
Sweet potato	70	–	–	–	34	40	–	24	32
Yams	66	–	–	60	65	80	45	50	65

*These products need to be sterilised at 121°C in glass jars.

APPENDIX 11.4: PREPARATION AND DRYING CONDITIONS

Because the drying circumstances always vary somewhat, the numbers in the Tables 11.9 to 11.11 should be seen as approximations rather than as absolute instructions. One must experiment to determine the best method for each situation and product.

Tray Capacity

The figures are based on the use of single racks and sun drying. The capacity for artificial drying will be the same or higher, depending on the relative humidity and airflow speed.

Characteristics of the Final Product

A description of the final product has been given to help determine when the product is sufficiently dry, since the moisture content itself is difficult to determine without expensive equipment. When in doubt, use the local standards, especially when these contradict the information in the Tables 11.9 to 11.11.

Maximum Temperature

The temperature of the product itself is difficult to measure, but the temperature of the drying air can be measured fairly easily. When the product contains much water the air temperature may be higher than the maximum given in the table, but at the end of the drying process this should be avoided. Measure the air temperature just above the product with a thermometer. Protect the thermometer against direct sunlight. Drying information is given in the following three Tables 11.9, 11.10 and 11.11.

Table 11.9. Fruit– preparation and drying conditions.

Product	Preparation	Drying conditions, remarks
Apples	Wash, peel, quarter and remove the core	–
Apricots	Wash, halve, remove pits	Spread on racks one layer thick with the cut side up
Bananas	Peel and cut in half length-wise or slice	–
Cherries	Wash and remove pits (this improves drying but decreases amount of juice)	–
Figs	Partly tree-dried, do not cut	–
Grapes	No usual preparation, sometimes a lye dip is given	–
Peaches and mangos	Wash, halve, remove pits	Spread on racks with the cut side up
Pears	Wash, cut in half, remove the core and stems	Spread on racks with the cut side up. Max. 2 days in full sun, thereafter shade
Pineapple	Peel and cut	Sulphite treatment maximum temp. 60°C
Plums	Sort by quality and size, immerse for 10 minutes in lye dip	Large plums should be turned occasionally

Table 11.10. Vegetables–preparation and drying conditions.

Product	Preparation	Blanching time (min.)	Remarks
Beans	Remove tops and strings, wash, break by hand	5–8 min.	Dried products should not be packed directly in tins or bags
Cabbage	Wash, cut (5 mm thick), blanch immediately	3–4 min.	Moderately long storage
Carrots	Use fresh, young roots, wash, remove tops and tips	None	Cut with stainless steel knife
Chillies capsicum	Select, remove stems; do not cut little chillies, cut big ones into 5–10 mm pieces	None	Sometimes blanched
Eggplant	Remove stem and flower parts, wash and cut in slices 3 mm thick	2–6 min.	–
Garlic	Peel (not necessary when making powder), cut slices 3 mm thick	None	Can be ground to powder
Greens	Select, cut, wash	2 min.	–
Okra	Select, wash, remove stems, slice 6 mm thick	4 min.	Rinse after blanching
Onions	Peel, cut slices 3 mm thick	None	Can be ground to powder
(Sweet) potatoes	Wash, peel, remove eyes, slice 2–3 mm thick, dip in lemon juice to prevent brown discolouration	4-6 min.	Irish potatoes can be ground to a powder to be used as a thickener

(Contd ...)

Product	Preparation	Blanching time (min)	Remarks
Pumpkin	Remove stem and flower parts, cut, remove seeds, peel, slice 3 mm thick	3–6 min.	Need to peel when making powder
Tomatoes	Wash, dip in boiling water, peel, cut in slices 7–10 mm thick	1½ min.	Rub paraffin oil on the rack to prevent sticking

Table 11.11. Fruits and vegetables—product information for drying.

Product	Tray capacity kg/m²	Max. air temp. °C	Yield (kg) per 100 kg fresh product		Final product	
			Prepared	Dried	Water content	Description
Apples	6	68	60	10	15–20%	Buoyant
Apricots	4–8	66	90	18	18%	Leathery
Bananas	6		85	18	12%	Hard
Beans	4	68	90	9–12	4%	Brittle, dark
Cabbage	4	55	85	6–9	4%	Tough, brittle
Carrots	4	71	80-85	8–9	5–7%	Brittle
Cherries	25	74	80	28	25%	Leathery
Chillies (capsicum)	6	60–65	85	10	5–7%	Tough, brittle
Eggplant	4	65	90	10	5%	Tough
Figs	6	71		20	15–20%	Can be kneaded, skin flexible
Garlic	4	63			5–7%	Brittle
Grapes	6	71	90	7	10–14%	Can be kneaded
Greens	2.5	65	60–75	8–10	4%	Brittle, crisp
Okra	4	65	90	9–12	5%	Brittle
Onions	4	60	90	9	5–7%	Brittle
Peaches/mangos	6	68	85–90	15–20	14%	Leathery
Pears	6	65	80–85	15–20	10–15%	Leathery
Plums	6	74	100	34	15–20%	Can be kneaded
Potatoes	5	65	74	11	5%	Hard, brittle
Pumpkin	4	70	70	7–12	5%	Tough, brittle
Sweet potatoes	5	71	80–85	27	7–8%	Hard, brittle
Tomatoes	5	65	70–90	4-5	5%	Tough, brittle

APPENDIX 11.5: PREPARATION OF VEGETABLES FOR SALTING

Table 11.12 has given preparation of vegetables for salting and the best method for each type of vegetable.

Table 11.12. Preparation of vegetables for salting and the best method for each type of vegetable.

Product	Preparation	Method
Beets	See green tomatoes	See green tomatoes
Beet tops	See kale	See kale

(Contd ...)

Product	Preparation	Method
Brown beans	See peas	See peas
Cabbage	Remove outer leaves and stalks; shred	Light salting
Cauliflower	Remove stalks and leaves; cut into small pieces; no cutting is needed with the heavy brine method	Light brine, heavy brine
Sweet corn	Boil the cobs for 10 minutes; remove kernels	Heavy salting
Green beans	Wash, cut off tips, blanch 5 minutes, cut into short pieces; whole beans can be used with the light brine method	Light salting, heavy salting, light brine
Kale	Trim leaves; wash well, use the whole leaves	Light brine
Lettuce	Wash, remove outer leaves and stalk; shred	Light salting
Okra	Cut ripe okra into small pieces	See peas
Onions	Remove dry skins	Heavy brine
Peas	Shell; with the heavy brine method, wait until repacking from big vats to small pots before shelling; do not use overripe peas with the heavy brine method; blanch 5 minutes	Heavy salting, heavy brine
Swedes and turnips	Wash well; remove tops and bottoms; cut into small pieces	Light salting
Sweet pepper	Cut length-wise, remove seeds and stem	Heavy brine
Green tomatoes	Wash well, do not slice	Light brine

APPENDIX 11.6: JUICE EXTRACTION METHODS

Sugar need only be added when a sweetened taste is desired. Table 11.13 has given methods of juice extraction from various types of fruit.

Table 11.13. Methods of juice extraction from various types of fruit.

Fruit	Preparation	Method	Sugar
Apples	Wash, use juice centrifuge, hand press or vegetable mill (fine)	Do not heat; press through a clean cloth or bag	none
Apricots/peaches	Use solid ripe fruit; wash, remove stems	Boil in a little water until soft, strain or use a juice steamer	1 part sugar + 4 parts water + 5 parts juice or 1 part juice + 1 part water
Berries	Wash and crush ripe berries, heat to 80°C	Press through cloth; filter or use a juice steamer	If desired: 1 part sugar + 1 part juice
Cherries (Morellos)	Wash, remove stems and pits, cut, heat to 80°C (not for morellos)	Press through cloth or filter	If desired: 1 part sugar + 9 parts juice
Citrus fruit	Remove navels and seeds, do not heat	Juice steamer, do not press peel, do not remove pulp, use a coarse sieve	None

(Contd ...)

Fruit	Preparation	Method	Sugar
Purple grapes	Wash, remove long stems, dip in a muslin bag in boiling water for 30 sec., chop, let stand for 10 min.	Press through cloth or cloth bag, filter or use a juice steamer	None
	Wash, crush		
Blue and green grapes	Wash, remove stems, chop, remove seeds; heat blue grapes to 71°C; do not heat green grapes	Press through cloth or cloth bag, filter	None
Mango	Wash and cut into pieces, boil for 5 minutes, separate seed from pulp	Mix pulp in blender/food processor or use a juice steamer	None
Plums	Use ripe plums, wash and crush, add 1 litre water to 1 kg of fruit, heat to 82°C until soft or wash, cut	Press through cloth or cloth bag or use a juice steamer	1 part sugar + 4 parts juice
Rhubarb	Wash and cut into pieces, add 2 litres water per kg fruit, heat until boiling or wash and cut	Press through cloth or cloth bag or use a juice steamer	1 part sugar + 8 parts juice
Straw berries	See berries	See berries	1 part sugar + 3 parts juice
Tomatoes	Use well-ripened fruit	Press through a fine sieve	None, salt to taste

Chapter 12

Contamination, Preservation and Spoilage of Fish and Meat

INTRODUCTION

Preservation is the processing of foods so that they can be stored longer. Man is dependent on products of plant and animal origin for food. Because most of these products are readily available only during certain seasons of the year and because fresh food spoils quickly, methods have been developed to preserve foods. Preserved foods can be eaten long after the fresh products would normally have spoiled. With the growth of towns, the need to preserve foods longer increased as some people could no longer grow their own vegetables nor keep animals.

Preservation must be seen as a way of storing excess foods that are abundantly available at certain times of the year, so that they can be consumed in times when food is scarce. Consumption of fresh foods is always preferable, however, as preservation usually decreases the nutritional value. In other words, preserved foods are not as healthy as fresh foods.

A number of simple preservation techniques suitable for small-scale preservation, such as at the household or village level, will be described in this chapter. The emphasis is on 'small-scale', to inform individuals how to process and store their surplus economically.

In times of scarcity, preserved foods can be a welcome addition to the diet. Through preservation, sales of out of season products are possible and prices asked are independent of the usually lower market prices during the harvest season. The following preservation methods are discussed: salting, drying and smoking of fish and meat, fermenting of fish, canning of fish and meat, and cooling and freezing of fish and meat.

STORAGE LIFE AND SPOILAGE

How Long can Fish or Meat be Kept?

Fresh fish will spoil very quickly. Once the fish has been caught, spoilage progresses rapidly. In the high ambient temperatures of the tropics, fish will spoil within 12 hours. Using good fishing techniques (to ensure the fish is barely damaged) and cooling the fish, with the help on ice on board, can increase the storage life of fresh fish.

The speed with which meat spoils not only depends on hygiene conditions and storage temperature, but also on the acidity of the meat and the structure of the muscular tissue. The firm muscular tissue of beef, for example, spoils less quickly than liver. Hygienic slaughtering and clean handling of the carcass have a positive effect on storage life. After slaughtering, one should preserve the meat as quickly as possible.

When has Fish or Meat Gone Bad?

Spoilage is the deterioration of food which makes it taste and smell bad (e.g. when it is sour, rotten or mouldy) and/or makes it a carrier of disease germs.

Properties of spoiled fish compared to fresh fish are:

1. Strong odour.
2. Dark-red gills with slime on them instead of bright red ones.
3. Soft flesh with brown traces of blood instead of firm flesh with red blood.
4. Red, milky pupils without slime instead of clear ones.

The onset of spoilage in meat is seen by changes in colour, among other things. Typical spoilage smells also develop (such as a rotten egg smell).

Spoiled food, when consumed, can cause symptoms such as diarrhoea, stomach pains, nausea and vomiting, and stomach infections or cramps. In very serious cases it can cause death.

In fish and meat the most important kinds of spoilage are:

1. Microbiological spoilage caused by bacteria.
2. Autolytic spoilage caused by enzymes.
3. Fat oxidation.

Bacteria are single-celled micro-organisms that are invisible to the naked eye. They break down the wastes and bodies of dead organisms. Some cause severe illness. Under favourable conditions microbiological spoilage starts quickly in fresh and non-acidic products such as fish and meat. Bacteria from the animal's skin or intestines can rapidly reproduce.

Enzymes are proteins which assist biological reactions, e.g. the conversion of certain organic substances into different ones. When fish or animals are killed, the enzymes inside them are still intact. Those enzymes start breaking down components into smaller parts. This affects smell, taste and texture. Several hours after death 'rigour mortis' occurs (a stiffening of the flesh). After that the flesh gets softer again due to enzymatic reactions (autolysis). Heat treatment (e.g. pasteurisation) can inactivate enzymes.

With fatty fish or meat, chemical reactions can take place between the fat and oxygen in the air (oxidation reactions). By exposing these products for a long time to air, e.g. during drying and smoking, the product acquires a rancid smell and taste. It is, therefore, better to use less fatty kinds or pieces of fish or meat for smoking and drying.

Which Micro-organisms Cause Spoilage?

Not all micro-organisms cause spoilage. Some cause desirable changes in fish and meat. An example of this is the fermentation of fish, for example resulting in fish pastes or sauces. These changes are caused by useful micro-organisms, of which there are thousands of kinds. Micro-organisms are usually not visible to the naked eye, which means that serious infections and food poisoning can be caused without the food being visibly changed.

Bacteria can grow in fresh foods (meat, fish, milk, vegetables) which are not acidic. Some bacteria can cause infections and poisoning as well as spoilage. A number of bacteria can form spores which are less easily destroyed by preservation techniques; they can start to grow again after insufficient heat treatment.

Spoilage and/or Fish and Meat Poisoning

Bacteria can only cause rotting if, after contamination of the fish and meat, the bacteria are also able to grow in the fish and meat. The following factors influence the growth of bacteria and the speed with which rotting takes place.

Damage

The skin of fish and meat, for example, is a protection against bacterial growth in the flesh. By damaging the skin, which functions as a barrier, nutrients are released. Bacteria can enter the flesh and start to grow.

Water content (internal water content and humidity)

Fish consists of on average 70 per cent water; in fatty fish this percentage is about 65 per cent and in lean fish about 80 per cent. Beef consists of 65 per cent and pork of 60 per cent water on average. With such high levels of internal moisture, bacteria can grow rapidly. Meat forms a protective layer on the flesh as a result of drying out at low humidity. A film of condensation is formed on cold meat lying in warm surroundings, which is a good medium for bacteria and moulds.

Oxygen content

Strictly aerobic micro-organisms need oxygen for their growth, while strictly anaerobic micro-organisms can only grow in the absence of oxygen. Minced meat, for example, spoils very quickly because a lot of air has been mixed into it.

Acidity

The acidity of a product is indicated by its pH. Fish and meat have a neutral pH, i.e. 7. Bacteria only grow between a minimum pH of 4.5 and a maximum of 8–9 with an optimum of 6.5–7.5. As a result, fish and meat are very susceptible to spoilage. When fermenting fish and meat, the pH is deliberately kept low so that only the desired micro-organisms affect the product and not those bacteria which cause spoilage.

Specific chemical composition

Bacteria need sources of energy and nitrogen. Minerals and vitamins are also important for growth. In meat, the first source of energy used by bacteria is sugar, then lactate, free amino acids and only then protein. Sources of nitrogen are nitrate, ammonia, peptides, amino acids or products of decomposition.

Temperature

The ideal temperature for the growth of micro-organisms is between 7° and 55°C (45°–131°F). The range within which bacteria grow is between –10°C and 70°C (14°–158°F), but the range within which they will survive is much greater.

With freezing, micro-organisms are inactivated, and with long-term heating all micro-organisms will eventually die. At temperatures above 80°C (176°F) they usually die. Spores are often resistant to temperatures above 100°C (212°F).

Apart from all these preconditions for growth, the time between contamination and processing or consumption is also of importance. Some micro-organisms grow faster than others. This means that the number of micro-organisms and the amount of toxins they produce can vary.

At 37°C (99°F) certain bacteria can multiply from 1000 to 100,00,000 individual organisms in seven hours. The actual rate at which bacteria grow depends on a combination of the factors mentioned above. A watery product at 25°C (77°F) will spoil much quicker than a dry, acidic product at 5°C (41°F).

How does Contamination Takes Place?

Contamination can come from people (germs on skin, intestines, cuts, throat or hands), soil, dust, sewage, surface water, manure and other spoiled foods. Contamination can also be caused by poorly cleaned apparatus, domestic animals, pets, vermin or unhygienic ally slaughtered animals.

Contamination after a preservation treatment has been carried out is especially dangerous. An example of this is the contamination of cooked meat by placing it on the same plate on which raw meat was kept.

Hygiene

1. Ensure good personal hygiene. Wash hands thoroughly with hot water and soap after using the toilet, handling cuts, cleaning infections and doing dirty work, and before touching fish and meat.
2. Change towels and wash clothes regularly.
3. Keep fish and meat on smooth surfaces which can be and are washed well (e.g. stainless steel kitchen block, tiles, stone).
4. Keep the places where fish and meat are stored clean by regularly washing with a kitchen soda solution.
5. Wash all tools used for fish and meat regularly.
6. Cover all foods well.
7. Try to keep all pests away from the places where foods are kept.
8. Never store leftovers at room temperature.
9. Ensure proper hygiene when animals are slaughtered.
10. Use clean water. If necessary, boil the water before use.

Prevention of Spoilage

Preservation can have two effects:

1. Retention of the original qualities and properties of the foods.
2. Radical changes which result in new products with completely new qualities and properties.

Preservation is based on slowing down or preventing spoilage by micro-organisms. The dangers of micro-organisms can be avoided in three ways.

Micro-organisms are removed

This is a very costly method which can only be used with liquids (e.g. filtering of drinking water).

Micro-organisms are killed

This is usually done with heat. When all the micro-organisms present are killed by a heat treatment, the process is called sterilisation and the product can be stored for a long time, if kept at the right temperature. When a short heat treatment at 80°C (176°F) is applied, so that not all micro-organisms are killed, the process is called pasteurisation and the product can be stored for only a limited time. Cured meat products contain salt and sometimes also nitrite. They therefore need less intense heat than is needed in the preservation of vegetables, for example.

Micro-organism activity is suppressed

An environment in which micro-organisms can no longer grow or can grow only very slowly, is created. There are various ways of doing this:

Lowering the temperature

Products remain fresh in the refrigerator (2°–4°C/35.5°–41°F) for 4–7 days; they can be stored much longer in the deep-freeze (–20°C/–4°F). Low temperatures must be maintained accurately and continuously and high demands are made on the freezer, energy supply and food quality. As this method requires a lot of energy and materials and a large investment, it will be only briefly described here.

Reducing the water content

Drying is the oldest way of preserving foods. When sufficient water is removed from a product, micro-organisms can no longer grow. The amount of water to be removed varies with the product. The simplest and cheapest method is to dry the product in the open air (with or without sun). Somewhat more expensive and difficult methods make use of driers in which the products are artificially dried using heated air. Sun-dried products are of slightly less quality due to the breakdown of certain vitamins in sunlight. Lengthy smoking is also based on the principle of reducing the internal water content. Smoke particles give an added taste to the product.

Increasing the osmotic pressure

In this technique, salt is added to stop the growth of micro-organisms. Examples are the salting of meat and fish. These preserved products keep well. The nutritional value of the final product is reasonable.

Adding preservatives

Addition of certain substances can partly prevent spoilage. In practice, this method is only used as an aid for other preservation methods and will therefore not be covered here. Because of the nature of the substances, the accompanying directions must be followed exactly.

Changing the foods

By preserving in liquids, by adding acid or through special microbial processes, 'new' foods can be made. These often have a very special odour and taste, such as smoked fish and many local fermented products.

Which Method should be Chosen?

The choice of a preservation method depends on the product, the desired properties of the product to be stored, the availability of energy sources (wood, gasoline, oil, electricity, sun), the storage facilities, possible packaging materials and the costs involved for each method. It is sometimes necessary to combine methods, such as salting and drying meat or adding acid and then sterilising. It is also desirable to conform to local customs if the products are to be acceptable to the local population.

A number of advantages and disadvantages of several methods are summarised below:

1. Salting fish and meat: inexpensive when salt is cheap; no energy required; storage at room temperature; reasonable quality; long storage life; nutritional value reasonable.
2. Drying fish and meat: inexpensive; no energy required; little equipment needed; dry and/or airtight storage required; quality and nutritional value reasonable with good storage.
3. Smoking fish and meat: inexpensive; little energy required; fuel must be present; little equipment needed; quality and nutritional value reasonable.
4. Fermentation of fish and meat: often cheap (local techniques); no energy needed; taste and odour often radically changed; storage life varies from short to long depending on the fermented product; nutritional value often high.
5. Canning fish and meat: fairly expensive; labour intensive; requires much energy and water; tins or jars with lids are needed; sterilisers or pressure cookers and canning machines are needed; packaging is expensive; storage is easy (below 25°C/77°F) and possible for long periods; the quality of the product and its nutritional value is good.
6. Cooling and freezing fish and meat: very expensive technique; uses much energy; large investments are needed; quality, nutritional value and storage life of the product are good.

PREPARATION

Catching and Cleaning Fish

Catching and preparing fresh fish

As fish spoils very quickly, measures must already be taken on board the fishing boat to limit spoilage. First of all, the fish must immediately be kept out of the salt water so that the fish does not get contaminated by bacteria in the salt water.

Apart from preventing contamination, one should also prevent outgrowth of bacteria which are already present. The best way is to remove the intestines and gills of the fish on board the fishing boat. After that the fish must be washed with clean water to rinse off any blood or other remains. It is recommended to transport the fish on ice to shore. However, cleaning and transporting the fish on ice is often difficult and expensive to realise. All that can be done then is to transport the fish as quickly and carefully as possible to the shore. To prevent the bacteria in the intestines, liver, gills and on the skin of the fish from increasing, the fish must be kept in a clean boat and in the shade.

Cleaning fish

To clean fish, first of all one needs good and clean tools. Personal hygiene is also important. It is important that the fish is not cleaned on the ground but on a clean table or bench. The table should be at working height and can be made of wood, metal or concrete. The surface of the table must be smooth and easy to clean. It is also handy to clean the fish on a cutting board so that the table is not damaged.

Knives are the most important tools for cleaning fish. Short knives are used for small kinds of fish, long flexible knives to fillet larger kinds of fish and a thick, strong knife to cut open large fish. The knives must be sharp.

To salt, dry and smoke fish, it is important that the surface area of the fish be increased. Then the salt and smoke particles can penetrate easily into the fish and moisture can work its way out. The method used to clean fish depends primarily on the size and kind of fish.

1. With very small kinds of fish, such as anchovies, sardines and others smaller than 10 cm, usually only the intestines are removed. Whether or not this is done depends on local customs and the purpose for which the fish is to be used. For some fermentation processes the intestines are not removed.
2. Fish larger than 15 cm are, apart from being cleaned, also cut crosswise so that the surface area of the fish is increased and the flesh becomes less thick. Preservation methods work faster with a larger surface area of the flesh.
3. In addition to cleaning and splitting fish that are larger than 25 cm, one also makes extra cuts in the flesh. Sometimes the fish are cut into chunks or completely filleted.

The way in which the fish are cleaned depends not only on the size of the fish but also on the wishes of the consumer. Some consumers, for example, want the fish with its head intact while others especially want it cut off. The last thing to be discussed is a brief description of how to gut, split and fillet fish.

Gutting and scaling

Gutting and scaling as shown in Fig. 12.1.

1. Place the fish on a clean board and hold it by its head. Scrape the scales off starting at the tail and working towards the head. Try not to damage the skin of the fish while doing so.
2. Wash the fish in clean (drinking) water and remove all loose scales.

3. Lay the fish on its side on a clean board and cut into the fish along its gills with a sharp knife. Do the same on the other side but do not cut the head off.
4. Cut the gills free by cutting the ends free from the head and body with the point of the knife.
5. Slit the abdominal wall open from the anal opening towards the head of the fish. Cut deep enough but try not to damage the intestines of the fish.
6. When the fish has been opened up, the gills and intestines can be removed by placing one's fingers under the gills and pulling everything out.
7. Scrape any remaining blood out with the knife.
8. Clean the abdominal wall with clean (drinking) water.

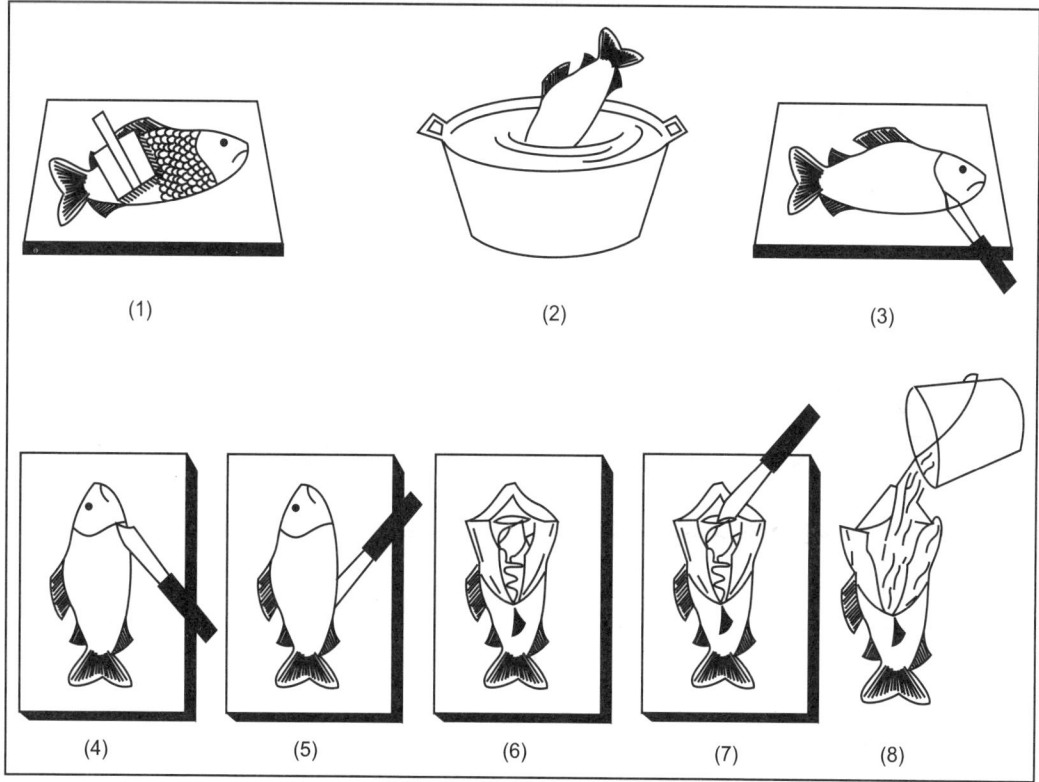

(1)　　　　　　(2)　　　　　　(3)

(4)　　　(5)　　　(6)　　　(7)　　　(8)

Fig. 12.1. Gutting and scaling of fish.

Splitting

Splitting is shown in Fig. 12.2.

Small and medium-sized fish

Small and medium-sized fish shown in Fig. 12.2(a).

1. Place the fish on a clean board with its back facing you and its head to the right if you are right-handed. Slit the fish open down the middle from the head to the tail, along the middle fish bone, but do not cut into the underbelly.
2. Open the fish and remove the intestines and gills. Wash the fish thoroughly with clean (drinking) water.

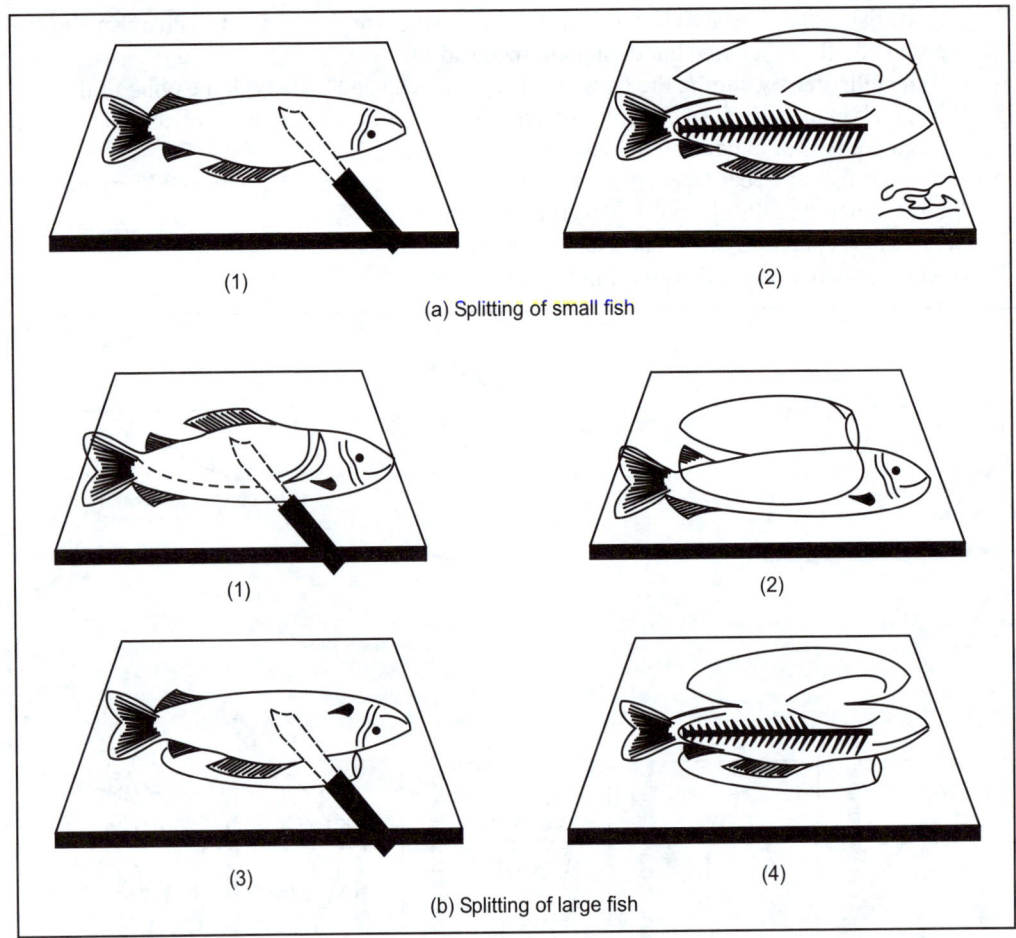

(1)   (2)

(a) Splitting of small fish

(1)   (2)

(3)   (4)

(b) Splitting of large fish

Fig. 12.2. Splitting of fish.

Large fish

Large fish shown in Fig. 12.2(b). Extra cuts are made in the flesh of large fish to increase the surface area and to decrease the thickness of the fish:

1. Place the fish on a clean board, with the abdominal side facing you and the head to the right if you are right-handed. Make a cut in the fish from the gill arch to the tail so that a strip of fish-flesh is left.
2. Turn the fish over and open it up. The strip of flesh must remain attached at the back.
3. Place the fish with its head to the right and the abdominal side facing you. Split the head open and cut towards the tail so that a second strip of flesh is formed. In doing so, the abdomen is also cut open.
4. Open the fish and remove its intestines and gills. Then wash with clean (drinking) water.

Filleting

Filleting is shown in Fig. 12.3.

Small fish

Small fish shown in Fig. 12.3(a).

One can use a fish which has not been cleaned for this.

1. Place the fish on a clean board with its back facing you. Place the head on the left if you are right-handed. Cut along the contours of the gill arches until you hit the backbone.
2. With one slice, cut the fillet loose from the backbone from the head to the tail. In doing so, the abdomen is cut open.
3. When the fillet is loose, you can see the intestines and other organs.
4. Turn the fish over so its abdominal side faces you.
5. Repeat steps 1, 2 and 3.
6. If necessary, cut the fins from the fillets. Then wash the fillets with clean (drinking) water.

Large fish

Large fish shown in Fig. 12.3(b).

1. Place the fish on a clean board with the stomach facing up. For right-handed people the head must be on the right. Cut along the contours of the gill arches.
2. Remove the head and intestines.
3. Place the fish on its side. For the first fillet, start at the head end and cut the fish in the direction of the tail to halfway along the backbone. Cut as close to the backbone as possible.
4. Also cut the other side of the fillet loose.
5. Turn the fish so that its tail is to the right.
6. Remove the other fillet from the backbone. If necessary, remove the fins from the fish. Wash the fillets with clean (drinking) water.

With all preservation methods it is important to use fish of the same size within one batch so that a uniform final product is made.

Butchering

Only a brief description of how to butcher livestock is given here. The storage life of consumer meat and meat products depends on the quality of the fresh meat. Meat must therefore be as clean as possible after being butchered so that microbial decay is avoided. The chemical reactions which occur are also important.

After being killed, the animal is hung upside down so that the blood can drain from the carcass. After bleeding dry, the head can be removed. Subsequently the hooves and the hide are removed from most kinds of animals. After a thorough inspection for visible abnormalities, the carcass can be divided into four parts and each part can be hung up.

Pigs, after being killed, hung up and bled, are heated so that the hide with the hairs can be scraped off. The butchering of sheep and goats is comparable to that of pigs.

It is best after butchering to store the parts of the carcass in cooling cells. However, as cooling facilities are often absent, the meat must be consumed or processed as quickly as possible (within several hours).

Cutting Meat into Pieces for Drying

After hanging up the carcass quarters, the meat is trimmed. This means the membranes within which the meat is enclosed are cut away.

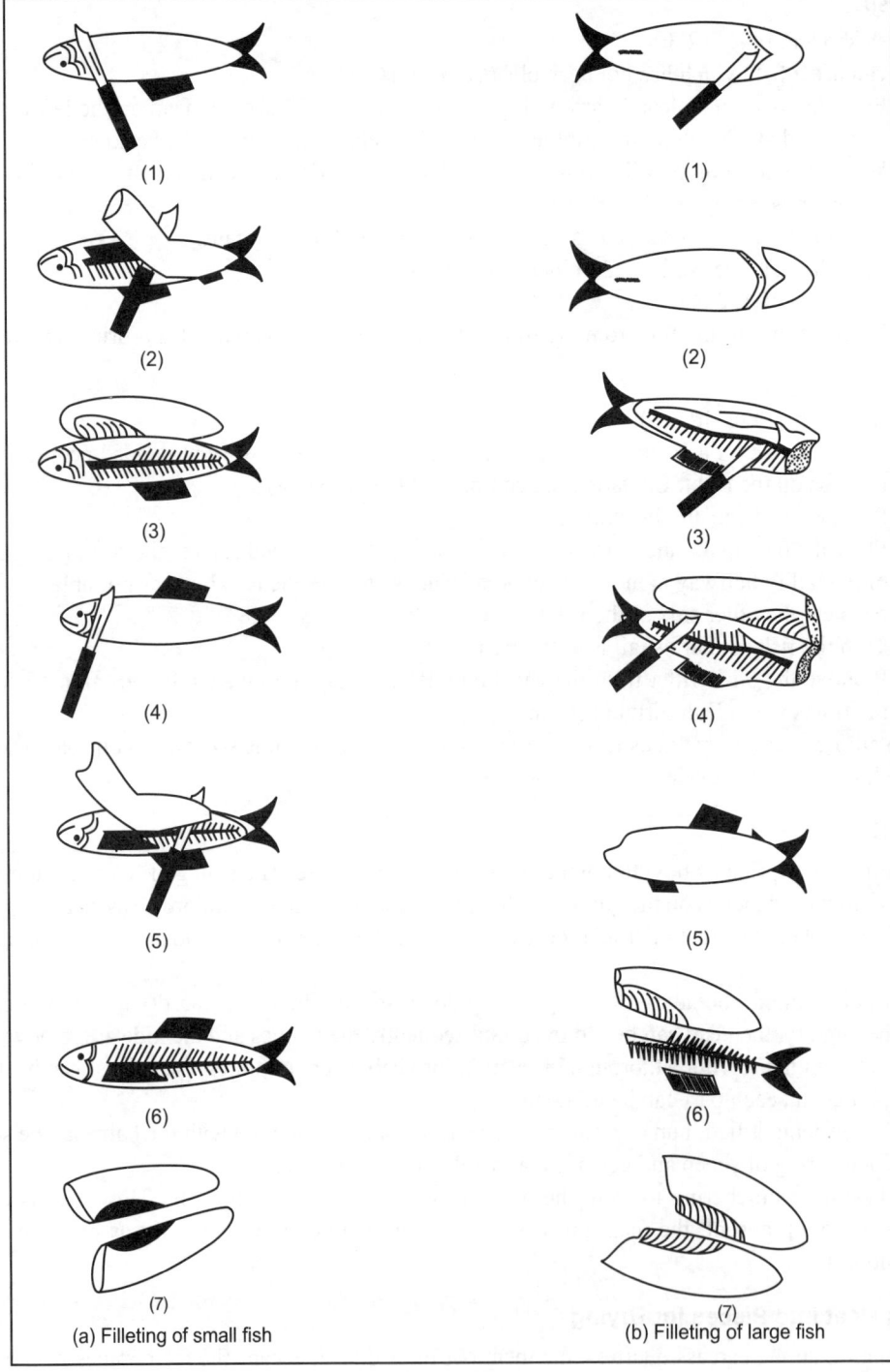

(a) Filleting of small fish

(b) Filleting of large fish

Fig. 12.3. Filleting of fish.

Bad parts in the meat such as damaged areas, discolourations, insect or parasite affected parts must also be cut away. After this the bones are cut out of the carcass, during which the flesh should be damaged as little as possible. Then pieces of meat of good quality must be selected for preservation. For the drying of meat, for example, one can best use lean meat of an animal which has been slaughtered when it is middle-aged. The larger pieces of meat are cut into smaller ones following the anatomical lines (Fig. 12.4).

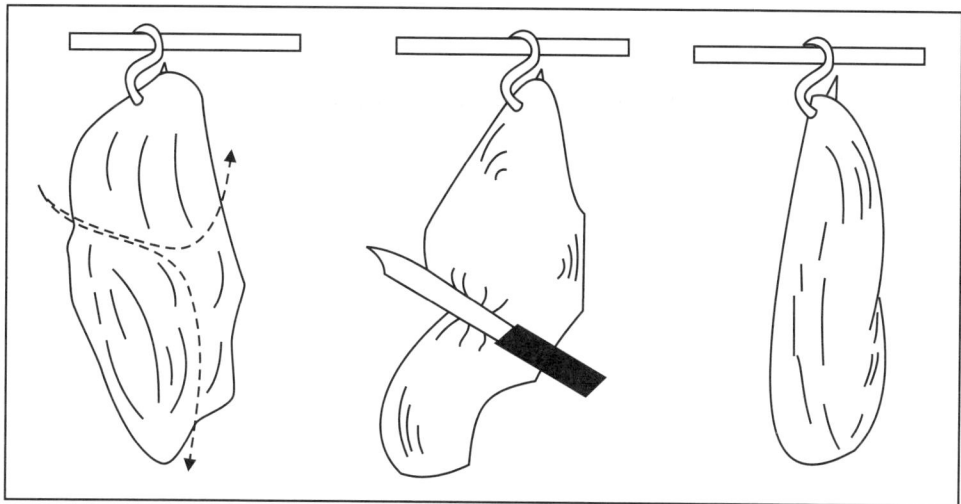

Fig. 12.4. Cutting meat into pieces.

The larger muscles are left in one piece but one piece of meat may contain a number of smaller muscles. Subsequently the pieces of meat are cut into strips. There are two ways to cut the pieces into strips:

1. Place the meat on a board and cut it into strips.
2. Hang the meat up and cut strips off it.

In both cases the meat must be cut in the direction of the muscular tissue (Fig. 12.5).

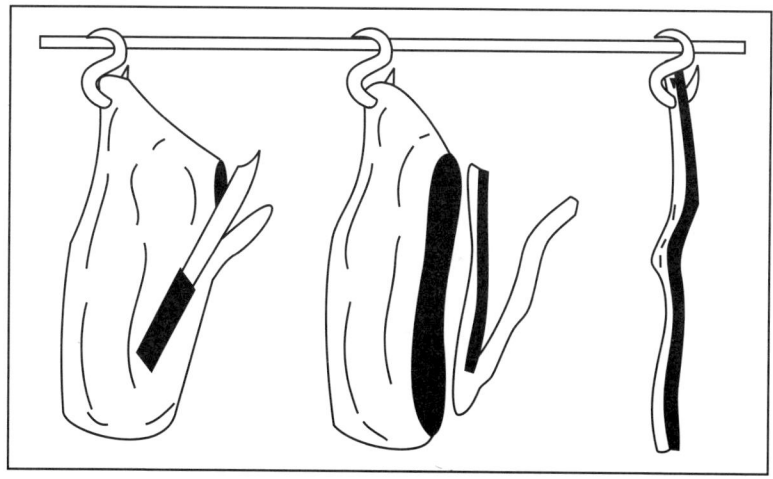

Fig. 12.5. Cutting meat into strips.

The length of the strip can vary from 20 to 70 cm. Short strips of meat take more time to be hung up, but longer strips can break under their own weight when drying.

The thickness of the meat is important in determining the necessary drying time of the meat. In one batch it is important that all the meat strips are equally thick so that after drying you are not left with too dry or not dry enough pieces of meat.

Examples of different thicknesses which are used are:

1. Strips of 1 × 1 cm.
2. Flat strips of 0.5 × (3, 4 or 5 cm).

The exact shape of the strips depends on the preservation method to be used.

It is very important that a clean working surface and knife are used so that the starting material for preservation is good. Personal hygiene is also very important. Further preparatory work such as salting is described under the appropriate preservation method in the following section.

SALTING

General Information

By salting food, storage life is prolonged. Salt absorbs much of the water in the food and makes it difficult for micro-organisms to survive. For salting, it is important that the fish or meat has been prepared in such a way that the salt added can quickly draw into the flesh and the moisture can leave the fish or meat. Large pieces of flesh must be cut into thin slices to allow this.

Fish are divided in half or even in quarters depending on their size. Fish smaller than 10 cm (anchovies, sardines) usually only have their intestines removed. Fish of ±15 cm are split open so that the surface area of the fish is increased, salt can penetrate better, and the flesh of the fish therefore becomes thinner. Large cuts can be made in fish 25 cm or longer, or these can be split a number of times.

To learn how to salt fish, for example the amount of salt needed and the effect of those quantities on the firmness and the taste of the fish, it is recommended at first to use small amounts of different kinds of fish that are easily available. It is easier to start with non-fatty kinds of fish. Lean fish is recognisable by its white or very pale flesh. More fatty fish usually have a darker colour.

The quality of the starting material to be used must be good. Old, rotten fish or fish of poor quality is not improved by salting it and is certainly not storable for longer. The same is true for meat. Salt intended for salting fish should be as clean as possible. The salt may not contain any dust, sand, etc. Salt can contain bacteria which can survive despite a very high salt concentration. These bacteria can therefore also cause salted fish or meat to spoil. Strongly contaminated salt can be recognised by a slightly pink colour. It can be heated on a metal plate over a fire to kill the bacteria. Salt can be very fine or have large chunks; a mixture of fine and coarse salt is best. During the salting of fish and meat in the tropics, attention must be paid to the following:

1. Use the cleanest salt available.
2. Use enough salt. Note that salting products is not the same as using a lot of salt. Large amounts of salt give fish and meat a very salty taste. At the same time many of the nutrients are lost if too much salt is used.
3. The water which is to be used must not be contaminated; it must be clean and clear (drinking water quality).
4. The most effective way of preserving fish and meat is to combine salting with smoking or drying.

Salting Fish

Three ways of salting fish are described here: dry and wet salting (in technical jargon: kench salting and pickle curing) and brining. The first two methods result in fish with a relatively high salt content, the third method is usually used if one wants fish with a relatively low salt content.

For kench salting and pickle curing, 30–40 kg of salt is used per 100 kg of cleaned fish. Using more salt does not improve the process and only leads to unnecessarily high costs: salt is expensive.

Dry salting fish: kench salting

Coarse salt is more suitable for dry (kench) salting. Fine salt will draw water too quickly from the outside of the fish, making the outside hard. As a result the water inside the fish cannot escape and the salt cannot penetrate deep into the fish. Therefore the fish spoils despite being salted. This is known as 'salt burn'. Coarse salt does not have this effect. Kench salting is very suitable for mainly lean kinds of fish.

You will need:

1. Split fish or fish fillets. If the flesh is thick, make cuts in it so the salt can penetrate well.
2. Salt: Use 30–35 kg of salt for 100 kg of cleaned fish. Use more salt where deep cuts have been made or where the flesh is thicker.
3. Baskets or other perforated containers from which moisture can drain.

Method of working (Fig. 12.6):

1. Split fish or fish fillets.
2. Rub the fish well with salt, especially in the deep cuts.
3. Put a thick layer of salt in the bottom of the basket or container.
4. Place one layer of fish with the skin facing up on the salt. The fish are not allowed to overlap.
5. Follow with one layer of salt, one layer of fish, etc. until the basket is full.
6. Cover the basket with a layer of plastic but do not put any weights on it.

By adding salt to fish, moisture is drawn out of the fish. This moisture, with the salt dissolved in it, is called brine. Place the basket on some stones so the brine can drain.

Take care with this method that the fish is piled in such a way that the brine can drain easily and will not collect in spots. If it does, it causes an uneven preservation. After a day the fish must be stacked anew so that the fish which was originally on the bottom now lies on top of the pile. The salt is thus distributed more evenly (replenish it if necessary) and you will not get the effect that the fish on the bottom of the pile has a different amount of salt than the fish on top.

After being salted, the fish must look clear and see-through. The fish must feel firm and have a whitish salt layer all over it. A fishy smell and the smell of brine must dominate.

Strongly salted fish, if it is properly covered, can be stored for a long time. A disadvantage of this method is that the brine drains away, leaving the fish standing dry. Fatty kinds of fish can then turn rancid as they are exposed to air. Scavengers can easily get to the fish and bacteria and moulds cause decay there where insufficient salt has been used.

Wet salting fish: pickle curing

Wet salting is a good way to preserve fatty fish such as herring, sardines, anchovies and mackerel. With this method the fish is better protected against vermin and a more uniform salt distribution is achieved. You will need:

1. A clean watertight barrel with a lid of a smaller diameter than the barrel itself. It must not be made of iron, zinc or aluminium because of corrosion. Plastic, wood, clay or stainless steel is acceptable.

2. Large stones washed clean to be used as weights.
3. Salt. Use one kg of salt for three kg of fish, which is equal to 30–35 kg of salt for 100 kg of fish.
4. A bucket or large pan in which to make brine.
5. Fish. With small fish (<10 cm): leave the fish whole.
6. With large fish (>10 cm): remove the intestines.

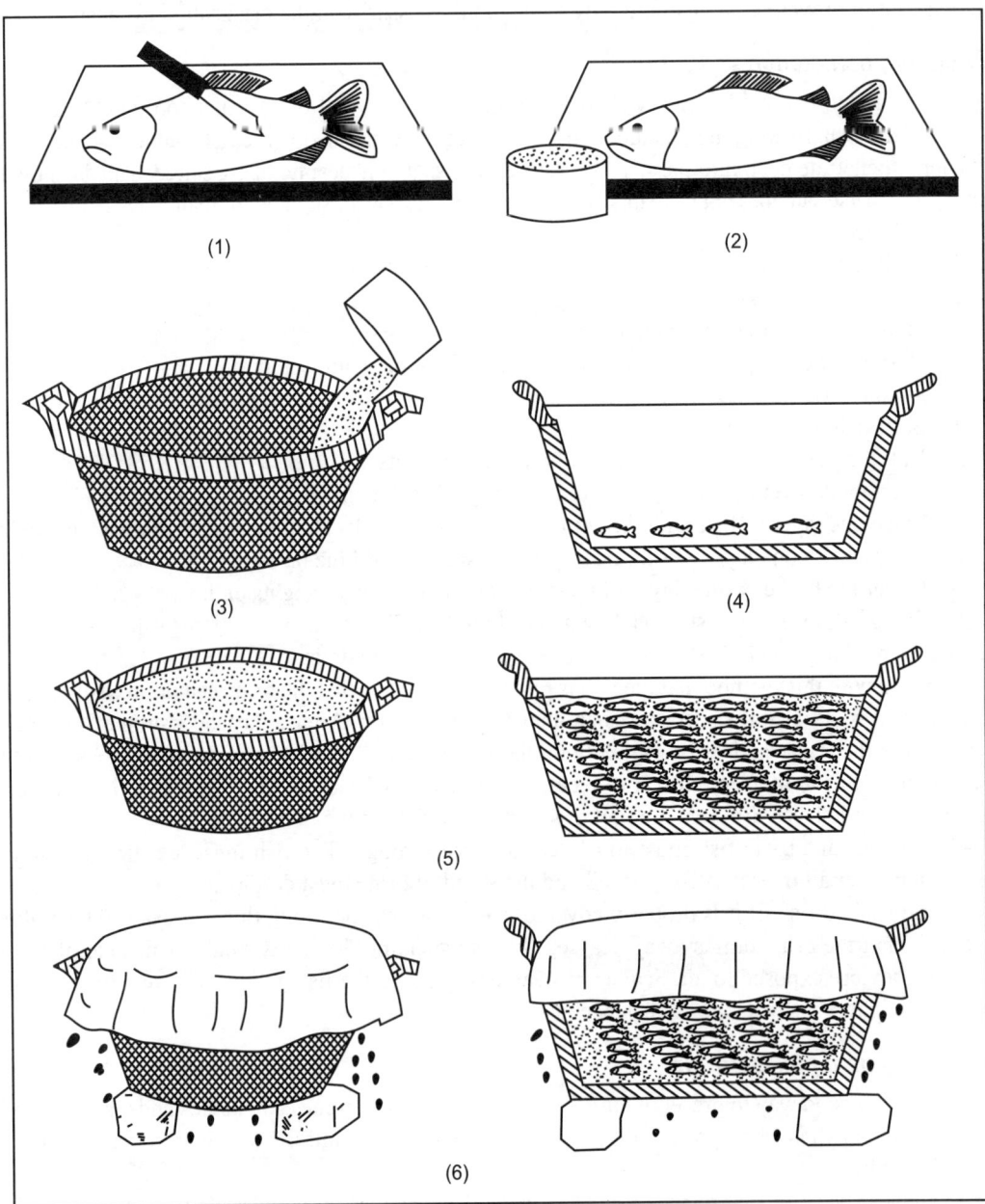

Fig. 12.6. Kench salting.

Method of working:

1. Put a thick layer of salt on the bottom of the barrel.
2. Put one layer of fish on the salt with the skin facing up.
3. Cover the fish with a layer of salt and make sure that no parts are left uncovered. Use more salt at deep cuts or thicker flesh.
4. Alternate one layer of salt, one layer of fish, etc. Make sure the fish do not overlap. Finish with a layer of fish with the skin facing up.
5. Cover the final layer of fish with a thick layer of salt.
6. Cover the barrel with the lid and distribute the weights evenly on top of it.
   As explained above, by adding salt to fish, moisture is drawn out of the fish. This moisture, with the salt dissolved in it, is called brine. Because more and more water is drawn out of the fish, the brine in this wet method becomes diluted. The brine must be topped up with salt to keep it saturated. This can be done by hanging a jute bag filled with fine salt in the brine (Fig. 12.7.).
7. Keep the brine saturated. This can be done by hanging a jute bag filled with fine salt in the brine (Fig. 12.7). Using unsaturated brine will lead to spoilage.
8. If, after several hours, the level of the created brine does not reach the lid, a saturated salt solution must be added.
9. The salt solution is made of at least 360 grams of salt dissolved in each litre of water. Heat the solution in a pan and let it boil for 10 minutes. Let the brine cool down until it is warm to the touch. Then add the brine to the barrel with fish until it reaches the lid.
10. Keep the barrel in as cool a place as possible.

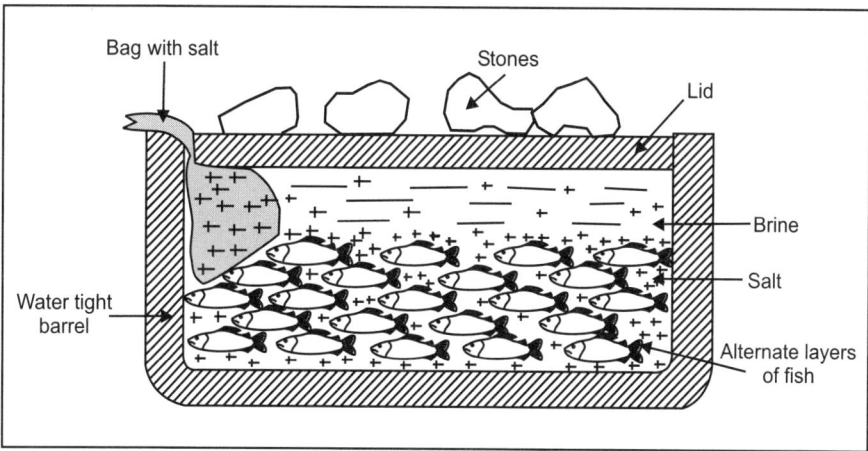

Fig. 12.7. Pickle curing.

After being salted, the fish must look clear and see-through. The fish must feel firm and have a whitish salt layer all over them. A fishy smell and the smell of brine must dominate. Check the container regularly. If foam appears on top of the brine (a result of fermentation), replace the old brine with a fresh brine solution.

Brining

With this method, fish is soaked in a solution of water and salt (brine). Brining is not used as such as a preservation method but as preparation for smoking or drying. The use of a light salt solution ensures a decrease in bacterial growth on the surface of the fish during the smoking or drying process. It also protects the fish against insects and other vermin; however the protection provided is not complete.

You will need:

1. A clean watertight barrel with a lid of a smaller diameter than the barrel itself. It must not be made of iron, zinc or aluminium. Plastic, wood, clay or stainless steel is acceptable.
2. Salt. To make brine, very fine salt is best. Use one kg of salt for three kg of fish.
3. A bucket or large pan in which to make brine.
4. Cleaned, washed large stones to be used as weights.
5. Chicken wire or a bamboo rack.
6. Small fish: Leave the fish whole but remove the intestines.
7. Large fish: Clean large fish and divide them in two. If the fish is larger than 30 cm, cut it into pieces. Make cuts in large, fatty fish.

Method of working:

1. Wash the fish with clear, clean water (preferably of drinking water quality).
2. Soak the fish for 30 minutes to 1 hour (1.5 hours for large fish) in not too strong brine. Make this brine by dissolving 300 grams of salt in every four litres of water. By submerging the fish in this brine, the blood and slime are removed.
3. Next, wash small fish with clear, clean water.
4. Do not wash large fish but let them drain briefly on a bamboo rack, keeping the fish from overlapping.
5. Next, place the fish in a saturated brine solution: 3.0–3.5 kg of salt in 10 litres of water.
6. Mix the brine well before the fish are put in it; all of the salt must be dissolved. If the fish sink, add more salt.
7. Cover the container with a clean board or mat and put clean washed stones on top of that until the fish are covered by the brine.
8. Leave the fish for 5–6 hours in this brine. Leave larger fish longer in the brine than smaller fish.
9. Take the fish out of the brine.
10. Put the fish on the chicken wire or bamboo rack to drain, taking care not to let the fish overlap.
11. Cover the fish with a clean white cloth or mosquito netting. Do not let the netting touch the fish.

The fish is now ready to be dried or smoked.

Salting Meat

The methods of salting meat are very comparable to those for fish. To get good results, one should start with fresh meat.

Dry salting meat

This method of salting is used for meat which is to be dried after being salted.

You will need:

1. Fresh, raw meat in long strips that weigh 1.5–2 kg and are about 1 cm thick.
2. Salt. Use 30–35 kg of salt for 100 kg of meat.
3. Clean wood or plastic sheets, perforated.
4. Heavy stones.

Method of working:

1. Always take care to work in a hygienic way; for example wash your hands well at every step of the process to prevent cross-contamination.

2. After cutting the meat, wash it in clean, running water and let the strips drain briefly in the shade.
3. Place the meat for 1 hour in a saturated salt solution (brine). This brine is made by dissolving at least 360 grams of salt in every litre of water. Dissolve the salt completely before placing the meat in the brine.
4. Next, hang the meat up above the brine to let it drip dry.
5. Rub the meat thoroughly with salt; use a total of 30–35 kg of salt for 100 kg of meat.
6. Put a 1–2 cm thick layer of salt on a (perforated) wooden or plastic board, or if possible, a concrete or stone slab with diagonal grooves.
7. Put the meat on top of this layer of salt. Put another 1–2 cm layer of salt on top of the layer of meat. Alternate one layer of meat, one layer of salt, etc. until the pile is about 1–1.5 metres high.
8. Cover the pile with a wood or plastic board on which there are several heavy, clean stones to weigh it down. The liquid which comes out of the meat must be able to drain away.
9. The next day, rotate the layers by putting the top layers on the bottom and the bottom layers of meat on top. Again, use salt. If after two days the liquid starts to come out of the pile, and no more liquid drips out of the meat, the process can be stopped. If this is not the case, keep on rotating the layers of meat until no more moisture comes out of the meat. Only then can the drying process start.

Wet salting meat

One can also wet salt meat by placing it in brine (pickling). In that case it is not necessary to dry the meat. This salting process gives the best results when the process and the storage of the final product take place at as low a temperature as possible.

Pickling

You will need:
1. Fresh, raw meat in strips that are 2–3 cm thick and weigh 0.5–1 kg.
2. Salt: Use 10 kg of salt for 100 kg of meat.
3. A clean watertight barrel, with a lid of a smaller diameter than the barrel itself. It must not be made of iron, zinc or aluminium because of corrosion. Plastic, wood, clay or stainless steel is acceptable.
4. Large stones.
5. A large pan in which to make brine.

Method of working (Fig. 12.8):
1. Cut raw meat in strips.
2. Spread a layer of salt on the bottom of the barrel and put a layer of meat on top of it. Alternate one layer of salt, one layer of meat until the barrel is full.
3. Place the lid on top of the meat and push it down using the stones. Let the meat stand for two weeks, during which time brine is formed from the salt and the moisture leaving the meat.
4. Take the meat out of the brine and rinse it with cold (drinking) water.
5. Make a brine solution of at least 360 grams of salt per litre of water.
6. Boil the brine for several minutes.
7. Let it cool until it is warm to the touch.
8. Put the rinsed meat in a clean, empty barrel. Fill the barrel with the boiled, saturated brine. In this way the meat is preserved for later consumption.

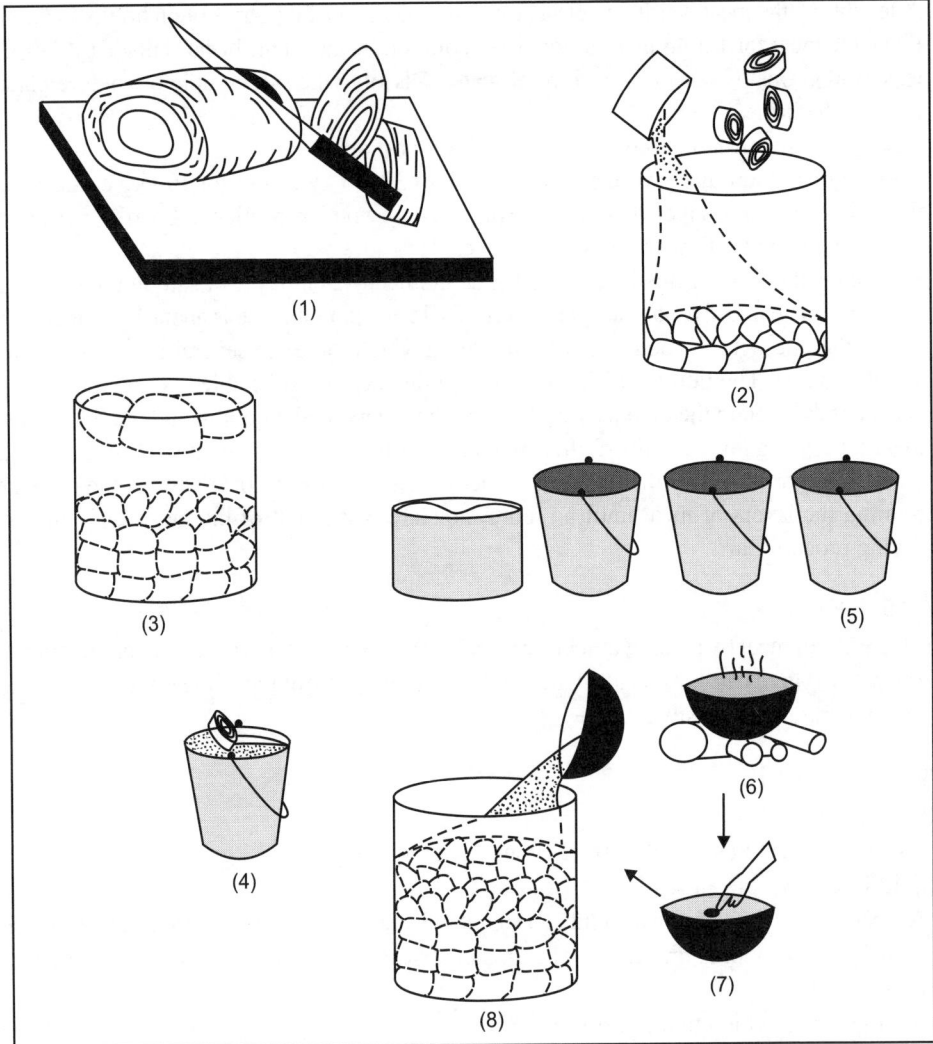

Fig. 12.8. Pickling.

Alternative method of pickle brining

Below an alternative pickling method is described which can be used as an initial preparation for drying meat.

For what you need (materials): Pickling.

Method of working:

1. Follow the method described above; let the meat cure for two weeks during which time a brine is formed from the salt and the moisture leaving the meat.
2. Soak the meat in boiled water for 2–3 hours to remove any excess salt. Refresh the water 2–3 times with clean, freshwater.
3. The meat is now ready to be sun-dried.

Brine salting

With this method, meat is soaked in a solution of water and salt (brine). Brining is not used as such as a preservation technique but as preparation for the smoking or drying of meat. The use of a light brine solution slows bacterial growth at the surface of the meat during the smoking or drying process. It also protects the meat against insects and other vermin; however, it does not provide complete protection.

You will need:

1. Fresh, raw meat in long strips of about 1 cm thick.
2. Salt: Use a 15 per cent salt solution (150 grams of salt per litre of water). Very fine salt is best for making brine.
3. A strainer.

Method of working:

1. Submerge the strips of meat in the brine as soon as the salt has dissolved in the water. Leave the meat in the brine for 5–10 minutes.
2. Let the meat drain in a strainer. Catch the brine for reuse. The meat can now be dried and/or smoked.

Preparing Salted Fish and Meat for Consumption

Fish

Before salted fish can be used it must first be soaked in clean, cold water for 48 hours. When the weather is very warm the fish must not be left any longer. The water must be replaced several times by clean, freshwater. Fish can also be broken up into pieces before being soaked. If the fish is very salty it can also be slowly heated in water (until just before boiling) for about 1 hour. However, the preserved fish, salted, dried and/or smoked, must eventually always be heated to 100°C (212°F) before being eaten.

Meat

Heavily salted meat must be soaked for at least a day prior to use in cold (drinking) water. The water must be replaced regularly by freshwater. One can also let the meat boil gently for several hours over a low fire. If the meat is very salty, soak it in (drinking) water and also boil it for about an hour. How long one should soak the meat or let it boil gently, depends on the final taste desired.

DRYING

General Information on Natural Drying

Spoilage of fish and meat is slowed when water is drawn from the fish or meat. This can be achieved by salting as described in section but also by naturally drying fish or meat. The best results are achieved by combining salting with drying. Salting the fish or meat is not essential but has great advantages and is therefore strongly recommended before drying. The salting ensures, among other things, that during drying the micro-organisms at the surface are inhibited and insects and other vermin are kept away. Thus the spoilage of material is slowed. After drying, salt gives a more stable product with a longer storage life. The use of salt before drying and the manner of salting depend on the availability of salt and local customs. Generally very small fish are dried unsalted. Large fish will spoil before the drying process is completed and therefore salting is necessary.

It is important that fish and meat be prepared in such a way that salt can be quickly drawn into the flesh and moisture can quickly leave. To achieve this, try to keep the flesh of the products thin and the surface area of the product as large as possible. Be sure to work as hygienically as possible.

Make sure that a batch of meat or fish to be dried is made up of pieces of roughly the same size. This ensures that the whole batch dries evenly and that after drying part of the product is not too dry or actually not dry enough.

Very fatty fish or meat is difficult to convert into a good salted and/or dried product. The problem is that the fat forms a barrier to salt penetration and/or loss of moisture.

Preparation

Salting is part of the preparation for drying, and depends among other things on the availability of salt and on local customs.

After salting, the excess water formed must be removed from the fish or meat. With meat, it can be done by passing the larger pieces of meat through a wringer (two wooden rolls 1.5–2.0 cm apart). In doing so, the surface area is also increased which reduces the time needed for drying. A somewhat simpler method for removing moisture is to press meat and (mainly whole) fish.

Put the fish on a clean, level surface and, using sheets of e.g. wood with weights on them, press the fish or meat as flat as possible. Subsequently the fish and meat is hung up before drying to speed up the drying process.

Hanging Fish and Meat up to Dry

Fish can be hung up in several ways on horizontal sticks to dry. It is advisable to hang fish on hooks or with string tied around the tails (Fig. 12.9).

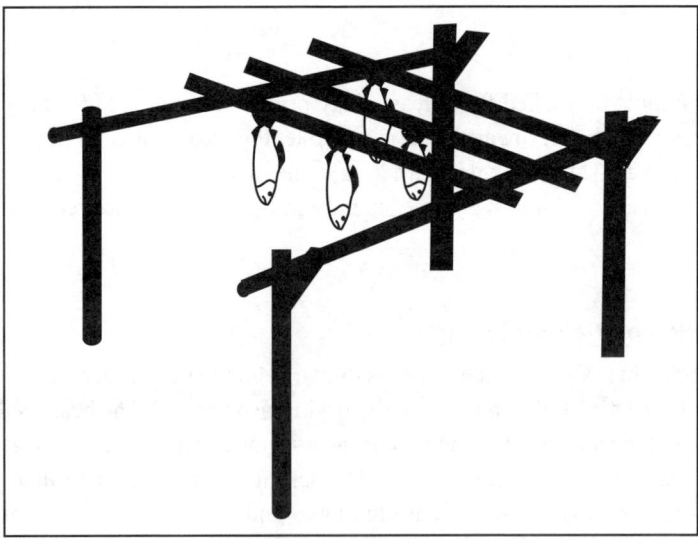

Fig. 12.9. Drying fish.

Meat to be dried is hung on hooks or on strings. The pieces of meat are then evenly spaced on sticks hanging horizontally in such a way that the pieces of meat do not touch (Figs 12.10 and 12.11).

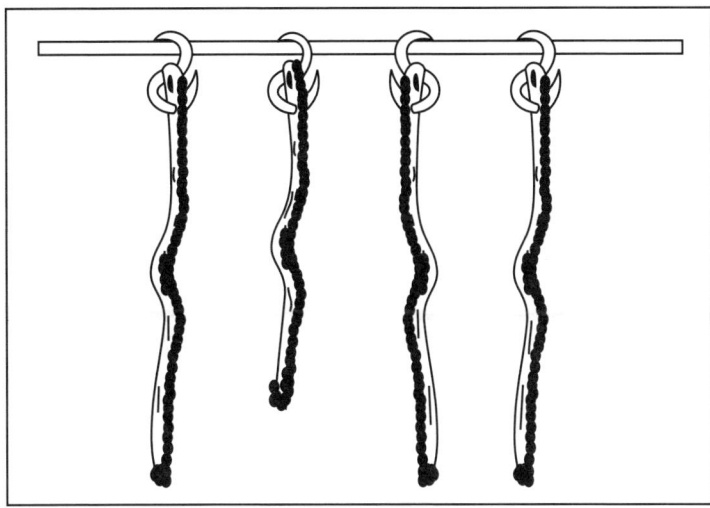

Fig. 12.10. Hanging up strips of meat on hooks and strings.

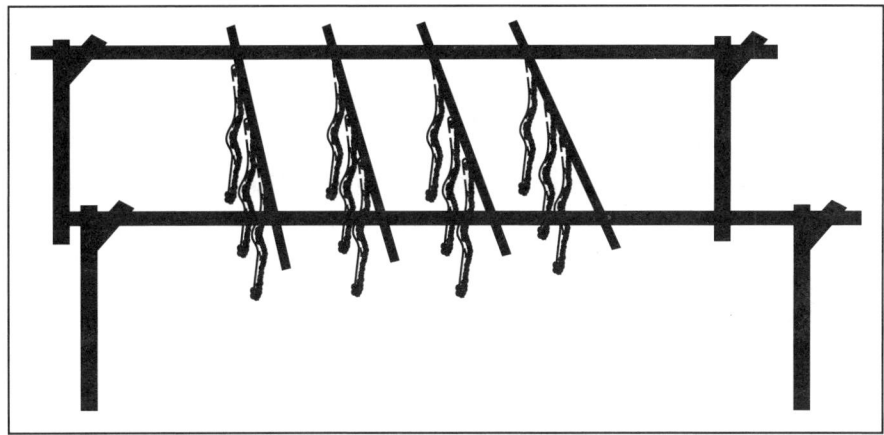

Fig. 12.11. Simple construction of wood for drying meat.

With this method of drying, air is free to circulate all-around the meat and the product will dry quickest and most uniformly. If there is no free air circulation, some parts will remain moist. Spoilage by bacteria or insect damage (they are carriers of bacteria) can especially start at such places.

Whole fish, fish fillets or meat can also be dried on drying racks made of chicken wire or bamboo poles (Fig. 12.12). The disadvantage of this method is that, due to the contact between the meat or fish and the poles or wire, there is a chance the product will remain moist in places and thus cannot dry completely.

Drying Process

Drying must take place carefully and uniformly. The best results are achieved in dry weather with a lot of wind. Take care that the meat or fish does not get so hot the fat starts to melt or that a crust is formed on the surface. The inside of the fish or meat would then stay moist which would make it spoil quickly. Therefore do not put the meat or fish to be dried directly in the sun at the start of the drying process. In the early morning or the late afternoon sun, the product to be dried will stay relatively cool, but in the middle of the day it must be protected against overheating by temporarily putting it in the shade. Experience will teach you what the best method is.

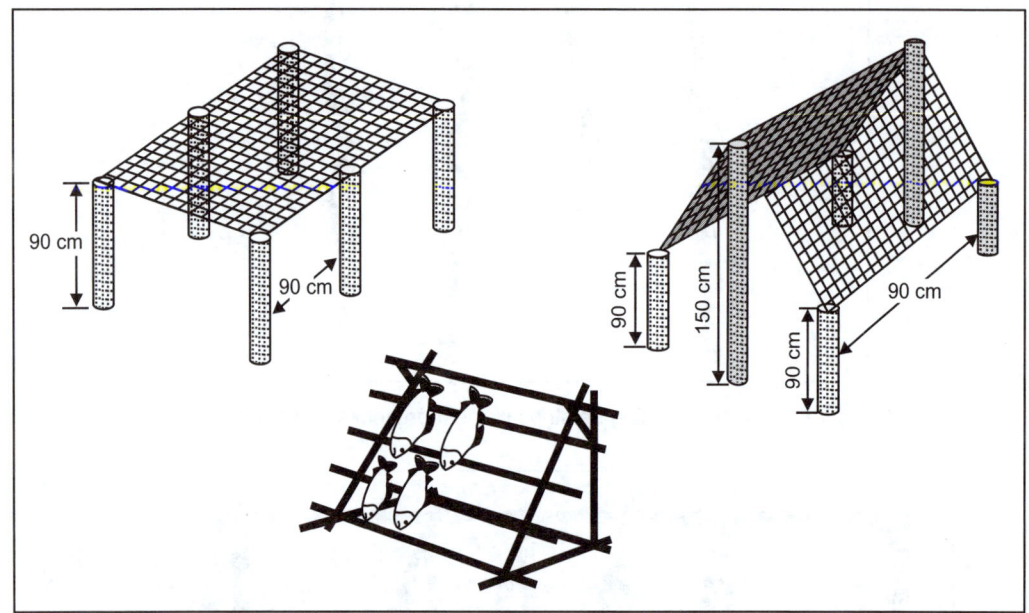

Fig. 12.12. Drying racks with horizontal and downward sloping drying surfaces.

If drying racks are used, the pieces of fish or meat must be turned every two hours so they dry uniformly. The product to be dried must be protected as much as possible against vermin and insects. Insects are carriers of various bacteria which can cause the product to spoil. Bluebottle or carrion flies lay their eggs on the still damp product and their larvae eat the flesh. Beetles of the species Dermestes lay their eggs especially in the already dried product. Try to prevent such insects from nestling in or near the material to be dried. To do so, remove all animal waste from the immediate vicinity. This is a highly suitable breeding place for these kinds of insects. Using a good salting technique helps to keep the insects at a distance during drying. Also use mosquito netting to keep insects, and especially the bluebottle/carrion flies, away. Do not let the netting touch the material to be dried.

Put the drying rack at least one metre above the ground so that other vermin do not get a chance to get to the product. Put the legs of the rack in a pan of water to which a little oil has been added.

The meat or fish must be protected against dusty wind, rain and dew. The products can be covered with banana or palm leaves or plastic. They can of course also be put under an awning or in a shed. However, put the products to be dried out in the sun again as soon as possible to let them dry further.

Dried Fish and Meat: Storage and Use

Fish

How long fish must dry depends on the type of fish, its size and the weather. The final moisture content must be less than 25 per cent to prevent microbial spoilage. Weighing the fish before and after the drying process can tell you whether the fish is dry enough. If during the drying process the weight of the fish does not decrease further, it is sufficiently dry. In general, naturally dried fish needs about 3–10 days to dry. After drying, the dried fish is difficult to bend. Some of the dried fish products are very crumbly and breakable and must be handled with care after being dried.

In dry climates it is possible to store dried fish in sealable, sturdy boxes or wooden crates in which ventilation holes have been made. The holes must be covered with mosquito netting to keep out insects and vermin.

In humid conditions dried fish can take up moisture from the air and must be packed airtight. An additional advantage of airtight packaging is a delay in the onset of rancidity in fatty fish. Strong plastic bags can be used which are then closed properly. These provide protection against insects and moisture. However, the bags should not be placed in the direct sun or in warm places. The product can then start sweating; there is, after all, some moisture left. This moisture can cause mould to grow on the fish. When such moisture is seen, the fish should be redried in the sun for several hours and re-packed.

Store the packed, dried fish in a cool, dry, well-ventilated and dark place. Before unsalted or salted dried fish can be eaten, it must first be soaked in clean, cold water for 48 hours. In very warm weather, the fish should not be left standing longer than that. The water must be replaced several times by clean, freshwater. Fish can also be broken into smaller pieces before being soaked. If the fish is very salty, it can be slowly heated in water (until just before boiling) for about 1 hour. However, preserved fish, whether salted, dried and/or smoked, must eventually always be heated to 100°C (212°F) before being eaten!

Meat

Experience will help you determine when meat is dry enough. Often this is after 5 days, depending on the weather. Well-dried meat has a uniform appearance after being broken. The colour is the same throughout the product and is often dark red. The consistency is hard and when it is pushed with a finger, it does not give. The smell and taste of dried meat is different to that of fresh meat. Light oxidation of the meat fats gives a typical dried meat taste. Meat which has any signs of spoilage should not be stored any longer nor eaten.

After drying, the meat can be packed and stored. In dry climates it is possible to store dried meat in sealable, sturdy boxes or wooden crates in which ventilation holes have been made. These holes must be covered with mosquito netting to keep out insects and vermin. One can also store-dried meat in closed (jute) bags hung from the ceiling to keep out any vermin. In humid conditions dried meat can take up moisture from the air and must be packed airtight. Strong plastic bags can be used which are then closed properly. Keep the packed meat in a cool, dry, well-ventilated and dark place. In such conditions, welldried meat can be kept for months.

Before using salted or unsalted dried meat, it must first be soaked in boiling water or be boiled gently. How long the meat is soaked or heated depends on the desired taste and consistency.

Solar Drying

Natural drying of fish and meat sometimes has disadvantages. Long periods of sunshine are required, the drying speed is slow and in areas with a relatively high humidity it is often difficult to dry the fish and meat adequately. An alternative for conventional sun drying is solar drying.

Improved sun drying for fish

A solar tent dryer can be used for solar drying. This is the simplest and cheapest way of solar drying. Solar dryers work by retaining the heat of the sun's rays. A higher drying temperature and thus greater drying speed can then be achieved. The moisture content of the final product is lower than that achieved with conventional sun drying. All this means that the chance of spoilage occurring during the drying process and storage is smaller. The higher temperatures in a tent dryer slow down bacterial growth on and in the product and kill insects and their larvae if they are present in the product. Product loss due to insect damage is thus less than with sun drying. A tent dryer (Fig. 12.13) is almost completely sealed so the product is protected against rain, dust, vermin, etc. Inlet and outlet openings can be covered with taped-on pieces of mosquito netting if necessary. All these factors ensure that the final product is of higher quality.

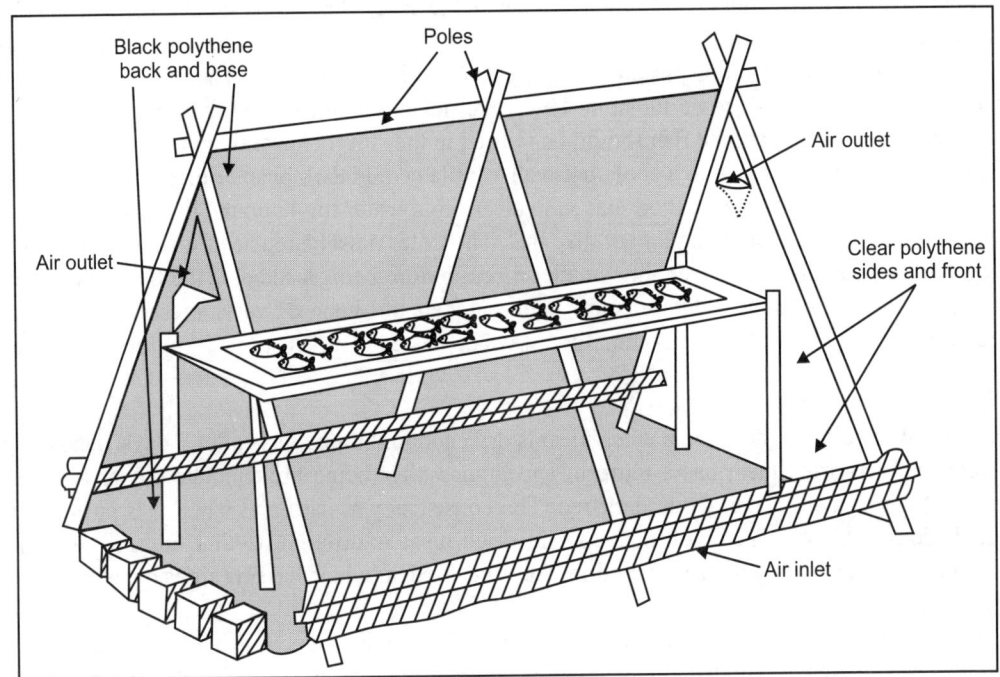

Fig. 12.13. Solar tent dryer.

It is relatively easy to make a tent dryer and it requires little material. The dryer consists of a tent-shaped frame of bamboo or wooden poles covered with a piece of strong plastic. For the sun side of the tent and the two sides, transparent plastic is used. For the shadow side and the ground, black plastic is used. The black plastic absorbs and retains the heat from the sun. Along the whole length in the middle of the tent a drying rack is placed on which the products are spread. Put the drying rack about 30 cm above the ground. By opening one side panel the drying rack can be put inside the tent. Close this side again well by putting sand or stones on the base of the plastic (Fig. 12.13).

The transparent plastic on the front side is wrapped around a stick at the bottom. In this way the plastic can be rolled up or let down to allow air into the tent and to regulate the temperature a bit. The air entering is heated in the tent and absorbs moisture when it flows past the fish on the rack. The humid air can leave the tent through both air outlets in the top of the tent.

A disadvantage of tent dryers is that they are light in weight which makes them susceptible to damage in windy weather. The tent dryer also requires the use of a lot of plastic, which can be costly.

Experience will help you determine when the fish is dry enough and can be packed. The drying time depends on the kind and the size of the fish.

SMOKING

General Information

Raw fish and meat can also be preserved by smoking. The preserving effect of the smoke is a result of drying (withdrawal of moisture) of the product during the smoking. The smoke particles, absorbed by the flesh, also have a preserving effect which, however, is less than the drying effect. The smoke particles, after being absorbed by the product, inhibit bacterial growth on the surface of the product. The smoke particles also have a positive effect on the taste and colour of the product.

The heat of the fire dries the fish or meat during the smoking process and if the temperature gets high enough, the flesh is cooked. This means that bacterial spoilage and spoilage due to enzyme activity is prevented. Drying and cooking of the flesh when being smoked play an important role in the preservation. If a product is well dried during smoking then it can be stored for a long time.

There are three ways of smoking:

Cold smoke method: The temperature during the smoking is at most 30°C (86°F) which means the product does not get cooked.

Hot smoke method: During this process the product does get cooked but not dried (temperature varies between 65° and ±100°C [149°–212°F]).

Smoke drying: During this process, the product is first hot smoked, so that it gets cooked, and then, with continued smoking the product is dried (temperatures vary between 45°–85°C [113°–185°F]).

Cold smoking gives a product which is not cooked. It is, therefore, susceptible to spoilage and must be kept cool. The storage life of a coldsmoked product is not greater than that of fresh fish or meat. Furthermore, it is difficult to control the process in high ambient temperatures; the temperature may not rise above 30°C (86°F). The process demands strict hygiene and the danger of spoilage occurring during the smoking process itself is present. Because of these disadvantages, this process will not be described further in this section. Hot smoking, during which the fish or meat is heated without being dried, extends the storage life of raw products by at most two days. Hot smoking will also therefore not be described further.

Most traditional smoked products in the tropics belong to the third category. They are hot smoked and subsequently dried under continued smoking (smoke drying). The process takes about 12–18 hours or even days, depending on the product. Sometimes the product is salted and/or pre-dried before being smoke dried. The smoke drying method will be described further below. Because smoking is virtually the same for meat and fish, no further distinction will be made between the two.

Preparation

Fish can be smoked whole, cleaned, split or filleted, depending on local preferences and the desired final product. Meat must be cut into strips 5 cm wide and 1 cm thick before being smoked. An important fact is that the greater the surface area of the meat or fish, the greater the amount of smoke particles which can be absorbed during smoking and the better the product can dry.

It is advisable to kench salt or brine the product in a saturated salt solution before smoking. This extends the storage qualities of the final product. Remove excess salt after salting by rinsing the raw material in clean (drinking) water, since salt can form a hard, impenetrable crust during smoking.

It is also advisable to dry the raw product for an hour in the sun before smoking it. This prevents the outer layer of the fish or meat from sealing shut (case hardening) during smoking. That would mean the outer layer (which in the case of fish is their skin) would no longer allow moisture to pass through and therefore the inside of the fish would not be able to dry properly. Insufficiently dried fish or meat cannot be stored long. Furthermore, pre-drying fish gives it a nice shiny surface layer. Whether or not a product is salted and/or dried before smoking depends on local customs and preferences.

The fish are threaded on stakes or tied to them using string or hooks. Meat is attached to sticks using string or hooks. Products which are hung up may not touch each other during smoking. The smoke would then not be able to reach everywhere and the product would not dry uniformly.

Wood

The best smoke production is obtained from a smouldering fire of wood shavings and hard wood blocks. One can best begin the smoking process by burning damp wood. After that, smoke with dry wood. Some kinds of wood (such as oleander) are not suitable for smoking as they contain poisonous substances.

All wood from deciduous trees and pines is reported to be safe. A disadvantage of smoking is that a lot of wood is needed. If wood is scarce, one can also use papyrus, palm kernels, peeled maize-cobs and coconut husks as fuel.

Smoking Ovens

The smoking process has the best results in a dry environment. It is therefore often better to work in a smoke house rather than in the open air. A few types of smoking ovens are described below.

Simple ovens

The simplest oven is open grating on which the meat or fish is placed with a smouldering fire underneath. The capacity is small, however, and there is much loss of smoke. An improvement is an oven made of layers of dried mud or clay or oil drums, with a grating on top [Figs 12.14(a) and 12.14(b)]. The grating is best made from wood; steel can scorch the fish. A number of these small ovens can be put in a hut.

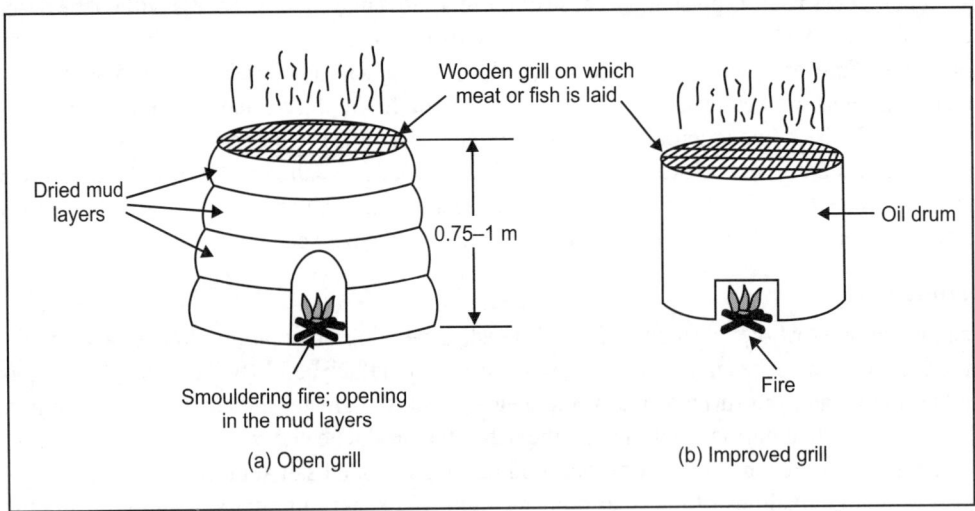

Fig. 12.14. Simple ovens.

Oil-drum smoking ovens

Another possible model is a few oil drums placed on top of each other. The rims must fit well. A damp sack is placed over the rim of the top drum. This system uses the smoke more efficiently. The order of the drums or of the meat in the drums, must be changed regularly as the lowest drum gets most of the heat and the smoke [Fig. 12.15(b)]. Oil drums and mud ovens can only be used to make smoked products.

One disadvantage of these kinds of oven is that the temperature is difficult to control and in the end the products are not equally or uniformly smoked. The ovens are sensitive to the influence of rain and wind. An advantage is, of course, the low cost of materials to make these ovens.

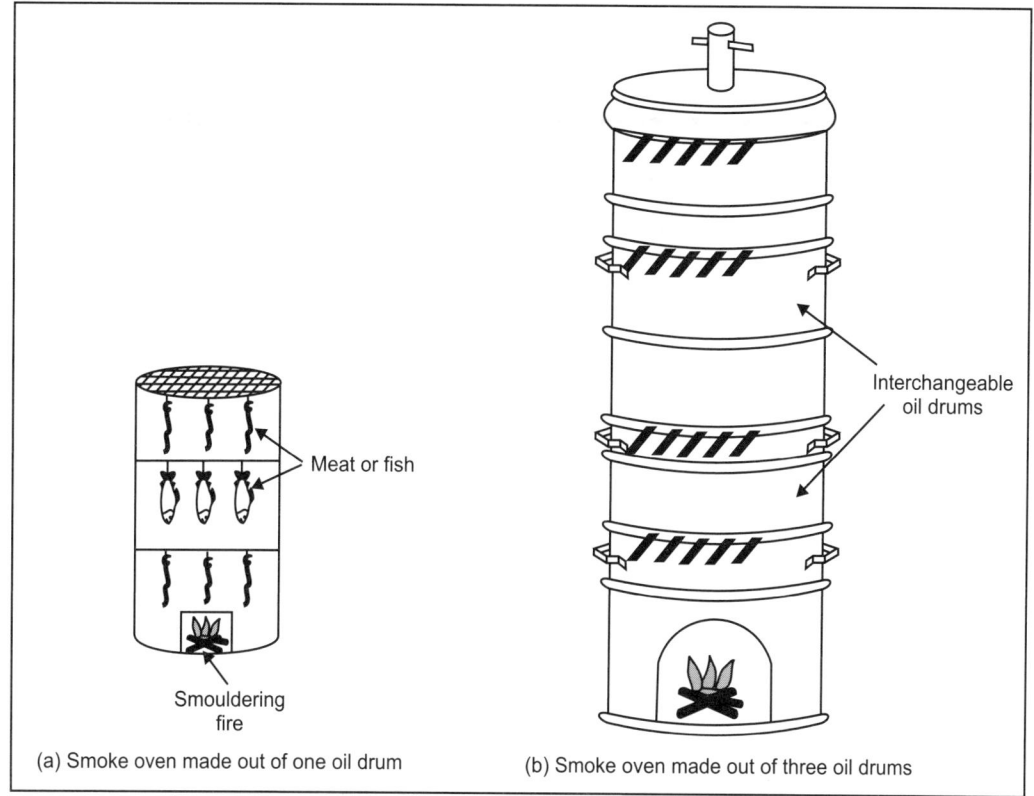

(a) Smoke oven made out of one oil drum

(b) Smoke oven made out of three oil drums

Fig. 12.15. Oil-drum smoking ovens.

Chorkor oven

The chorkor oven is shown in Fig. 12.16. This large, rectangular smoking oven is especially suited for smoking smaller fish. It consists of a rectangular fire box onto which a number of shallow wooden framed wire mesh trays are stacked. Fish are placed on the trays and firewood is burnt in the fire box. The fire box can be constructed in different ways:

1. Clay and mud shaped by hand.
2. Packed mud faced with cement.
3. Clay mud blocks and mortar.
4. Cement blocks with mortar.

The use of cement is more expensive, but the oven will last longer (Fig. 12.16). The stoke holes should be arched for structural strength. The oven should be low, for ease of stacking up to 15 trays, but the flames of the fire should be at least 50 cm removed from the lowest tray, hence a 10–20 cm fire pit is required for each stoke hole. The smoker is designed so that wooden trays will rest along the midlines of the oven walls.

The top tray may be covered by a sheet of plywood or corrugated iron. During the smoking process trays can be exchanged. This way the fish are smoked more uniformly.

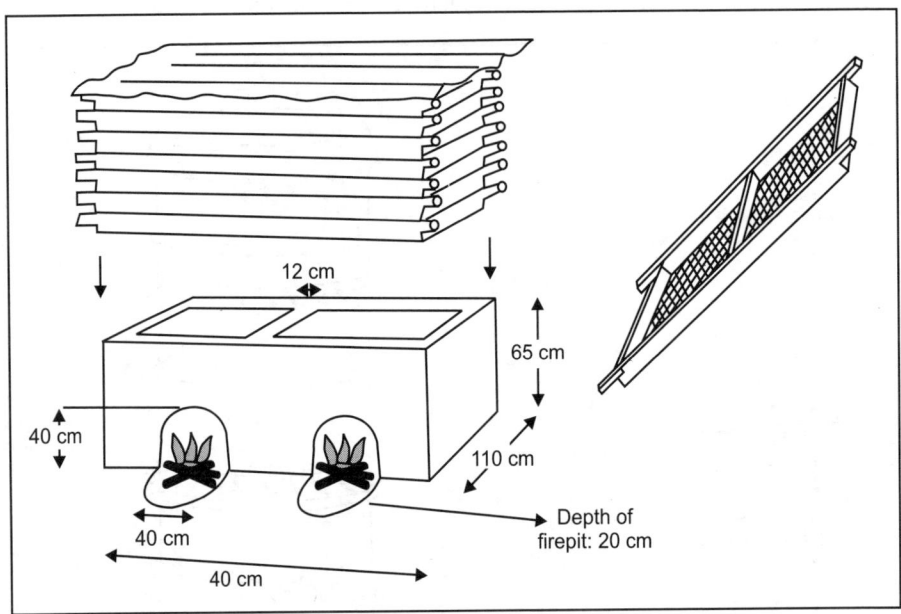

Fig. 12.16. Chorkor oven.

Smokehouse

The last suggestion is to build a smokehouse. This house should have a floor space of about 2 by 2 metres. Place an oil drum on an earthen or stone floor. Fire proof the place where the drum stands with stone walls. Remove the bottom from the drum and build a grate for the fire a little above the bottom. Make a door in the drum to regulate the oxygen flow and cut smoke holes in the top. Build shelves above the drum on which to put the meat. Leave enough room to let the smoke permeate the house. Instead of shelves, the walls can have supports to rest removable beams on. The meat and fish can be hung from these beams. The walls and the roof must be closed so that the smoke cannot escape. Build a ventilation valve or flap into the roof. This can be used to control the smoke circulation (Fig. 12.17). When one builds a completely closed smokehouse, the fire can be made directly on the floor. Hang the meat on ropes or hooks above the oven.

Smoke-drying Process

Start the smoking process with a smouldering fire using some damp wood so that a lot of smoke (at ±45°C/113°F) is produced. This damp smoke forms a layer of moisture on the surface of the product which allows smoke particles to be absorbed quicker.

Next, slowly raise the temperature (to ±85°C/185°F) by allowing more oxygen to enter. With fish do not allow the temperature to rise too quickly as the skin may split and case hardening can occur. Case hardening can also occur during the smoking of meat. The product is then cooked for a short time

(2–4 hours) at ±85°C (185°F). It must be remembered that at such temperatures fat will leak from the product and be lost. You will, therefore, be left with a final product which has a lower fat content.

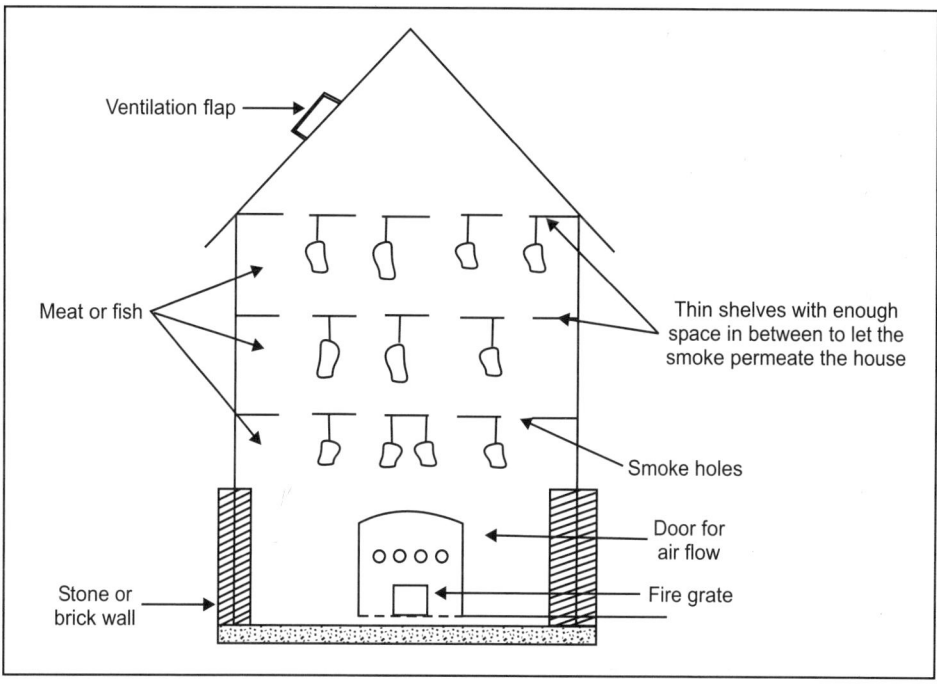

Fig. 12.17. Smokehouse.

If the smoking is continued after 2–4 hours at a lower temperature (±50°C/122°F) for several hours, the product will slowly dry further. Lower the temperature of the smoke by reducing the oxygen flow to the fire. Smoke the products at this temperature until they are sufficiently dried. A cheaper alternative is to do all or part of the drying using solar energy.

The smoked and dried final product should be clearly brown, nice and dry and have a hard structure. If the final product is well dried, it can be kept for several months.

Experience will help you determine when the fish or meat has been properly smoked and dried. The total smoking time also depends on the oven used and the kind of fish or meat. Smoke-dried fish or meat can be stored in the same way as dried fish or meat, as already described in this chapter. The final product can be eaten dry or cooked well in clean (drinking) water.

FERMENTING FISH

General Information

Fish is an important source of protein in the daily diet. However, fish also has the disadvantage that it spoils quickly. If fish is not boiled, salted, dried, smoked or preserved in some other way, it will quickly spoil. In South-East Asia, fermentation is the most important way of preserving fish. Fermented fish pastes and sauces have a much more important place in the daily diet than salted or dried fish. Fish sauces and pastes provide a welcome variation in the monotonous South-East Asian diet which often consists mainly of rice. Although fermented fish products are a good source of protein, they can be consumed only in limited quantities because of the high salt content of these products. Fermentation of fish is especially used in situations where drying of fish is not possible because the climate is too wet and where cooling and sterilisation of the product is too expensive.

Fermentation

During the fermentation of fish, protein is broken down in the presence of a high salt concentration. The fish protein is mainly broken down by enzymes which come from the fish itself. These enzymes are mainly present in the gut. In the traditional fermentation methods in which the intestines are removed from the fish, fermentation will often be slower as there are fewer enzymes present in the flesh.

Role of micro-organisms

Micro-organisms probably play no role in the breaking down of protein during fermentation. However, micro-organisms which can tolerate salt (because of the high concentrations of salt which are used during fermentation of fish) do seem to contribute to the specific taste and smell of the fermented product.

In some traditional fermentation techniques, such as in the production of sushi, a fermentable source of carbohydrates such as boiled rice is added to the fermented fish product. This combination stimulates the growth of lactic acid bacteria. The rice is a source of sugars for the lactic acid bacteria. Due to the formation of lactic acid, which is desirable in these products, the pH of the fish mixture is lowered making the product safer and easier to keep.

Salt

Salt is used to draw liquid out of the fish and to control the fermentation. Thus, the high salt content (20–30 per cent) ensures that spoilage due to bacteria is prevented and that the number of bacteria present drops as quickly as possible during fermentation. From a nutritional point of view, however, it would be best to use as little salt as possible. The high salt concentration also slows down the fermentation speed.

Traditional Fermentation Methods

The fermentation methods described in this section are traditional methods. That is to say that the fermentation is allowed to take place by chance and is guided by experience. No control is exerted over the fermentation. If enough salt is added, some 30 per cent by weight of fish, and there is no influx of air during the fermentation process (anaerobic environment), the fermentation will proceed by itself. The fermentation methods are more or less standard for a given region. Local adaptations or changes in the procedure can, of course, be found.

Experience will help determine whether or not the fermentation has gone well. If the product is different than normal, for example if it has a different colour or smell, the product should not be eaten.

Traditional products are divided into two groups:
1. Products which, in the presence of salt, are fermented by the enzymes present in the fish flesh and intestines.
2. Products which are fermented in the presence of boiled or roasted rice.

Usually in South-East Asia boiled rice is added to the fish-salt mixture.

There are three kinds of fermented fish products:
1. The fish flesh is converted into a liquid fish sauce.
2. The fish is converted into a paste.
3. The fish, whole or in pieces, retains as much as possible of its own structure.

Fermented fish products are eaten mainly in South-East Asia. Protein consumption is relatively low in those countries and the most important sources of protein are fish and fish products. Fermented fish products are an important protein supplement. They contain a number of essential amino acids which can form an important addition to the daily diet. For example, fish sauce contains a lot of the amino acid lysine. This amino acid is found only in small quantities in rice.

The quality of the resulting product depends on the fat content of the fish, the enzyme activity in the fish flesh, contaminations in the salt used and the temperature. Contaminated salt can be recognised by its slightly pink colour and can be purified by heating the salt on a metal sheet over a fire. If the same fermentation process takes place at a higher temperature, a completely different product results.

Fish used

Often the surplus or the side catch of the main catch are fermented. These fish would otherwise be lost to spoilage. Mainly small kinds of fish are used. Table 12.1 lists the different kinds of fish used in South-East Asia for fermentation.

Table 12.1. Saltwater and freshwater fish and crustaceans which are mainly used in the fermentation methods of South-East Asia.

Product group	Species
Saltwater fish	Anchovies, herring, deep-bodied herring, Fimbriated herring, mackerel, round scad, slipmouth
Freshwater fish	Carp, catfish, climbing perch, gourami, mudfish
Shellfish and crustaceans	Shrimp, mussels, oysters, octopus

Fermented Fish Sauce with 20–25 per cent Salt

Fish are washed and left intact. The fish are then packed with large quantities of salt in earthenware or wooden containers. Usually 1 kg of salt is used for 3 to 4 kg of fish. The containers are filled to the rim so that no air is present and sealed so as to create an anaerobic environment. The fish protein is broken down as a result of the activity of the enzymes present in the fish. After several months a clear, amber coloured liquid will have been formed which is separated from the residue by squeezing it out. Sometimes a fish sauce can also be made during the preparation of fish paste. Fermentation of fish sauce takes longer than that of fish paste because all of the flesh must be broken down to create a clear liquid. A number of methods are given below for making the most common fish sauces.

South-East Asia

Nuoc-mam

The basic principle of nuoc-mam preparation is the breaking down of fish protein by enzymes in the presence of large amounts of salt. The fish, usually anchovies or mackerel, which are not cleaned, are kneaded by hand and mixed with salt (1 kg of salt to 3 kg of fish). The mixture is put in an earthenware pot. The pot is filled to the rim so that no air is present. The pot is then closed carefully and put in the ground. After several months the pot is dug up and opened. The liquid thus made is nuoc-mam.

On a larger scale the fresh, not cleaned fish are mixed with salt and put in bamboo vats fitted with a tap. 4 to 5 kg of salt are used for 6 kg of fish. The fish are put in the vats in alternating layers with the salt, the final layer being salt. After 3 days a cloudy and bloody liquid, 'nuoc-boi', can be tapped. After tamping the fish-salt mixture down, the nuoc-boi is again added to the vat so that the fish is 10 cm underwater. The vat is covered and stones are put on top of it so that the mass is put under pressure.

After months of fermentation, several months for small fish and 12 to 18 months for large fish, the nuoc-mam can be tapped. Figure 12.18 illustrates a vat for the preparation of nuoc-mam. After the first nuoc-mam has been taken, lower-quality products can be made by extracting more from the residue using boiling water.

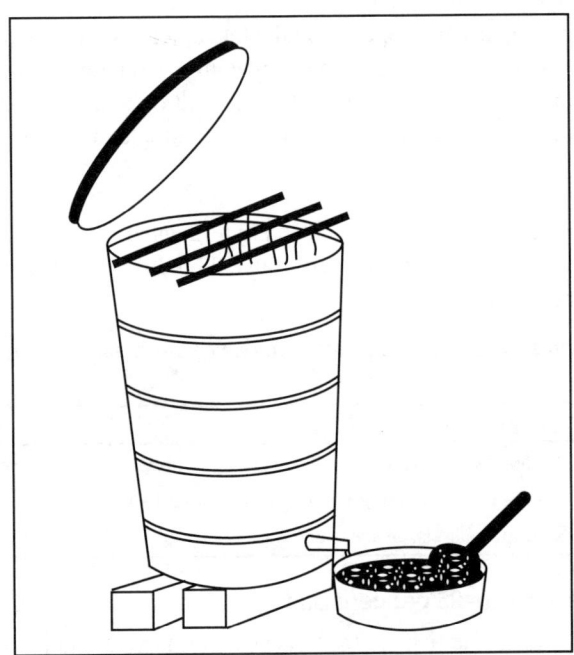

Fig. 12.18. Vat for the preparation of nuoc-mam.

Sometimes caramel, roasted rice or molasses are added to fish to get a dark colour and a certain taste. This improves the keeping qualities of the qualitatively inferior nuoc-mam. At a fermentation temperature higher than 45°C (113°F), the nuoc-mam loses its characteristic taste. It is, therefore, best to keep the vats somewhere cool.

Nampla

This product from Thailand is made in the same way as nuoc-mam. The ratio of salt:fish is 1 kg of salt to 4 kg of fish. The fermentation time is 6 to 12 months. The sauce is ripened for another 1 to 3 months in the sun.

Patis

In the Philippines a sauce comparable to nuoc-mam is made. The procedure for making patis is more or less the same as that for nuoc-mam. After the first patis yield, which has a characteristic taste, a saturated brine solution is used to obtain the second yield of patis of an inferior quality. Patis is usually made of small fish. Small shrimp or alamang, goby fry, herring fry and anchovies give the best results. Enough salt must be added to saturate the moisture which oozes from the fish. One kg of salt to 3.5–4 kg of fish gives a final product with 20 to 25 per cent salt content. Patis is also a by-product of the preparation of the fish paste bagoong (described further on).

Japan

Shottsuru

A Japanese variation of the nuoc-mam of South-East Asia is soyasauce, made from soyabeans. However, another sauce, shottsuru, is also made in Japan from sandfish. Sardines, anchovies and molluscs can also be used as starting material. The fluid is filtered and boiled and can be kept for years. Soyabean sediment or 'koji', which is fermented with wheat, can be added to shottsuru.

Fish Pastes and Whole Fish

A considerable part of the protein consumption in a number of Asian countries comes from the consumption of fish pastes, which are of greater importance from a nutritional point of view than fish sauces.

There are two kinds of fish pastes in South-East Asia:
1. Fish-salt mixtures.
2. Products which are fermented in the presence of cooked or roasted rice on which yeasts and moulds are present.

The general method of preparation of fish pastes is the same as that described for fish sauces. Only the fermentation time is shorter, as not all of the fish flesh needs to be broken down. Fish paste must be mixed regularly to keep the salt evenly distributed.

South-East Asia

Bagoong

Bagoong, a fish paste from the Philippines, is made by fermenting well-cleaned whole or minced fish, shrimp, fish or shrimp eggs in the presence of salt (1 kg of salt to 3 kg of fish). The salt-fish mixture is put into earthenware pots and covered with cheesecloth for 5 days. The covered pots are then put in the sun for 7 days. After that, the product is fermented for a further 3 to 12 months. As a by-product, the fish sauce patis can be harvested by separating the liquid above from the paste. The paste is sometimes coloured by adding 'angkak', rice which has been treated with the red yeast-like organism Monascus purpureus. Bagoong can be stored for several years.

Balao-balao

Balao-balao, which comes from the Philippines, is a fermented riceshrimp product. Balao-balao is made by mixing boiled rice, whole raw shrimp and salt (20 per cent of the weight of the shrimp). The product is stored in jars and is fermented for 7 to 10 days. The mixture becomes less sour the longer the fermentation takes place. The shells of the shrimp become red and soft and the mixture, including the rice, becomes liquid. In the general preparation it is fried with garlic and onion after fermentation. It is eaten as a sauce or as a complete meal in itself.

Belachan

Belachan is a paste made of small shrimp to which a relatively small amount of salt has been added (4 to 5 kg per 100 kg of shrimp). The mixture is dried on mats on the ground in the sun. After 4 to 8 hours of drying, during which 50 per cent of the moisture is lost, any contaminants in the shrimp are removed. The shrimp are then chopped up and squeezed into wooden vats so that no more air is present. The paste which results is fermented for 7 days. After 7 days the substance is taken out of the barrel and is dried for 3 to 5 hours in the sun. The paste is again ground up after which it is put back in the wooden vats. The paste should now be fermented for one month.

Ngapi

Small anchovies are washed with salt water and dried in the sun for 2 days. One kg of salt is added to 6 kg of dried fish in bamboo baskets. The mixture is pounded until it is fine and is then packed into wooden crates, after which fermentation takes place for a period of 7 days. Next, the mixture is again ground up and the same amount of salt is added. The mixture is dried in the sun for 3 to 5 hours. Further fermentation takes place for 1 month in wooden crates.

Prahoc

In Kampuchea, prahoc is prepared as follows: after the fish (cyprinids) are beheaded they are kneaded by hand so that the scales and intestines come loose. The fish are then washed in drinking water, during which care is taken to remove all scales. The fish are placed in a basket and covered with banana leaves and stones for 24 hours in order to drain. The fish are salted and, after leaving them for half an hour, they are dried on mats for 1 day in the sun. The fish are then pounded into a paste. The paste is put into open jars and placed in the sun. At night, the jars are closed so that insects cannot get at the fish. Fermentation now takes place. The liquid which appears on top is removed. The paste can be eaten when no more liquid comes out.

Trassi

Trassi is a fish paste made in Indonesia. Trassi udang is made of shrimp and trassi ikan of fish. The fresh shrimp or fish are mixed with 15 per cent salt. The mixture is spread out on mats and is dried for 1 to 3 days in the sun. The moisture content of the fish or shrimp drops from 80 to 50 per cent. The substance is kneaded and pounded until it is a paste. The paste is dried in thin layers in the sun. It is then packed in cylinders made of bamboo or nipa leaves after which it is allowed to ripen as long as is needed to get a typical trassi smell. Three kg of shrimp give 2 to 2.5 kg of trassi. Rice and potato peelings are sometimes added. Trassi must never be eaten raw but must always be heated in some way, such as boiling or frying, before consumption. Trassi is used as a seasoning. As a supplement to fish sauces and fish pastes, entire fish are also fermented in South-East Asia.

Colombo cure

The intestines and gills are removed from mackerel or non-fatty sardines after which the fish are washed in drinking water. The fish are mixed with salt (1 kg of salt to 3 kg of fish) and put into jars. Dried fruit pulp or tamarind (a tropical fruit) is added to the salt and fish to lower the pH (8 kg of tamarind to 100 kg of fish). The fish are kept covered with brine with the help of weighted mats and are fermented for 2 to 4 months. They are transferred to wooden barrels and care is taken to keep them covered with brine. The fermented fish can be kept for one year.

Pedah-siam

This product is made of salted mackerel. During the preparation, the intestines are removed through the mouth. The fish are then salted, 3 kg of fish to 1 kg of salt, and stored for 24 hours. Ripening takes place under anaerobic conditions. The brine formed is removed regularly. A red colour appears after ripening.

Japan

Sushi

Sushi is a group of preserved fish products which are formed through the addition of boiled rice to fermented fish and salt. The low pH which results from the growth of lactic acid bacteria contributes to the preserving effect. The general preparation is as follows. The intestines of the fish are removed and the fish is mixed with 20 to 30 per cent salt. After being stored for 1 to 2 months the fish are de-salted and the liquid is removed. Boiled rice and 'koji' (fermented wheat) are placed on the bottom of a basket and the de-salted fish are alternated in layers with boiled rice or 'koji'. The amount of boiled rice added is equal to 40 or 50 per cent of the weight of the fish, the amount of 'koji' is half the amount of boiled rice (rice: fish:koji = 2:4:1). The fermentation continues for another 10 days.

South America

Anchoa

Anchoa is a product found in a few South American countries, including Peru, Chili and Argentina. Whole anchovies are mixed with 35 per cent salt and placed in barrels. The fermentation, a result of enzyme activity, takes place for a period of 3 to 4 months.

Africa

Momone

Momone is product from Ghana. In its general preparation, the intestines and gills of the fish are removed and the fish are washed in water. They are then rubbed with salt and packed in layers in barrels, alternating with layers of salt. The salt:fish ratio is 1:9. Fermentation takes place for 7 days. After that the fish are dried for 1 to 3 days on mats in the sun.

CANNING

General Information

First, some general information about canning of fish and meat will be given. This covers the advantages and disadvantages of the process, packaging materials and materials needed. After this general introduction, the following will be described: preparation of fish and meat, processing techniques and storage of the product.

A lot of canning equipment is manufactured in the US. Therefore, pressures and temperatures will be given both in metric and American measuring units (e.g. pounds/inch^2 and degrees Fahrenheit).

Principle and limitations

The canning process involves placing foods in cans or jars and heating them to a temperature that destroys micro-organisms that could be a health hazard or cause the food to spoil. Canning also inactivates enzymes that could cause the food to spoil. As the cans or jars are sealed hermetically, re-contamination from outside is prevented. In general, canned products can be stored for a long time without refrigeration. Chemical quality loss (in taste, colour and amount of certain essential nutrients) will slowly continue though.

Not all products can be heated in the same way. The amount of time and the temperature needed depends on:

1. The number and kinds of micro-organisms and the form (active cells or spores) in which they are present.
2. Water content of the product.
3. Acidity of the product.
4. Presence of salt and/or other inhibitors of bacterial growth.
5. Fat content of the product.

6. Shape and size of the tin can or glass jar.
7. Storage temperature.

In fish and meat the number of micro-organisms initially present may be large, the internal water content is high and the pH is close to neutral. It is, therefore, difficult to kill all micro-organisms present and to get a safe product. The only safe way to sterilise low acid products such as fish and meat is by prolonged heating in a pressure canner or steriliser in which temperatures higher than 100°C (212°F) can be reached.

The main reason pressure canning is necessary is the hazard of the *Clostridium botulinum* bacterium. Though the bacterial cells are killed at boiling temperatures, they can form spores that can withstand these temperatures. The spores grow well in low acid foods, in the absence of air, such as in canned low acid foods (vegetables and meats). When the spores germinate and grow to high numbers, they produce the deadly botulinum toxins (poisons). The spores can be destroyed by canning the food at a temperature of 115°–121°C (240°–250°F) for the correct length of time. This temperature can only be reached in a pressure canner.

As the canning of fish and meat requires a lot of energy, clean water and a large investment in equipment, usually it can only be done at a small-scale industrial level. It is less suited for household-level preservation.

Advantages and Disadvantages of the Canning Process

Advantages of canning

1. The product can be stored longer and more safely.
2. A good-quality product is ensured with fish and meat; it is better than that of foods preserved by other methods like drying in the sun. The best quality is achieved by using fresh, healthy products and by exactly following the heating specifications for that product.

Disadvantages of canning

1. The high price of the preserved foods due to the following:
   (a) Glass or tinned steel packaging materials must be used, and may be expensive and difficult to obtain. Glass can be reused.
   (b) The processing equipment is, when compared with sun drying or smoking, very expensive. The costs for canning in glass jars are less.
   (c) The process requires a lot of fuel.
2. The process requires more clean water than other methods do.
3. The extended heating at high temperatures causes both a decrease in taste and vitamin losses. The nutritional value of the food, compared to the fresh product, is therefore, somewhat lower. Nutrients dissolving in the brine are lost if these juices are not consumed.

In this chapter, the methods for canning and sterilising a variety of fish and meats are given. Because the packaging materials are very important in the procedures, these will be discussed first.

Packaging Materials

General

Cans made of tinned steel plate are especially used to store fish and meat products. Sometimes it is better to use glass; acid products, for example, corrode cans and are therefore better packed in glass.

The shape and volume of the vessels must be chosen according to the quantity to be processed. Big bulky products such as pieces of meat must be sterilised in small or flat tin cans or jars which allow the heat to penetrate quickly to the centre of the product. Small products and products in brine, etc. can be packed in all shapes and types of tin cans or jars.

The contents of an opened tin can or jar must be consumed as quickly as possible (in any case within 24 hours), which implies that the amount of food put in one can or jar should be adjusted to the amount of food consumed during one meal or in one day. Of course, it is true that the larger the tin cans or jars, the cheaper the packaging material will be per kilo of processed product. But in general, larger tin cans or jars with meat must be heated longer (Table 12.2), which means that the quality is usually somewhat lower than that of meat in smaller tin cans or jars.

Tin cans

Tin cans are steel cans which are covered with a thin layer of tin. They are used especially for sterilising and are very suitable for sterilising larger amounts. Unfortunately they can only be used once. There are many different types of tin cans available with varying capacities and shapes (cylindrical = long and thin, flat = wide and shallow). Tin cans can also vary according to the presence or absence of a layer of varnish on the inside. For fish and meat unvarnished tin cans are often suitable (Fig. 12.19).

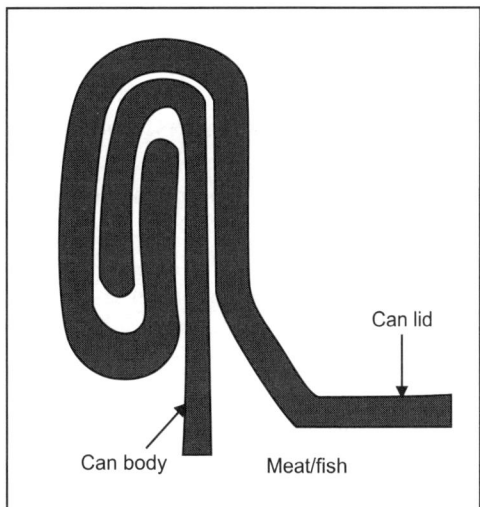

Fig. 12.19. Can seam.

Every tin can has a lid which can be hermetically sealed with a tin can seamer. Various types of seamers are available, ranging from simple hand-operated tools to new, automatic machines. The seam must be made correctly so as to prevent leakage. This can be checked by closing the tin can with a little amount of water and immersing it in boiling water. If, after a few minutes, steam escapes, the seaming machine must be readjusted and a newly seamed can must be checked again, as described before.

New tin cans delivered from the factory are fairly clean and do not require extra washing. However, do check that they were not contaminated during storage. Do not use damaged or corroded cans. Store them upside down to keep dirt out. If they are not clean, wash them in hot soda water (1.5 wt% sodium carbonate), rinse with hot water and let them drip dry on a clean cloth. The lids must also be clean.

Glass jars

Glass jars can be used for sterilising under pressure and for bottling. Glass is used less frequently for fish and meat as large pieces of fish or meat are difficult to get out and the product does not look as nice. However, glass is a good option for small and acidic products. Furthermore, at the (large) household level sterilising products in glass jars in a pressure canner may be an economically feasible option. Glass has the advantages that it can be reused after the product has been consumed and it does not affect the product. The fragility of glass, its weight, poor heat conduction and the fact that light can get to the product are some disadvantages.

Jars and lids must be cleaned before use with soap (soda) and hot water. Keep clean jars in hot water until they are needed. Jars come in different sizes. Manufacturers have their own rings, lids and sometimes clamps which fit on jars. The best results are achieved when all parts are obtained from the same manufacturer.

Processing Equipment

The items needed for the whole process are:
1. Tubs for washing and rinsing fish, meat, tin cans, jars, etc.
2. Cutting equipment: tables, knives.
3. Kettles for heating, boiling, pre-boiling, processing.
4. Shallow open pans for sterilising at 100°C (212°F) for acid products like fish in tomato sauce.
5. A steriliser (autoclave, Fig. 12.20) or pressure canner for sterilising at temperatures higher than 100°C (212°F) for 'low acid' products. These include almost all meat and fish products.
   Note: There are various types of pressure canners. Not all pressure cookers are suitable as canners. In a good canner a pressure of at least 1 atmosphere (101.3 kPa or 14.7 pounds per square inch) above atmospheric level should be attainable.
6. A thermometer to check the temperature.
7. Cans or glass jars with lids.
8. (Hand-operated) seaming machine for seaming tin cans.

Preparation

Clean and tidy work pays off in lower levels of micro-organisms and a greater chance the process will be successful. A few remarks are made below about preparations specific to the canning of fish and meat.

Fish

For the canning of fish, it is also important that the fish to be canned is brought ashore as quickly as possible. The mechanisation of fishing boats, transporting on ice and cooling facilities are useful for that. Especially fatty kinds of fish spoil quickly, due to oxidative rancidity. Good personal hygiene among fishermen and processors and hygienic conditions in harbours and factories are also necessary for the proper processing of the fish.

Not all kinds of fish are suitable for canning. When boiling fish with white flesh, the flesh will rapidly fall apart leaving hard bones. Thus these kinds of fish are unsuitable for canning. Fish with a high fat content (usually fish which swim in schools such as herring, mackerel, tuna and sardines) have much firmer flesh and softer bones. When cooking such fish, the bones get soft before the flesh starts to fall apart. The fish thus retain their original shape and are very suitable for canning. Another advantage of canning fatty kinds of fish is that the oxygen entrapped in the can will be consumed during sterilisation and this will prevent fat oxidation and rancidness, which is not achieved with simpler preservation methods such as drying, etc.

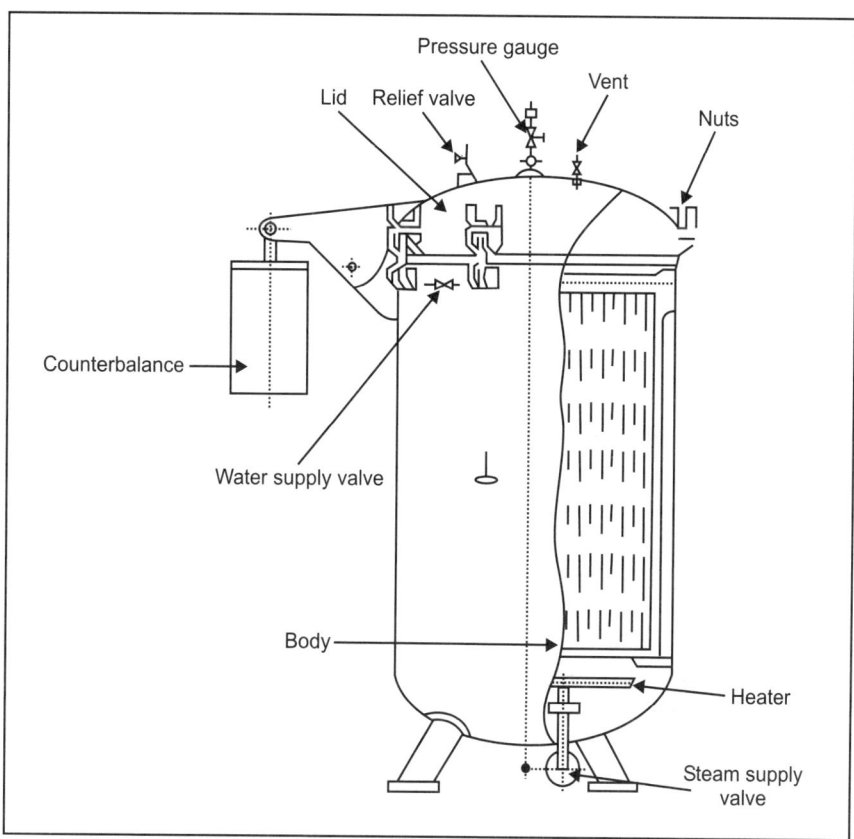

Fig. 12.20. A steam-heated autoclave.

Start with fresh, healthy fish. Wash them and gut them in such a way that the intestines do not touch the flesh while being removed. Remove the head and tail, and the bones of large fish, then wash the fish thoroughly in cold water. The fish can be tinned raw, but preferably fried or cooked. Fish is often also salted, pickled, smoked, etc. after being cleaned and before canning. The protein thus denatures which makes the flesh stay firm and not shrink after canning.

Use as little herbs and spices as possible. These are often a source of contamination with bacterial spores. Put small fish straight up in flat oval cans (herring). Big fish have to be cut into smaller pieces to get them into small tin cans.

Meat

Bottling meat at 100°C (212°F) is not advisable but sterilising it at 115°–121°C (240°–250°F) is possible. Use only clean, fresh pieces of meat. Remove the bones, cut the meat into smaller pieces (a few cm thick) and season as desired. Brown the meat by roasting or frying; big pieces should be partially cooked before frying. For small pieces in sauce, stock or brine, various sizes of tins and jars can be used. For bigger pieces, use flat tin cans.

In general, almost all meat products are suitable for canning. Only products which are eaten raw such as raw dry-cured ham or dry sausage are not suitable.

Processing Techniques

A simple description of the process of canning fish or meat is given below:
1. Prepare fish or meat.
2. Precook (or roast/smoke) meat and fish; this reduces volume and makes the flesh firmer.
3. Fill tin can with fish or meat and filling liquid.
4. Remove excess air from can, but keep the required headspace.
5. Seal can shut with seamer.
5. Apply heat treatment (115°–121°C/240°–250°F for most fish and meat products or 100°C/212°F for sour products).
6. Cool can, wash it and affix label.

Filling and closing containers

After initial preparation, the products, which are still warm or heated to the filling temperature, are put into tin cans or glass jars as quickly as possible. These are then filled with hot water, hot broth, hot salt solution or hot oil to about half a centimetre under the rim. This is called the headspace; it is needed to give the food inside the jar room to expand during heating and to create a vacuum in the jar after cooling. Take care that no air pockets are sealed in with the product.

Glass jars can be closed at this point. The lid should fit well, but (for example in the case of a screw cap) it should not be twisted tightly closed, because some air should be allowed to escape while the jar is being heated. Immediately after the heating process the lid should be closed tightly. This way a vacuum will develop in the jar as the product cools and the food inside has no more chance of coming in contact with outside air and becoming contaminated.

Tin cans can be sealed after adding the liquid, as long as the middle of the product has reached the sealing temperature. Always measure the temperature in the middle of the tin can. The sealing temperature must not be lower than 60°–80°C (140°–176°F), depending on the product and the size of the can. If it is lower, the cans must be quickly reheated in a shallow water bath until the temperature in the middle of the tin can is equal to or higher than the indicated temperature. This procedure ensures that the can will not deform at the sterilising temperature and that a proper vacuum is created after cooling. The time between filling, sealing and sterilising must be as short as possible. Never use damaged cans or jars.

Sterilising using an autoclave or pressure canner

In low acid products spores of pathogenic (disease causing) micro-organisms, which are not killed at 100°C/212°F can grow and multiply. To kill those spores sterilisation for 60 minutes or longer at 121°C (250°F) may be necessary. At 115°C (240°F) spores will be killed too, but it takes longer (Table 12.3). Sterilising below 115°C (240°F) is generally not safe.

To sterilise at temperatures higher than 100°C (212°F), a pressure canner or autoclave is needed. These high temperatures can be reached only through increased pressure. At sea level water boils at 121°C (250°F) when the pressure inside an autoclave is one atmosphere (equivalent to 101.3 kilopascal) above atmospheric pressure. At 0.7 atmospheres above atmospheric pressure, water boils at 115°C (239°F). In higher areas, greater pressure is needed to attain the required temperature. As a rule of thumb, 0.1 atmospheres (1.5 pound/square inch) of extra pressure is needed per 1000 metres above sea level (Table 12.2).

Table 12.2. Pressure required to reach canning temperature.

| | Required canning pressure | | | |
| | for 115°C/240°F | | for 121°C/250°F | |
Altitude	Pounds/inch²	Kilo-pascal	Pounds/inch²	Kilo-pascal
Sea level	10	68.9	15	103.4
2000 ft (609 m)	11	75.8	16	110.3
4000 ft (1219 m)	12	82.7	17	117.2
6000 ft (1829 m)	13	89.6	18	124.1

Many household canners are fitted with counterweights of 5, 10 and 15 pounds as pressure regulators. Above 300 m (1000 ft) the 15 pound weight should be used.

The general method of working is as follows:

1. Cover the bottom of the pressure canner with water.
2. Place the basket with the jars in the pressure canner. The holes in the basket must not all be blocked, as steam must be able to pass through. Remember to unscrew the jar lids a little bit.
3. Seal the pressure canner and open the ventilation system. Apply heat. The autoclave may be heated by gas or by electricity and in an industrial setting frequently saturated steam is directly injected in the retort.
4. After steam has escaped for 10 minutes, close the ventilation system (the air has by then been evacuated) and let the pressure build up.
5. When the required temperature is reached, the cooking time starts. Cooking times depend on the product, can shape and size, temperature and pressure. For any specific situation consult experts like research institutes, can manufacturers or manufacturers of sterilising equipment. In Table 12.3 some indicative values are given for safe processing at household level. Keep the temperature and pressure as constant as possible during cooking by regulating the heat source.
6. Tin cans: After the process, let the steam escape slowly. This can be done faster with small tin cans than with bigger ones, but nonetheless should be done slowly and carefully as the cans can deform or even burst. When the pressure is again normal, the lid of the canner can be opened. Remove the tin cans and immerse them in cold water, replacing the water now and then to keep it cold. When the tin cans have cooled down enough (i.e. when they feel hand-warm), they still contain sufficient heat to dry by themselves if stored in the open air.
7. Glass jars: Wait until the pressure canner cools down and the pressure inside has gone down before opening the lid. Remove the jars and tighten the lids immediately. A disadvantage of glass jars is that they cannot be cooled quickly. The safest way to cool them is to leave them in open air until they are hand-warm and then to put them in cold water.

A second technique for sterilisation with an autoclave uses more energy and water but gives a slightly better product. The autoclave is completely filled with water and the tin cans and jars are put in it. The process proceeds as above. The cooling can be quickened by slowly removing the hot water and adding cold water to the autoclave after sterilisation. During cooling, the pressure in the autoclave must be reduced gradually.

Sterilising sour products in a boiling water bath

Sour fish products, such as fish in tomato sauce, are barely heated (e.g. 5 minutes at 100°C/212°F) as most micro-organisms will not survive in an acidic environment anyway. A boiling water bath is used to preserve sour products.

Table 12.3. Indicative cooking times.

Product	Can size (litre)	Processing time (minutes)	
		115°C (240°F)	*121°C (250°F)*
Chicken	0.5	95	75
	1.5	155	125
Beef, pork	0.5	90	75
	1	120	90
Fish	0.25	75	60
	0.5	105	85
	1.5	220	180
Meat stock	0.5	30	20
	1	40	25

To prevent glass jars from breaking, start with hot but not yet boiling water. Tin cans can go straight into boiling water. Cans or jars should be completely under water. Start timing the process from the moment the water boils again, making sure that the water remains at a rolling boil during the entire sterilisation period.

An open water bath boils at 100°C (212°F) at altitudes of up to 300 metres above sea level. At greater altitudes, water boils at a lower temperature and the products must be sterilised longer to achieve the same effect, as shown in Table 12.4.

Table 12.4. Time needed for sterilisation at different altitudes.

Altitude (metres)	Sterilisation time (minutes) (for example when a = 20 min.)	
0–300	a	20 min
300–600	a + 1/5*a	24 min
600–900	a + 2/5*a	28 min
900–1200	a + 3/5*a	32 min

After heating, the cans can be cooled in cold water, which should be changed occasionally to speed up the cooling. Glass jars should be put into cold water only when they are lukewarm. The cooling can be speeded up by gradually adding cold water to the hot water in the steriliser. When doing so, one should use chlorinated water (water containing 0.01 wt% chloride of lime = bleaching powder, available worldwide) so that the cans with possible micro leaks are not contaminated.

Storage

Store the canned foods in a cool place. Label them so that you know the contents. The storage temperature should preferably stay below 20°C (68°F); the cooler the better, as chemical quality degradation still continues after canning. With conventional canning techniques as described in this chapter not all bacterial spores may be killed. Fortunately, these heat resistant survivors do not grow at temperatures below 35°C. If you want to store the product for a long time (up to 2 years) in tropical conditions with higher temperatures (of 35°C or more), than a much more intensive heat treatment at 121°C (250°F) is necessary so that all micro-organism spores are inactivated. This is expensive in terms of fuel and will lower the quality of the canned product. Do not pile the preserved foods too close to each other; air should be able to circulate. The storeroom should also be dry and kept at a constant temperature. Only ventilate with dry air; avoid ventilation in warm, humid weather, as condensation could rust the tin cans. Always consume the oldest preserved foods first. Check each product for spoilage. Pasteurised meat products (heat treatment at 80°C/176°F) can be kept in cooling cells (2–4°C/35.5–39°F) for up to 6 months.

Setting up a Small-scale Canning Factory: Prerequisites

Apart from the materials that are needed, there are also a number of other prerequisites to be met to ensure the success of a small-scale fish or meat canning factory.

Some important prerequisites are:
1. Sufficient clean water and energy.
2. Good infrastructure (roads, cooling facilities, harbours, slaughterhouses, etc.).
3. Financial feasibility: Is there a sound business plan?
4. Sufficient trained personnel to operate machines and the right level of skills for bookkeeping and management.
5. Technical support: Machine maintenance and supply of spare parts.
6. Regular supply of fish or meat at a reasonable price (Certain kinds of fish are not available at certain times of the year).
7. Good temperature control during the process.
8. Testing of chemical and micro-biological quality after the process (Laboratory facilities are needed for this).
9. A good market for canned fish or meat. If export is also possible, apart from local trading, the cost of a can of fish or meat can be lowered.

Unless all of the above prerequisites for canning are satisfied, it is better not to set up a fish or meat canning factory. Canning of meat under primitive conditions is not to be recommended. However, if one can meet all the necessary requirements and canning fish or meat proves to be economically feasible, then the local canning of fish or meat will certainly make a positive contribution to the diet of the local population.

COOLING AND FREEZING

General Information

The storage life of fish or meat, or of a fish or meat product, depends on the acidity and water content of the product. External influences such as oxygen (from the air), micro-organisms, storage temperature, light and water secretion are all also important determining factors.

Fresh fish and meat spoil very quickly in the high ambient temperatures of the tropics. If you want to keep fish or meat more than one day, you will have to preserve it. Another preservation method is to cool or freeze the products.

There are two possibilities for storing fresh fish or meat at low temperatures:
1. Cooling at –1° to +4°C/30° to 39°F, which inhibits the growth of micro-organisms.
2. Freezing at –18° to –30°C/–0.5° to –22°F, which completely stops bacteria from growing.

Because of the low temperatures, all (bio)chemical, physical and microbiological processes are slowed down so decaying does not occur. To increase the storage life of the product, it is important to lower the temperature very quickly so as to preserve its quality. If the freezing goes too slowly, large ice crystals are formed which affect the structure of the product.

To cool meat, one needs a large cooling cell. Cooling of fish is often done by keeping it on ice. This requires ice-making machines. Very expensive and advanced freezing equipment is needed for the freezing of fresh fish or meat. Furthermore, these preservation methods require a lot of energy and a large investment in the necessary materials. The supply of fish or meat must be large to cover these costs and there must also be a good market for cooled or frozen fish or meat. Therefore, cooling and freezing can only be done at an industrial level. As we are mainly focusing on preservation methods which are feasible at household level, these methods will be described only very briefly. For further information, please read other relevant literature. In the following, an indication will be given of the relationship between storage temperature and storage time for fish and meat so as to give an impression of the effectiveness of these methods. The installation of an ice factory and/or cooling or freezing facility will not be discussed.

Cooling and Freezing Fish

Whole fish, with the intestines and gills removed, and fish fillets are often cooled (at 0°C/32°F) by putting ice on them. Alternating layers of fish and ice are put in a box. Be sure to use at least as much ice as fish. One should always end with a layer of ice. When the ice has melted, new ice must be added to keep the fish at 0°C (32°F). Especially with fatty fish it is important to cool quickly so that oxidation of the fat is slowed down. Fish can also be stored in cooling cells. The temperature there is just above freezing point, so ice lying on the fish melts and the fish stay fresh. This way fish will not freeze. The boxes in which the product are kept must not be kept on the ground, against a wall or against each other, but in clusters on pallets and slightly away from walls so that air can circulate freely. If one wishes to store fish for more than 2 or 3 weeks, it must be frozen. For the freezing of fish in freezing cells, a temperature of –30°C/–22°F is recommended. If good quality fish is frozen at –30°C/–22°F quickly after being caught, then it can be stored for a very long time. Table 12.5 gives examples of the storage life of different kinds of fish using the cooling/freezing method. The storage life which one achieves depends on the quality of the fish and the storage conditions (e.g. how constant the temperature is).

Table 12.5. Storage life of fish at different temperatures.

Product	Temperature (°C/F)	Storage life
Cooling		
Cod fillets	0/32	11 days
	3/37	5 days
	10/50	25 hours
Bred trout (cleaned and vacuum packed)	0/32	18 days
	5/41	10 days
South American hake (cleaned)	0/32	11 days
	5/41	5 days
Freezing		
Cod	–30/–22	8 months–4 years
Herring	–30/–22	6 months–1 year

Cooling and Freezing Meat

Cooling and freezing is also used for the storage of meat as well. With meat it is important to quickly lower the temperature of the carcass (±40°C/104°F) down to 0°–5°C (32°–41°F) to prevent microbiological spoilage at the surface of the meat. After this initial rapid cooling, the meat is kept cool or frozen.

Preparations for cooling consist of slaughtering and quartering the carcass. Under optimal cooling of a quarter carcass, the meat loses 1–3 per cent of its moisture in the first 24 hours. Cooling at –1°C (30°F) to +3°C (37°F) may be necessary during the period between slaughter and sale or during long transport. Cooling of meat is also used to ripen the meat: it makes it softer. This is frequently done, especially with beef. The air circulation in meat cooling cells is also very important.

Sometimes quarter carcasses are frozen but sometimes their volume is decreased by boning the quarters and cutting the meat into large chunks. At –10°C (14°F) to –18°C (–0.5°F), freezing a quarter carcass of beef takes 4 to 6 days. Storage of frozen meat usually takes place at –12°C (10°F) to –20°C (–4°F). At such temperatures beef can be kept for 1 year while pork has a shorter storage life. This is due to oxidation of the fat in pork. Examples of the storage life of different kinds of meat at different temperatures are given in Table 12.6. The actual storage life attained depends on the quality of the meat and the storage conditions.

Table 12.6. Storage life of meat at different temperatures.

Product	Temperature (°C/F)	Storage life
Cooling		
Beef	–1/30	3–5 weeks
Pork	–1/30	1–2 weeks
Freezing		
Beef	–18/–0.5	12 months
	–30/–22	24 months
Pork	–18/–0.5	6 months
	–30/–22	15 months

Chapter 13

Contamination, Preservation and Spoilage of Eggs

INTRODUCTION

The spoilage of uneviscerated and eviscerated poultry is somewhat different from the spoilage of canned meat. Various parts of world is eviscerated, only this type of poultry is considered in this section. Uneviscerated poultry is discussed by Barnes and Shrimpton.

Immediately after processing, any of several hundred species of micro-organisms might be found. However, as the poultry is chilled and held in cold storage, psychrotrophic micro-organisms predominate and cause deterioration.

The main defects are off-odour, which appears at a bacterial load between 10^6 and $10^8/m^2$, and slime formation, which occurs soon after off-odour is noted. As the number of bacteria increases, the flavour score decreases, species of *Pseudomonas* are the principal spoilage organisms. Besides *Pseudomonas*, other organisms, similar to those in fresh red meat spoilage, are found on spoiled poultry (Table 13.1). These include *Aeromonas*, *Moraxella*, *Alcaligenes*, *Flavobacterium*, and *Micrococcus*.

Table 13.1. Microbial defects of poultry and poultry products.

Product	Defect	Micro-organism
Poultry meat	Off-odour, slime	*Pseudomonas, Acinetobacter, Moraxella, Alcaligenes, Aeromonas, Alteromonas*
Shell eggs	Black rot	*Proteus, Aeromonas*
	White rot (colourless)	*Citrobacter, Alcaligenes*
	Sour	*Pseudomonas*
	Green white	*P. fluorescens*
	Musty	*Pseudomonas*
	Mouldy	Many types of moulds
	Red rot	*Serratia marcescens*
	Custard rot	*Citrobacter, Proteus, Enterobacter*
	Yellow and green rot	*Alcaligenes, Flavobacterium, Cytophaga*
Liquid whole egg	Fishy	*Pseudomonas, Flavobacterium, Chromobacterium*
	Off-odour, sour	*Proteus, Alcaligenes, Escherichia, Flavobacterium, Pseudomonas, Bacillus*
Liquid albumen	Off-odour	*Pseudomonas, Acinetobacter, Enterobacter*

When antibiotics were used on poultry, yeasts became the important spoilage micro-organisms. However, yeasts are not important on normally processed and eviscerated poultry.

Daud, McMeekin, and Thomas studied the flora of chicken meat held at 2°C. Before storage, the flora included species of *Micrococcus, Flavobacterium, Cytophaga, Acinetobacter, Moraxella*, and *Pseudomonas*, as well as enterics. During storage, the off-odour producers (principally *Pseudomonas* II) became dominant, accounting for 62 per cent of the population after twelve days.

At this time, species of *Pseudomonas* accounted for 98 per cent of the bacterial population. Nonpigmented strains of pseudomonads produce more intense odours than do pigmented strains. Off-odours of poultry have been listed as sulphidelike, fruity, fishy, and like evaporated milk.

The chemicals produced by pseudomonads grown in chicken meat include acetone, 2-butanone, 2-pentanone, toluene, dimethyl benzenes, ethyl methyl disulphide, 2-heptanone, and dimethyl trisulphide. Some of the more important volatile sulphur-containing compounds are dimethyl disulphide, dimethyl sulphide, methanethiol and propylene sulphide.

Packaging poultry in oxygen-impermeable film or vacuum packaging it causes inhibition of pseudomonads so that the predominant flora at spoilage consists of lactic and enteric types of bacteria.

EGGS

It is generally accepted that, when an egg is laid, its contents are free from bacteria. But there are exceptions because of ovarian infections. The egg contents are protected by the shell and associated membranes and chemical inhibitors in the egg albumen. This means that micro-organisms must penetrate these barriers and then be able to grow inside the egg to cause spoilage. Penetration of eggs is aided by moisture on the shell. If the eggs are not properly stored or washed, penetration may be quite rapid, and spoilage can occur. For egg products, the shell and membranes are removed. During processing, the liquid egg is subject to contamination from organisms on the egg shell, equipment, humans, added ingredients, and the final container.

Bacterial analysis of shell eggs during storage has revealed moulds (*Penicillium, Aspergillus, Cladosporium, Rhizopus*, and *Mucor*), yeasts (*Rhodotorula*), and bacteria (*Pseudomonas, Micrococcus, Bacillus, Proteus, Alcaligenes, Flavobacterium, Citrobacter, Escherichia*, and *Enterobacter*).

As with other protein foods, species of *Pseudomonas* are the main spoilage organisms of shell eggs and egg products. When bacteria grow within the egg, they decompose the contents and form by-products. This results in characteristic odours, appearance or colours from which the various rots acquire their name (Table 13.1).

The United States Department of Agriculture (USDA) described a loss egg as 'an egg that is inedible, smashed or broken so that the contents are leaking, frozen, contaminated or containing bloody whites large blood spots, largely unsightly meat spots, or other foreign material'. Inedible eggs are due to nonmicrobial defects as well as microbial defects. An egg with a blood ring, embryo or stuck yolk is inedible. Besides these loss types, shell eggs will absorb odours from the storage atmosphere. Most vegetables and fruits will impart flavours and odours to shell eggs. If stored with apples, the eggs will be bitter and have a cardboard flavour and odour. If stored near gasoline or kerosene, the shell eggs will taste and smell like these compounds.

Eggs that become inedible due to microbial growth are listed by USDA as black rots, white rots, sour eggs, eggs with green whites, mixed rots, musty eggs, and mouldy eggs. Other designations for rotten eggs are fluorescent green, red, custard, colourless, green and yellow, mixed, and rusty red rots.

Black rots: When viewed with a candling light, black rot eggs are virtually opaque. When broken out, the egg content has a muddy (dark brown) appearance and a repulsive putrid odour, and H_2S is evident. In many eggs, an internal gas pressure develops. The bacteria associated with this type of spoilage are species of *Proteus* and *Aeromonas*. Rots of this type are more likely to occur at room temperature (20°C) than in cold storage (4°C or less).

White rot: Threadlike shadows may be seen in the thin white, and in later stages the yolk appears severely blemished when the shell egg is viewed with the candling light. When opened, the egg yolk shows a crusted appearance and frequently has a fruity odour. This type of inedible egg sometimes is referred to as a colourless rot. Various organisms have been associated with this rot, including *Citrobacter*, *Salmonella*, and *Alcaligenes*.

Sour eggs: These eggs are difficult to detect by ordinary candling, but they usually show a weak white and murky shadow around an off-center, swollen yolk. These eggs also are called fluorescent and are quite readily detected by observing with UV light. A green sheen is produced by species of *Pseudomonas*. Since a green fluorescence is observed, these inedible eggs also have been termed fluorescent green rots.

Green whites: This defect is caused mainly by *Pseudomonas fluorescens*. Green whites of broken-out eggs fluoresce when observed with UV light. Eggs with green whites may or may not have a sour odour, since the green fluorescence can be observed long before any odour can be detected.

Musty eggs: These frequently appear clear and free from foreign material when candled. The musty odour may be caused by odours in the atmosphere being absorbed by the egg contents. Also, some micro-organisms occasionally invade shell eggs and produce a musty odour.

Mouldy eggs: Mould growth is visible as spots on the shell, in checked areas of the shell or inside the egg. The mould contamination of eggs seems to be due to the reuse of mouldy packing materials. Several moulds, such as *Penicillium*, *Alternaria*, and *Rhizopus* can grow on eggs. However, moulds are not a prominent cause of egg spoilage.

Red rot: These eggs are distinguished by a red discolouration of the albumen and the surface of the yolk. An ammoniacal to putrid odour may occur. *Serratia marcescens* has been considered as the cause of red rot.

Custard rot. In this rot, the yolk is encrusted with custardlike material and occasionally flecked with olive-green pigment. The albumen becomes thin with an orange tint. There may be a slightly putrid to putrid odour. *Citrobacter* and *Proteus vulgaris* have been associated with this type of spoilage.

Mixed rot: These addled eggs occur when the vitelline membrane of the yolk breaks and the yolk mixes with the white, resulting in a murkiness throughout the interior of the egg when viewed with a candling light. With no off-odour, these are referred to as odourless mixed rots.

Other rots: *Alcaligenes* has been accused of causing both yellow rots and green rots. These rots are similar in odour and in the appearance of albumen. However, the yolk is dark yellow in the former and dark green to black in the latter case. Rust red rot is associated with growth of *P. vulgaris*.

Egg products: The spoilage of egg products is evidenced by off-odours described as sour, fecal or fishy. Organic acids (lactic, succinic) are recognised as indices of decomposition of egg products.

COMPOSITION OF AN EGG

Hen's egg consists of three main parts, the shell, the egg white and the egg yolk. The shell consists of calcite crystals embedded in a matrix of proteins and polysachharide complex. Inside the shell the viscous colourless liquid called the egg white accounts for about 60 per cent of the total egg weight.

Eggs have high nutritional value, moreover egg, eggs may be used as thickening agents, binding and coagulating agents, coatings, foaming agents, emulsifiers, shortening agents, flavouring agents and colourant in a variety of food products.

Percentage distribution of weight:

Part	Weight%
Shell	8–11
White	56–61
Yolk	27–32

Percentage composition of egg white and yolk:

Nutrients	Egg white	Egg yolk
Water	88.0	48.0
Protein	11.0	17.5
Fat	0.2	32.5
Minerals	0.8	2.0

Egg white is composed of thin and thick portions. 20–25 per cent of the total white of fresh eggs (1–5 days old) is thin white. The chief constituents of egg white besides water are proteins. Different types of proteins are present in egg white.

Ovalbumin: This constitutes 55 per cent of the proteins of egg white. This is a phosphoglycoprotein and is composed of three components A1, A2, and A3, which differ only in phosphorus content.

Conalbumin: This constitutes 13 per cent protein of the egg albumin. It consists of two forms neither of which contains phosphorus nor sulphur.

Ovamucoid: It is a glycoprotein. This constitutes about 10 per cent of the egg white proteins.

Ovomucin: This protein is responsible for the jelly like character of egg white and the thickness of the albumin. It contains 2 per cent of the egg white. Its content in the thick layers of albumin is about 4 times more than in thin layers. It is insoluble in water but soluble in dilute salt solution.

Lysozyme: 3.5 per cent of the egg white protein is lysozyme. This is an enzyme capable of lysing or dissolving the cell of wall of bacteria. It is composed of 3 components A, B and C. It binds biotin and makes the vitamin unavailable.

Avidin: Avidin is 0.05 per cent of the egg white protein. It is denatured by heat and cooked eggs do not affect the availability of biotin.

Ovoglobulin: It is a protein consisting of two components G1 and G2 and both are excellent foaming agents.

Ovoinhibitor: 0.1 per cent of egg protein is made up of ovoinhibitor. It is another protein capable of inhibiting trypsin and chymotrypsin.

Egg yolk: Solid content of yolk is about 50 per cent.

Percentage composition of egg yolk on dry weight basis:

Nutrient	Granules	Plasma
Lipid	34	77–81
Protein	60	18
Ash	66	2

The major proteins in egg yolk are lipoproteins, which include lipovitellins and lipovitellinin. The lipoproteins are responsible for the excellent emulsifying properties of egg yolk, when it is used in such products as mayonnaise.

Fatty acid composition of egg yolk:

Fatty acid	% of total fatty acids
C16:0 Palmitic acid	23.5
C18:0 Stearic acid	14.0
C18:1 Oleic acid	38.4
C18:2 Linoleic acid	16.4
C18:3 Linolenic acid	1.4
C18:4 Arachidonic acid	1.3

Nutritive Value of Eggs

Table 13.2 shows nutritive value of eggs/100 g.

Table 13.2. Nutritive value of eggs/100 g

Nutrient	Amount	Nutrient	Amount
Energy (K cal)	173.0	Carotene (μ/g)	600*
Protein (g)	13.3	Thiamine (mg)	0.1
Fat (g)	13.3	Riboflavin (mg)	0.4
Calcium (mg)	60.0	Niacin (mg)	0.1
Phosphorus (mg)	220.0	Folic acid (μ/g)	78.3
Iron (mg)	2.1		

*+360 mg of vitamin A.

Evaluation of Egg Quality

Candling

The quality of the egg in the shell is evaluated by candling. The egg is held up to an opening behind which is a source of strong light. Candling will reveal:

1. A crack in the shell.
2. The size of the air cell.
3. The firmness of albumin.
4. The position and mobility of yolk.
5. The possible presence of foreign substances like blood spots, moulds and developing embryo.

Floating in water

If the egg sinks it is considered as good. Poor quality egg floats (due to increase in air cell). It shows that the egg floating in water has lost in weight due to dehydration.

Haughs unit

Good quality egg has 72 haugh units and as the quality deteriorates it comes down to 36–60.

White index

The height of the thickest portion of the white is divided by the diameter of the egg gives white index.

Yolk index

Measurement of the height of the yolk in relation to the width of the yolk gives the yolk index.

Grading

The interior quality of the egg deteriorates from the time it is said to until it is consumed. With proper care, however, this decline in quality can be minimised.

DETERIORATION DURING STORAGE

1. Fertile eggs get deteriorated more rapidly than infertile eggs. Deterioration takes place as physical and chemical changes takes place.
2. Egg white becomes less viscous and spreads rapidly.
3. The size of the air cell and volume increases.
4. Loss of water, carbon dioxide, protein break down, egg flavour deteriorates.
5. Bacterial decomposition takes place.

EFFECT OF HEAT ON THE EGG PROTEINS

Upon heating the egg proteins are denatured and then gradually aggregate to form a three-dimensional get network. Ovalbumin the main protein in egg white is a globular protein denatured by heat. The range in temperatures over which coagulation takes place varies with the rate of heating. Heating on egg much beyond this temperature shrinks and toughens the coagulum of the white.

CHANGES DURING STORAGE

The changes that take place in eggs while they are being held or stored may be divided into those due to noumicrohial causes and those resulting from the growth of micro-organisms.

Changes Not Caused by Micro-organisms

Untreated eggs lose moisture during storage and hence lose weight. The amount of shrinkage is shown to the candler by the size of the air space or air cell at the blunt end of the egg, a large cell indicating much shrinkage. Of more importance is the change in the physical state of the contents of the egg, as shown by candling or by breaking out the egg. The white of the egg becomes thinner and more watery as the egg ages, and the yolk membrane becomes weaker. The poorer the egg, the more movement there is of the yolk and the nearer it approaches the shell when the egg is twirled during candling. When an old egg is broken onto a flat dish, the thinness of the white is more evident and the weakness of the yolk membrane permits the yolk to flatten out or even break. By contrast, a broken fresh egg shows a thick white and a yolk that stands up strongly in the form of a hemisphere. During storage, the alkalinity of the white of the egg increases from a normal pH of about 7.6 to about 9.5. Any marked growth of the chick embryos in fertilised eggs also serves to condemn the eggs.

Changes Caused by Micro-organisms

To cause spoilage of an undamaged shell egg, the causal organisms must do the following: (i) contaminate the shell, (ii) penetrate the pores of the shell to the shell membranes (usually the shell must be moist for this to occur), (iii) grow through the shell membranes to reach the white (or to reach the yolk if it touches the membrane), (iv) grow in the egg white, despite the previously mentioned unfavourable conditions there, to reach the yolk, where they can grow readily and complete spoilage of the egg. Bacteria unable to grow in the white can reach the yolk and flourish there only when the yolk touches the inner cell membrane. The time required for bacteria to penetrate the shell membranes varies with the organisms and the temperature but may take as long as several weeks at refrigerator temperatures. The special set of environmental conditions, the selective egg-white medium, and the low storage temperature of about 0°C combine to limit the number of kinds of bacteria and moulds that can cause spoilage chiefly to those to be mentioned.

In general, more spoilage of eggs is caused by bacteria than by moulds. The types of bacterial spoilage or 'rots', of eggs go by different names. Alford list five groups of rots that are found in Australian eggs for export. Among the three chief ones are the green rots, caused chiefly by *Pseudomonas fluorescens*, a bacterium that grows at 0°C; the rot is so named because of the bright-green colour of the white during early stages of development. This stage is noted with difficulty in candling but shows up clearly when the egg is broken.

Later the yolk may disintegrate and blend with the white so as to mask the green colour. Odour is lacking or is fruity or 'sweetish'. The contents of eggs so rotted fluoresce strongly under ultraviolet light. A second important group of rots are the colourless rots, which may be caused by *Pseudomonas*, *Acinetobacter*, *Alcaligenes*, certain coliform bacteria, or other types of bacteria. These rots are detected readily by candling, for the yolk usually is involved, except in very early stages, and disintegrates or at least shows a white incrustation. The odour varies from a scarcely detectable one to fruity to 'highly offensive'. The third important group of rots are the black rots, where the eggs are almost opaque to the candling lamp because the yolks become blackened and then break down to give the whole-egg contents a muddy-brown colour.

The odour is putrid, with hydrogen sulphide evident, and gas pressure may develop in the egg. Species of *Proteus* most commonly cause these rots, although some species of *Pseudomonas* and *Aeromonas* can cause black rots. *Proteus melanovogenes* causes an especially black colouration in the yolk and a dark colour in the white. The development of black rot and of red rot usually means that the egg has at some time been held at temperatures higher than those ordinarily used for storage. Pink rots occur less often, and red rots are still more infrequent. Pink rots are caused by strains of *Pseudomonas* and may at times be a later stage of some of the green rots. They resemble the colourless rots, except for a pinkish precipitate on the yolk and a pink colour in the white. Red rots, caused by species of *Serratia*, are mild in odour and are not offensive.

Florian and Trussell have listed rots by ten different species of the genera *Pseudomonas*, *Alcaligenes*, *Proteus*, *Flavobacterium*, and *Paracolobactrum*. These rots have been characterised as fluorescent, green and yellow, custard, black, red, rusty red, colourless, and mixed. These authors also list secondary invaders in the genera *Enterobacter*, *Alcaligenes*, *Escherichia*, *Flavobacterium*, and *Paracolobactrum*. These bacteria can grow in the egg but cannot initiate penetration.

The spoilage of eggs by fungi goes through stages of mould growth that give the defects their names. Very early mould growth is termed pin-spot moulding because of the small, compact colonies of moulds appearing on the shell and usually just inside it.

The colour of these pin spots varies with the kind of mould; *Penicillium* species cause yellow or blue or green spots inside the shell, *Cladosporium* species give dark-green or black spots, and species of *Sporotrichum* produce pink spots. In storage atmospheres of high humidity a variety of moulds may cause superficial fungal spoilage, first in the form of a fuzz or 'whiskers' covering the shell and later as more luxuriant growth. When the eggs are stored at near-freezing temperatures, as they usually are, the temperatures are high enough for slow mycelial growth of some moulds but too low for sporulation, while other moulds may produce asexual spores. Moulds causing spoilage of eggs include species of *Penicillium, Cladosporium, Sporotrichum, Mucor, Thamnidium, Botrytis, Alternaria*, and other genera. The final stage of spoilage by moulds is fungal rotting, after the mycelium of the mould has grown through the pores or cracks in the egg.

Jellying of the white may result, and coloured rots may be produced, e.g. fungal red rot by *Sporotrichum* and a black colour by *Cladosporium*, the cause of black spot of eggs as well as of other foods. The hyphae of the mould may weaken the yolk membrane enough to cause its rupture, after which the growth of the mould is stimulated greatly by the food released from the yolk.

Off-flavours sometimes are developed in eggs with little other outward evidence of spoilage. Thus mustiness may be caused by any of a number of bacteria, such as *Achromobacter perolens, Pseudomonas graveolens*, and *P. mucidolens*. The growth of *Streptomyces* on straw or elsewhere near the egg may produce musty or earthy flavours that are absorbed by the egg. Moulds growing in the shell also give musty odours and tastes.

A hay odour is caused by *Enterobacter cloacae*, while fishy flavours are produced by certain strains of *Escherichia coli*. The 'cabbage-water' flavour mentioned in connection with type II black rot of Haines may appear before rotting is obvious. Off-flavours, such as the 'cold-storage taste', may be absorbed from packing materials.

PROTECTIVE BARRIERS

Some foods are protected from direct contact with micro-organisms by a natural cover or barrier. Examples of barriers are the shell and shell membrane of eggs, the testa of seeds, and the cuticle of intact plant organs.

Egg Shell and Membranes

An invisible, natural, proteinlike film on the egg shell, called the cuticle or bloom, is considered by some to be the first line of defense against microbial penetration of the egg. The second physical barrier is the egg shell. Inside the shell are two membranes, the outer and inner shell membranes, which are the third and fourth barriers to microbial penetration. The structure of the egg and egg shell is shown in Fig. 13.1.

Cuticle

Washing of eggs and the use of abrasives to remove dirt disrupt the cuticle layer and allow easier penetration by micro-organisms. There is a diversity of opinion on the effect of washing eggs on the resultant contamination of the interior. The cuticle tends to crack and deteriorate with time. Hence, it is not much of a barrier for stored eggs.

Egg shell

The egg shell is not a homogeneous structure. It consists of an organic framework of fibres and an interstitial substance of inorganic material. The two main layers of the shell are the outer or spongy layer and the inner or mammillary layer. The outer layer is thicker and contains most of the minerals.

The shell contains from 6000 to 8000 microscopic pores. These pores allow the exchange of water vapour and gases between the contents of the shell and the outer atmosphere. The pores vary in size, with extremes being reported as 1.6 to 7.47 µm. The average pore size is probably between 20 and 45 µm. The size of most pores will allow the passage of many micro-organisms. Even yeast cells can be forced through pores, and mould mycelia grow through the pores. There is a linear relationship between shell porosity and infection of the eggs.

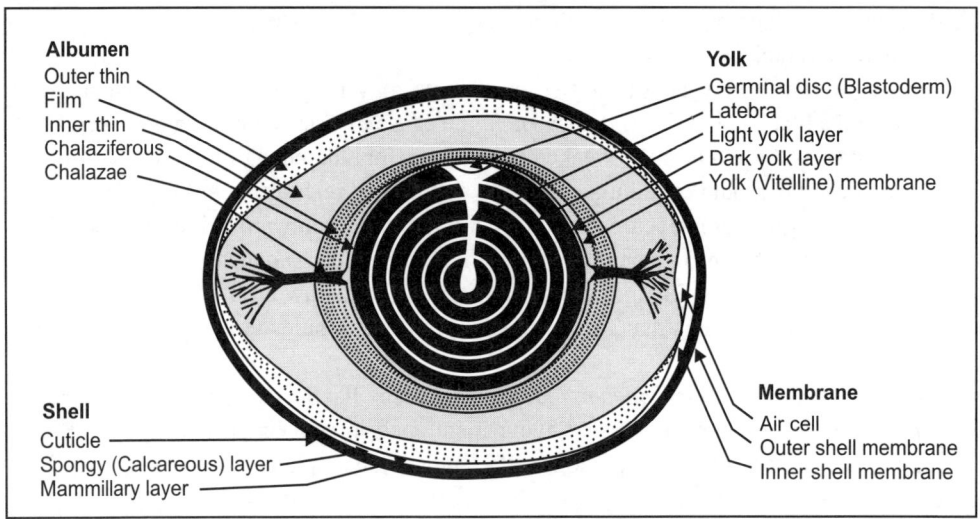

Fig. 13.1. The parts of an egg.

Shell weight and shell thickness do not correlate with penetration of micro-organisms. However, thin shells have a tendency to crack more readily than thicker shells. Eggs with damaged shells are more subject to penetration of bacteria and egg spoilage.

If the temperature of the egg is higher than the surroundings, a condition that exists when the egg is laid, there is a greater possibility of penetration and, as the temperature differential increases, the potential for infectivity increases. As the egg contents cool, they contract, which results in a higher pressure outside the shell than inside. This pressure differential will force micro-organisms through the pores of the shell.

Moisture on the egg shell, such as occurs during washing of eggs or when a cold egg is brought into a warm and humid room, increases the potential for microbial infection of the egg.

Shell membranes

The outer shell membrane is in contact with the egg shell, and the inner shell membrane, sometimes called the egg membrane, is in contact with the albumen. They are composed mainly of protein fibres (fibrin and mucin) strengthened with an albuminous cementing material. The membranes have been considered effective bacterial filters. The inner membrane is more effective than the outer membrane because of its closely knit fibres. Organisms inoculated onto the shell surface are found on the membranes almost instantly, but micro-organisms inoculated into the air cell and onto the inner membranes are not recoverable from the albumen for several days. This apparent retention of bacteria on the inner membrane may be partly due to conalbumin in the albumen, since adding iron to the inoculum or to the interior albumen of the egg hastens the penetration of the bacteria through the inner membrane. Wedral, Vadehra, and Baker found no difference in the permeability of the inner shell membrane before and after passage of either *Pseudomonas aeruginosa* or *Salmonella typhimurium*, indicating that no enzymatic activity is needed for penetration. With the conditions of their experiment, both bacterial species were able to penetrate from the shell surface through the inner membrane within two hours. By 36 hr after shell inoculation, all except one egg showed contaminated albumen. Although there are no pores, *per se*, in the membranes, there are apparently openings between the intermeshed fibres similar to a maze, which allow passage of bacteria through the membranes.

Even if bacteria can penetrate these barriers, they are confronted with the antimicrobial mechanisms of the albumen before they can attack the nutrients in the yolk.

When an egg is laid, it is essentially sterile. Some bacteria (salmonellae) and avian viruses may invade the ovaries of hens and contaminate the yolk before the egg is formed. Even for those few eggs that might be contaminated, the bacterial number is relatively low. Most of the contaminants on the egg shells are of intestinal origin.

Other sources of organisms are nesting material, feather dust, the feet and body of the bird, as well as subsequent handling and storage. Eggs obtained from poultry flocks on wire have less bacterial contamination than do eggs from flocks in houses with floor litter. This is because nesting material, including feces, has less chance of coming into contact with the shell.

PASTEURISATION

The heat treatment of foods below temperatures needed for sterilisation may be referred to as pasteurisation. Quite often, a temperature below 100°C is called pasteurisation, while above 100°C, the process is sterilisation. In most of the pasteurisation processes, the food is heated to between 60° and 85°C for a few seconds up to an hour. Generally, the heat treatment given to a food is designed to inactivate specific types or groups of micro-organisms. With pasteurisation, some organisms are killed and some are attenuated (sublethal injury), while the spores may be stimulated to germinate. The lethal effect depends upon the heat resistance of the organisms. Pasteurisation can be used for foods in which quality is affected adversely by a more severe heat treatment.

The pasteurisation process is named for Louis Pasteur, the French chemist who found that heating wine to 50° or 60°C for a short time inactivated spoilage micro-organisms without seriously affecting the quality of the wine. Since his work, the main objective of pasteurisation has evolved to destroy certain pathogenic micro-organisms in specific foods. When spoilage organisms are not very heat resistant, pasteurisation can extend the storage life of products, especially if the treated food is refrigerated, frozen, or otherwise treated to control surviving micro-organisms.

Pasteurisation is used to control micro-organisms in foods such as liquid egg products, dairy products, alcoholic beverages (beer, wine), crab, smoked fish, and certain high-acid products (fruit juice, pickles, sauerkraut, vinegar).

Egg Products

The USDA regulations stipulate that all liquid, frozen, and dried whole egg, yolk, and white be pasteurised or otherwise treated to destroy all viable salmonellae. Depending on the nature of the liquid egg product, various times and temperatures are used, as listed in Table 13.3. Salmonellae are less heat resistant in egg white than in whole egg or egg yolk. Higher temperatures are needed to pasteurise egg yolk products than liquid whole egg. A variety of egg products are produced, and they have different degrees of heat sensitivity. Salted eggs used in salad dressings do not have to be pasteurised. They must be properly labelled, and the salad dressing must contain not less than 1.4 per cent acetic acid and have a pH of 4.1 or lower. The final product must be held for 72 hr. Salmonellae will die at room temperature under these conditions.

Table 13.3. Pasteurising conditions for egg products.

Product		Temperature (°C)	Average holding time (min.)
Whole egg, plain		60	3.5
Yolk			
Plain		60	7.0
	or	62.2	3.5
Sugared or salted		62.2	7.0
	or	64.4	3.5
Egg white			
Plain, pH 9.0		65.7	3.5
Plain, pH 9.0, treated with H_2O_2		51.7	3.5
Stabilised with $Al_2(SO_4)_3$ at pH 7.0		50	3.5

These pasteurisation conditions ordinarily will reduce the standard plate count by about 99.9 per cent and the number of salmonellae essentially to zero. The heat sensitivity of salmonellae is affected by the pH. When 60°C is used, the D value at pH 9.0 is about 0.1 min. and at pH 5.5, it is about 1.0 min. Hence, pasteurisation of egg white at pH 9 requires less heat treatment than at lower pH levels. The addition of 10 per cent salt or sugar to egg yolk increases the heat stability of salmonellae by five to ten times. Fortunately, the stability of the egg proteins to heat also is increased by sugar or salt.

Successful pasteurisation is based on a critical time-temperature relationship. If the temperature is lowered by 1°C, the efficiency of pasteurisation is decreased. If the temperature is allowed to increase, there is danger of coagulating the egg, forming a film on the heat-exchanger surfaces or damaging the functional properties of the treated egg.

As liquids flow through the holding tubes, the flow may be laminar, turbulent or transitional. The latter has some characteristics of both laminar and turbulent flow. In any flow, the material in the center of the tube is flowing at a faster rate than that near the side of the tube. Hence, not all of the liquid egg passes through the pasteuriser at the same rate. Researchers suggested that the holding tube requirements should be based on the fastest, rather than the average, particle to traverse the tube.

The pasteurisation specifications (USDA) requires that every particle be held for at least a specified time and temperature. The normal control of plant operations uses the average holding times. These times are considered to be twice that of the fastest particle time. Hence, the minimum time for whole egg at 60°C would be 1.75 min., and the average time 3.5 min.

Liquid egg white is more heat sensitive than whole egg or yolk. If egg white is heated above 56° to 57°C, there are problems of coagulation. The addition of hydrogen peroxide to egg white reduces the heat resistance of the salmonellae so that lower pasteurisation temperatures can be used.

Except for conalbumin, the proteins in egg white are sufficiently heat stable at pH 7.0. Adding an aluminium salt such as aluminium sodium sulphate stabilises the conalbumin so that it can be heated to 60°C without coagulation.

Shafi, Cotterill, and Nichols found *Micrococcus, Alcaligenes, Pseudomonas, Bacillus*, and unidentified bacteria in pasteurised egg white. These genera, as well as species of *Staphylococcus, Streptococcus, Arizona (Salmonella)* and unidentified yeasts and moulds, were reported in pasteurised whole egg. The researchers reported similar types in pasteurised egg yolk. Payne, Gooch, and Barnes found

Microbacterium, various cocci and coccobacilli, and some *Bacillus* in pasteurised (65°C for 3 min.) whole egg. The presence of egg yolk protected *S. aureus* from the effects of heat.

PRESERVATION OF EGGS

The spoiling of eggs is due to the entrance of air carrying germs through the shells. Normally the shell has a surface coating of mucilaginous matter, which prevents for a time the entrance of these harmful organisms into the egg. But if this coating is removed or softened by washing or otherwise the keeping quality of the egg is much reduced. These facts explain why many methods of preservation have not been entirely successful, and suggest that the methods employed should be based upon the idea of protecting and rendering more effective the natural coating of the shell, so that air bearing the germs that cause decomposition may be completely excluded.

Eggs are often packed in lime, salt or other products, or are put in cold storage for winter use, but such eggs are very far from being perfect when they come upon the market. German authorities declare that water glass more closely conforms to the requirements of a good preservative than any of the substances commonly employed. A 10 per cent solution of water glass is said to preserve eggs so effectually that at the end of three and one-half months eggs still appeared to be perfectly fresh. In most packed eggs the yolk settles to one side, and the egg is then inferior in quality. In eggs preserved in water glass the yolk retained its normal position in the egg, and in taste they were not to be distinguished from fresh, unpacked store eggs.

Of twenty methods tested in Germany, the three which proved most effective were coating the eggs with vaseline, preserving them in limewater, and preserving them in water glass. The conclusion was reached that the last is preferable, because varnishing the eggs with vaseline takes considerable time, and treating them with limewater is likely to give the eggs a limy flavour.

Other methods follow:

1. Method I: Eggs can be preserved for winter use by coating them, when perfectly fresh, with paraffine. As the spores of fungi get into eggs almost as soon as they are laid, it is necessary to rub every egg with chloroform or wrap it a few minutes in a chloroform soaked rag before dipping it into the melted paraffine. If only a trace of the chloroform enters the shell the development of such germs as may have gained access to freshly laid eggs is prevented. The paraffine coating excludes all future contamination from germ-laden air, and with no fungi growing within, they retain their freshness and natural taste.

2. Method II: Preserving with lime—Dissolve in each gallon of water 12 ounces of quicklime, 6 ounces of common salt, 1 drachm of soda, 0.5 drachm saltpeter, 0.5 drachm tartar, and 1.5 drachms of borax. The fluid is brought into a barrel and sufficient quicklime to cover the bottom is then poured in. Upon this is placed a layer of eggs, quicklime is again thrown in and so on until the barrel is filled so that the liquor stands about 10 inches deep over the last layer of eggs. The barrel is then covered with a cloth, upon which is scattered some lime.

3. Method III: Melt 4 ounces of clear beeswax in a porcelain dish over a gentle fire, and stir in 8 ounces of olive oil. Let the solution of wax in oil cool somewhat, then dip the fresh eggs one by one into it so as to coat every part of the shell. A momentary dip is sufficient, all excess of the mixture being wiped off with a cotton cloth. The oil is absorbed in the shell, the wax hermetically closing all the pores.

4. Method IV: The Reinhard method is said to cause such chemical changes in the surface of the eggshell that it is closed up perfectly airtight and an admittance of air is entirely excluded, even

in case of long-continued storing. The eggs are for a short time exposed to the direct action of sulphuric acid, whereby the surface of the eggshell, which consists chiefly of lime carbonate, is transformed into lime sulphate. The dense texture of the surface thus produced forms a complete protection against the access of the outside air, which admits of storing the egg for a very long time, without the contents of the egg suffering any disadvantageous changes regarding taste and odour. The egg does not require any special treatment to prevent cracking on boiling, etc. Some object to this on the ground that sulphuric acid is a dangerous poison that might, on occasion, penetrate the shell.

5. Method V: Take about half a dozen eggs and place them in a netting (not so many as would chill the water below the boiling point, even for an instant), into a boiling solution of boric acid, withdraw immediately, and pack. Or put up, in oil, carrying 2 or 3 per cent of salicylic acid. Eggs treated in this way are said to taste, after six months, absolutely as fresh as they were when first put up. The eggs should be as fresh as possible, and should be thoroughly clean before dipping. The philosophy of the process is that the dipping in boiling boric acid solution not only kills all bacteria existing on, or in, the shell and membrane, but reinforces these latter by a very thin layer of coagulated albumen; while the packing in salicylated oil prevents the admission of fresh germs from the atmosphere. Salicylic acid is objected to on the same grounds as sulphuric acid.

6. Method VI: Dissolve sodium silicate in boiling water, to about the consistency of a syrup (or about 1 part of the silicate to 3 parts water). The eggs should be as fresh as possible, and must be thoroughly clean. They should be immersed in the solution in such manner that every part of each egg is covered with the liquid, then removed and let dry. If the solution is kept at or near the boiling temperature, the preservative effect is said to be much more certain and to last longer.

USES OF PRESERVATIVES

Preservatives may be used on the shells of eggs, in the atmosphere around them, or on wraps or containers for eggs. An enormous number of different substances have been applied to the surface of the shells of eggs or used as packing material about eggs to aid in their preservation. Some of these substances are used primarily to keep the shell dry and reduce penetration of oxygen into the egg and passage of carbon dioxide and moisture out; waxing, oiling the shells, and otherwise sealing are examples. Other materials inhibit the growth of micro-organisms, and some are germicidal. Materials used for the dry packing of eggs in the home include salt, lime, sand, sawdust, and ashes. Immersion in water glass, a solution of sodium silicate, long has been a successful home method of preservation. The solution is inhibitory because of its alkalinity.

Other inhibitory chemicals that have been tried are borates, permanganates, benzoates, salicylates, formates, and a host of other compounds. The utilisation of warm or hot solutions of germicides in the washing of eggs has been mentioned, such as solutions of hypochlorites, lye, acids, formalin, quaternary ammonium compounds, and detergent-sanitiser combinations. Sealing the shell with a solution of dimethylolurea has been found effective in inhibiting mould growth.

Some attempts have been made to reduce spoilage of eggs by moulds during storage by treatment of the flats and fillers of storage cases with a mycostatic or mould-inhibiting chemical. Sodium pentachlorophenate and related compounds have been used with some success. Fumigation of eggs with gaseous ethylene oxide before storage has been reported to protect them against bacterial spoilage.

The only two gases that are added to the atmosphere about eggs to improve their keeping quality are carbon dioxide and ozone, although nitrogen has been used experimentally. Recommendations vary concerning the optimal concentration of carbon dioxide in the air for this purpose. A low concentration, 2.5 per cent, for example, slows physical and chemical changes in the egg that accompany the rise in pH as carbon dioxide escapes from the egg but has little effect on microbial growth, particularly of moulds. Concentrations as high as 60 per cent will markedly delay microbial spoilage, especially if the temperature is near freezing, even if the relative humidity approaches saturation, but the white becomes thinner and an unpleasant flavour develops. Thus the recommendations vary from 0.5 to 0.6 per cent at −1°C and from 2.5 to 5 per cent at 0°C up to a 15 per cent maximum. There has been some disagreement about the effectiveness of ozone. It has been claimed that from 0.6 ppm of ozone (for clean eggs) to 1.5 ppm (for dirty eggs) at −0.55°C and 90 per cent relative humidity will keep eggs fresh for 8 months and that 3.5 ppm will not injure them, but some workers claim that 0.5 to 1.5 ppm have little effect on micro-organisms. Low concentrations of ozone are reported to improve the flavour of stored eggs because of the deodourising effect of the gas.

Chapter 14

Contamination, Preservation and Spoilage of Milk Products

INTRODUCTION

Milk is brought from the farm to the dairy for processing. When received at the dairy, the following information on the milk is required:

1. Quality: Before weighing the milk, its quality should be checked. Taste and smell are good preliminary indicators of milk quality, and visual observation can also be useful. If the person receiving the milk suspects that it is of poor quality, he or she can carry out one of the following tests: acidity, pH, alcohol and clot-on-boiling. These will determine the quality of the milk. Once the person receiving the milk is satisfied with its quality, it can be weighed and the weight recorded.

2. Weight: The quantity of milk received can be estimated either volumetrically or gravimetrically. Milk processors usually base payments for milk on its solids content, and hence it is more appropriate to use weight to estimate the quantity of milk being tendered. In a small-scale processing centre a spring balance and a stainless-steel bucket can be used to weigh milk. The milk weight must be recorded accurately as losses can be incurred or underpayments made to suppliers if care is not taken at this stage.

3. Composition of milk and presence of additives: A dairy engaged in butter-making will need to base its payments on the butterfat content of the milk. The milk received will have to be sampled for butterfat analysis. The procedure for this is dealt with below. Spot checks can also be carried out to test for added water and the presence of neutralisers if malpractice is suspected.

WHAT IS MILK SPOILAGE?

This is contamination of milk with foreign substances and harmful bacteria that can cause illness to consumers. Contamination and spoilage occurs from before milking up to the time of consumption. Contaminated milk is rejected by processors, dairy societies and consumers leading to loss of farmers' income. Spoilt milk has various characteristics which include:

1. Has clots or yellow brownish colour.
2. Clots on boiling.
3. Bad smell.
4. Appears watery.

Causes of Milk Spoilage

Various factors may contribute towards milk spoilage. These include:

1. The cow: The cow may collect mud, straw or dung from a poorly constructed or dirty shed which may contaminate milk. Cow diseases like mastitis as well as antibiotic residues may also contaminate milk.

2. The milker: If proper hygiene is not observed by the milker, spoilage can occur. Poor hygiene may be failure to wash hands before milking and use of dirty and inappropriate utensils among others.

3. Environment: Disease pathogens, flavours in feeds as well as straw, dung and soil from the cow sheds environment may also contaminate milk.

4. Environmental saprophytic micro-organisms: From teat canal, teat and udder skin, dust, manure, bedding material, feed, water, milking system, cooling tanks.

5. Pathogenic micro-organisms: From diseased cows—80 per cent of inflamed quarter milk samples contain pathogenic bacteria.

Preventive measures to minimise or evade spoilage are shown in the Table 14.1.

Table 14.1. Spoilage factors, sources and prevention.

Factor	Source of spoilage	Prevention
The cow	Soil, dust, mud, dung	Wash mud off the cow.
		Wash udder with clean cloth dipped in warm water.
	Disease, e.g. Mastitis	Cut udder hair short.
		Maintain cleanliness.
		Treat cows.
		Cull cows which do not respond to avoid infection of others.
	Antibiotic residue in treatment of sick cows	Observe drug withdrawal period.
The milker	Inadequate hygiene	Wash hands before milking and ensure nails are short.
		Cut nails short.
		Do not milk when you are sick.
		Do not sneeze, cough, spit, and smoke over the milk.
Milk utensils	Unsuitable utensil type and cleanliness	Wash milking utensils in clean hot water.
Bacteria, yeasts and moulds	Dirty housing of cow	Good roofing and concrete floor for cow shed.
	Plastic milk utensils	Clean metal cans for milk storage.
		Cool milk in refrigerator, water basin or wet charcoal cooler.
Impurities	Soil, straw, dung	Maintain clean cow shed.
Off-flavours	Feed sources with odours, inadequate cleansing of detergents and/or pesticides	Avoid strong smelling fodder or silage two hours before milking.
		Avoid milk storage near wet paint.

Steps to Minimise Spoilage

1. Always use boiled water to wash your hands, udder and teats before milking.
2. Use clean cloth to wash, clean and dry the udder.
3. Milk the first drop from each of the quarters into a black gum boot to check for clots and reddish brown colour which are indicators of mastitis.
4. Sieve the milk with a strainer or muslin cloth into an appropriate container to remove particles (Fig. 14.1).

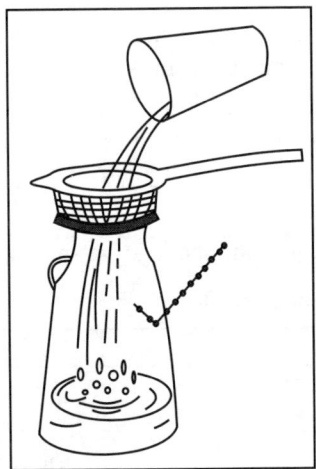

Fig. 14.1. Container to remove particles.

5. Cover the milk and transport it to a clean and cool place.
6. Milk mastitis infected cows last after milking clean cows and thereafter dip teats in an antiseptic teat dip and discard such milk.

Testing the Quality of Milk

If you suspect that your cow has mastitis but you are not observing the symptoms: Take a sample of milk from an affected quarter of the udder and send to the nearest veterinary investigation or research laboratory.

BASIC MICROBIOLOGY

Micro-organism

Micro-organisms are living organisms that are individually too small to see with the naked eye. The unit of measurement used for micro-organisms is the micrometre (μ m); 1 μm = 0.001 millimetre; 1 nanometer (nm) = 0.001 μm. Micro-organisms are found everywhere (ubiquitous) and are essential to many of our planets life processes. With regards to the food industry, they can cause spoilage, prevent spoilage through fermentation or can be the cause of human illness.

There are several classes of micro-organisms, of which bacteria and fungi (yeasts and moulds) will be discussed in some detail. Another type of micro-organism, the bacterial viruses or bacteriophage, will be examined in a later section.

Bacteria

Bacteria are relatively simple single-celled organisms. One method of classification is by shape or morphology:

1. Cocci: spherical shape, –0.4–1.5 μm, e.g. staphylococci—form grape-like clusters; streptococci—form bead-like chains.
2. Rods: –0.25–1.0 μm width by 0.5–6.0 μm long, e.g. bacilli—straight rod; spirilla—spiral rod.

There exists a bacterial system of taxonomy or classification system, that is internationally recognised with family, genera and species divisions based on genetics.

Some bacteria have the ability to form resting cells known as endospores. The spore forms in times of environmental stress, such as lack of nutrients and moisture needed for growth, and thus is a survival strategy. Spores have no metabolism and can withstand adverse conditions such as heat, disinfectants, and ultraviolet light. When the environment becomes favourable, the spore germinates and giving rise to a single vegetative bacterial cell. Some examples of spore-formers important to the food industry are members of *Bacillus* and *Clostridium* generas.

Bacteria reproduce asexually by fission or simple division of the cell and its contents. The doubling time, or generation time, can be as short as 20–20 min. Since each cell grows and divides at the same rate as the parent cell, this could under favourable conditions translate to an increase from one to 10 million cells in 11 hours! However, bacterial growth in reality is limited by lack of nutrients, accumulation of toxins and metabolic wastes, unfavourable temperatures and dessication.

Note: Bacterial populations are expressed as colony forming units (CFU) per gram or millilitre.

Bacterial growth generally proceeds through a series of phases:

1. Lag phase: time for micro-organisms to become accustomed to their new environment. There is little or no growth during this phase.
2. Log phase: bacteria logarithmic, or exponential, growth begins; the rate of multiplication is the most rapid and constant.
3. Stationary phase: the rate of multiplication slows down due to lack of nutrients and build-up of toxins. At the same time, bacteria are constantly dying so the numbers actually remain constant.
4. Death phase: cell numbers decrease as growth stops and existing cells die off.

The shape of the curve varies with temperature, nutrient supply, and other growth factors. This exponential death curve is also used in modelling the heating destruction of micro-organisms.

Yeasts

Yeasts are members of a higher group of micro-organisms called fungi. They are single-cell organisms of spherical, elliptical or cylindrical shape. Their size varies greatly but are generally larger than bacterial cells. Yeasts may be divided into two groups according to their method of reproduction:

1. Budding: Called fungi imperfecti or false yeasts.
2. Budding and spore formation: Called ascomycetes or true yeasts.

Unlike bacterial spores, yeast form spores as a method of reproduction.

Moulds

Moulds are filamentous, multi-celled fungi with an average size larger than both bacteria and yeasts (10 × 40 μm). Each filament is referred to as a hypha. The mass of hyphae that can quickly spread over a food substrate is called the mycelium.

Moulds may reproduce either asexually or sexually, sometimes both within the same species. Asexual reproduction:

1. Fragmentation—hyphae separate into individual cells called arthropsores.
2. Spore production—formed in the tip of a fruiting hyphae, called conidia, or in swollen structures called sporangium.

Sexual reproduction: sexual spores are produced by nuclear fission in times of unfavourable conditions to ensure survival.

Microbial Growth

There are a number of factors that affect the survival and growth of micro-organisms in food. The parameters that are inherent to the food, or intrinsic factors, include the following:

1. Nutrient content.
2. Moisture content.
3. pH.
4. Available oxygen.
5. Biological structures.
6. Antimicrobial constituents.

Nutrient requirements

While the nutrient requirements are quite organism specific, the micro-organisms of importance in foods require the following:

1. Water.
2. Energy source.
3. Carbon/nitrogen source.
4. Vitamins.
5. Minerals.

Milk and dairy products are generally very rich in nutrients which provides an ideal growth environment for many micro-organisms.

Moisture content

All micro-organisms require water but the amount necessary for growth varies between species. The amount of water that is available in food is expressed in terms of water activity (a_w), where the a_w of pure water is 1.0. Each micro-organism has a maximum, optimum, and minimum a_w for growth and survival. Generally bacteria dominate in foods with high a_w (minimum approximately 0.90 a_w) while yeasts and moulds, which require less moisture, dominate in low a_w foods (minimum 0.70 a_w). The water activity of fluid milk is approximately 0.98 a_w.

pH

Most micro-organisms have approximately a neutral pH optimum (pH 6–7.5). Yeasts are able to grow in a more acid environment compared to bacteria. Moulds can grow over a wide pH range but prefer only slightly acid conditions. Milk has a pH of 6.6 which is ideal for the growth of many micro-organisms.

Available oxygen

Micro-organisms can be classified according to their oxygen requirements necessary for growth and survival:
1. Obligate aerobes: oxygen required.
2. Facultative: grow in the presence or absence of oxygen.
3. Microaerophilic: grow best at very low levels of oxygen.
4. Aerotolerant anaerobes: oxygen not required for growth but not harmful if present.
5. Obligate anaerobes: grow only in complete absence of oxygen; if present it can be lethal.

Biological structures

Physical barriers such as skin, rinds, feathers, etc. have provided protection to plants and animals against the invasion of micro-organisms. Milk, however, is a fluid product with no barriers to the spreading of micro-organisms throughout the product.

Antimicrobial constituents

As part of the natural protection against micro-organisms, many foods have antimicrobial factors. Milk has several nonimmunological proteins which inhibit the growth and metabolism of many micro-organisms including the following most common:
1. Lactoperoxidase.
2. Lactoferrin.
3. Lysozyme.
4. Xanthine.

Where the intrinsic factors are related to the food properties, the extrinsic factors are related to the storage environment. These would include temperature, relative humidity, and gases that surround the food.

Temperature

As a group, micro-organisms are capable of growth over an extremely wide temperature range. However, in any particular environment, the types and numbers of micro-organisms will depend greatly on the temperature. According to temperature, micro-organisms can be placed into one of three broad groups:
1. Psychrotrophs: Optimum growth temperatures 20° to 30°C capable of growth at temperatures less than 7°C. Psychrotrophic organisms are specifically important in the spoilage of refrigerated dairy products.
2. Mesophiles: Optimum growth temperatures 30° to 40°C; do not grow at refrigeration temperatures.
3. Thermophiles: optimum growth between 55° and 65°C.

It is important to note that for each group, the growth rate increases as the temperature increases only up to an optimum, after which it rapidly declines.

Detection and Enumeration of Micro-organisms

There are several methods for detection and enumeration of micro-organisms in food. The method that is used depends on the purpose of the testing.

Direct enumeration

Using direct microscopic counts (DMC), coulter counter, etc. allows a rapid estimation of all viable and nonviable cells. Identification through staining and observation of morphology also possible with DMC.

Viable enumeration

The use of standard plate counts, most probable number (MPN), membrane filtration, plate loop methods, spiral plating, etc. allows the estimation of only viable cells. As with direct enumeration, these methods can be used in the food industry to enumerate fermentation, spoilage, pathogenic, and indicator organisms.

Metabolic activity measurement

An estimation of metabolic activity of the total cell population is possible using dye reduction tests such as resazurin or methylene blue dye reduction, acid production, electrical impedance, etc. The level of bacterial activity can be used to assess the keeping quality and freshness of milk. Toxin levels can also be measured, indicating the presence of toxin producing pathogens.

Cellular constituents measurement

Using the luciferase test to measure ATP is one example of the rapid and sensitive tests available that will indicate the presence of even one pathogenic bacterial cell. Isolation of micro-organisms is an important preliminary step in the identification of most food spoilage and pathogenic organisms. This can be done using a simple streak plate method.

MICRO-ORGANISMS IN MILK

Milk is sterile at secretion in the udder but is contaminated by bacteria even before it leaves the udder. Except in the case of mastisis, the bacteria at this point are harmless and few in number. Further infection of the milk by micro-organisms can take place during milking, handling, storage, and other preprocessing activities.

Lactic acid bacteria: This group of bacteria are able to ferment lactose to lactic acid. They are normally present in the milk and are also used as starter cultures in the production of cultured dairy products such as yogurt. Note: many lactic acid bacteria have recently been reclassified; the older names will appear in brackets as you will still find the older names used for convenience sake in a lot of literature. Some examples in milk are:

1. Lactococci:
    (a) *L. delbrueckii* subsp. *lactis* (*Streptococcus lactis*).
    (b) *Lactococcus lactis* subsp. *cremoris* (*Streptococcus cremoris*).
2. Lactobacilli:
    (a) *Lactobacillus casei.*
    (b) *L. delbrueckii* subsp. *lactis* (*L. lactis*).
    (c) *L. delbrueckii* subsp. *bulgaricus* (*Lactobacillus bulgaricus*).
3. Leuconostoc.

Coliforms: Coliforms are facultative anaerobes with an optimum growth at 37°C. Coliforms are indicator organisms; they are closely associated with the presence of pathogens but not necessarily pathogenic themselves. They also can cause rapid spoilage of milk because they are able to ferment lactose with the production of acid and gas, and are able to degrade milk proteins. They are killed by HTST treatment, therefore, their presence after treatment is indicative of contamination. *Escherichia coli* is an example belonging to this group.

Significance of Micro-organisms in Milk

1. Information on the microbial content of milk can be used to judge its sanitary quality and the conditions of production.
2. If permitted to multiply, bacteria in milk can cause spoilage of the product.
3. Milk is potentially susceptible to contamination with pathogenic micro-organisms. Precautions must be taken to minimise this possibility and to destroy pathogens that may gain entrance.
4. Certain micro-organisms produce chemical changes that are desirable in the production of dairy products such as cheese, yogurt.

Spoilage Micro-organisms in Milk

The microbial quality of raw milk is crucial for the production of quality dairy foods. Spoilage is a term used to describe the deterioration of a foods' texture, colour, odour or flavour to the point where it is unappetising or unsuitable for human consumption. Microbial spoilage of food often involves the degradation of protein, carbohydrates, and fats by the micro-organisms or their enzymes. In milk, the micro-organisms that are principally involved in spoilage are psychrotrophic organisms. Most psychrotrophs are destroyed by pasteurisation temperatures, however, some like *Pseudomonas fluorescens*, *Pseudomonas fragi* can produce proteolytic and lipolytic extracellular enzymes which are heat stable and capable of causing spoilage. Some species and strains of *Bacillus*, *Clostridium*, *Cornebacterium*, *Arthrobacter*, *Lactobacillus*, *Microbacterium*, *Micrococcus*, and *Streptococcus* can survive pasteurisation and grow at refrigeration temperatures which can cause spoilage problems.

Pathogenic Micro-organisms in Milk

Hygienic milk production practices, proper handling and storage of milk, and mandatory pasteurisation has decreased the threat of milkborne diseases such as tuberculosis, brucellosis, and typhoid fever. There have been a number of foodborne illnesses resulting from the ingestion of raw milk or dairy products made with milk that was not properly pasteurised or was poorly handled causing post-processing contamination. The following bacterial pathogens are still of concern today in raw milk and other dairy products:

1. *Bacillus cereus*.
2. *Listeria monocytogenes*.
3. *Yersinia enterocolitica*.
4. *Salmonella* spp.
5. *Escherichia coli* O157:H7.
6. *Campylobacter jejuni*.

It should also be noted that moulds, mainly of species of *Aspergillus*, *Fusarium*, and *Penicillium* can grow in milk and dairy products. If the conditions permit, these moulds may produce mycotoxins which can be a health hazard.

HAZARD ANALYSIS AND CRITICAL CONTROL POINTS (HACCP)

Raw and end-products may be tested for the presence, level, or absence of micro-organisms. Traditionally these practices were used to reduce manufacturing defects in dairy products and ensure compliance with specifications and regulations, however, they have many drawbacks:

1. Destructive and time consuming.
2. Slow response.

3. Small sample size.
4. Delays in the release of the food.

In the 1960's, the Pillsbury Company, the US Army, and NASA introduced a system for assuring pathogen-free foods for the space program. This system, called Hazard Analysis and Critical Control Points (HACCP), is a focus on critical food safety areas as part of total quality programs. It involves a critical examination of the entire food manufacturing process to determine every step where there is a possibility of physical, chemical or microbiological contamination of the food which would render it unsafe or unacceptable for human consumption. These identified points are the critical control points (CCP). There are seven principles to HACCP:

1. Analyse hazards.
2. Determine CCPs.
3. Establish critical limits.
4. Establish monitoring procedures.
5. Establish deviation procedures.
6. Establish verification procedures.
7. Establish record keeping procedures.

Before these principles can be put into place, a prerequisite program and preliminary setup is necessary.

Prerequisite Program

1. Premise control.
2. Receiving and storage control.
3. Equipment performance and maintenance control.
4. Personnel training.
5. Sanitation.
6. Recall procedure.

Preliminary Setup

1. Assemble team.
2. Describe the product.
3. Identify intended use.
4. Construct flow diagram and plant schematic.
5. Verify the diagram on-site.

Food Safety Enhancement Program-FSEP is The Canadian Food Inspection Agency's HACCP initiative. There is extensive information at their Website regarding FSEP, including implementation manuals, HACCP curriculum guidelines, and generic models.

STARTER CULTURES

Starter cultures are those micro-organisms that are used in the production of cultured dairy products such as yogurt and cheese. The natural microflora of the milk is either inefficient, uncontrollable, and unpredictable, or is destroyed altogether by the heat treatments given to the milk. A starter culture can provide particular characteristics in a more controlled and predictable fermentation. The primary function of lactic starters is the production of lactic acid from lactose.

Other functions of starter cultures may include the following:
1. Flavour, aroma, and alcohol production.
2. Proteolytic and lipolytic activities.
3. Inhibition of undesirable organisms.

There are two groups of lactic starter cultures:
1. Simple or defined: single strain, or more than one in which the number is known.
2. Mixed or compound: more than one strain each providing its own specific characteristics.

Starter cultures may be categorised as mesophilic or thermophilic:

Mesophilic

1. *Lactococcus lactis* subsp. *cremoris*.
2. *L. delbrueckii* subsp. *lactis*.
3. *L. lactis* subsp. *lactis* biovar *diacetylactis*.
4. *Leuconostoc mesenteroides* subsp. *cremoris*.

Thermophilic

1. *Streptococcus salivarius* subsp. *thermophilus* (*S. thermophilus*)
2. *Lactobacillus delbrueckii* subsp. *bulgaricus*.
3. *L. delbrueckii* subsp. *lactis*.
4. *L. casei*.
5. *L. helveticus*.
6. *L. plantarum*.

Mixtures of mesophilic and thermophilic micro-organisms can also be used as in the production of some cheeses.

Bacteriophage

Bacteriophages are viruses that require bacteria host cells for growth and reproduction. Initially, the bacteriophage attaches itself to the bacteria cell wall and injects nuclear substance into the cell. Inside the cell, the nuclear substance produces shells or phage coats, for the new bacteriophage which are quickly filled with nucleic acid. The bacterial cell ruptures and dies as the new bacteriophage are released.

Bacteriophages are ubiquitous but generally enter the milk processing plant with the farm milk. They can be inactivated heat treatments of 30 min. at 63° to 88°C or by the use of chemical disinfectants.

Bacteriophages are of most concern in cheese making. They attack and destroy most of the lactic acid bacteria which prevents normal ripening known as slow or dead vat.

Starter Culture Preparation

Commercial manufacturers provide starter cultures in lyophilised (freeze-dried), frozen or spray-dried forms. The dairy product manufacturers need to inoculate the culture into milk or other suitable substrate. There are a number of steps necessary for the propagation of starter culture ready for production:
1. Commercial culture.
2. Mother culture—first inoculation; all cultures will originate from this preparation.
3. Intermediate culture—in preparation of larger volumes of prepared starter.
4. Bulk starter culture—this stage is used in dairy product production.

PATHOGENIC BACTERIA IN MILK

Raw milk obtained from cows is complete nutrition that can fulfil a person's needs. It contains helpful lactobacillus acidophilus bacteria that are useful for maintaining the healthy gastrointestinal tract along with many other useful things. Normally, these bacteria contain and even kill the pathogenic bacteria and yeast that are found in the gut. However, during the milking process, presence of mastitis in the udder can cause the pathogenic bacteria in the milk. Bacteria present on the outside skin of the udders and unhygienic milking practices which allows the milk to come in contact with contaminants like feces may also cause pathogenic bacteria in the milk. During the process of pasteurisation, which is performed to cure and extend the milk's shelf-life, the probiotic lactobacillus bacteria are killed along with pathogenic bacteria in the milk. However, the process fails to eradicate all of the pathogenic bacteria. Because of this one may find, through laboratory tests, different types of pathogenic bacteria in milk.

Types of Pathogenic Bacteria in Milk

The presence of these pathogenic bacteria, as you may have guessed, is a threat to its consumer's digestive health and may cause various types of food allergies. The following is the information about the few of them from the pathogenic bacteria list which may prove useful to all.

Enteropathogenic Escherichia coli (EPEC)

This micro-organism can gain entry into the human body through contaminated food items. The presence of this pathogenic bacteria in milk is a clear indication that during the milking process there was a lack of sanitary measures followed. The milk, during the process, has come into the contact with feces contaminated with this pathogen. *E. coli* (*Escherichia coli*) which is rod-shaped and typed as a gram negative bacteria that is classified under the family *Enterobacteriaceae*. These are known to produce enterotoxins and cause gastroenteritis in their victims. Infection of *E. coli* leads to watery or bloody diarrhea and most of the time, is the cause of infantile diarrhea.

Campylobacter jejuni

Campylobacter jejuni or *C. jejuni* is a Gram negative, curved and motile rod like bacteria. The presence of this pathogenic bacteria in milk causes gastroenteritis or *Campylobactor enteritis* in the consumer. Alternatively, the illness is called as *Campylobacteriosis* which can cause fever, abdominal pain, headache or muscle pain in an infected person. *C. jejuni* infection is often a cause of diarrhea which can be watery, bloody or sticky. It may also contain fecal leukocytes. The transmission of this pathogen in humans can occur from healthy livestock, chicken and raw milk. Research on *C. jejuni* shows that this pathogenic bacteria causes more bacterial diarrheal illness in the United States than any other microbe.

Yersinia enterocolitica

Yersinia enterocolitica or *Y. enterocolitica* is pathogenic bacteria that is typed as Gram negative and is small rod-shaped. The entry of this bacteria in the body of its victim can occur through contaminated milk and ice cream. The infection of the *Y. enterocolitica* can cause gastroenteritis in the its victim. He may suffer due to intestinal infection symptoms such as fever, abdominal pain, diarrhea or vomiting along with the gastroenteritis. In addition to food stuff such as pork, beef and fish, raw milk also act as the vehicle of the transmission of this pathogenic bacteria. The detection of this pathogenic bacteria in milk is thought to be because of poor sanitation, improper sterilisation technique and improper storage of milk.

Listeria monocytogenes

Listeria monocytogenes or *L. monocytogenes* is one of the most prevalent Gram negative bacteria in mammals, birds, fish, shellfish and feral. It is believed that 1–10 per cent of humans carry this bacterium in their intestine. Dealing with the infection of this bacterium is considered to be difficult because it is quite hardy. Because of its ability to adapt itself to extreme conditions, the presence of this pathogenic bacteria in milk is quite harmful.

It may enter its victim's body after consumption of raw milk, cheese and even, through pasteurised milk and is really dangerous. The diseases that are caused by the *L. monocytogenes* are covered under an umbrella term of listeriosis.

The infection by this pathogen can cause septicemia, meningitis, and encephalitis in the infected person. In case of pregnant women, it may cause intrauterine or cervical infections which may result in an abortion or still birth. *L. monocytogenes* has the capacity to overcome the victim's monocytes, macrophages, or polymorphonuclear leukocytes which forms the defense against pathogens.

For thousands of year people have used milk as a source of nutritional supplement and have obtained raw milk benefits. However, when it comes to supplying milk to people on a large scale, as it is done today, improper practices or ignorance at the time of handling it, can cause this source to get contaminated. To avoid such a waste of this valuable food source and health complications because of pathogenic diseases in consumers, proper training, and sanitary methods must be employed. Tests, to ensure quality and food safety, must be conducted to detect pathogenic bacteria in milk before it is passed on to consumers.

Comparison of the composition of cow's, goat's, and human's milk is given in Table 14.2.

Table 14.2. Compounds in cow's milk, goat's milk and human milk.

Compounds	Cow's milk (%)	Goat's milk (%)	Human milk (%)
Fat	3.90	3.80	3.30
Milk-sugar	4.90	4.50	6.50
Proteins, combined with calcium	3.20	3.10	1.50
Salts	0.901	0.939	0.313
Di-calcium phosphate	0.175	0.092	0.000
Tri-calcium	0.000	0.062	0.000
Mono-magnesium phosphate	0.103	0.000	0.027
Di-magnesium	0.000	0.068	0.000
Tri-magnesium	0.000	0.024	0.000
Mono-potassium	0.000	0.073	0.069
Di-potassium	0.230	0.000	0.000
Potassium citrate	0.052	0.250	0.103
Sodium	0.222	0.000	0.055
Potassium chloride	0.000	0.160	0.000
Sodium	0.000	0.095	0.000
Calcium	0.119	0.115	0.059

Composition of Milk

Phosphates

Cow's milk

The insoluble phosphate is di-calcium phosphate; tri-calcium, di- and tri-magnesium phosphates do not appear to be present. The soluble phosphates are mono-magnesium and di-potassium, which constitute about two-thirds of the total phosphates.

Goat's milk

This differs from cow's milk: (i) in containing tri-calcium, di- and tri-magnesium, and mono-potassium phosphates, and (ii) in containing no mono-magnesium or di-potassium phosphates.

Human milk

This differs noticeably from both cow's milk and goat's milk in containing no insoluble phosphates, but only the soluble compounds, mono-magnesium and mono-potassium phosphates. The phosphates in human milk are much less in amount than in cow's or goat's milk.

Citrates

All three milks contain potassium citrate, while cow's milk and human milk contain sodium citrate also.

Chlorides

Chlorides are present in goat's milk in much larger amounts than in cow's milk or human milk; the amount in cow's milk is considerably larger than in human milk. In cow's milk and human milk the chloride appears to be calcium chloride, while in goat's milk potassium and sodium chlorides are also present.

Total salts

The total amount of salts in human milk is about one-third that in cow's milk or goat's milk. The number of different salts appears to be greatest in goat's milk and least in human milk.

EFFECT OF BACTERIA ON MILK

The first and most universal change effected in milk is its souring. So universal is this phenomenon that it is generally regarded as an inevitable change which cannot be avoided, and, as already pointed out, has in the past been regarded as a normal property of milk. Today, however, the phenomenon is well understood. It is due to the action of certain milk bacteria upon the milk sugar which converts it into lactic acid, and this acid gives the sour taste and curdles the milk. After this acid is produced in small quantity its presence proves deleterious to the growth of the bacteria, and further bacterial growth is checked. After souring, therefore, the milk for some time does not ordinarily undergo any further changes.

Milk souring has been commonly regarded as a single phenomenon, alike in all cases. When it was first studied by bacteriologists it was thought to be due in all cases to a single species of micro-organism which was discovered to be commonly present and named *Bacillus acidi lactici*. This bacterium has certainly the power of souring milk rapidly, and is found to be very common in dairies in Europe.

As soon as bacteriologists turned their attention more closely to the subject it was found that the spontaneous souring of milk was not always caused by the same species of bacterium. Instead of finding this *Bacillus acidi lactici* always present, they found that quite a number of different species of bacteria have the power of souring milk, and are found in different specimens of soured milk. The number of species of bacteria which have been found to sour milk has increased until something over a hundred are known to have this power. These different species do not affect the milk in the same way. All produce some acid, but they differ in the kind and the amount of acid, and especially in the other changes which are effected at the same time that the milk is soured, so that the resulting soured milk is quite variable. In spite of this variety, however, the most recent work tends to show that the majority of cases of spontaneous souring of milk are produced by bacteria which, though somewhat variable, probably constitute a single species, and are identical with the *Bacillus acidi lactici*. This species, found common in the dairies of Europe, according to recent investigations occurs in this country as well. We may say, then, that while there are many species of bacteria infesting the dairy which can sour the milk, there is one which is more common and more universally found than others, and this is the ordinary cause of milk souring.

When we study more carefully the effect upon the milk of the different species of bacteria found in the dairy, we find that there is a great variety of changes which they produce when they are allowed to grow in milk. The dairyman experiences many troubles with his milk. It sometimes curdles without becoming acid. Sometimes it becomes bitter or acquires an unpleasant 'tainted' taste, or, again, a 'soapy' taste. Occasionally a dairyman finds his milk becoming slimy, instead of souring and curdling in the normal fashion. At such times, after a number of hours, the milk becomes so slimy that it can be drawn into long threads. Such an infection proves very troublesome, for many a time it persists in spite of all attempts made to remedy it.

Again, in other cases the milk will turn blue, acquiring about the time it becomes sour a beautiful sky-blue colour. Or it may become red, or occasionally yellow. All of these troubles the dairyman owes to the presence in his milk of unusual species of bacteria which grow there abundantly.

Bacteriologists have been able to make out satisfactorily the connection of all these infections with different species of the bacteria. A large number of species have been found to curdle milk without rendering it acid, several render it bitter, and a number produce a 'tainted' and one a 'soapy' taste. A score or more have been found which have the power of rendering the milk slimy. Two different species at least have the power of turning the milk to sky blue colour; two or three produce red pigments, and one or two have been found which produce a yellow colour. In short, it has been determined beyond question that all these infections, which are more or less troublesome to dairymen, are due to the growth of unusual bacteria in the milk.

These various infections are all troublesome, and indeed it may be said that, so far as concerns the milk producer and the milk consumer, bacteria are from beginning to end a source of trouble. It is the desire of the milk producer to avoid them as far as possible—a desire which is shared also by everyone who has anything to do with milk as milk. Having recognised that the various troubles, which occasionally occur even in the better class of dairies, are due to bacteria, the dairyman is, at least in a measure, prepared to avoid them. The avoiding of these troubles is moderately easy as soon as dairymen recognise the source from which the infectious organisms come, and also the fact that low temperatures will in all cases remedy the evil to a large extent.

With this knowledge in hand the avoidance of all these troubles is only a question of care in handling the dairy. It must be recognised that most of these troublesome bacteria come from some unusual sources of infection. By unusual sources are meant those which the exercise of care will avoid. It is true that the souring bacteria appear to be so universally distributed that they cannot be avoided by any ordinary means. But all other troublesome bacteria appear to be within control. The milkman must remember that the sources of the troubles which are liable to arise in his milk are in some form of filth: either filth on the cow, or dust in the hay which is scattered through the barn, or dirt on cows' udders or some other unusual and avoidable source. These sources, from what we have already noticed, will always furnish the milk with bacteria; but under common conditions, and when the cow is kept in conditions of ordinary cleanliness, and frequently even when not cleanly, will only furnish bacteria that produce the universal souring. Recognising this, the dairyman at once learns that his remedies for the troublesome infections are cleanliness and low temperatures. If he is careful to keep his milk vessels scrupulously clean; if he will keep his cow as cleanly as he does his horse; and if he will use care in and around the barn and dairy, and then apply low temperatures to the milk, he need never be disturbed by slimy or tainted milk, or any of these other troubles or he can remove such infections, speedily should they once appear. Pure sweet milk is only a question of sufficient care. But care means labour and expense. As long as we demand cheap milk, so long will we be supplied with milk procured under conditions of filth. But when we learn that cheap milk is poor milk, and when we are willing to pay a little more for it, then only may we expect the use of greater care in the handling of the milk, resulting in a purer product.

Bacteriology has therefore taught us that the whole question of the milk supply in our communities is one of avoiding the too rapid growth of bacteria. These organisms are uniformly a nuisance to the milkman. To avoid their evil influence have been designed all the methods of caring for the dairy and the barn, all the methods of distributing milk in ice cars. Moreover, all the special devices connected with the great industry of milk supply have for their foundation the attempt to avoid, in the first place, the presence of too great a number of bacteria, and in the second place, the growth of these bacteria.

PASTEURISATION

Pasteurisation is not just a simple case of heat stroke. To understand what heat does to a bacterium, we need to know about its structure. A bacterium is a single-celled organism. Think of it like a studio apartment, one room containing all the things a person needs to live: food, water, air. The walls of the apartment enclose the electrical wiring and gas pipes that deliver energy, along with the sewage pipes that get rid of waste products. In contrast to the size of this single-celled organism, even an animal as small as a mouse would be like a huge city with thousands of buildings and extensive infrastructure to keep it 'alive'.

In more scientific terms, a bacterium is made up of the cell envelope, the cytoplasm and, often, the flagella. Besides holding in the cytoplasm, the cell envelope is where energy-generating functions like photosynthesis and respiration happen. The cytoplasm refers to everything inside the cell envelope, a mixture of water, ribosomes, chromosomes, nutrients and enzymes—all the things that keep the bacterium alive and kicking. Enzymes are especially important because they cause the chemical reactions that make up the cell's metabolism. The flagella are tiny appendages on the outside of the bacterium that help it move around, attach to surfaces or fend off enemies.

Now that we've set the scene and introduced the characters, here comes the dramatic climax. When the temperature gets hot enough, the enzymes in the bacterium are denatured, meaning they change shape. This change renders them useless, and they're no longer able to do their work. The cell simply ceases to function.

Heat can also damage the bacterium's cell envelope. Proteins and fatty acids making up the envelope lose their shape, weakening it. At the same time, fluid inside the cell expands as the temperature rises, increasing the internal pressure. The expanding fluid pushes against the weakened wall and causes it to burst, spilling out the guts of the bacterium.

Thermoduric bacteria are more heat-resistant and harder to kill. In terms of our apartment analogy, thermoduric bacteria have reinforced walls, double-paned windows, insulated pipes and an emergency supply of water and food. These heat-defying bacteria have to be kept under control by refrigeration, which keeps them from multiplying.

Thermal Processing and Pasteurisation

The term thermal processing applies to a range of heat treatments used for food processing. In general, the point of thermal processing is to kill pathogens and inactivate enzymes that cause negative changes to the food during storage. The most common type of thermal processing is the kind that happens in the kitchen at mealtime. Even the most domestically challenged among us have heated something in the microwave and have therefore 'thermally processed' something.

Pasteurisation constitutes one of the milder forms of thermal processing. Ultra-high temperature (UTH) and sterilisation methods kill all micro-organisms in the food, while milder heat treatments like thermisation and pasteurisation only kill some of them. Why not use a higher temperature if it will kill more pathogens? The answer is that higher temperatures change the characteristics of the food. Since milk is what most people think of in relation to pasteurisation, we'll use the pasteurisation of milk throughout the rest of this article to show how pasteurisation works.

At higher temperatures, as with UHT, several things happen to milk that make it less desirable to consumers:

1. The proteins in milk are altered, changing how the milk acts when used to make other foods like cheese.
2. Protective enzymes in milk are inactivated, making it more susceptible to spoilage.
3. The Maillard reaction, a chemical reaction between proteins and sugars, occurs at higher heats and causes browning, discolouring the milk.
4. The milk may taste 'cooked'.

If you look at the sidebar, you'll notice that each method of thermal processing requires a certain length of time. For example, HTST pasteurisation takes 15 seconds. This minimum time requirement is based on the thermal death kinetics of the bacteria. No, that's not the name of a death metal band; it's a way to describe the conditions needed to kill bacteria. The D-value is the amount of time it takes to kill 90 per cent of one type of bacteria at a particular temperature. The higher the temperature is, the lower the D-value, and vice versa.

The pasteurisation of milk kills off the most heat-sensitive pathogens but retains the qualities of milk that consumers expect: creamy texture, fresh flavour and milky-white colour.

Methods of Pasteurisation

Batch (or 'vat') pasteurisation

Batch (or 'vat') pasteurisation is the simplest and oldest method for pasteurising milk. Milk is heated to 154.4°F (63°C) in a large container and held at that temperature for 30 minutes. This process can be carried out at home on the stovetop using a large pot or for small-scale dairies, with steam-heated kettles and fancy temperature control equipment. In batch processing, the milk has to be stirred constantly to make sure that each particle of milk is heated.

High-temperature short-time (HTST) pasteurisation,

High-temperature short-time (HTST) pasteurisation or flash pasteurisation, is the most common method these days, especially for higher volume processing. This method is faster and more energy efficient than batch pasteurisation. Though the higher temperature may give the milk a slightly cooked flavour, HTST pasteurisation has been used for so long that people are used to the flavour.

Here are the basics of HTST:

1. Cold raw milk (39.2°F and 4°C) is fed into the pasteurisation plant.
2. The milk passes into the regenerative heating section of the plate heat exchanger. The plate heat exchanger is basically a series of stainless steel plates stacked together with some space in between, forming chambers to hold the milk as it passes through. Let's call the odd-numbered chambers 'A' chambers, and the even-numbered chambers, 'B' chambers. In the regenerating section, cold milk is pumped through the A chambers, while milk that has already been heated and pasteurised is pumped through the B chambers. The heat from the hot milk passes to the cold milk through the steel plates. This warms the milk to 134.6° to 154.4°F (57° to 68°C).
3. Next, the milk passes into the heating section of the plate heat exchanger. Here, hot water in the B chambers heats the milk to at least 161.6°F (72°C). This is the goal temperature for HTST pasteurisation.
4. The hot milk is then passed through a holding tube. It takes the milk about 15 seconds to pass through the tube, fulfilling the time requirement for this method of pasteurisation (remember the D-values?). The milk has been officially pasteurised once it passes through the holding tube.
5. Now the pasteurised milk is sent back through the regenerative section, where it warms the incoming cold milk. This cools the pasteurised milk to about 89.6°F (32°C).
6. In the last part of the process, the cooling section of the plate heat exchanger uses coolant or cold water to bring the milk to 39.2°F (4°C).

Milk Contamination

Why doesn't pasteurisation make our milk completely safe? Pasteurised milk still causes outbreaks of foodborne illness. In this section, we will look at the many ways milk can become contaminated on its journey from the cow to the table.

1. The cow: Before the cow is even milked, pathogens in the surrounding environment can get into the cow's feed or water. During milking, bacteria on the inside or outside of the cow's udder can get into the milk. If the milking device (human or mechanical) hasn't been properly sanitised it may contaminate the raw milk.
2. Storage and transfer of raw milk: Any time the milk is transferred or stored, all equipment and containers must be sterile to prevent contamination. The storage temperature must be low enough (usually 4°C) to keep any bacteria remaining in the milk from growing.
3. Pasteurisation: We know that pasteurisation does not kill all the bacteria in milk, but it won't even kill the ones it's supposed to if the guidelines for time and temperature are not met. One way the dairy industry checks milk to make sure it has been properly pasteurised is by testing for alkaline phosphatase. This enzyme has the same D-value as the tuberculosis bacterium, so if it's found in pasteurised milk, that means that time and temperature requirements were not met.
4. Equipment: Postpasteurisation contamination (PPC) because of flaws in equipment or poor sanitation practices is the most common reason for pasteurisation failures.

5. Equipment has to be properly maintained and tested, and cleaned and sterilised between uses.
6. The plate heat exchanger is one potential source of PPC, since cold raw milk and hot pasteurised milk pass each other on opposite sides of the heat exchange plates. If the plates have leaks or cracks, the raw milk can contaminate the pasteurised milk.
7. Storage and transfer after pasteurisation: Milk is vulnerable to what the industry calls time-temperature abuse whenever the milk is transferred or stored. This includes all points at or between the processing plant, the warehouse, the store and your home. The weak link in the overall cold chain is usually that indeterminate period after (the milk) leaves the retail outlet and reaches the consumer's refrigerator.
8. Now that it's been brought to your attention, the pressure is on to get the milk home and into the fridge as quickly as possible. Check the temperature of your refrigerator regularly, too. It should always be less than 41°F.

Food Safety and Raw Milk

The debate over which is better—raw milk or pasteurised—is a hot topic right now. Besides being a matter of public health, it's a politically and emotionally charged issue for many people. In the United States, the sale of raw milk is currently legal in 28 states though it can't be transported over state lines. Here are the highlights of both sides of the argument.

The main argument in support of the pasteurisation of milk is that it protects the public from foodborne illness. It's also believed to extend the shelf-life of milk while maintaining its flavour, texture and nutritional content.

The US Centres for Disease Control and Prevention, and the US Food and Drug Administration take the position that pasteurisation should be mandatory for all milk products due to its potential for causing foodborne illness. In her food politics blog, nutrition expert Marion Nestle writes that while she supports the right to drink raw milk, she also believes that raw milk carries inherent dangers of which we should all be aware.

The Weston A. Price Foundation is the most outspoken proponent of raw milk. This organisation makes a very in-depth argument for raw milk. It claims that enzymes and other milk components that naturally protect the milk from spoilage and help humans digest milk are deactivated by pasteurisation. The group presents research that shows that heat treatment causes significant changes in the nutritional content of milk—especially vitamin C, some B vitamins and several minerals, such as calcium and magnesium. It also objects to conventional dairy practices and believes that producers of raw milk are much better caretakers of the cows, the land and the milk.

The organisation also emphasises the fact that pasteurising milk does not prevent outbreaks of disease from pasteurised milk. Whichever side of this debate you take, the type of milk you drink is still a matter of personal choice as long as you live in a state that allows the sale of raw milk.

SPRAY DRYING AND SPRAY DRYERS

Spray drying has become the most important method for dehydration of fluid foods in the Western world. The development of the process has been intimately associated with the dairy industry and the demand for drying of milk powders. However, the technology has been expanded to cover a large food group which now is being successfully spray dried.

Applications

Spray drying applications are given in Table 14.3.

Table 14.3. Spray drying applications.

Bananas	Egg (whole)	Proteins (animals)
Blood	Egg (white)	Proteins (milk)
Cake mixes	Egg (yolk)	Proteins (plants)
Citrus juice	Fish concentrates	Shortening (bakery)
Coffee	Infant formulas	Starch derivatives
Corn syrup	Milk (whole)	Tea
Cream	Milk (skim)	Tomato puree
Creamers (coffee)	Milk (replacers)	Yeast
Cremes (pharmac.)	Potatoes	Yogurt

Unit Operations

Spray drying consists of the following unit operations:

1. Pre-concentration of liquid.
2. Atomisation (creation of droplets).
3. Drying in stream of hot, dry air.
4. Separation of powder from moist air.
5. Cooling.
6. Packaging of product.

Relatively high temperatures are needed for spray drying operations. However, heat damage to products is generally only slight, because of an evaporative cooling effect during the critical drying period and because the subsequent time of exposure to high temperatures of the dry material may be very short. The typical surface temperature of a particle during the constant drying zone is 45°–50°C. For this reason, it is possible to spray dry some bacterial suspensions without destruction of the organisms. The physical properties of the products are intimately associated with the powder structure which is generated during spray drying. It is possible to control many of the factors which influence powder structure in order to obtain the desired properties.

Typical Spray Drying Systems

The Fig. 14.2 shows a schematic representation of a typical spray drying system for milk powder. For spray drying, it is usual to pump a concentrate of the liquid product to the atomising device where it is broken into small droplets. These droplets meet a stream of hot air and they loose their moisture very rapidly while still suspended in the drying air. The dry powder is separated from the moist air in cyclones by centrifugal action. The centrifugal action is caused by the great increase in air speed when the mixture of particles and air enters the cyclone system. The dense powder particles are forced toward the cyclone walls while the lighter, moist air is directed away through the exhaust pipes. The powder settles to the bottom of the cyclone where it is removed through a discharging device. Sometimes the air-conveying ducts for the dry powder are connected with cooling systems which admit cold air for transport of the product through conveying pipes. Cyclone dryers, such as shown here have been designed for large production schedules capable of drying ton-lots of powder per hour.

Cyclone spray dryer

The following Fig. 14.2 is a diagram of a typical spray drying operation utilising a centrifugal atomiser and a cyclone separator.

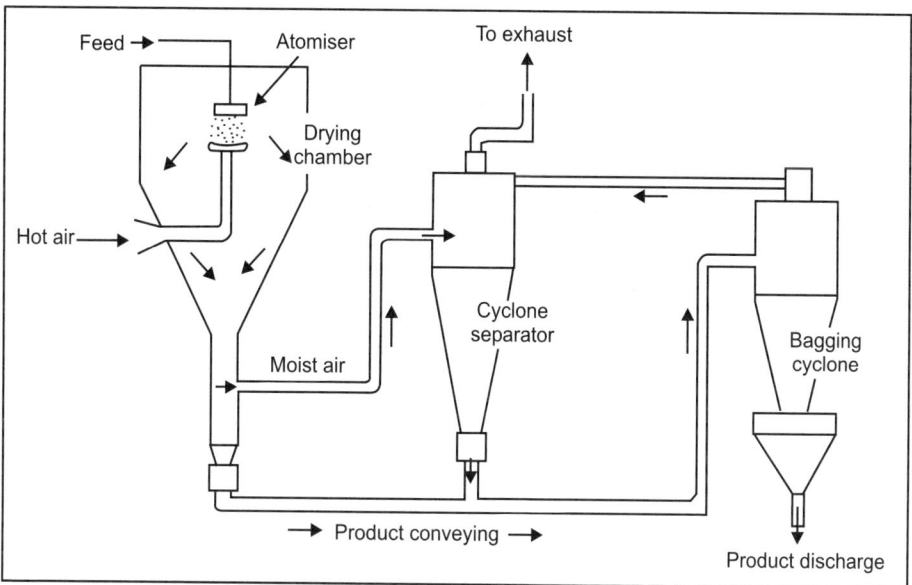

Fig. 14.2. Cyclone spray dryer.

Box spray dryer

A different system, known as the 'Rogers process' is shown in Fig. 14.3. This design has been popular for relatively small production schedules and for physically sensitive powder material which may not withstand the friction generated by the cyclone action. In this process, filtered air is preheated with steam or gas and is blown into ductwork (A) and then into the specially proportioned distributing head (B), passing through air inlets to the drying chamber (C).

The hot air absorbs the moisture from the finely divided, atomised liquid spray and passes under air baffle (D) to cloth filter bags (E) where 100 per cent of any remaining powder is trapped from the exhaust air. The filter bags are intermittently shaken by a mechanical device to release any adhering powder which then drops to the floor and blends in with the remaining powder.

Rogers spray drying process

The moist air is then exhausted to the atmosphere through the exhaust fan (F). Liquid to be dried is preheated in heater (G), passing to a high pressure pump (H), through the high pressure line (I) to spray nozzles located in air inlets (C). The atomised liquid droplets are dried while suspended in the chamber and the powder settles to the floor where it is conveyed by a reciprocating scraper (J) to the screw conveyor (K). The powder moves to the chamber outlet (L) where it is may be removed manually or picked up by an optional pneumatic system to a cyclone separator (M) which cools the powder with fresh air. A sifter is located below the cyclone discharge (Fig. 14.3).

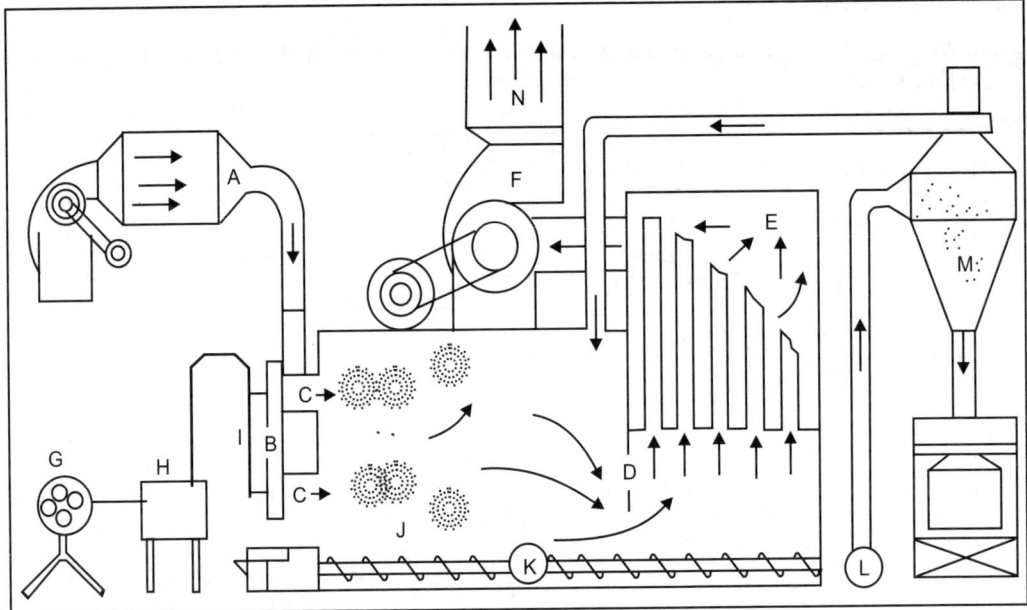

Fig. 14.3. Rogers spray drying process.

Preconcentration of Liquid Feed

For operation of a spray dryer it is usual practice to pre-concentrate the liquid as much as possible. There are several reasons for this:

1. Economy of operation (evaporation is less expensive).
2. Increased capacity (amount of water evaporation is constant).
3. Increase of particle size (each droplet contains more solids).
4. Increase of particle density (reduction of vacuole size).
5. More efficient powder separation (related to increased density).
6. Improved dispersibility of product (reduction in surface area).

First, it must be recognised that water removal in a vacuum evaporator and in a spray dryer are two very different processes. Evaporation under vacuum is a process which takes place at a much lower temperature than spraydrying.

Generally, the temperature of the first stage is only 65°C and subsequent stages even less. For this reason, vacuum evaporation in multiple stages permits the use of low-cost energy and regeneration of the energy contained in the vapour removed from the product. In principle, very little heat energy is used or lost during vacuum evaporation. In contrast, spray drying takes place at atmospheric pressure; therefore, the drying air needs to be heated to high temperatures, generally around 150°–175°C. This requires high-cost fuel in the form of gas or oil. Besides, there is almost no opportunity to regenerate the energy from the vapour phase. Thus, for efficient industrial spray drying operation, it is usual to combine the two processes.

Next, it must be recognised that the performance of a spray dryer is rated according to the maximum amount of water which can be removed per hour by that system. For example, a spray dryer rated at 1000 kg/hr water evaporation will produce only 111 kg/hr of bone-dry powder from a liquid of 10 per cent total solids. If that liquid is concentrated to 45 per cent total solids, the powder production increases to 818 kg/hr of bone-dry powder.

Finally, the powder structure and, therefore, the physical properties of a powder is very dependent upon the total solids concentration of the liquid which is being dried. If the droplets are maintained at a constant size, then, the amount of solids will affect both the size and the density of the dry particles. The structure of a spray-dried particle is a hollow sphere, with the solids being a shell which surrounds a central vacuole. As the total solids of the feed increases, the shell becomes thicker and, as a consequence, the particle does not shrink as much during drying.

Similarly, as the air-filled vacuole decreases in size, the particle density increases. The increase in particle density has a pronounced influence on the efficiency of powder separation/collection by the cyclones, because these operate on the principle of a difference in the buoyant density difference between air and particles.

It is well-known in the spraydrying industry that drying a liquid of low solids content is the cause of very fine particles which are difficult to collect. This results in product losses as well as environmental pollution when they are discharged into the atmosphere.

Limitations on preconcentration

The limit on the extent of preconcentration of the feed is dictated by the viscosity of the liquid, which must not be so high, that the product cannot be pumped or atomised. For milk powder manufacture, it is common to preconcentrate the milk (9 per cent total solids in skim milk; 13 per cent total solids in whole milk) to 45 per cent in an evaporator. For many protein isolates, such a high concentration cannot be used, because most protein solutions are very viscous. In this case, spraydrying must be done with a concentrate of about 25 per cent total solids concentration. This practice, however, causes the powder particles to have a lower density. Therefore, these products are typically very light and fluffy and the unit cost of operation increases dramatically.

Atomisation

The size and uniformity of droplets are determined by the atomisation. Karel has described this operation as the most important feature of a spray dryer. Two different principles are illustrated in the Figs 14.4 and 14.5.

Centrifugal atomiser

This is a spinning disk assembly with radial or curved vanes which rotates at high velocities (2000–20,000 rpm). The feed is delivered near the center and spreads between the two plates and is accelerated to high linear velocities before it is thrown off the disk in the form of thin sheets, ligaments or elongated ellipsoids. However, the subdivided liquid immediately attains a spherical shape under the influence of surface tension. The atomising effect is dependent upon centrifugal force but also must depend upon the frictional influence of the external air.

Centrifugal atomisers have the great advantage of less tendency to become clogged. For this reason, they are preferred for spray drying of non-homogeneous foods.

Centrifugal Atomiser for Cyclone Spray Dryers

Figure 14.4 shows centrifugal atomiser for cyclone spray dryers.

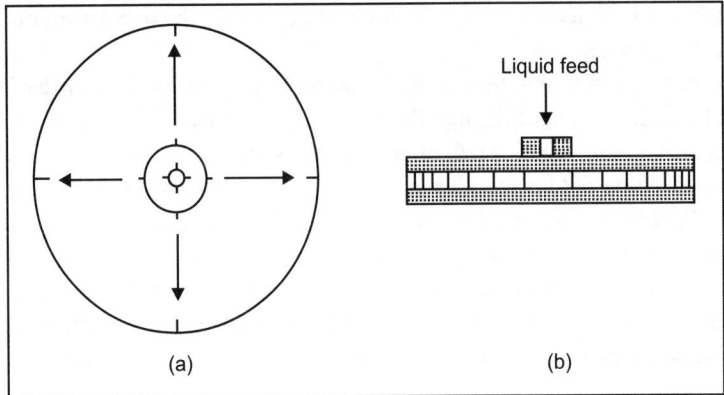

Fig. 14.4. Centrifugal atomiser for cyclone spray dryers (a) top view, and (b) side view.

High Pressure Spray Jets

High pressure jets are alternative atomising systems in which a fluid acquires a high-velocity tangential motion while being forced through the nozzle orifice. The fluid emerges with a swirling motion in a cone shaped sheet, which breaks up into droplets (Fig. 14.5).

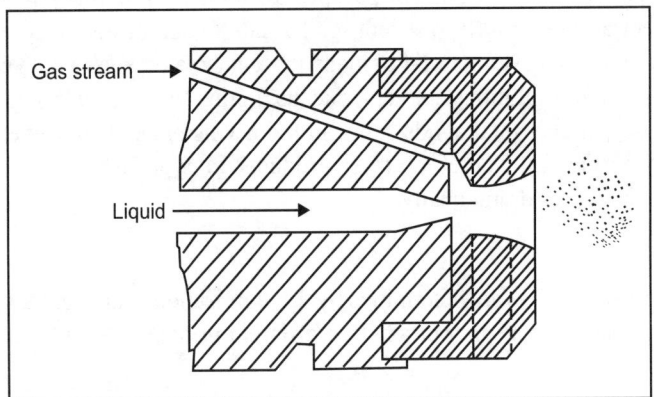

Fig. 14.5. High pressure spray jets.

The nozzle shown in the Fig. 14.5 is an atomiser with internal mixing of gas and liquid. The design permits air or steam to break up the stream of liquid into a mist of fine droplets. The action of many jet-spray nozzles is similar to the spray formed by a common garden hose; only the design and construction are made with greater care.

Heat and Mass Transfer in the Dryer

There are only few details known about actual heat- and mass-transfer processes in the drying chamber. However the history of drying in a single droplet can be constructed.

Drying of a droplet

1. In the initial period, the temperature increases to the wet bulb temperature.

2. In the second period, a concentration gradient builds up in the drop and water activity at the surface decreases, thus causing the surface temperature to rise above that of the wet bulb temperature.

3. In the third period, internal diffusion becomes limiting. A critical moisture content is eventually reached below which the surface becomes impenetrable.

The drying time for a single droplet may be estimated by the following equation:

$$t = [r^2 d_L \mathit{Æ}H_V] \times [m_i - m_f]/[3h(\mathit{Æ}T)] \times [1 + m_i]$$

where, t = time (hr); r = radius of droplet; d_L = density of liquid (lb/ft³); $\mathit{Æ}H_V$ = latent heat of vapourisation (Btu/lb); m_i = initial moisture content (lb H_2O/lb dry food); m_f = final moisture content (lb H_2O/lb dry food); h = film coefficient for heat transfer (Btu/ft²/hr/°F); $\mathit{Æ}T$ = temperature difference between initial and final stages (°F).

The typical drying time for an average milk droplet of 40 μ is only a fraction of a second. However, because of the great initial velocity, the particle will have travelled a considerable distance from the atomiser before it is dry (13.5 cm for average conditions). It should be noted, that the drying time is proportional to the square of the radius; thus, for larger droplets the drying time may become so long that the droplet reaches the wall of the dryer while still wet. This problem is often encountered in small scale dryers.

The above equation also stresses that the drying time can be shortened by reducing the initial moisture content by preconcentration of the liquid.

Separation of Dry Particles

Separation is carried out partly within the drying chamber itself and partly in secondary separation equipment. In general, it is easy to remove 90 per cent or more of the powder, but removal of the remainder becomes problematic. Cyclone separators operate on the 'momentum separation' principle (centrifugal action) and are extensively used in large scale dryers for removal of fines.

Charm has given an equation which relates the dimensions of a cyclone to the smallest particle (D_p) which can be separated:

$$D_p^2 = (3.6 \, A_i \, D_0 \, \mu)/(^1 Z D V_0 d_s)$$

where, D_p = diameter of particle; A_i = inlet cross sectional area of cyclone; D_0 = diameter of outlet of cyclone; μ = viscosity of the fluid; Z = depth of the separator; D = diameter of the separator; V_0 = velocity of air/powder mixture entering the cyclone; and d_s = density of the particle.

From the equation it appears that in designing a cyclone the depth and diameter should be as large as possible. Increasing the air velocity is also important. Industrial experience has shown that efficiency is also affected by the powder concentration in the air stream. For this reason, it is better to use several cyclones in parallel than just one single separator. Since cyclones do not always allow complete separation of 'fines' other systems are also in use, including filters, scrubbers or electrostatic precipitation equipment. Cloth-bag filters are very effective systems but are expensive in labour cost to maintain. Besides, the fabric is weakened by high temperatures.

Cyclone Separator

Figure 14.6 shows a cyclone separator.

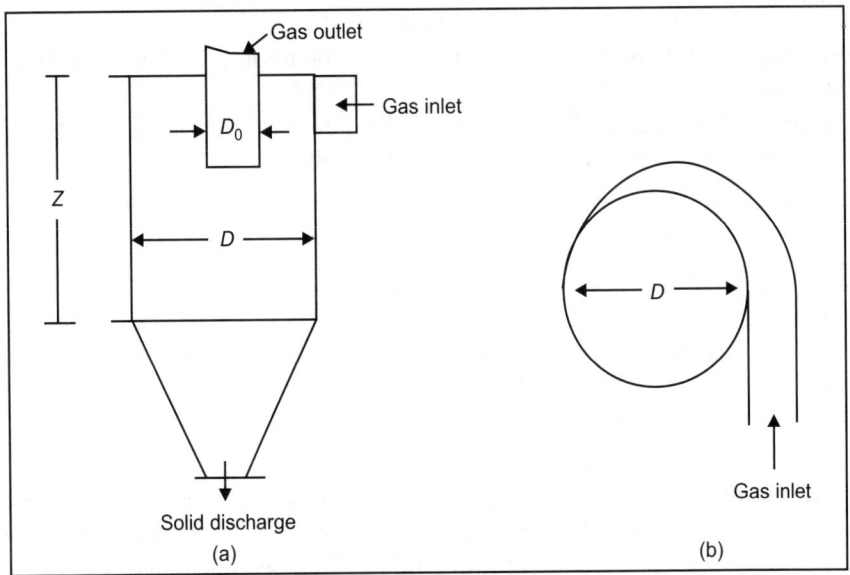

Fig. 14.6. Diagram of cyclone separator.

Structure of Spray Dried Powder Particles

Buma has used scanning electron microscopy to study the particle structure and the distribution of free fat in the particles. He has shown that spray drying results in hollow particles, the shells of which have a glassy structure, primarily of amorphous (non-crystalline) lactose. Pure lactose dries into spherical particles with no dents or folds, whereas skim milk, caseinates and other proteins always give rise to surface folds. Buma and Henstra have explained that proteins, unlike lactose and other sugars, shrink unevenly during drying. The physical properties of spray dried powders is related to the characteristics of the matrix of the shells and to the size of the vacuole. The presence of the vacuole causes the particles to have a lower density than the solid itself (0.33 g/cc versus 1.6 g/cc). Generally, powders with low density are fluffy and do not wet or sink readily when brought in contact with water. Sugars, such as lactose in milk powder, do not crystallise during drying but are present in an amorphous state. Such amorphous sugars are very hygroscopic and readily absorb moisture and eventually recrystallise. This is the cause for many powders caking during storage. Recrystallisation is usually accompanied by changes in colour and development of off-flavours.

Dispersion Characteristics of Spray Dried Powders

Many spray-dried powders do not disperse readily in water. The difficulties are associated with the exterior of the powder absorbing water very rapidly and forming lumps, dry on the inside but covered with a viscous layer through which water penetrates very slowly. The problem arises particularly in products which contain soluble proteins, such as milk powder and flour. Karel has discussed the requirements for rapid dispersibility of powders in cold water. The following properties are desired:
1. A large wettable surface.
2. Sinkability (must not float on surface).
3. Solubility.
4. Resistance to sedimentation.

The wettability is crucial and depends upon the total surface area of the powder and on the surface properties of the powder particles. The spray drying industry in Western countries have improved the dispersibility characteristics of their products by a combination of surface treatments (for example addition of lecithin) and 'instantising' (agglomeration).

Instantising is an aggregation process which is intended to prevent powder particles from sticking together and becoming lumpy during rehydration.

Instantised Powders

'Instant' powders are usually produced by processes in which the spray-dried powder is first wetted and then redried. The degree of rewetting is closely controlled (15 per cent) to permit the particles to stick together and form aggregates before redrying. In these products the small particles are fused together but the points of contact are so few that practically all of the surfaces are available for wetting. The aggregates, however, are sufficiently stable to prevent lumping when stirred into water. During the rewetting procedure, lactose will partly crystallise.

Therefore, instant powder is less hygroscopic. The flow diagram (Fig. 14.7) of the instantising process and a schematic representation of particle agglomeration.

Instantising process

Figure 14.7 shows instantising process.

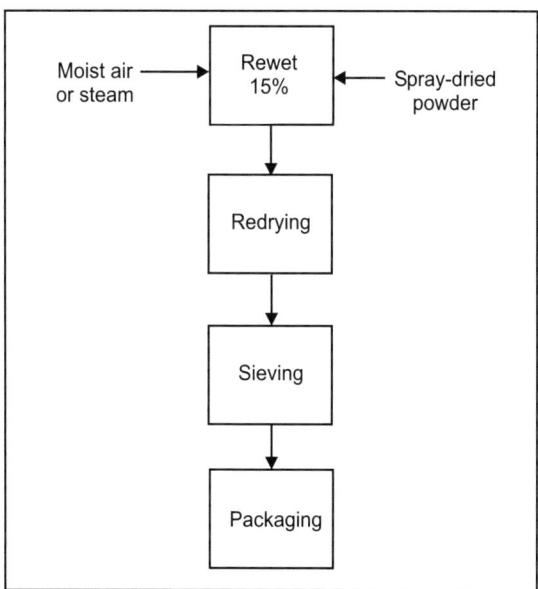

Fig. 14.7. Instantising process.

Particle agglomeration after instantising process

In the Fig. 14.8, (a) is a representation of regular powder, and (b) represents aggregates from drying a rewetted powder.

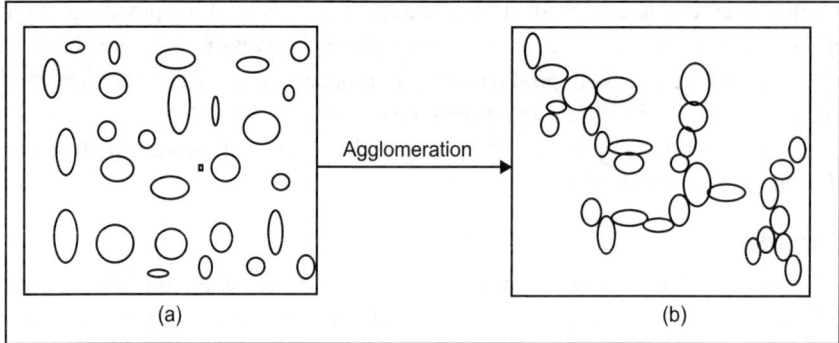

Fig. 14.8. Particle agglomeration after instantising process.

Selection of Operating Conditions

The most important responsibility for an operator of a spray drier is to maintain a constant moisture content of the powder. This is required to meet legal standards and for maintaining a uniform quality. Average operating conditions for spray drying of milk powder will vary somewhat depending upon the dryer system used and must be adjusted to produce the desired uniform moisture content. It is important to understand how the final moisture content can be controlled by changing the conditions. But first, it should be noted that the final moisture content is controlled by the relative humidity of the outlet air. If that value is too high, then the powder particles will absorb moisture rather than give moisture away. The primary conditions which may be controlled directly by the operator are:

1. Inlet temperature (setting of thermostat).
2. Flow rate of liquid feed (pump speed; pump pressure).
3. Air flow rate (fan speed; position of baffles).
4. Particle size (adjustment of atomiser).

Among other operating conditions, outlet temperature and relative humidity of the outlet air are particularly important and need careful attention. However, these can only be indirectly controlled by adjusting the primary conditions.

For outlet temperature, the condition is dependent upon liquid feed intake. If the feed intake is increased, the outlet temperature will drop. If the intake is reduced, the outlet temperature will increase and approach the inlet temperature. The outlet temperature will also be affected by the air flow rate. For a constant inlet temperature and constant feed intake, an increase in the air flow will raise the outlet temperature.

Average Spray Drying Conditions for Milk

1. Temperature of air (ambient) 25.0°C.
2. Temperature of feed: 60.0°C.
3. Temperature of inlet air: 150.0°C.
4. Temperature of outlet air: 82.0°C.
5. Temperature of drop surface (const. zone) 45.0°C.
6. Relative humidity (ambient air) 55.0 per cent.
7. Relative humidity (inlet air, psychrom.) 0.3 per cent.
8. Relative humidity (outlet air, psychrometric) 12.0 per cent.

9. Moisture content of milk: 87.0 per cent.
10. Moisture content of concentrate: 45.0 per cent.
11. Moisture content of powder: 4–5.0 per cent.
12. Droplet size (initial), av. diameter: 40.0 μ.
13. Particle size (final) , av. diameter: 20.0 μ.
14. Density of milk 1.33 g/ccm.
15. Density of milk powder (bulk): 0.33 g/ccm velocity of air: 61.0 metres/sec.
16. Velocity of droplet (initial): 17,000.0 cm/sec.
17. Velocity of droplet (free fall): 1.0 cm/sec.
18. Drying time (constant rate zone): 0.0023 sec.
19. Drying time (falling rate zone): 0.0014 sec.
20. Drying time (total): .0037 sec.
21. Travel distance for drying: 13.5 cm.

For relative humidity of outlet air, the value is dependent upon the psychrometric relationship between the conditions of the ambient air and the conditions in the dryer. It is controlled by establishing the correct outlet temperature.

FACTORS AFFECTING MILK COMPOSITION

Milk composition is affected by genetic and environmental factors.

Genetic

Breed and individual cow

Milk composition varies considerably among breeds of dairy cattle: Jersey and Guernsey breeds give milk of higher fat and protein content than Shorthorns and Friesians. Zebu cows can give milk containing up to 7 per cent fat.

Variability among cows within a breed

The potential fat content of milk from an individual cow is determined genetically, as are protein and lactose levels. Thus, selective breeding can be used to upgrade milk quality. Heredity also determines the potential milk production of the animal. However, environment and various physiological factors greatly influence the amount and composition of milk that is actually produced. Herd recording of total milk yields and fat and SNF percentages will indicate the most productive cows, and replacement stock should be bred from these.

Environmental

Interval between milkings

The fat content of milk varies considerably between the morning and evening milking because there is usually a much shorter interval between the morning and evening milking than between the evening and morning milking.

If cows were milked at 12-hour intervals the variation in fat content between milkings would be negligible, but this is not practicable on most farms. Normally, SNF content varies little even if the intervals between milkings vary.

Stage of lactation

The fat, lactose and protein contents of milk vary according to stage of lactation. Solids-not-fat content is usually highest during the first 2 to 3 weeks, after which it decreases slightly. Fat content is high immediately after calving but soon begins to fall, and continues to do so for 10 to 12 weeks, after which it tends to rise again until the end of the lactation. The variation in milk constituents throughout lactation is shown in Fig. 14.9.

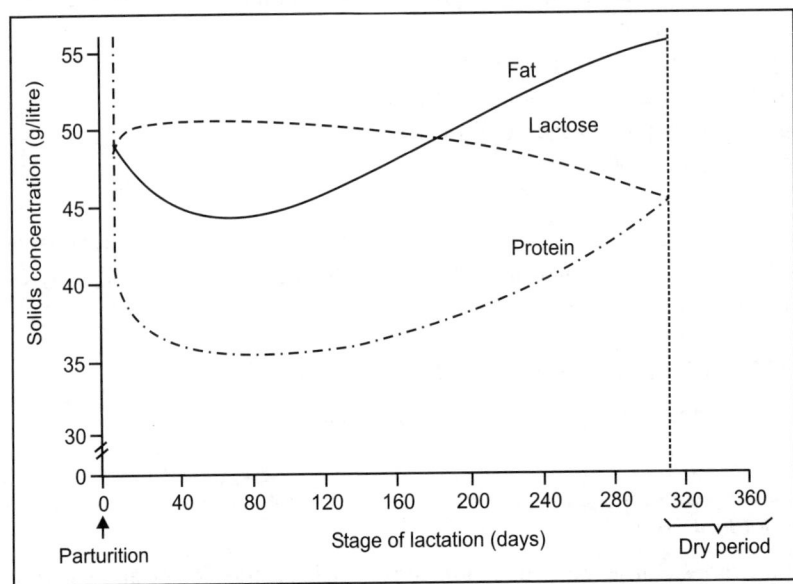

Fig. 14.9. Changes in the concentrations of fat, protein and lactose over lactation of a cow.

Age

As cows grow older the fat content of their milk decreases by about 0.02 percentage units per lactation. The fall in SNF content is much greater.

Feeding regime

Underfeeding reduces both the fat and the SNF content of milk produced, although SNF content is more sensitive to feeding level than fat content. Fat content and fat composition are influenced more by roughage (fibre) intake.

The SNF content can fall if the cow is fed a low-energy diet, but is not greatly influenced by protein deficiency, unless the deficiency is acute.

Disease

Both fat and SNF contents can be reduced by disease, particularly mastitis.

Completeness of milking

The first milk drawn from the udder is low in fat while the last milk (or strippings) is always quite high in fat. Thus it is essential to mix thoroughly all the milk removed, before taking a sample for analysis.

The fat left in the udder at the end of a milking is usually picked up during subsequent milkings, so there is no net loss of fat.

MANAGING LACTOSE INTOLERANCE

For persons living in societies where the diet contains relatively little dairy, lactose intolerance is not considered a condition that requires treatment. However, those living among societies that are largely lactose-tolerant may find lactose intolerance troublesome. Although there are still no methodologies to reinstate lactase production, some individuals have reported their intolerance to vary over time (depending on health status and pregnancy).

Lactose intolerance is not usually an all-or-nothing condition: the reduction in lactase production—and hence, the amount of lactose that can be tolerated—varies from person to person. Since lactose intolerance poses no further threat to a person's health, managing the condition consists of minimising the occurrence and severity of symptoms. Berdanier and Hargrove recognise four general principles: avoidance of dietary lactose, substitution to maintain nutrient intake, regulation of calcium intake, and use of enzyme substitute.

Avoiding Lactose-containing Products

Since each individual's tolerance to lactose varies, according to the US National Institute of Health, 'Dietary control of lactose intolerance depends on people learning through trial and error how much lactose they can handle.' Label reading is essential, as commercial terminology varies according to language and region.

Lactose is present in two large food categories: conventional dairy products, and as a food additive (in dairy and non-dairy products).

Dairy products

Lactose is a water-soluble molecule. Therefore, fat percentage and the curdling process have an impact on which foods may be tolerated. After the curdling process, lactose is found in the water portion (along with whey and casein), but is not found in the fat portion. Dairy products which are 'fat reduced' or 'fat free' generally have a slightly higher lactose percentage. Additionally, low fat dairy foods also often have various dairy derivatives such as milk solids added to them to enhance sweetness, increasing the lactose content.

Milk

Human milk has the highest lactose percentage at around 9 per cent. Unprocessed cow milk has 4.7 per cent lactose. Unprocessed milk from other bovids contains similar lactose percentages (goat milk 4.7 per cent, buffalo 4.86 per cent, yak 4.93 per cent, sheep milk 4.6 per cent).

Butter

The butter-making process separates the majority of milk's water components from the fat components. Lactose, being a water soluble molecule, will still be present in small quantities in the butter unless it is also fermented to produce cultured butter.

Yogurt, frozen yogurt and kefir

People can be more tolerant of traditionally made yogurt than milk, because it contains lactase enzyme produced by the bacterial cultures used to make the yogurt. Frozen yogurt, if cultured similarly to its unfrozen counterpart, will contain similarly reduced lactose levels. However, many commercial brands contain milk solids, increasing the lactose content.

Cheeses

Traditionally made hard cheese (such as Emmental) and soft ripened cheeses may create less reaction than the equivalent amount of milk because of the processes involved. Fermentation and higher fat content contribute to lesser amounts of lactose. Traditionally made Emmental or Cheddar might contain 10 per cent of the lactose found in whole milk. In addition, the traditional ageing methods of cheese (over 2 years) reduces their lactose content to practically nothing. Commercial cheese brands, however, are generally manufactured by modern processes that do not have the same lactose reducing properties, and as no regulations mandate what qualifies as an 'aged' cheese, this description does not provide any indication of whether the process used significantly reduced lactose.

Sour cream

Sour cream if made in the traditional way, may be tolerable, but most modern brands add milk solids. Consult labels.

Examples of lactose levels in foods

As scientific consensus has not been reached concerning lactose percentage analysis methods (nonhydrated form or the monohydrated form), and considering that dairy content varies greatly according to labelling practices, geography and manufacturing processes, lactose numbers may not be very reliable. The following are examples of lactose levels in foods which commonly set off symptoms. These quantities are to be treated as guidelines only (Table 14.4).

Table 14.4. Examples of lactose levels in foods.

Dairy product	Serving size	Lactose content
Milk, regular	250 ml	12 g
Milk, reduced fat	250 ml	13 g
Yogurt, plain, regular	200 g	9 g
Yogurt, plain, low-fat	200 g	12 g
Cheddar cheese	30 g	0.02 g
Cottage cheese	30 g	0.1 g
Butter	1 tsp	0.03 g
Ice cream	50 g	3 g

Lactose in non-dairy products

Lactose (also present when labels state lactoserum, whey, milk solids, modified milk ingredients, etc.) is a commercial food additive used for its texture, flavour and adhesive qualities, and is found in foods such as processed meats (sausages/hot dogs, sliced meats, pâtés), gravy stock powder, margarines sliced breads, breakfast cereals, potato chips, processed foods, medications, pre-prepared meals, meal replacement (powders and bars), protein supplements (powders and bars) and even beers in the 'milk stout' style.

Kosher products labelled pareve or fleishig are free of milk. However, if a 'D' (for 'Dairy') is present next to the circled 'K', 'U' or other hechsher, the food likely contains milk solids (although it may also simply indicate that the product was produced on equipment shared with other products containing milk derivatives).

Alternative products

Plant-based milks and derivatives are inherently lactose free: soya milk, rice milk, almond milk, hazelnut milk, oat milk, hemp milk, peanut milk, horchata. The dairy industry has created low-lactose or lactose-free products to replace regular dairy. Lactose-free milk can be produced by passing milk over lactase enzyme bound to an inert carrier; once the molecule is cleaved, there are no lactose ill-effects. Forms are available with reduced amounts of lactose (typically 30 per cent of normal), and alternatively with nearly 0 per cent. The only noticeable difference from regular milk is a slightly sweeter taste due to the generation of glucose by lactose cleavage. It does not however contain more glucose, and is nutritionally identical to regular milk. Finland, where approximately 17 per cent of the Finnish-speaking population has hypolactasia, has had 'HYLA' (acronym for hydrolysed lactose) products available for many years. Lactoce of low-lactose level cow's milk products, ranging from ice cream to cheese is enzymatically hydrolysed into glucose and galactose. The ultra-pasteurisation process, combined with aseptic packaging, ensures a long shelf-life. In 2001, Valio launched a lactose-free milk drink which is not sweet like HYLA milk but has the fresh taste of ordinary milk. Valio patented chromatographic separation method to remove lactose. Valio also markets these products in Sweden, Estonia, Belgium and the US.

In the UK, where an estimated 15 per cent of the population are affected by lactose intolerance, Lactofree produces milk, cheese, and yogurt products which contain only 0.03 per cent lactose.

Alternatively, a bacterium such as *L. acidophilus* may be added, which affects the lactose in milk the same way it affects the lactose in yogurt.

Lactase supplementation

When lactose avoidance is not possible, or on occasions when a person chooses to consume such items, then enzymatic lactase supplements may be used.

Lactase enzymes similar to those produced in the small intestines of humans are produced industrially by fungi of the genus *Aspergillus*. The enzyme, β-galactosidase, is available in tablet form in a variety of doses, in many countries without a prescription. It functions well only in high-acid environments, such as that found in the human gut due to the addition of gastric juices from the stomach. Unfortunately, too much acid can denature it, and it therefore should not be taken on an empty stomach. Also, the enzyme is ineffective if it does not reach the small intestine by the time the problematic food does. Lactose-sensitive individuals can experiment with both timing and dosage to fit their particular needs.

While essentially the same process as normal intestinal lactose digestion, direct treatment of milk employs a different variety of industrially produced lactase. This enzyme, produced by yeast from the genus *Kluyveromyces*, takes much longer to act, must be thoroughly mixed throughout the product, and is destroyed by even mildly acidic environments. Its main use is in producing the lactose-free or lactose-reduced dairy products sold in supermarkets.

Enzymatic lactase supplementation may have an advantage over avoiding dairy products, in that alternative provision does not need to be made to provide sufficient calcium intake, especially in children.

Rehabituation to dairy products

For healthy individuals with secondary lactose intolerance, it may be possible in some cases for the bacteria in the large intestine to adapt to an altered diet and break down small quantities of lactose more effectively by habitually consuming small amounts of dairy products several times a day over a period of time. Reintroducing dairy in this way to people who have an underlying or chronic illness, however, is not recommended, as certain illnesses damage the intestinal tract in a way which prevents the lactase enzyme from being expressed.

Some studies indicate that environmental factors (more specifically, the consumption of lactose) may 'play a more important role than genetic factors in the etiopathogenesis of milk intolerance', but some other publications suggest that lactase production does not seem to be induced by dairy/lactose consumption.

Nutritional Concerns

Primary lactose intolerance

Populations where primary lactose intolerance is the norm have demonstrated similar health levels to westerners or better health.

Secondary lactose intolerance

Dairy products are relatively good and accessible sources of calcium and potassium and many countries mandate that milk be fortified with vitamin A and vitamin D. Consequently, in dairy-consuming societies, dairy is often a main source of these nutrients and, for lacto-vegetarians, a main source of vitamin B_{12}. Individuals who reduce or eliminate consumption of dairy must obtain these nutrients elsewhere. However, Asian populations for whom dairy is not part of their food culture do not present decreased health and sometimes present above average health, as in Japan.

Plant based milk substitutes are not naturally rich in calcium, potassium, or vitamins A or D (and, like most non-animal products, contain no vitamin B_{12}). However, prominent brands are often voluntarily fortified with many of these nutrients.

An increasing number of calcium-fortified breakfast foods — such as orange juice, bread, and dry cereal—have been appearing on supermarket shelves. Many fruits and vegetables are rich in potassium and vitamin A; animal products like meat and eggs are rich in vitamin B_{12}, and the human body itself produces some vitamin D from exposure to direct sunlight. Finally, a dietitian or physician may recommend a vitamin or mineral supplement to make up for any remaining nutritional shortfall.

Most infants with gastroenteritis due to rotavirus do not develop lactose intolerance, so these infants do not benefit from being put on a lactose-free diet unless symptoms of lactose intolerance are severe and persistent.

Buttermaking with Fresh Milk or Cream

Butterfat can be recovered from milk or cream and converted to a number of products, the most common of which is butter. Butter is an emulsion of water in oil and has the following approximate composition:

Fat	80%
Moisture	16%
Salt	2%
Milk SNF	2%

In good butter the moisture is evenly dispersed throughout in tiny droplets. In most dairying countries legislation defines the composition of butter, and buttermakers conform to these standards insofar as possible. Butter can be made from either whole milk or cream, however, it is more efficient to make it from cream.

Buttermaking theory

To make butter, milk or cream is agitated vigorously at a temperature at which the milk fat is partly solid and partly liquid. Churning efficiency is measured in terms of the time required to produce butter granules and by the loss of fat in the buttermilk. Efficiency is influenced markedly by churning temperature and by the acidity of the milk or cream. In churning, cream is agitated in a partly filled chamber. This incorporates a large amount of air into the cream as bubbles. The resultant whipped cream occupies a larger volume than the original cream. As agitation continues the whipped cream becomes coarser and eventually the fat forms semisolid butter granules that rapidly increase in size and separate sharply from the liquid buttermilk. The remainder of the buttermaking process consists of removing the buttermilk, kneading the butter granules into a homogeneous mass and adjusting the water and salt contents to the levels desired.

Theory of the mechanism of churning

In considering the mechanism of churning the following factors must be taken into account:
1. The function of air.
2. The release of the stabilising membrane surrounding the fat globules into the buttermilk.
3. The differences in structure between butter and cream.
4. The temperature dependence of the process.

Air is thought to be necessary for the process, but some workers have demonstrated that milk or cream can be churned in the absence of air, although it takes longer. About one half of the stabilising material surrounding the fat globule is liberated into the buttermilk during churning. It is thought that during churning the fat globule membrane substance spreads out over the surface of the air bubbles, partly denuding the globules of their protective layer, and that a liquid portion of the fat exudes from the globule and partly or entirely covers the globule, rendering it hydrophobic. In this condition the globules tend to stick to the air bubbles. Free fat destabilises the foam, causing it to collapse. The partly destabilised globules clinging to the air bubbles thus collect in clusters cemented together by free fat. These clusters appear as butter grains. Cream prepared by gravitational or mechanical separation can be used to make butter. Good butter can be made in any type of churn provided it is clean and in good repair.

Churn preparation

The churn is prepared by rinsing with cold water, scrubbing with salt and rinsing again with cold water. Alternatively, it can be scalded with water at 80°C. After the butter has been removed, the churn should be washed well with warm water, scalded with boiling water and left to air. When not in use wooden churns should be soaked occasionally with water. A new churn should first be washed with tepid water, scrubbed with salt and then washed with hot water until the water comes away clear. A hot solution of salt should then be allowed to stand in the churn for about ten minutes. After rinsing again with hot water the churn should be left to air for at least one day before being used.

Churning temperature

The temperature of the cream during churning is of great importance. If too cool, butter formation is delayed and the grain is small and difficult to handle. If the temperature is too high, the butter yield will be low because a large proportion of the fat will remain in the buttermilk, and the butter will be spongy and of poor quality. Cream should be churned at 10°–12°C in the hot season and at 14°–17°C in the cold season. The temperature may be raised by standing the vessel containing the cream in hot water, and lowered by standing the vessel in cold spring water for a few hours before the cream is churned. The churning temperature may also be adjusted by the water used to dilute the cream. In the hot season, the coldest water available should be used, preferably water that has been stored in a refrigerator.

The amount of cream to be churned should not exceed one half the volumetric capacity of the churn. An airtight churn should be ventilated frequently during the first 10 minutes of churning to release gases driven out of solution by the agitation. If butter is slow in forming, adding a little water which is warmer than the churning temperature, but never over 25°C, usually causes it to form more quickly. When the butter appears like wet maize meal, water (1 litre per 4 litres of cream) at 2°C below the churning temperature should be added. It may be necessary to add water a second time to maintain butter grains of the required size. Churning should cease when the butter grains are the size of small wheat grains.

Washing the butter

When the desired grain size is obtained, the buttermilk is drained off and the butter washed several times in the churn. Each washing is done by adding only as much water as is needed to float the butter and then turning the churn a few times. The water is then drained off. As a general rule two washings are enough but in very hot weather three may be necessary before the water comes away clear. In the hot season the coldest water available should be used for washing, and in the cold season water about 2° to 3°C colder than the churning temperature should be used.

Salting, working and packing the butter

Equipment for working may consist of a butter worker or a tub or keeler. Good-quality spatulas are important, and a sieve and scoop facilitate the removal of butter from the churn. This equipment must be clean. The butter is spread on the worker which has been previously soaked with water of the same temperature as the washing water. If salted butter is required, it should be salted before working at a rate of 16 g salt/kg or according to taste. Salt is added to butter most commonly using the dry-salting method in which dry salt is sprinkled evenly over the butter and worked in. The salt used should be dry and evenly ground and of the best quality available.

The butter is then either rolled out 8 to 10 times or ridged with the spatulas to remove excess moisture. Adding salt to butter disturbs the equilibrium of the emulsion (the butter). This in turn changes the character of the body and alters its colour. Unless the butter is subjected to sufficient working to regain the original equilibrium of the emulsion, it will tend to have a coarse, leaky body and uneven colour. The butter should be worked until it seems dry and solid, but it must not be worked too much or it will become greasy and streaky.

Butter must be adequately worked if it is to be stored for a long time. First, working distributes the salt uniformly in the moisture and this helps inhibit microbial growth. Secondly, it distributes the salt solution into many tiny droplets rather than fewer large ones. For a given level of microbial contamination, the microbes will be more isolated in small droplets and will have less of the butter's nutrients available to them for growth.

Surplus good-quality butter can be stored, but should contain more salt than usual—at least 30 g/kg and a low moisture content (14–15 per cent). The butter must be packed in clean containers, such as seasoned boxes or glazed crocks, and stored in a cold room or in a cold, airy place. If a box is used, it should be lined with good-quality polythene. The container should be filled to capacity from one churning. The more firmly butter is packed, the better; it may be covered with a layer of salt, but this is not essential. The container should be securely covered with a lid or a sheet of strong paper and stored in a cool, dark place.

Washing the churn and buttermaking equipment after use

The churn and buttermaking equipment should be washed as soon as possible, preferably while the wood is still damp. Wash the inside of the churn thoroughly with hot water. Invert the churn with the lid on to clean the ventilator; this should be pressed a few times with the back of a scrubbing brush to allow water to pass through. The ventilator should be dismantled occasionally for complete cleansing.

Remove the rubber band from the lid and scrub the groove. Scald the inside of the churn with boiling water, invert and leave to air. Dry the outside and treat the steel parts with vaseline to prevent rusting. The rubber band should not be placed in boiling water; dipping in warm water is sufficient. Place the sieve, scoop and spades on the butter worker or keeler and clean in the same way as the churn.

Overrun and produce in buttermaking

Two criteria that are used to check the efficiency of converting milk or cream into butter are 'overrun' and 'produce'. Produce or butter ratio is the ratio of milk used to butter obtained from it. Overrun, which is usually calculated as per cent overrun, is the excess of butter made over butterfat used per 100 kg butter or the percentage increase of butter over butterfat.

Overrun

An enterprise engaged in buttermaking must be able to measure the efficiency of the process, i.e. by measuring the yield of butter from the butterfat purchased. First, the theoretical yield of butter has to be estimated. Butter contains an average of 80 per cent butterfat. Thus, for every 80 kg of butterfat purchased 100 kg of butter should be produced, or for every 100 kg of butterfat purchased 125 kg of butter should be produced. The difference between the number of kilograms of butterfat churned and the number of kilograms of butter made is known as the overrun. This difference is due to the fact that butter contains non-fatty constituents such as moisture, salt, curd and small amounts of lactic acid and ash in addition to butterfat. The overrun is financially important to the milk processor and constitutes the margin between the purchase price of butterfat and the sale price of butter. The dairy unit depends largely on overrun to cover manufacturing costs and to defray expenses incurred in the purchase of milk.

The maximum legitimate overrun is 25 per cent. In commercial operation, however, it is not possible to establish the degree of accuracy that is assumed in the calculation of theoretical overrun. The actual overrun shows the difference between the amount of butter churned out and the amount of butterfat bought. Overrun is affected by:

1. Accuracy of weighing milk received.
2. Accuracy of sampling and testing milk for fat.
3. Losses during separation.
4. Efficiency of churning.
5. Percentage of fat in the butter.
6. Amount of salt and water in the butter.
7. Amount of product loss throughout the process.

Butter quality

The first step the producer can take to ensure a high-quality product is to make sure the manufacturing process is hygienic. This results in fewer spoilage organisms in the butter. Another step is to take care in the handling and storage of the butter. Using permitted preservatives is by far the most effective means of maintaining butter quality when used in conjunction with the above precautions. Salt is an excellent preservative, and salting butter to 3 per cent extends its storage life; salted butter can be stored for up to four months without significant deterioration. An added advantage of adding salt is that it also increases overrun. A salt concentration in excess of 3 per cent gives little advantage and can adversely affect the flavour of the butter. Butter quality can be discussed under two main headings:

1. Compositional quality.
2. Organoleptic quality.

The compositional quality of butter can be further divided into two subsections, namely chemical and bacteriological.

Compositional quality

The chemical composition of butter is determined at the processing stage when the salt, moisture, curd and fat contents of the product are regulated. Once these parameters have been set there is little one can do to change them. The microbiological quality of butter is also determined during the production and processing stages.

Chemical composition affects butter yield, while butter of poor microbiological quality will deteriorate rapidly and become unacceptable to consumers. Cleanliness at all stages of production is, therefore, essential, to preserve the quality and wholesomeness of butter.

Organoleptic quality

The organoleptic quality of butter can be described as the customer's reaction to its colour, texture and flavour. It has been said that the consumer tastes with his or her eyes, and it is true that a person's initial impression of a food will often determine whether or not he or she will buy it. It is important, therefore, to produce butter that has an even colour, clean flavour and close texture. It is also important that it is free from defects such as loose moisture. It should be packed attractively, both to attract customer attention and to retain its quality. Butter produced carelessly and without salt may have a very short shelf-life. Preservation of butter quality can assist the smallholder in two ways. The less perishable the product the longer the smallholder can retain it to obtain a good price and the surplus made during the production season can be stored for consumption during the season in which butter is not being produced.

Buttermaking with Sour Whole Milk

Smallholder milk processing is based on sour milk. This is due to a number of reasons including high ambient temperatures, small daily quantities of milk, consumer preference and increased keeping quality of sour milk.

Products made from sour milk include fermented milks, concentrated fermented milks, butter, ghee, cottage cheese and whey. Other products are made by mixing fermented milk with boiled cereals. The equipment required for processing sour milk is simple and available locally. Milk vessels can be made from clay, gourds and wood, and can be woven from fibre, such as the *gorfu* container used by the Borana pastoralists in Ethiopia. The products and by-products of buttermaking from sour whole milk are shown in Fig. 14.10.

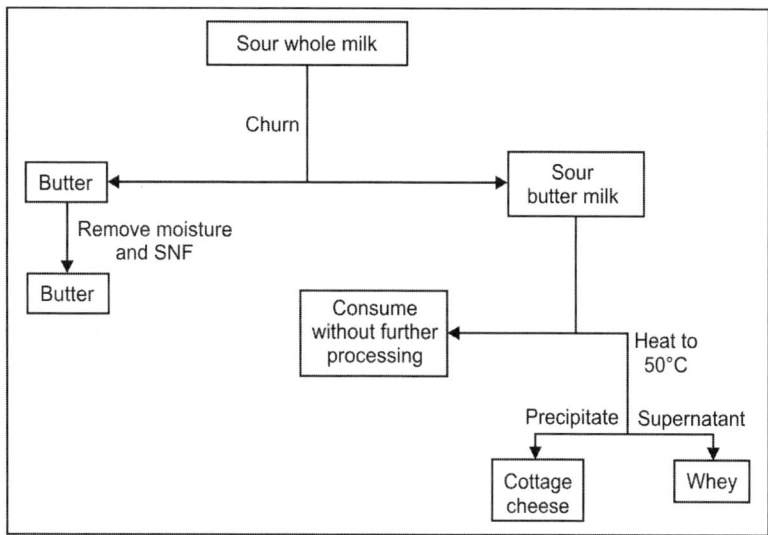

Fig. 14.10. Products and by-products of buttermaking from sour whole milk.

Buttermaking

This is a very important process in many parts of Africa and countries with a developing dairy industry. Smallholders produce one to four litres of milk per day for processing. Under normal storage conditions the milk becomes sour in four to five hours. Souring milk has a number of advantages. It retards the growth of undesirable micro-organisms, such as pathogens and putrefactive bacteria and makes the milk easier to churn.

Milk for churning is accumulated over several days by adding fresh milk to the milk already accumulated. The churn may hold up to 20 litres and the amount of milk churned ranges from 4 to 10 litres. Butter is made by agitating the milk until butter grains form. The churn is then rotated slowly until the fat coalesces into a continuous mass. The butter thus formed is taken from the churn and kneaded in cold water.

The milk is usually agitated by placing the churn on a mat on the floor and rolling it to and fro. It can also be agitated by shaking the churn on the lap or hung from a tripod. The International Livestock Centre for Africa (ILCA) has developed a wooden agitator that fits inside a clay pot which is the traditional type of churn in many parts of Africa. Using this internal agitator cuts churning time in half and increases recovery of butterfat as butter.

A number of factors influence churning time and recovery of butterfat as butter:

1. Milk acidity.
2. Churning temperature.
3. Degree of agitation.
4. Extent of filling the churn.

Effect of acidity

Fresh milk is difficult to churn—churning time is long and recovery of butterfat is poor—however, milk containing at least 0.6 per cent lactic acid is easier to churn. Acidity higher than 0.6 per cent does not significantly influence churning time or fat recovery.

Effect of temperature

Sour milk is normally churned at between 15° and 26°C, depending on environmental temperature. At low temperatures churning time is long; butter-grain formation can take five hours or longer. As churning temperature increases churning time decreases. ILCA trials have shown that when churning sour whole milk using the traditional method, fat recovery values of 67 and 44 per cent were obtained with churning temperatures of 18° and 25°C, respectively. Controlling the temperature is therefore critical. The optimum churning temperature is between 15° and 17°C.

Degree of agitation

Increasing agitation reduces churning time. Fitting an agitator to a traditional churn reduces churning time and increases butter yield. The percentage of fat recovered as butter is increased, with as little as 0.2 per cent fat remaining in the buttermilk. The advantage of using the ILCA internal agitator was demonstrated when churning sour whole milk at 18°C. Using the traditional clay pot a fat recovery of 67 per cent was obtained compared to a 76 per cent fat recovery when using the clay pot fitted with the internal wooden agitator.

Extent of filling the churn

Churns should be filled to between a third and half their volumetric capacity. Filling to more than half the volumetric capacity increases churning time considerably but does not reduce fat recovery. Thus, when churning whole milk, the following conditions should be adhered to:

1. Milk acidity should be greater than 0.6 per cent.
2. The temperature should be adjusted to about 18°C.
3. Internal agitation should be used to reduce churning time and increase fat recovery.
4. The churn should not be filled to more than half its volumetric capacity.

Once the fat has been recovered by churning the buttermilk contains casein, whey proteins, milk salts, lactic acid, lactose, the unrecovered fat and some fat globule membrane constituents. Buttermilk is suitable, and is often used, for direct consumption. It is also used to inoculate fresh milk to encourage acid development and for cheesemaking.

Ghee, Butter Oil and Dry Butterfat

These products are almost entirely butterfat and contain practically no water or milk solids-not-fat (SNF). Ghee is made in eastern tropical countries, usually from buffalo milk. An identical product called *samn* is made in Sudan. Much of the typical flavour comes from the burned milk SNF remaining in the product. Butter oil or anhydrous milk fat is a refined product made by centrifuging melted butter or by separating milk fat from high-fat cream.

Ghee is a more convenient product than butter in the tropics because it keeps better under warm conditions. It has low moisture and milk SNF contents, which inhibits bacterial growth.

Milk or cream is churned as described in the sections dealing with churning of sour whole milk or cream. When enough butter has been accumulated it is placed in an iron pan and the water evaporated at a constant rate of boiling. Overheating must be avoided as it burns the curd and impairs the flavour. Eventually a scum forms on the surface and can be removed using a perforated ladle. When all the moisture has evaporated the casein begins to char, indicating that the process is complete. The ghee can then be poured into an earthenware jar for storage.

A considerable amount of moisture and milk SNF can be removed before boiling by melting the butter in hot water (80°C) and separating the fat layer. The fat can be separated either by gravity or using a hand separator. The fat phase yields a product containing 1.5 per cent moisture and little fat is lost in the aqueous phase.

Alternatively, the mixture of butter and hot water can be allowed to settle in a vessel similar to that used in the deep-setting method for separating whole milk. Once the fat has solidified the aqueous phase is drained. The fat is then removed and heated to evaporate residual moisture. Products made using these methods have excellent keeping qualities with a shelf-life of about six months at ambient temperature.

Cheesemaking Using Fresh Milk

Cheese is a concentrate of the milk constituents, mainly fat, casein and insoluble salts, together with water in which small amounts of soluble salts, lactose and albumin are found. To retain these constituents in concentrated form, milk is coagulated by direct acidification, by lactic acid produced by bacteria, by adding rennet or a combination of acidification and addition of rennet.

Rennet coagulation theory

Rennet, a proteolytic enzyme extracted from the abomasum of suckling calves, was traditionally used for coagulating milk. Originally the abomasum was itself immersed in milk. The extraction of rennet which could be stored as a liquid was the first step towards refining this procedure. This was followed by purification and concentration of the enzyme. The purified enzyme was originally called rennin and is now called chymosin.

On weaning the chymosin of the suckling calf is replaced by bovine pepsin. With the decrease in the practice of slaughtering calves chymosin became scarce resulting in a search for chymosin substitutes. Rennet is a general term currently used to describe a variety of enzymes of animal, plant or microbial origin used to coagulate milk in cheesemaking.

Rennet transforms liquid milk into a gel. While the process is not fully understood, rennet coagulation is thought to take place in two distinct phases, the first of which is regarded as being enzymatic, the second nonenzymatic. The first, or primary phase, can be illustrated as:

$$\text{Casein} \xrightarrow[\text{rennet}]{\text{Water}} \text{para casein} + \text{glycomacropeptide}$$

Since k-casein stabilises the other caseins and its hydrolysis leads to the coagulation of the casein fraction, the primary phase can also be expressed as:

$$k\text{-Casein} \xrightarrow[\text{rennet}]{\text{Water}} \underset{\text{(insoluble)}}{\text{para casein}} + \underset{\text{(soluble)}}{\text{glycomacropeptide}}$$

The effect of milk coagulants on the other caseins is thought to be negligible at this stage.

The second, or secondary, phase is the nonenzymatic precipitation of para casein by calcium ions. Para-casein, in association with the calcium ions, is thought to produce a lattice structure throughout the milk. This traps the fat and whey is gradually exuded. The coagulum then contracts, a process known as syneresis. This is accelerated by increasing the temperature and reducing pH to as low as pH 4.6.

Rennet also has a tertiary action on milk proteins. This occurs during cheese ripening when rennet hydrolyses milk proteins. If the desired hydrolysis is not obtained, the cheese becomes bitter. While a wide variety of proteolytic enzymes coagulate milk, the tertiary action of many of these on milk proteins causes undesirable flavours in cheese, which limits the range of coagulants that can be used.

Cheese varieties

Many cheese varieties are manufactured around the world but they are all broadly classified by hardness, i.e. very hard, hard, semi-soft and soft, according to their moisture content. Cheese is usually made from cow milk, although several varieties are made from the milk of goats, sheep or horses.

White cheese

Queso blanco (white cheese) is of Latin American origin. It is usually made from milk containing about 3 per cent fat. Starter or rennet is not used and curd precipitation is brought about by an organic acid usually in the form of lemon juice. *Queso blanco* is a pressed cheese (it contains less moisture than unpressed cheese) and therefore has a longer shelf-life than soft curd cheese. The milk is heated to a high temperature (over 80°C) and this also contributes to the increased shelf-life of the cheese. *Queso blanco* is an ideal cheese for manufacture by smallholders as all the materials required may be obtained or made locally. The expected yield is one kilogram of cheese from eight litres of milk.

Halloumi

Halloumi is a firm pickled cheese with its origins in Cyprus where it is made from sheep or goat milk or a mixture of both. It can also be made from cow milk. Starter is not used. The cheese may be eaten fresh or after storage in a cool store. If it is stored at below 12°C it will keep for several months. After salting the cheese pieces may also be stored in plastic bags without brining; if stored at about 10°C the cheese has a shelf-life of two to three months. About one kilogram of cheese will be obtained from nine litres of milk.

Gybna beyda

Gybna beyda is a hard white cheese made in Sudan. It is similar to *Domiati* which is made in Egypt. Starter is not used. The storage life of the cheese may be more than one year. About one kilogram of cheese will be obtained from seven litres of milk.

Cheddar

Cheddar cheese has its origins in Britain. Traditionally the cheese was made in different sizes from about 0.5 to 25 kg. The procedure for making Cheddar may be considered difficult and tedious by the inexperienced but the resultant mature cheese with its characteristic nutty flavour and close texture makes the task worthwhile. The Cheddar cheese recipe can be manipulated to give a cheese which may be consumed in four weeks or stored for up to two years. Therefore Cheddar offers the opportunity to preserve milk constituents in times of surplus milk production.

In order to obtain a cheese of good body and texture it is necessary to use milk with about 3.3 per cent fat. If milk with excess fat content is used there will be high losses of fat in the whey and the cheese will have a weak, pasty body.

Cheese yield

In cheesemaking, the milk fat and casein are recovered with some moisture. The cheese yield can be expressed in kilograms of cheese obtained per 100 kg of milk processed. Cheese yield is influenced by milk composition, the moisture content of the final cheese and the degree of recovery of fat and protein in the curd during cheesemaking.

Milk low in total solids will give a low cheese yield, while milk high in total solids will give a high cheese yield. To predict the theoretical yield of cheese, the fat and casein content of the milk must be known. Because of difficulties encountered in estimating casein content, the following formula, derived from results of experiments on Cheddar cheese, is often used to estimate cheese yield:

$$(2.3 \times \text{fat}\%) + 1.4 = \text{cheese yield (kg/100 kg milk)}$$

Therefore, with milk containing 4 per cent fat the expected yield would be:

$$(2.3 \times 4) + 1.4 = 10.6 \text{ kg/100 kg milk}$$

This formula gives an estimate of cheese yield and is applied most often to Cheddar cheese. It is useful as an immediate check on efficiency, but a universal yield factor for cheese varieties is unrealistic. If the cheese yield is less than expected, the following checks should be made:

1. Weigh and record milk received.
2. Sample and analyse milk received.
3. Weigh, store and record cheese made.
4. Sample and analyse whey.

The fat content of whey should be analysed for each batch of cheese made. In estimating the profitability of cheesemaking enterprises, an average annual yield of 9.5 per cent, i.e. 9.5 kg of cheese per 100 kg of milk, is used. Milk may be standardised to increase cheese yield, particularly with high-fat milk. Standardisation also gives a good return for skim milk, however, over-standardising (reducing the fat content to below 3 per cent) results in coarse-textured cheese with poor flavour.

High moisture content increases cheese yield, but reduces keeping quality. Cheese loses moisture during storage if it is not properly wrapped, thus reducing yield. Waxing reduces moisture loss, as does storing cheese in brine.

Cheesemaking with Sour Skim Milk

The casein and some of the unrecovered fat in skim milk and buttermilk can be heat-precipitated as cottage cheese, known in Ethiopia as *ayib*.

The defatted milk is heated to about 50°C until a distinct curd mass forms. It is then allowed to cool gradually and the curd is ladled out. Alternatively, the curd can be recovered by filtering the cooled mixture through a muslin cloth. This facilitates more complete recovery of the curd and also allows more effective moisture removal. Temperature of heating can be varied between 40° and 70°C without markedly affecting product composition and yield. Heat treatments between 70° and 90°C do not appear to affect yield but give the product a cooked flavour.

The whey contains about 0.75 per cent protein, indicating near-complete recovery of casein. Whey may be consumed by humans or fed to animals. The approximate composition of cottage cheese made at smallholder level is 76 per cent water, 14 per cent protein, 7 per cent fat and 2 per cent ash. It has a short shelf-life because of its high moisture content. The shelf-life can be increased by adding salt, reducing the moisture content of the cheese or by storing the product in an airtight container.

Skim milk can be heated in any suitably sized vessel that is able to withstand heat. Heating can be direct or indirect. A ladle or muslin cloth can be used for product recovery. The yield depends on milk composition and on the moisture content of the product, but should be at least 1 kg of cottage cheese from 8 litres of milk (12.5 per cent).

MICROBIOLOGY OF BUTTER

Butter is made as a means of extracting and preserving milk fat. It can be made directly from milk or by separation of milk and subsequent churning of the cream.

Sources of Contamination

In addition to bacteria present in the milk other sources of bacteria in butter are: (i) equipment, (ii) wash water, (iii) air contamination, (iv) packing materials, and (v) personnel.

Equipment

In smallholder butter-making, bacterial contamination can come from unclean surfaces, the butter maker and wash water. Packaging materials, cups and leaves are also sources of contaminants. Washing and smoking the churn reduces bacterial numbers. But traditional equipment is often porous and is therefore a reservoir for many organisms. When butter is made on a larger processing scale, bacterial contamination can come from holding-tank surfaces, the churn and butter-handling equipment.

A wooden churn can be a source of serious bacterial, yeast and mould contamination since these organisms can penetrate the wood, where they can be destroyed only by extreme heat. If a wooden churn has loose bands, cream can enter the crevices between the staves, where it provides a growth medium for bacteria which contaminate subsequent batches of butter. However, if care is taken in cleaning a wooden churn this source of contamination can be controlled. Similar care is required with scotch hands and butter-working equipment.

Wash water

Wash water can be a source of contamination with both coliform bacteria and bacteria associated with defects in butter. Polluted water supplies can also be a source of pathogens.

Air

Contamination from the air can introduce spoilage organisms: mould spores, bacteria and yeasts can fall on the butter if it is left exposed to the air. Moulds grow rapidly on butter exposed to air.

Packaging

Care is required in the storage and preparation of packaging material. Careless handling of packaging material can be a source of mould contamination.

Personal hygiene

A high standard of personal hygiene is required from people engaged in butter-making. For example, in New Zealand the 1938 dairy produce regulations stated 'no person shall permit his bare hands to be brought in contact with any butter at any time immediately following manufacture or during the wrapping, packaging, storage and transport of such butter'.

Personal pass organisms to butter via the hands, mouth, nasal passage and clothing. Suitable arrangements for disinfecting hands should be provided, and clean working garments should not have contact with other clothes.

Control of Micro-organisms in Butter

Salting effectively controls bacterial growth in butter. The salt must be evenly dispersed and worked in well. Salt concentration of 2 per cent adequately dispersed in butter of 16 per cent moisture will result in a 12.5 per cent salt solution throughout the water-in-oil emulsion.

Washing butter does little to reduce microbiological counts. It may be desirable not to wash butter, since washing reduces yield. The acid pH of serum in butter made from ripened cream or sour milk may control the growth of acid-sensitive organisms. Microbiological analysis of butter usually includes some of the following tests: total bacterial count, yeasts and moulds, coliform estimation and estimation of lipolytic bacteria.

Yeast, mould and coliform estimations are useful for evaluating sanitary practices. The presence of defect producing types can be indicated by estimating the presence of lipolytic organisms. All butter contains some micro-organisms. However, proper control at every stage of the process can minimise the harmful effects of these organisms.

PRODUCTION AND USE OF MICROBIAL ENZYMES FOR DAIRY PROCESSING

For improving the quality of milk and milk products, a number of different enzymes from microbial as well as from nonmicrobial sources have potential applications in dairy processing, principal among some enzymes that have important and growing applications are lipases and β-galactosidases. Enzymes with limited applications include glucose oxidase, superoxide dismutase, sulphydryl oxidase, etc.

India being the highest producer of milk in the world, and consequently the surplus availability of milk in our country has triggered the food and dairy industry to convert the liquid milk into value-added products using biochemical and enzymatic processes.

Microbial Rennets in Dairy Applications

Animal rennet (bovine chymosin) is conventionally used as a milk-clotting agent in dairy industry for the manufacture of quality cheeses with good flavour and texture. Rennin acts on the milk protein in two stages, by enzymatic and by nonenzymatic action, resulting in coagulation of milk. In the enzymatic phase, the resultant milk becomes a gel due to the influence of calcium ions and the temperature used in the process. Many micro-organisms are known to produce rennet-like proteinases which can substitute the calf rennet. Micro-organisms like *Rhizomucor pusillus*, *R. miehei*, *Endothia parasitica*, *Aspergillus oryzae*, and *Irpex lactis* are used extensively for rennet production in cheese manufacture.

Extensive research that has been carried out so far on rennet substitutes has been reviewed by several authors. Different strains of species of Mucor are often used for the production of microbial rennets. Whereas best yields of the milk-clotting protease from *Rhizomucor pusillus* are obtained from semisolid cultures containing 50 per cent wheat bran, *R. miehei* and *Endothia parasitica* are well suited for submerged cultivation.

Using the former, good yields of milk-clotting protease may be obtained in a medium containing 4 per cent potato starch, 3 per cent soyabean meal, and 10 per cent barley. During growth, lipase is secreted together with the protease. Therefore, the lipase activity has to be destroyed by reducing the pH, before the preparation can be used as cheese rennet.

Microbial rennets from various micro-organisms (marketed under the trade names such as Rennilase, Fromase, Marzyme, Hanilase, etc.) being marketed since the 1970s have proved satisfactory for the production of different kinds of cheese. The molecular and enzymatic properties of chymosins have been studied extensively. Although the proteolytic specificities of the three commonly used fungal rennets are considerably different from those of calf chymosin, these rennets have been used to produce acceptable cheeses.

Recently Novo Nordisk has succeeded in expressing just one proteolytic enzyme from the fungus *R. miehei* in the well-known organism *A. oryzae*. This host organism is able to produce the single protease that cleaves the casein into a glycomacropeptide and para *k*-casein by hydrolysing only at the phe105–met106 peptide bond between phenyl alanine and methionine. This monocomponent enzyme product has the trade name Novoren. One major drawback of microbial rennet use in cheese manufacture, is the development of off flavour and bitter taste in the nonripened as well as in the ripened cheeses. The rennets from microbial sources are more proteolytic in nature in comparison to rennet from animal sources, resulting in production of some bitter peptides during the process of cheese ripening. Hence, attempts have been made to clone the gene for calf chymosin, and to express it in selected bacteria, yeasts, and moulds.

Recombinant Rennets for Cheese Manufacture

Due to shortage of calf stomachs and the economic value of cheese rennet, gene for calf chymosin was one of the first genes for mammalian enzymes that was cloned and expressed in micro-organisms. Many different laboratories have cloned the gene for calf prochymosin in *Escherichia coli*, and analysed the structure of the gene as well as the properties of the recombinant chymosin. The expressed proenzyme in *E. coli*, is present mainly as insoluble inclusion bodies, comprised of reduced prochymosin as well as molecules that are interlinked by disulphide bridges. After disintegration of the cells, inclusion bodies are harvested by centrifugation.

The individual laboratories have reported some differences in the procedure for renaturation of prochymosin from the inclusion bodies, but all have followed the same general scheme. The enzymatic properties of recombinant *E. coli* chymosin are indistinguishable from those of native calf chymosin. The enzymes were identical when observed by immunodiffusion in gels, but a slight difference was observed by enzyme linked immunosorbent assay (ELISA).

The gene for prochymosin has also been cloned in *Saccharomyces cerevisiae*; the levels of expression have been reported to be 0.5 to 2.0 per cent of total yeast protein. In yeast, about 20 per cent of the prochymosin can be released in soluble form which can be activated directly; the remaining 80 per cent is still associated with the cell debris. The cloning of chymosin was carried out without the prosequence. Though the level of chymosin mRNA was similar to that of prochymosin mRNA, no milk-clotting activity was observed in clones containing the chymosin gene only. The results suggest that the prosequence is essential for correct folding of the polypeptide chain. The zymogen for the aspartic proteases from *R. pusillus*, also called mucor rennin, has likewise been cloned and expressed in yeast. Studies on its conversion to active form showed that secretion of *R. pusillus* protease from recombinant yeast was dependent on glycosylation of the enzyme.

Compared to yeast, the filamentous fungi generally secrete larger quantities of proteins into the culture medium. Furthermore, filamentous fungi secrete the heterologous proteins with correct folding of the polypeptide chain, and process correct pairing of sulphydryl groups. The gene for *R. miehei* protease has been expressed in *A. oryzae*.

Prochymosin has been expressed in *Kluyveromyces lactis*, *A. nidulans*, *A. niger*, and *Trichoderma reesei*. In most of the cases, the reported yields of the model systems were about 10–40 mg of enzyme per litre of culture medium. However, 3.3 g of enzyme per litre has also been achieved. Yeast, *Kluyveromyces lactis*, has recently been used as an efficient host for the secretion of recombinant chymosin, which has led to the development of large-scale production process for chymosin. If produced on an industrial scale, the yields will perhaps be of the latter magnitude.

Since most of the rennet (>90 per cent) added to cheese milk is lost in the whey, immobilisation would considerably extend its catalytic life. Several rennets have been immobilised, but their efficiency as milk coagulants has been questioned. So, there is a fairly general support for the view that immobilised enzymes cannot coagulate milk properly owing to inaccessability of the Phe–Met peptide bond of *k*-casein, and that the apparent coagulating activity of immobilised rennets is due to leaching of the enzyme from the support.

Different types of conventional cheeses have been successfully made by using recombinant rennet on an experimental or pilot scale. No major differences have been detected between cheeses made with recombinant chymosins or natural enzymes, regarding cheese yield, texture, smell, taste and ripening. The recombinant chymosins are identical with calf rennet according to the report on biochemical and genetic evidences.

Lactase in Dairy Industry

Lactose, the sugar found in milk and whey, and its corresponding hydrolase, lactase or β-galactosidase, have been extensively researched during the past decade. This is because of the enzyme immobilisation technique which has given new and interesting possibilities for the utilisation of this sugar. Because of intestinal enzyme insufficiency, some individuals, and even a population, show lactose intolerance and difficulty in consuming milk and dairy products. Hence, low-lactose or lactose-free food aid program is essential for lactose-intolerant people to prevent severe tissue dehydration, diarrhoea, and, at times, even death. Another advantage of lactase-treated milk is the increased sweetness of the resultant milk, thereby avoiding the requirement for addition of sugars in the manufacture of flavoured milk drinks. Manufacturers of ice cream, yoghurt and frozen desserts use lactase to improve scoop and creaminess, sweetness, and digestibility, and to reduce sandiness due to crystallisation of lactose in concentrated preparations. Cheese manufactured from hydrolysed milk ripens more quickly than the cheese manufactured from normal milk.

Technologically, lactose crystallises easily which sets limits to certain processes in the dairy industry, and the use of lactase to overcome this problem has not reached its fullest potential because of the associated high costs. Moreover, the main problem associated with discharging large quantities of cheese whey is that it pollutes the environment. But, the discharged whey could be exploited as an alternate cheap source of lactose for the production of lactic acid by fermentation. The whey permeate, which is a by-product in the manufacture of whey protein concentrates, by ultrafiltration could be fermented efficiently by *Lactobacillus bulgaricus*.

Lactose can be obtained from various sources like plants, animal organs, bacteria, yeasts (intracellular enzyme) or moulds. Some of these sources are used for commercial enzyme preparations. Lactase preparations from *A. niger*, *A. oryzae*, and *Kluyveromyces lactis* are considered safe because these sources already have a history of safe use and have been subjected to numerous safety tests. The most investigated *E. coli* lactase is not used in food processing because of its cost and toxicity problems.

Properties of lactase

The properties of the enzyme depend on its source. Temperature and pH optima differ from source to source and with the type of particular commercial preparation. Immobilisation of the enzymes, method of immobilisation, and type of carrier can also influence these optima values. In general, fungal lactase have pH optima in the acidic range 2.5–4.5, and yeast and bacterial lactases in the neutral region 6–7 and 6.5–7.5, respectively. The variation in pH optima of lactases makes them suitable for specific applications, for example fungal lactases are used for acid whey hydrolysis, while yeast and bacterial lactases are suitable for milk (pH 6.6) and sweet whey (pH 6.1) hydrolysis. Product inhibition, e.g. inhibition by galactose, is another property which also depends on the source of lactase. The enzyme from *A. niger* is more strongly inhibited by galactose than that from *A. oryzae*.

This inhibition can be overcome by hydrolysing lactose at low concentrations by using immobilised enzyme systems or by recovering the enzyme using ultrafiltration after batch hydrolysis. Lactase from *Bacillus* species are superior with respect to thermostability, pH operation range, product inhibition, and sensitivity against high-substrate concentration. Thermostable enzymes, able to retain their activity at 60°C or above for prolonged periods, have two distinct advantages viz. they give higher conversion rate or shorter residence time for a given conversion rate, and the process is less prone to microbial contamination due to higher operating temperature. *Bacillus* species have a pH optima of 6.8 and a temperature optima of 65°C. Its high activity for skim milk, and less inhibition by galactose has made it suitable for use as a production organism for lactase.

The enzymatic hydrolysis of lactose can be achieved either by free enzymes, usually in batch fermentation process, or by immobilised enzymes or even by immobilised whole cells producing intracellular enzyme. Although numerous hydrolysis systems have been investigated, only few of them have been scaled up with success and even fewer have been applied at an industrial or semi-industrial level. Several acid hydrolysis systems have been developed to industry-scale level. Large-scale systems which use free enzyme process have been developed for processing of UHT-milk and processing of whey, using *K. lactis* lactase (Maxilact, Lactozyme). Several commercial immobilised systems have been developed for commercial exploitation. Snamprogretti process of industrial-scale milk processing technology in Italy is one such working systems. They make use of fibre-entrapped yeast lactase in a batch process, and the milk used is previously sterilised by UHT. For pilot plants, there are three other processes designed and developed to handle milk; (i) by Gist-Brocades, Rohm GmbH (Germany), and (ii) by Sumitomo, Japan.

These are continuous processes with short residence times. Processing of whey UF-permeate is accomplished by the system developed by Corning Glass, Connecticut, Lehigh, Valio and Amerace corp. The process by Corning Glass is being applied at commercial scale in the bakers yeast production using hydrolysed whey.

Microbial Enzymes in Accelerated Cheese Ripening

Cheese ripening is a complex process mediated by biochemical and biophysical changes during which a bland curd is developed into a mature cheese with characteristic flavour, texture, and aroma. The desirable attributes are produced by the partial and gradual breakdown of carbohydrates, lipids, and proteins during ripening, mediated by several agents, viz. (i) residual coagulants, (ii) starter bacteria and their enzymes, (iii) nonstarter bacteria and their enzymes, (iv) indigenous milk enzymes, especially proteinases, and (v) secondary inocula with their enzymes.

Proteolysis occurs in all the cheese varieties and is a prerequisite for characteristic flavour development that can be regulated by proper use of the above agents. Cheese ripening is essentially an enzymatic process which can be accelerated by augmenting activity of the key enzymes. This has the advantage of initiating more specific action for flavour development compared to use of elevated temperatures that can result in accelerating undesirable nonspecific reactions, and consequently off flavour development. Enzymes may be added to develop specific flavours in cheeses, for example lipase addition for the development of Parmesan or Blue-type cheese flavours. Attempts to accelerate the multiple secondary flavour-forming-reactions, e.g. strecker degradation, have been scarce.

The pathways leading to the formation of flavour compounds are largely unknown, and therefore the use of exogenous enzymes to accelerate ripening is mostly an empirical process. Different microbial enzymes used to accelerate cheese ripening are presented in Table 14.5.

Table 14.5. Microbial enzymes used to accelerate cheese ripening.

Enzyme	Source
Microbial lipases	*Aspergillus niger*
	A. oryzae
	Rhizomucor miehei
Lactases	*Streptococcus lactis*
	Kluyveromyces sp.
	Escherichia coli
Microbial serine proteinases	*A. niger*
Neutral proteinases	*Bacillus subtilis*
	A. oryzae

Studies on the hydrolysis of whole casein and isolated casein components to observe the kinetics and specificity of aspartic proteases in rennin, pepsin, and four microbial rennet substitutes indicated the considerable differences in the reaction velocity and the extent of hydrolysis on the rennet curd yield. The rennet enzymes were active even in the later phases of cheese-ripening.

Proteinases and peptidases

Proteolysis is characteristic of most cheese varieties and is indispensable for good flavour and textural development. Proteinases used in cheese processing include: (i) plasmin, (ii) rennet, and (iii) proteinases (cell wall and/or intracellular) of the starter and nonstarter bacteria. Approximately 6 per cent of the rennet added to cheese milk remains in the curd after manufacture and contributes significantly to proteolysis during ripening. Combinations of individual neutral proteinases and microbial peptidases intensified cheese flavour, and when used in combinations with microbial rennets reduced the intensity of bitterness caused by the latter.

Acid proteases in isolation cause intense bitterness. Various animal or microbial lipases gave pronounced cheese flavour, low bitterness and strong rancidity, while lipases in combination with proteinases and/or peptidases give good cheese flavour with low levels of bitterness. In a more balanced approach to the acceleration of cheese ripening using mixtures of proteinases and peptidases, attenuated starter cells or cell-free extracts (CFE) are being favoured.

Proteolytic Enzymes of Lactic Acid Bacteria in Fermented Milk Products

The proteolytic system of lactic acid bacteria is essential for their growth in milk, and contributes significantly to flavour development in fermented milk products. The proteolytic system is composed of proteinases which initially cleaves the milk protein to peptides; peptidases which cleave the peptides to small peptides and amino acids; and transport system responsible for cellular uptake of small peptides and amino acids. Lactic acid bacteria have a complex proteolytic system capable of converting milk casein to the free amino acids and peptides necessary for their growth. These proteinases include extracellular proteinases, endopeptidases, aminopeptidases, tripeptidases, and proline-specific peptidases, which are all serine proteases. Apart from lactic streptococcal proteinases, several other proteinases from nonlactostreptococcal origin have been reported. There are also serine type of proteinases, e.g. proteinases from *Lactobacillus acidophillus*, *L. plantarum*, *L. delbrueckii* sp. *bulgaricus*, *L. lactis*, and *L. helveticus*. Aminopeptidases are important for the development of flavour in fermented milk products, since they are capable of releasing single amino acid residues from oligopeptides formed by extracellular proteinase activity.

Other Dairy Enzymes

Other enzymes used for dairy food application include: (i) proteases to reduce allergic properties of cow milk products for infants, and (ii) lipases for development of lipolytic flavours in speciality cheeses. The functional properties of milk proteins may be improved by limited proteolysis through the enzymatic modification of milk proteins. An acid-soluble casein, free of off flavour and suitable for incorporation into beverages and other acid foods, has been prepared by limited proteolysis. The antigenicity of casein is destroyed by proteolysis, and the hydrolysate is suitable for use in milk-protein-based foods for infants allergic to cow milk.

Lipolysis makes an important contribution to swiss cheese flavours, due mainly to the lipolytic enzymes of the starter cultures. The characteristic peppery flavour of Blue cheese is due to short-chain fatty acids and methyl ketones. Most of the lipolysis in Blue cheese is catalysed by *Penicillium roqueforti* lipase, with a lesser contribution from indigenous milk lipase.

Chapter 15

Spoilage of Heated Canned Foods

INTRODUCTION

Canning is a method of preserving food in which the food contents are processed and sealed in an airtight container, providing a typical shelf-life ranging from 1 year to 5 years and under specific circumstances a freeze dried canned product can last as long as 30 years and can still be safely consumed. The process was first developed as a French military discovery by Nicolas Appert in 1810. The packaging prevents micro-organisms from entering and proliferating inside.

To prevent the food from being spoiled before and during containment, quite a number of methods are used: pasteurisation, boiling (and other applications of high temperature over a period of time), refrigeration, freezing, drying, vacuum treatment, antimicrobial agents that are natural to the recipe of the foods being preserved, a sufficient dose of ionising radiation, submersion in a strong saline solution, acid, base, osmotically extreme (for example very sugary) or other microbe-challenging environments.

Other than sterilisation, no method is perfectly dependable as a preservative. For example, the micro-organism *Clostridium botulinum* (which causes botulism), can only be eliminated at temperatures above the boiling point. From a public safety point of view, foods with low acidity (a pH more than 4.6) need sterilisation under high temperature (116°–130°C). To achieve temperatures above the boiling point requires the use of a pressure canner. Foods that must be pressure canned include most vegetables, meat, seafood, poultry, and dairy products. The only foods that may be safely canned in an ordinary boiling water bath are highly acidic ones with a pH below 4.6, such as fruits, pickled vegetables or other foods to which acidic additives have been added.

SPOILAGE OF CANNED FOODS

Canned foods may spoil either due to biological or chemical reasons. We would discuss only the biological spoilage as it is the point at issue.

Biological Spoilage of Canned Foods

Biological spoilage of canned foods occurs due to the action of various micro-organisms. Spore forming bacteria, e.g. *Clostridium*, *Bacillus* represent the most important group of canned food spoiling micro-organisms because of their heat resistant nature (thermophilic nature). In addition, there are other micro-organisms which are not heat resistant (mesophilic) but enter through the leakage of the container during cooling and spoil the food. In this way, we can divide biological spoilage of canned into following two categories.

Biological spoilage by thermophilic bacteria

Underprocessing of canned foods results in spoilage by thermophilic bacteria, the bacteria that grow best at temperature of 50°C or higher. Five types of this spoilage can be recognised.

Flat sour spoilage

In canned foods, production of acid and no gas is referred to as flat sour spoilage because the food becomes sour, but the can shows no evidence of food spoilage because no gas is produced, i.e. the can remains flat. Thus, the spoilage cannot be detected unless the can is opened. The spoilage is caused by *Bacillus* spp. such as *B. coagulans* and *B. stearothermophilus* resulting in sour, abnormal odour, sometimes cloudy liquor in food content of the can.

Thermophilic anaerobic (TA) spoilage

Clostridium thermosaccharolyticum, an obligate thermophile, causes spoilage. The can swells and may burst due to production of CO_2 and H_2. The food becomes fermented sour, cheesy, and develops butyric odour.

Sulphide spoilage

Clostridium nigricans is involved in this spoilage. It produces H_2S gas which is absorbed by the food product. The latter becomes usually blackened and gives 'rotten egg' odour.

Putrefactive anaerobic spoilage

Clostridium sporogenes causes spoilage through putrefaction. The can swells and may burst. Putrefaction may result from partial digestion of the food. The latter develops typical 'putrid' odour.

Aerobic sporeformer's spoilage

Bacillus spp., the aerobic bacteria, cause spoilage. If the canned food is cured meat, swelling of the can is observed.

Biological spoilage by mesophilic micro-organisms

Bacillus spp., *Clostridium* spp., yeasts, and other fungi which are mesophilic (an organism growing best at moderate temperature range of 25° to 400°C) are mainly responsible for this type of canned food spoilage. As stated earlier, these organisms enter through the leakage of the container during cooling.

Clostridium butyricum and *C. pasteurianum* result in butyric acid type of fermentation in acidic (tomato juice, fruits, fruit juices, etc.) or medium acidic (corn, peas, spinach, etc.) food with swelling of the container due to the production of CO_2 and H_2.

Bacillus subtilis and *B. mesenteroides* have been reported as spoiling canned sea-foods, meats, etc. Other mesophilic bacteria which have been reported in cans are *Bacillus polymixa*, *B. macerans*, *Streptococcus* sp., *Pseudomonas*, *Proteus*, etc. Yeasts and moulds have also been found present in canned foods. Yeasts result in CO_2 production and swelling of the cans.

Microbiology of Canned Foods

One method of preserving canned food is by the use of heat which destroys most, if not all the micro-organisms. The type of heat treatment will however, depend on the nature of the food material and varies from pasteurisation for milk, juices and other liquids to sterilisation by steam under pressure for canned vegetables or soups.

At milder heat treatment: a number of heat resistant organisms survive and these may subsequently grow and cause spoilage if conditions are favourable. Following heating, the canned or bottled food is then stored at a low temperature. Some foods which are processed at high temperatures can be stored at room temperature.

Heated canned foods may undergo spoilage either due to chemical or biological reasons. The most important chemical spoilage of canned foods is the 'hydrogen swell' produced as a result of the action of the food acid with the metal can. Such spoilage occurs mostly due to imperfect tinning and lacquering of the interior of the can used for canning acidic foods.

Biological spoilage of canned' foods by micro-organisms may result either from the survival of organisms after the heat treatment or leakage of the container permitting entrance of micro-organisms. Surviving organisms may be vegetative cells or spore formers depending on the heat treatment. Acid foods are processed at temperatures around 100°C which results in the killing of all vegetative cells of bacteria, yeasts and moulds.

Only bacterial spores may survive but these do not grow in acid foods. On the other hand, meat, vegetables and milk are processed at lower temperatures. This may eliminate vegetative cells but not the spores, which germinate later. Micro-organisms that enter through leaks during cooling need not necessarily be heat resistant.

Normally, the two ends of the food can should be flat indicating partial vacuum. If pressure develops inside, the ends bulge and the extent of bulging can lead to a 'flipper', a 'springer', soft swell or a hard swell depending on the pressure inside the can.

Canned foods can be grouped as follows on the basis of acidity:

1. Group I: Low acid foods, pH 5.3, vegetables such as peas, corn, beans, etc. and meat, fish and poultry.
2. Group II: Medium acid foods, pH 5.3–5.5, beets, pumpkin, spinach, etc.
3. Group III: Acid foods, pH 4.5-5.7, tomatoes, pears, etc.
4. Group IV: High acid foods, pH 3.7, berries, etc.

The type of microbial spoilage of canned foods is divided into those caused by thermophilic bacteria and those caused by mesophilic organisms and the kind of spoilage is classified as putrefaction, acid production, gas formation, blackening, etc.

SAFE CANNING METHODS

Proper canning practices in the home insure a safe, high-quality product every time. However, it is vital to carefully follow guidelines for preparation, packing and processing foods to achieve a wholesome, safe canned food product.

Reasons for Spoilage

Micro-organisms

The major cause of food spoilage is microbial growth. Canning is a method of food preservation involving heat. Canning a food increases the length of time that a food can be stored at room temperature. During the heating process certain micro-organisms that cause food spoilage are destroyed. The types of micro-organisms that cause spoilage in foods are bacteria, yeasts and moulds. They contaminate food through air, soil, water or via the food handler. The growth of micro-organisms is affected by temperature, amount of water, amount of acid in the food and the presence of oxygen (air).

Canned foods provide a moist, yet oxygen-free environment that favours the growth of certain micro-organisms. While most micro-organisms are destroyed in the heating process, the organism that can survive in a moist, oxygen-free environment and which is of most concern in home canning is *Clostridium botulinum*. This organism causes the often fatal disease known as botulism.

C. botulinum is able to grow without oxygen (air) and thrives where there is little acid available. This particular micro-organism exists as a bacterial vegetative cell under favourable growth conditions, but reverts to a spore stage under unfavourable conditions. The spores are very heat-resistant, yet can be destroyed during the canning process. If the temperatures reached during the canning process are inadequate, the spores will change into cells, begin to grow inside the closed jar and produce the toxin that can be fatal. Times and temperatures for canning are based on those needed for the destruction of botulinum spores in the specific food product.

Enzymes

Chemical changes in food can also cause food spoilage. Such changes in canned foods are often caused by the action of enzymes which are not destroyed during heating. Enzymes are proteins which are naturally present in plants and animals. In living plants or animals they are important because they help speed up the ripening and maturing processes. However, when plants have been harvested or animals slaughtered, enzyme reactions often continue causing undesirable changes in a food product. Most enzymes deteriorate a food product under the same conditions which promote microbial growth. Canning, or an equivalent heat treatment, stops enzymes from causing undesirable chemical changes in a food.

Food Acidity Affects Canning Method

Foods are divided into two groups for canning based on the amount of acid they contain. Most foods have a neutral pH or are slightly acidic. In food preservation, a food with a pH of 4.6 or lower is considered to be a high-acid food, while one with a pH above 4.6 is a low-acid food.

Directions for proper canning have been developed on the basis of low- and high-acid foods. Because micro-organisms are easily destroyed by heat when acid is present, high-acid foods can be canned in boiling water at a temperature of 212°F. High-acid foods include fruit and fruit juices; jams, jellies and preserves; and pickles and pickled products. Tomatoes were once considered to be a high-acid food; however, because of problems in recent years with botulism in home-canned tomato products, new recommendations have been made.

Temperatures higher than 212°F are required to destroy the spores of *Clostridium botulinum* in low-acid feds, which include vegetables, red meat, poultry, fish and wild game. To reach temperatures higher than the boiling point of water (212°F), use a pressure canner. A temperature of at least 240°F is needed for the destruction of *C. botulinum* spores. Therefore, canning of low-acid foods is done in a pressure canner at 10 or 11 pounds of pressure (240°F) or at 15 pounds of pressure (250°F). Adjustments in canner pressure are made according to elevation above sea level.

Practices to avoid

The only safe way to can food at home is to match the food product to the correct method, use safe recipes and follow recommended procedures. Here are some practices and procedures to avoid:

Do not open-kettle can

This method involves pouring hot food into jars and sealing without further heat processing. As the jar and its contents cool, a vacuum forms to seal the product. This method is not recommended for home canning of fruits, vegetables or meats. Without sufficient heat to destroy bacteria, moulds and yeasts in food, microbial growth is likely and the product will spoil, even though it is sealed. Open-kettle canning directions are still included in some recipes for jellies. In Wisconsin, the method is not recommended for any product, including jelly.

Do not oven can

This method involves placing filled jars in the oven set at a specific temperature and 'processing' for a certain period of time. This method has never been recommended as a safe procedure for a variety of reasons. There are no safe and reliable processing times or temperature settings established for home canning in an oven. Also, dry heat, or hot air, is not as efficient as steam or boiling water for the transfer of heat to the center of the food in the jar. Oven temperatures vary considerably between the 'on' and 'off' cycles, so heating is uneven. Also, the temperature of the food does not correspond to the oven setting. In an oven, excess pressure can build up inside the jar, causing it to explode. The sudden temperature changes that occur when the oven is opened and the jars are removed could also cause the jars to break. Finally, besides the fact that oven canning can be dangerous, the end product would be underprocessed and thus could allow the growth of dangerous spoilage organisms, particularly *C. botulinum*.

Do not can in the microwave or dishwasher

Canning in the microwave oven or dishwasher is not recommended. Microwave ovens do not provide temperatures above 212°F for long enough periods of time to make certain the *C. botulinum* spores are destroyed. Similarly, temperatures in dishwashers are not high enough to sterilise food. (Jams and jellies can be cooked in a microwave, but must then be processed in a boiling water-bath canner after jars are filled.)

Do not steam can

There are several brands of steam canners available on the market. These are not the same steam pressure canners used for canning low-acid foods. They are also different from the water-bath canners. In the steam canner, the jars are not immersed in water as they are in the water-bath canner; therefore, heat flow inside the steam canner may be uneven. The end result would be underprocessed food that would be susceptible to microbial spoilage and chemical changes. Use of the steam canner is not recommended.

Do not use chemicals or preserving powders unless recommended

Chemicals such as aspirin should never be used as a substitute for heat treatment in home canning of food and cannot be relied upon to prevent spoilage or yield a satisfactory product. There is no safe ingredient that could destroy micro-organisms and extend the shelf-life of a food as heat processing does. The use of aspirin in food products is prohibited by state and federal laws. There is no evidence of its acceptability for use in protecting against hazardous spoilage. However, crystalline citric acid monohydrate, lemon juice from concentrate, tomato acidification tablets and ascorbic/citric acid mixtures can be added to tomato products prior to processing. The addition of these chemicals has been shown to cause an increase in acidity. Adding any chemical to a food product and omitting the heat treatment totally will result in the growth of spoilage organisms and the possible production of toxin by *C. botulinum*.

Do not take shortcuts or experiment in home canning

Use only tested, currently approved methods. The only safe canning method is a boiling water-bath for high-acid foods and a pressure canner for low-acid foods. Use only tested recipes and follow processing times exactly.

Do not use jars, cans and lids which are not made especially for home canning

Jars designed for commercial products such as peanut butter, coffee, pickles or vegetables may not withstand the heat treatment without breaking or may not accommodate standard two-piece canning lids. Mayonnaise or salad dressing jars that accommodate standard canning lids can be used for foods processed in boiling water canners but should not be used in a pressure canner.

Do not reuse or use zinc lids

Rubber rings used with zinc lids are not manufactured today. Old ones should not be used. Get new metal two-piece lids with sealing compound for safe products.

Do not use overripe food

Products change in chemical composition with age and lose acidity. Make sure the food is of good quality, with no bruises or soft spots.

Do not overpack foods

Trying to get too much food into one jar may result in underprocessing and spoilage. Leave recommended amount of headspace when jars are filled.

Do not use canned foods showing signs of spoilage

Watch for bulging lids, leaks, off-odours or mould. If in doubt, don't taste. Dispose of the food so that it cannot be consumed by humans or animals.

FISH SPOILAGE MECHANISMS

Fish spoilage results from three basic mechanisms: Enzymatic autolysis, oxidation, microbial growth.

Autolytic Enzymatic Spoilage

Shortly after capture, chemical and biological changes take place in dead fish due to enzymatic breakdown of major fish molecules autolytic enzymes reduced textural quality during early stages of deterioration but did not produce the characteristic spoilage off-odours and off-flavours. This indicates that autolytic degradation can limit shelf-life and product quality even with relatively low levels of spoilage organisms. Most of the impact is on textural quality along with the production of hypoxanthine and formaldehyde.

The digestive enzymes cause extensive autolysis which results in meat softening, rupture of the belly wall and drain out of the blood water which contains both protein and oil. Peptides and free amino acids can be produced as a result of autolysis of fish muscle proteins, essential, which lead towards the spoilage of fish meat as an outcome of microbial growth and production of biogenic amines.

Oxidative Spoilage

Lipid oxidation is a major cause of deterioration and spoilage for the pelagic fish species such as mackerel and herring with high oil/fat content stored fat in their flesh. Lipid oxidation involves a three stage free radical mechanism: initiation, propagation and termination. Initiation involves the formation of lipid free radicals through catalysts such as heat, metal ions and irradiation. These free radicals which react with oxygen to form peroxyl radicals. During propagation, the peroxyl radicals reacting with other lipid molecules to form hydroperoxides and a new free radical. Termination occurs when a buildup of these free radicals interact to form nonradical products. Oxidation typically involves the reaction of oxygen with the double bonds of fatty acids. Therefore, fish lipids which consist of polyunsaturated fatty acids are highly susceptible to oxidation. Molecular oxygen needs to be activated in order to allow oxidation to occur. Transition metals are primary activators of molecular oxygen.

In fish, lipid oxidation can occur enzymatically or non-enzymatically. The enzymatic hydrolysis of fats by lipases is termed lipolysis (fat deterioration). During this process, lipases split the glycerides forming free fatty acids which are responsible for: (i) common off-flavour, frequently referred to as rancidity, and (ii) reducing the oil quality.

The lipolytic enzymes could either be endogenous of the food product (such as milk) or derived from psychrotrophic micro-organisms. The enzymes involved are the lipases present in the skin, blood and tissue. The main enzymes in fish lipid hydrolysis are triacyl lipase, phospholipase A2 and phospholipase B. Nonenzymatic oxidation is caused by haematin compounds (haemoglobin, myoglobin and cytochrome) catalysis producing hydroperoxides. The fatty acids formed during hydrolysis of fish lipids interact with sarcoplasmic and myofibrillar proteins causing denaturation.

Microbial Spoilage

Composition of the microflora on newly caught fish depends on the microbial contents of the water in which the fish live. Fish microflora includes bacterial species such as *Pseudomonas*, *Alcaligenes*, *Vibrio*, *Serratia* and *Micrococcus*. Microbial growth and metabolism is a major cause of fish spoilage which produce amines, biogenic amines such as putrescine, histamine and cadaverine, organic acids, sulphides, alcohols, aldehydes and ketones with unpleasant and unacceptable off-flavours. Trimethylamine (TMA) levels are used universally to determine microbial deterioration leading to fish spoilage.

MEAT SPOILAGE

Meat is considered to be spoiled when it is unfit for human consumption. A variety of factors can cause meat to spoil including micro-organisms, exposure to air, and improper freezing techniques. Spoiled meat may be inedible due to unpleasant tastes and odours or may be unsafe for consumption especially when micro-organisms have caused the meat to spoil.

Meat Spoilage by Bacteria, Yeasts and Moulds

Although a number of factors may contribute to meat spoilage, the most common cause of meat spoilage is the deterioration of meat caused by micro-organisms (bacteria, yeasts, and moulds). Beware! Foods can contain dangerous bacteria and micro-organisms but still have a normal appearance. Food which has not been handled or stored properly should not be eaten even if it has no apparent indications of spoilage. Table 15.1 shows some of the common indications that meat has spoiled.

Table 15.1. Some of the common indications that meat has spoiled.

Indication of spoilage	Cause
Ammonia or sulphur smell, bad odour, tallow or chalky taste.	Degradation of proteins, lipids (fats) and carbohydrates caused by bacteria and/or enzymes naturally present in meat.
Slime formation, bad odour and rancid flavour, colour change (such as grey, brown, or green)	Bacterial and yeast spoilage

(Contd ...)

Indication of spoilage	Cause
Sticky meat surface	Mould spoilage
'Whiskers'	Mould spoilage
Surface colourations such as creamy, black or green	Growth of mould colonies
Tainting, souring, and putrefaction	Anaerobic bacterial spoilage of meat interiors, vacuum packed products, and sealed containers

Other Types of Spoilage

There are factors other than micro-organisms which can cause meat to spoil. They results from improper handling of meat (Table 15.2).

Table 15.2. Other types of spoilage.

Indication of spoilage	Cause
Oxidative rancidity (rancid flavour and odour)	Oxidation of meat fats due to improperly wrapped meat.
Brown or grey discolouration	Protein denaturation caused by heat, salts, ultraviolet light, low pH, and surface dehydration
Dehydration and discolouration during freezing resulting in dryness of cooked meat, nutrient loss, and sometimes a bitter flavour.	Freezer burn and drip which occurs during slow freezing.
Absorption of off-flavours	Storage of meat next to foods such as apples and onions which give off strong odours

Thus, spoilage can be prevented in home-canned products by adequately heat processing foods in a boiling water-bath or steam pressure canner for a specified period of time. The method used for processing depends on whether the food is high- or low-acid. For safety, use approved recipes that are based on scientific principles. Any practice that does not involve adequate processing may be potentially dangerous and should be avoided.

Chapter 16

Miscellaneous Foods

INTRODUCTION

The miscellaneous foods discussed in this chapter are fatty foods, salad dressings, essential oils, bottled soft drinks, spices and other condiments, salt, and nutmeats.

Food products compounded from combinations of the different groups of foods also would combine their microbial contents, and the new product may furnish a good culture medium for micro-organisms that previously had little chance to grow. Thus, yeasts from sugar added to bottled soft drinks may spoil the product. The water and flavouring materials also are potential source of contamination. Spices and other condiments added to foods may be important sources of micro-organisms, although spices may be treated with propylene oxide gas or may be irradiated to give them a low microbial content. Micro-organisms are added to salad dressings by ingredients such as spices, condiments, eggs and pickles. Salt (sodium chloride), especially solar salt, may add halophilic and salt-tolerant bacteria to salted fish and other salted or brined products.

FATTY FOODS

Fats and Oils

Fat is a nutrient that is an important source of calories. One gram of fat supplies 9 calories—more than twice the amount we get from carbohydrates or protein. Fat also is needed to carry and store essential fat-soluble vitamins, like vitamins A and D. There are two basic types of fat. They are grouped by their chemical structure. Each type of fat is used differently in our bodies and has a different effect on our health. When we eat a lot of high fat foods, we get a lot of calories. With too many calories, we may gain weight. Eating too much fat may also increase the risk of getting diseases like cancer, heart disease, high blood pressure or stroke. Health experts recommend that we should get no more than 30 per cent of our calories from fat to reduce our risk of getting these diseases.

Fat is found in many foods. Some of the fat that we eat comes from the fat we add in cooking or spread on breads, vegetables or other foods. A lot of fat is hidden in foods that we eat as snacks, pastries or prepared meals. We can reduce the amount of fat we eat by cutting down on the fat that we add in cooking or spread on foods. We can eat skim milk and low fat cheeses instead of whole milk and cheese. We can also use less fat, oil, butter, and margarine. Another way to cut down on fat is to drain and trim meats and take the skin off poultry. We can also read labels and compare the amount of fat in foods to make lower fat choices.

Fatty acids benefit the body in the following ways:

1. Elevate mood, resulting in less depression.
2. Improve cognitive function in the elderly.
3. Improve learning and attention span in schoolchildren.
4. Improve vision, especially night vision.
5. Lower the risk of cardiovascular disease.
6. Lowers the risk of breast and colon cancer.
7. Promote healthy skin.

Types of fats

Dietary fats are concentrated source of food energy. They are also the source of linoleum acid, an essential nutrient, and the fat-soluble vitamins A, D, E and K. While we all need some dietary fat each day, a tablespoon is generally sufficient when cutting back on fats, it is helpful to know which the most dietary culprits are.

Saturated fats

Saturated fats are the only fatty acids that raise blood cholesterol levels. Saturated fats are found in meats and whole dairy products like milk, cheese, cream and ice cream. Some saturated fats are also found in plant foods like tropical oils (coconut or palm kernel oil). When margarine or vegetable shortening is made from corn oil, soyabean oil or other vegetable oils, hydrogen atoms are added making some of the fat molecules 'saturated'. This also makes the fat solid at room temperature. Butter, margarine, and fats in meat and dairy products are all especially high in saturated fat.

We can reduce the saturated fats in our diets by using skim milk and low fat cheeses instead of whole milk and cheese. We can also use less fat, oil, butter, and margarine. At the table, use tub margarine instead of butter. Another way to cut down on fat is to drain and trim meats and take the skin off poultry. Simply reducing the total amount of fat we eat goes a long way toward reducing saturated fats.

Unsaturated fats

Unsaturated fats are usually liquid at room temperature. They are found in most vegetable products and oils. An exception is a group of tropical oils like coconut or palm kernel oil which is highly saturated. Using foods containing 'polyunsaturated' and 'monounsaturated' fats does not increase our risk of heart disease. However, like all fats, unsaturated fats give us 9 calories for every gram. So eating too much of these types of fat may also make us gain weight.

We can reduce the fat and unsaturated fats in our diets by using less fat, oil, and margarine. We can also eat more low-fat foods like vegetables, fruits, breads, rice, pasta and cereals.

Cholesterol

Cholesterol is an essential fat made by the liver. Many people get additional cholesterol by eating meat and dairy products. Too much dietary intake may raise blood cholesterol levels, and lead to heart disease. Cholesterol is transported through the bloodstream by lipoproteins.

Knowing the facts about cholesterol can reduce your risk for a heart attack or stroke. But understanding what cholesterol is and how it affects your health are only the beginning. To keep your cholesterol under control:

1. Schedule a screening.
2. Eat foods low in cholesterol and saturated fat.

3. Maintain a healthy weight.
4. Exercise regularly.
5. Follow your healthcare professional's advice.

Trans fats

Trans fats are produced when liquid oil is made into a solid fat. This process is called hydrogenation. Trans fats act like saturated fats and can raise your cholesterol level. Trans fats are listed on the label, making it easier to identify these foods. Unless there is at least 0.5 grams or more of trans fat in a food, the label can claim 0 grams. If you want to avoid as much trans fat as possible, you must read the ingredient list on food labels. Look for words like hydrogenated oil or partially hydrogenated oil. Select foods that either does not contain hydrogenated oil or where liquid oil is listed first in the ingredient list. Sources of trans fat include:

1. Processed foods like snacks (crackers and chips) and baked goods (muffins, cookies and cakes) with hydrogenated oil or partially hydrogenated oil.
2. Stick margarines.
3. Shortening.
4. Some fast food items such as French fries.

Why do we need fats?

Although fats have received a bad reputation for causing weight gain but still some fat is essential for survival. According to the Dietary Reference Intakes published by the USDA 20–35 per cent of calories should come from fat. We need this amount of fat for:

1. Body to use vitamins: Vitamins A, D, E, and K are fat-soluble vitamins, meaning that the fat in foods helps the intestines absorb these vitamins into the body.
2. Brains development: Fat provides the structural components not only of cell membranes in the brain, but also of myelin, the fatty insulating sheath that surrounds each nerve fibre, enabling it to carry messages faster.
3. Energy: Gram for gram fats is the most efficient source of food energy. Each gram of fat provides nine calories of energy for the body, compared with four calories per gram of carbohydrates and proteins.
4. Healthier skin: One of the more obvious signs of fatty acid deficiency is dry, flaky skin. In addition to giving skin its rounded appeal, the layer of fat just beneath the skin acts as the body's own insulation to help regulate body temperature.
5. Healthy cells: Fats are a vital part of the membrane that surrounds each cell of the body. Without a healthy cell membrane, the rest of the cell couldn't function.
6. Making hormones: Fats are structural components of some of the most important substances in the body, including prostaglandins, hormone-like substances that regulate many of the body's functions. Fats regulate the production of sex hormones, which explains why some teenage girls who are too lean experience delayed pubertal development and amenorrhea.
7. Pleasure: Besides being a nutritious energy source, fat adds to the appealing taste, texture and appearance of food. Fats carry flavour.
8. Protective cushion for our organs: Many of the vital organs, especially the kidneys, heart, and intestines are cushioned by fat that helps protect them from injury and hold them in place.

Rancidity

Fats are added directly to many products such as crackers, cookies, and cake because of their shortening power; they are added to other products in the form of such ingredients as nut meats, coconut, fatty seeds, milk, and cheese. Prevention of rancidity may become a problem in such baked goods as crackers, cookies, and fruit cake which may be stored for longer or shorter periods; in the cereal industry; in the confectionery industry; in dairy products; in the fat and oil industry; in salad dressings; and in storage of meats, particularly cured meats such as bacon and ham, and in stored frozen fresh meats. Meat, the fat of which contains more unsaturated glycerides, is subject to the development of rancidity more rapidly than fat containing greater percentages of saturated glycerides. Thus frozen poultry and pork present more problems when stored for long periods than beef and mutton.

Types of fat spoilage

The chemical change that needs to occur in a fat before taint is detectable organoleptically is very small. Davies states that butyric and capric acids are detectable by smell and taste in concentrations of less than 80 parts per million parts of fat. Changes in fats can be detected by smell and taste before they can be detected by chemical tests. An isolated fat possessing excellent keeping qualities may show deterioration rapidly after it is combined with other ingredients, and vice versa; but, in general, the fresher the fat and the better its keeping quality, the better the keeping quality of the product with which it is combined.

Different types of spoilage may occur in fats. Davies says 'mustiness' is due to micro-organic breakdown of higher fatty acids and is accelerated by moisture. Mustiness is common in cereal products, particularly maize. Davies states it is accompanied by an increase in acidity of water extracts, matting of the product because of mould growth, and local spontaneous heating. It is prevented by keeping the humidity sufficiently low.

'Fishiness', according to Davies, is due to the production of trimethylamine in the presence of catalysts from lecithin, before the auto-oxidation of the fat proper. Fishiness occurs most commonly in butter. The presence or absence of other products can alter the fishy odour. The term rancidity is used by the homemaker to designate the development of any disagreeable odour and flavour in fats and oils. But in the fat and oil industry the term is often restricted to the oxidative changes in fats and oils. Different investigators classify the disagreeable odours and flavours according to their production in different ways. Davies gives three types of rancidity as follows: (i) acid, (ii) oxidative, and (iii) ketonic. Triebold's classification is: (i) hydrolytic, (ii) oxidative, and (iii) ketonic.

Hydrolytic rancidity

Hydrolytic or the acid rancidity of Davies is brought about by the action of lipase enzymes which by hydrolysis split the fat into glycerol and fatty acids. Davies adds that free fatty acids may also be liberated by a relatively high hydrogen-ion concentration in contact with the fat. Lipases are associated with fats in their natural state, i.e. nuts, seeds, milk, and fat of meat. Since lipase enzymes are destroyed by heat, this type of rancidity is encountered in products which are not heated to a high enough temperature to destroy the enzyme. The flavours developed by lipase action depend upon the composition of the fat. Thus flavours caused by butyric acid will be found only in products containing butter fat. Davies states that lipase activity in itself is of no great economic importance, except in the fats rich in the lower fatty acids, but secondary reactions associated with oleic acid introduce another aspect. The free fatty acids act as catalysts for oxidative changes. Greenbank says that lard with a low free fatty acid content keeps well, even when stored for long periods, and butter from sweet cream does not become rancid as rapidly as butter from sour cream. The better-keeping quality of the sweet-cream butter is attributed to its lower free fatty acid content.

Chemical and physical changes in fats with development of oxidative rancidity. Among the changes which occur when a fat or oil becomes rancid are the following: the iodine value decreases, whereas the specific gravity, acid value, and peroxide value increase. Smith states that numerous investigations have shown that when an oil or fat is protected from light by means of a green wrapper or container it may have a peroxide value equal to or even greater than an unprotected fat that has become rancid and still be organoleptically free from rancidity. From this Smith concludes that the reaction that gives rise to the rancid taste and odour has no connection with formation of peroxides.

Oxidative rancidity

Oxidative rancidity occurs through the taking up of oxygen at the double bonds of the unsaturated glycerides. Many oxidative decomposition products may be formed, though Kerr states the exact nature of these changes is not always clear. These products include aldehydes, ketones, fatty acids of lower molecular weight, hydroxy acids, oxy acids, and gases. Andrews has reported that among the gaseous decomposition products of rancid fats are carbon dioxide, carbon monoxide, hydrogen, nitrogen, oxygen, and other gases. Triebold gives a good summary of the products formed in development of rancidity.

Induction period

There is a period before the uptake of oxygen by a fat becomes appreciable which is known as the induction period. During this period the fat is still fresh and 'sweet'. The induction period varies for different fats and oils and for different samples of the same fat or oil. But oxidation products act as catalysts so that oxygen uptake receives increased momentum as these products are formed. Reports in the literature indicate that the first compounds formed in oxidation of unsaturated fatty acids are not oxides or peroxides. These compounds have never been isolated and have been given the name 'moloxides'. Exclusion of air or oxygen from a fat may retard but not inhibit its oxidation. It has been suggested that the source of this oxygen is oxygen in loose combination with the fat. It is sometimes suggested that loosely bound oxygen is the source of oxygen for the moloxides.

Salad Dressing Characteristics

A salad dressing is an 'oil in water' emulsion, where oil is the discontinuous phase and water is the continuous phase. Salad dressing is defined by the FDA as a semisolid emulsified food with the same ingredients and optional ingredients as mayonnaise with the exception of the inclusion of a cooked or partially cooked starch paste. The typical ingredients of salad dressing are acetic acid, salt, sugar, water and vegetable oil. There are two types of salad dressing, pourable and spoonable.

The original spoonable dressing was mayonnaise, which must contain at least 75 per cent oil. These two types of salad dressings vary in flavour, chemical and physical properties (especially viscosity). The pourable dressing may either be sold in a homogeneous phase or in two phases. The two-phase salad dressings are separated by water and oil and will require shaking prior to use. The typical pH of these products ranges from 3.5 to 3.9. However, 'spoonable' salad dressings contain less acid than the pourable salad dressings, causing less microbial stability. The primary preservatives used to control microbial spoilage are sodium benzoate and/or potassium sorbate. Refrigerating the spoonable salad dressing will also help control microbial contamination. Aseptic processing and packaging also play a major role in the prevention of contamination. However, in most salad dressings, microbial spoilage is not a major issue.

The production of a salad dressing requires the use of a colloid mill or a homogeniser (low fat dressings). The colloid mill uses the shear and turbulence of liquid passing between two surfaces that are closely spaced, to mix the ingredients. A colloid mill is used to mix high viscous materials, while a pressure homogeniser is used to mix lower viscous materials. The ingredients of the fluid are thoroughly mixed by a homogeniser when it passes through an orifice at high pressures and speeds.

In the production of standard salad dressing, the vinegar, salt, starch and water are heated to approximately 90°C. Once a starch paste has formed, this mixture is cooled and then eggs, sugar, spices and oil are added. This mixture is then passed through the colloid mill prior to packaging.

Formulations for pourable dressings of different fat contents

Pourable dressings have less oil than spoonable dressings and generally contain xanthan gum as a replacement for oil in Mayonnaise and starch in salad dressing. Table 16.1 shows some typical formulations.

Table 16.1. Some typical formulations of salad dressing.

Ingredient	40% fat pourable dressing	30% fat pourable dressing	20% fat pourable dressing
Oil (%)	40	30	20
Water (%)	35.2	45.2	55.2
Vinegar (%)	8	10	10
Sugar (%)	10	10	10
Salt (%)	2	2	2
Xanthan gum (%)	0.3	0.3	0.3
Egg yolk solids (%)	4.5	4.5	4.5

Spices are added to taste depending on the type of dressing.

Microbiological spoilage of mayonnaise and salad dressing

Spoilage in mayonnaise and salad dressings results from a variety of causes including separation of the emulsion, oxidation and hydrolysis of the oils by chemical or biological action, and growth of micro-organisms that produce gas or off-flavours.

Microbiological spoilage of these products is generally caused by yeasts and bacteria. Williams and Mrak reported gassy spoilage of a starch-based salad dressing to be caused by a yeast similar to *Zygosaccharomyces globiformis*. Fabian and Wethington found samples of salad dressing and French dressing to be spoiled by an unidentified species of *Zygosaccharomyces*.

Similarly, Appleman observed large numbers of an unidentified species of *Saccharomyces* in spoiled mayonnaise but also found *Bacillus subtilis* to be abundant. Pederson reported *B. vulgatus* to be responsible for spoilage in a Thousand Island dressing. The work of Charlton appears to be the first report of salad dressing spoiled by lactobacilli. The species involved was considered new and described as *Lactobacillus fructivorans*.

The question of survival of pathogenic bacteria in mayonnaise and salad dressings has previously been investigated, and the studies indicate that the products themselves generally represent no health hazard because of survival or multiplication of pathogenic bacteria.

SPICES AND OTHER CONDIMENTS

A spice is a dried seed, fruit, root, bark or vegetative substance used in nutritionally insignificant quantities as a food additive for flavour, colour, or as a preservative that kills harmful bacteria or prevents their growth. Flavouring may be to hide other flavours. In the kitchen, spices are distinguished from herbs, which are leafy, green plant parts used for flavouring.

Many spices are used for other purposes, such as medicine, religious rituals, cosmetics, perfumery or for eating as vegetables. For example, turmeric is also used as a preservative; liquorice as a medicine; garlic as a vegetable.

Salt

Salt, also known as table salt, or rock salt, is a mineral that is composed primarily of sodium chloride. It is essential for animal life in small quantities, but is harmful to animals and plants in excess. Salt is one of the oldest, most ubiquitous food seasonings and salting is an important method of food preservation. The taste of salt (saltiness) is one of the basic human tastes. Salt for human consumption is produced in different forms: unrefined salt (such as sea salt), refined salt (table salt), and iodised salt. It is a crystalline solid, white, pale pink or light gray in colour, normally obtained from seawater or rock deposits. Edible rock salts may be slightly greyish in colour because of mineral content.

Chloride and sodium ions, the two major components of salt, are needed by all known living creatures in small quantities. Salt is involved in regulating the water content (fluid balance) of the body. The sodium ion itself is used for electrical signalling in the nervous system. However, too much salt increases the risk of health problems, including high blood pressure. Therefore health authorities have recommended limitations of dietary sodium.

Antimicrobial Effects of Spices and Herbs

Spices and herbs have been used for thousands of centuries by many cultures to enhance the flavour and aroma of foods. Early cultures also recognised the value of using spices and herbs in preserving foods and for their medicinal value. Scientific experiments since the late 19th century have documented the antimicrobial properties of some spices, herbs, and their components.

Antimicrobial effectiveness of spices and herbs

Table 16.2 describes the relative antimicrobial effectiveness of some spices and herbs.

Table 16.2. Antimicrobial effectiveness of spices and herbs.

Spices and herbs	*Inhibitory effect*
Cinnamon, cloves, mustard	Strong
Allspice, bay leaf, caraway, coriander, cumin, oregano, rosemary, sage, thyme	Medium
Black pepper, red pepper, ginger	Weak

Studies in the past decade confirm that the growth of both gram-positive and gram-negative foodborne bacteria, yeast and mould can be inhibited by garlic, onion, cinnamon, cloves, thyme, sage, and other spices. Effects of the presence of these spices/herbs can be seen in food products such as pickles, bread, rice, and meat products. The fat, protein, water, and salt contents of food influence microbial resistance. Thus, it is observed that higher levels of spices are necessary to inhibit growth in food than in culture media. Table 16.3 is a list of various spices and herbs and their inhibitory effect on various micro-organisms.

Table 16.3. Inhibitory effects of spices and herbs.

Spice/Herb	Micro-organisms
Garlic	*Salmonella typhymurium, Escherichia coli, Staphylococcus aureus, Bacillus cereus, Bacillus subtilis,* mycotoxigenic *Aspergillus, Candida albicans*
Onion	*Aspergillus flavis, Aspergillus parasiticus*
Cinnamon	Mycotoxigenic *Aspergillus, Aspergillus parasiticus*
Cloves	Mycotoxigenic *Aspergillus*
Mustard	Mycotoxigenic *Aspergillus*
Allspice	Mycotoxigenic *Aspergillus*
Oregano	Mycotoxigenic *Aspergillus, Salmonella* spp., *Vibrio parahaemolyticus*
Rosemary	*Bacillus cereus, Staphylococcus aureus, Vibrio parahaemolyticus*
Bay leaf	*Clostridium botulinum*
Sage	*Bacillus cereus, Staphylococcus aureus, Vibrio parahaemolyticus*
Thyme	*Vibrio parahaemolyticus*

Microbial contamination of spices

Spices and herbs may be contaminated because of conditions in which they were grown and harvested. Spores of both *Clostridium perfringens* and *Bacillus cereus* have been found to be present in spices and herbs. Contaminated spices have been reported to have been causes of foodborne illness and spoilage. Fewer micro-organisms are present in spices with higher antimicrobial activity such as sage, cloves, and oregano. However, all spices and herbs should be cleaned and decontaminated with ethylene oxide, irradiation or other acceptable methods.

Antimicrobial compounds in spices and herbs

Essential oils extracted from spices and herbs are generally recognised as containing the active antimicrobial compounds. Table 16.4 is a list of the proximate essential oil content of some spices and herbs and their antimicrobial components.

Table 16.4. Antimicrobial components of spices and herbs.

Spice/Herb	Proximate essential oil content (%)	Antimicrobial component(s)
Garlic	0.3–0.5	Allicin
Mustard	0.5–1.0	Allyl isothiocyanate
Cinnamon	0.5–2.0	Cinnamaldehyde, eugenol
Cloves	16–18	Eugenol
Sage	0.7–2.0	Thymol, eugenol
Oregano	0.8–0.9	Thymol, carvacrol

Allicin and allyl isothiocyanate are sulphur-containing compounds. Allicin, isolated from garlic oil, inhibits the growth of both gram-negative and gram-positive bacteria. Sulphur-containing compounds are also present in onions, leeks, and chives.

Eugenol, carvacrol, and thymol are phenol compounds and, as Table 16.4 indicates, are found in cinnamon, cloves, sage, and oregano. The essential oil fraction is particularly high in cloves, and eugenol comprises 95 per cent of the fraction. The presence of these compounds in cinnamon and cloves, when added to bakery items, function as mould inhibitors in addition to adding flavour and aroma to baked products. Paster have shown that essential oils of oregano and thyme (which contain carvacrol and thymol) are effective as fumigants against fungi on stored grain. These investigators have proposed using them as an alternative to chemicals for preserving stored grains.

Antioxidant action

Spice extractives, such as oleoresin of rosemary, can provide inhibition of oxidative rancidity and retard the development of 'warmed-over' flavour in some products. Thus, some spices not only provide flavour and aroma to food and retard microbial growth, but are also beneficial in prevention of some off-flavour development. These attributes are useful in the development of snack foods and meat products.

Summary: Although the antimicrobial activity of some spices and herbs is documented, the normal amounts added to foods for flavour is not sufficient to completely inhibit microbial growth. The antimicrobial activity varies widely, depending on the type of spice or herb, test medium, and micro-organism. For these reasons, spice antimicrobials should not be considered as a primary preservative method. However, the addition of herbs and spices can be expected to aid in preserving foods held at refrigeration temperatures, at which the multiplication of micro-organisms is slow.

Zaika has given an excellent summary of the antimicrobial effectiveness of spices and herbs. A partial listing of this summary is as follows:

1. Micro-organisms differ in their resistance to a given spice or herb.
2. A given micro-organism differs in its resistance to various spices and herbs.
3. Bacteria are more resistant than fungi.
4. The effect on spores may be different than that on vegetative cells.
5. Gram-negative bacteria are more resistant than gram-positive bacteria.
6. The effect of a spice or herb may be inhibitory or germicidal.
7. Spices and herbs harbour microbial contaminants.
8. Spices and herbs may serve as substrates for microbial growth and toxin production.
9. Amounts of spices and herbs added to foods are generally too low to prevent spoilage by micro-organisms.
10. Active components of spices/herbs at low concentrations may interact synergistically with other factors (NaCl, acids, preservatives) to increase preservative effect.
11. Nutrients present in spices/herbs may stimulate growth and/or biochemical activities of micro-organisms.

Thus, food product safety and shelf-life depend in some part on the type, quantity, and character of spices and herbs added to the products.

SECTION IV

Food and Enzymes Produced by Micro-organisms

Chapter 17

Production of Cultures for Food Fermentations

INTRODUCTION

In simple terms, an organism is cultured or grown under conditions which are typically controlled. Microbiologists utilise a growth medium (generally an agar) which supplies nutrients and moisture for the organism. Numerous types of media are available and some may include added compounds to enhance growth or suppress competing organisms. In most cases the growth media is placed in a petri-dish to contain and protect the specimen.

Special media-coated strips inside of tubes are also commercially available. Once transferred to the media, the organism is allowed to grow and then observed both macroscopically and microscopically. Since the microbiologist can see what the organism looks like undisturbed, a more accurate identification is possible.

In some instances, the quantity of colonies formed on the culture plate relative to the size of the field specimen are reported. In these cases, microbiologists report 'Colony Forming Units' per unit of measure of the field specimen (i.e. cubic meters of air, square centimetres, grams, etc.). Quantified results are, therefore, listed as CFU/m^3; CFU/cm^2; CFU/g, etc.

TYPICAL VARIABLES OF CULTURING

The following variables highlight some of the issues encountered when growth of the organisms on culture plates under laboratory conditions are compared to conditions of the environment from which the specimen was obtained:

1. Contamination: Contamination of the media during field use can result in a false positive and generally requires additional specimens (control blanks) to be submitted to the laboratory.
2. Spore viability: The viability of mould spores is dependent on many factors; especially when considering field environmental conditions. Since nonviable spores will not grow on the media, the results are subject to significant false negatives (remember, nonviable spores still retain their adverse health properties and may outnumber the viable types on many projects).
3. Media compatibility: Fungi grow best on media that provides optimum nutrition which can vary by species (some species grow well on one type of media, but poorly on others). In addition, the media's water activity and pH also impact growth. During preliminary assessments, multiple genera are usually present and it is often important to identify all of them. Since there is no 'perfect' media for all types of mould, multiple types of media are typically required.

4. Competition: Competition exists at the micro-organism level and some fungi may overgrow or inhibit competing species. In addition, many fungal organisms are susceptible to infestation by mites which can completely strip a colony from the culture plate.

5. Temperature: Temperature impacts a number of species of fungi and temperature conditions in the field environment are seldom static. Since laboratories typically incubate culture specimens at a specific temperature, the resulting growth may not accurately reflect field conditions.

6. Light: Many species of fungi grow well in the dark, others tolerate daylight, and some sporulate best under cycles of light including near ultraviolet. The light/dark conditions used by the laboratory can have an impact on field-comparative growth.

7. Time: Some types of fungi grow faster than others; therefore, the duration of culture must be sufficient to identify all types present.

8. Handling: Most laboratories will emphasise the importance of temperature control and expedited shipping when dealing with specimens on culture media to avoid exposing the specimen to unknown conditions that may dramatically influence growth results.

Culture-based testing can provide specific information concerning fungal organisms, however, its use in obtaining the best overall view of conditions is severely limited due to the introduction of numerous variables leading to false negative and false positive results.

Micro-organisms necessary in food fermentation may be added as pure cultures or mixed cultures or in some instances, no cultures may be added if the desired micro-organisms are known to be present in sufficient numbers in the original raw material. In the food fermentations for the manufacture of sauerkraut, fermented pickles, and green olives and in the processing of cocoa, coffee, poi, and citron, the original raw product carries enough of the desired organisms, which will act in proper succession if favourable environmental conditions are provided and maintained. Therefore, the addition of pure or mixed cultures of the organisms responsible for the fermentations has not been found necessary, although in some of the fermentations, e.g. pickles and green olives, it is advantageous. On the other hand, controlled 'starter' cultures, pure or mixed, usually are employed in the manufacture of certain dairy products, such as fermented milks, some kinds of butter, and most types of cheese, and in most of the other food fermentations, e.g. bread, malt beverages, wines, distilled liquors, and vinegar.

GENERAL PRINCIPLES OF CULTURE MAINTENANCE AND PREPARATION

Selection of Cultures

Cultures for food fermentations are selected primarily on the basis of their stability and their ability to produce desired products or changes efficiently. These cultures may be established ones obtained from other laboratories or may be selected after the testing of numerous strains. Stability is an important characteristic; yields and rates of changes must not be erratic. Some cultures may be improved by breeding, e.g. the sporogenous yeasts, but selection is the most commonly used method for the improvement of strains. Selection of cultures with desirable traits can be made from new strains isolated from the environment, from existing strains or following mutation of strains by various means.

Refinement of plasmid transfer systems in the lactic acid bacteria will allow for gene cloning or gene amplification of a highly desirable trait such as lactic acid production. Since the gene responsible for lactese fermentation in some lactic streptococci is located on plasmids, the trait can be easily lost. Stabilising these industrially important traits has been demonstrated to be possible. McKay and coworkers have cloned the *lac*$^+$ genes of *S. lactis* and incorporated them into *S. sanguis*. The *lac*$^+$ genes, via a vector plasmid and transformation, were integrated into the chromosome of the host cell. As an integrated part of the chromosome, the lac^+ gene is much more stable than it is when it is plasmid-borne.

Maintenance of Activity of Cultures

Once a satisfactory culture has been obtained, it must be kept pure and active. Usually this objective is attained by periodic transfer of the culture into the proper culture medium, incubation until the culture reaches the maximal stationary phase of growth, and then storage at temperatures low enough to prevent further growth. Too frequent transfer of an unstable culture may lead to undesirable changes in its characteristics.

Stock cultures should be prepared for storage of cultures over long periods without transfer. Such cultures tend to remain stable and serve as a source of culture if the active culture deteriorates or is lost. Lyophilisation (freeze drying) and freezing in liquid nitrogen (–196°C) are now frequently used to prepare stock cultures, although some use still is made of a paraffin-oil seal over ordinary tube cultures. Bacterial cultures have been preserved for months to years at room temperature on slants of agar in which 1 per cent NaCl had been incorporated. A dry spore stock on sterilised soil can be used to preserve spores of bacteria or moulds for long periods.

Maintenance of Purity of Cultures

To ensure the purity of cultures, they should be obtained periodically from a culture laboratory or be checked regularly for purity. Methods for testing a culture for purity vary with the type of culture being tested. Microscopic examination will indicate contamination only if the contaminant differs from the desired organism in appearance and is high in numbers. Another method is to plate the culture with an agar medium that will grow contaminants but not the desired organism. Tests may be made for the presence of substances not produced by the desired organism, e.g. for catalase in a culture of catalase-negative lactic acid bacteria as indicative of the presence of catalase-positive contaminants.

Preparation of Cultures

Mother culture is usually prepared daily from a previous mother culture and originally from the stock culture. These mother cultures can be used to inoculate a larger quantity of culture medium to produce the mass or bulk culture to be used in the fermentation process. Often, however, the fermentation is on such a large scale that several intermediate cultures of increasing size must be built up between the mother culture and the final bulk or mass culture. Culture makers attempt to produce and maintain a culture that (i) contains only the desired micro-organism(s), (ii) is uniform in microbial numbers, proportions (if a mixed culture), and activity from day-to-day, (iii) is active in producing the products desired, and (iv) has adequate resistance to unfavourable conditions if necessary, e.g. heat resistance, if it has to take heating in a cheese curd. They try to maintain uniformity by standardising methods of preparation and sterilisation of the culture medium, inoculation, and incubation temperature and time. The stage of growth to which they will grow the culture depends on the purpose for which it is to be used. If they wish prompt and rapid growth, they use a culture that is late in its logarithmic phase of growth. If they want more resistance to heat or other unfavourable conditions, they use a culture that has just entered the maximal stationary phase. The temperature of incubation usually is somewhere near the optimal temperature for the organism, although there are exceptions. Temperature and time of incubation often are adjusted so that the culture will be ready at the time it is needed. Otherwise, it may have to be cooled to stop further development.

Activity of Culture

The activity of a culture is judged by its rate of growth and production of products. It should be good if the mother or the intermediate culture is satisfactory and culture medium, incubation time, and temperature are optimal. Deterioration of cultures may result from improper handling and cultivation, frequent transfer over long periods in an inadequate culture medium, selection, variation or mutation, or attack of bacteria by a bacteriophage.

Mixed Cultures

Known mixtures of pure cultures sometimes are prepared, being grown together continuously or grown separately and mixed at the time of use. The so-called butter or lactic, culture used in the dairy industry is an example of a mixture of several species of bacteria growing together and sometimes several strains of individual species. When different strains of the same species or different species are grown together, these organisms must be compatible, i.e. grow well together without causing the elimination of others. The maintenance of the desired balance of kinds of organisms within these mixed cultures is difficult. Unknown mixtures of organisms are present in starters used in some food products. Examples are the dough carried over from one lot of special French bread to a succeeding lot and the mixture of yeasts and bacteria carried from the surface smear of one Limburger cheese to the surface of another.

MICROBIOLOGICAL CULTURE

A microbiological culture or microbial culture, is a method of multiplying microbial organisms by letting them reproduce in predetermined culture media under controlled laboratory conditions. Microbial cultures are used to determine the type of organism, its abundance in the sample being tested, or both. It is one of the primary diagnostic methods of microbiology and used as a tool to determine the cause of infectious disease by letting the agent multiply in a predetermined medium. For example, a throat culture is taken by scraping the lining of tissue in the back of the throat and blotting the sample into a medium to be able to screen for harmful micro-organisms, such as *Streptococcus pyogenes*, the causative agent of strep throat. Furthermore, the term culture is more generally used informally to refer to 'selectively growing' a specific kind of micro-organism in the laboratory.

Microbial cultures are foundational and basic diagnostic methods used extensively as a research tool in molecular biology. It is often essential to isolate a pure culture of micro-organisms. A pure (or *axenic*) culture is a population of cells or multicellular organisms growing in the absence of other species or types. A pure culture may originate from a single cell or single organism, in which case the cells are genetic clones of one another.

For the purpose of gelling the microbial culture, the medium of agarose gel (agar) is used. Agar is a gelatinous substance derived from seaweed. A cheap substitute for agar is guar gum, which can be used for the isolation and maintenance of thermophiles.

Bacterial culture: Microbiological cultures use petri dishes of differing sizes that have a thin layer of agar-based growth medium in them. Once the growth medium in the petri dish is inoculated with the desired bacteria, the plates are incubated in an incubator (usually set at 37°C for cultures from humans or animals, or lower for environmental cultures). Another method of bacterial culture is liquid culture, in which the desired bacteria are suspended in liquid broth, a nutrient medium. These are ideal for preparation of an antimicrobial assay. The experimenter would inoculate liquid broth with bacteria and let it grow overnight in a shaker for uniform growth, then take aliquots of the sample to test for the antimicrobial activity of a specific drug or protein (antimicrobial peptides).

Virus and phage culture: Virus or phage cultures require host cells in which the virus or phage multiply. For bacteriophages, cultures are grown by infecting bacterial cells. The phage can then be isolated from the resulting plaques in a lawn of bacteria on a plate. Virus cultures are obtained from their appropriate eukaryotic host cells.

Lactic Acid Bacteria

The lactic acid bacteria (LAB) comprise a clade of Gram-positive, low-GC, acid-tolerant, generally non-sporulating, nonrespiring rod or cocci that are associated by their common metabolic and physiological characteristics. These bacteria, usually found in decomposing plants and lactic products, produce lactic acid as the major metabolic end-product of carbohydrate fermentation. This trait has, throughout history, linked LAB with food fermentations, as acidification inhibits the growth of spoilage agents. Proteinaceous bacteriocins are produced by several LAB strains and provide an additional hurdle for spoilage and pathogenic micro-organisms.

Furthermore, lactic acid and other metabolic products contribute to the organoleptic and textural profile of a food item. The industrial importance of the LAB is further evinced by their generally recognised as safe (GRAS) status, due to their ubiquitous appearance in food and their contribution to the healthy microflora of human mucosal surfaces. The genera that comprise the LAB are at its core *Lactobacillus, Leuconostoc, Pediococcus, Lactococcus*, and *Streptococcus* as well as the more peripheral *Aerococcus, Carnobacterium, Enterococcus, Oenococcus, Sporolactobacillus, Tetragenococcus, Vagococcus*, and *Weisella*; these belong to the order *Lactobacillales*.

The lactic acid bacteria (LAB) are rod-shaped bacilli or coccus. LAB are characterised by an increased tolerance to a lower pH range. This aspect partially enables LAB to outcompete other bacteria in a natural fermentation, as they can withstand the increased acidity from organic acid production (e.g. lactic acid). Laboratory media used for LAB typically includes a carbohydrate source as most species are incapable of respiration. LAB are catalase negative. LAB are amongst the most important groups of micro-organisms used in the food industry.

There are two main hexose fermentation pathways that are used to classify LAB genera. Under conditions of excess glucose and limited oxygen, homolactic LAB catabolise one mole of glucose in the Embden-Meyerhof-Parnas (EMP) pathway to yield two moles of pyruvate. Intracellular redox balance is maintained through the oxidation of NADH, concomitant with pyruvate reduction to lactic acid. This process yields two moles ATP per glucose consumed. Representative homolactic LAB genera include *Lactococcus, Enterococcus, Streptococcus, Pediococcus*, and group I *lactobacilli*.

Heterofermentative LAB use the pentose phosphate pathway, alternatively referred to as the pentose phosphoketolase pathway. One mole Glucose-6-phosphate is initially dehydrogenated to 6-phospho-gluconate and subsequently decarboxylated to yield one mole of CO_2. The resulting pentose-5-phosphate is cleaved into one mole glyceraldehyde phosphate (GAP) and one mole acetyl phosphate. GAP is further metabolised to lactate as in homofermentation, with the acetyl phosphate reduced to ethanol via acetyl-CoA and acetaldehyde intermediates. In theory, end-products (including ATP) are produced in equimolar quantities from the catabolism of one mole of glucose. Obligate heterofermentative LAB include *Leuconostoc, Oenococcus, Weissella*, and group III *lactobacilli*.

Propionic Culture

Spray-dried or lyophilised cultures of *Propionibacterium freudenreichii* are added to milk used in the manufacture of Swiss cheese to improve the flavour and assist eye formation.

Cheese Smear Organisms

Most cheese makers inoculate the surfaces of smear-ripened cheese from previous cheeses, shelves, cloths, brine tank, hands, and other sources in the plant. The micrococci, *Brevibacterium linens*, and film yeasts important in the smear have been isolated and used in pure or mixed cultures to wash cheese surfaces, thereby inoculating them.

Acetic Acid Bacteria

For most of human history, acetic acid, in the form of vinegar, has been made by acetic acid bacteria of the genus *Acetobacter*. Given sufficient oxygen, these bacteria can produce vinegar from a variety of alcoholic foodstuffs. Commonly used feeds include apple cider, wine, and fermented grain, malt, rice, or potato mashes. The overall chemical reaction facilitated by these bacteria is:

1. A high concentration of acetic acid in wine is a strong indication that the grapes have been contaminated. The culprit of contamination is usually acetic acid or lactic acid bacteria. Winemakers and viticulturalists will pay the utmost attention to make sure that this does not occur.

2. Dilute solutions of acetic acids are used for their mild acidity. Examples in the household environment include the use in a stop bath during the development of photographic films, and in descaling agents to remove limescale from taps and kettles. The acidity is also used for treating the sting of the box jellyfish by disabling the stinging cells of the jellyfish, preventing serious injury or death if applied immediately, and for treating outer ear infections in people in preparations such as Vosol. Equivalently, acetic acid is used as a spray-on preservative for livestock silage, to discourage bacterial and fungal growth. Glacial acetic acid is also used as a wart and verruca remover.

YEAST

Yeasts are eukaryotic micro-organisms classified in the kingdom Fungi, with the 1500 species currently described estimated to be only 1 per cent of all yeast species. Most reproduce asexually by budding, although a few do so by mitosis. Yeasts are unicellular, although some species with yeast forms may become multicellular through the formation of a string of connected budding cells known as pseudohyphae or false hyphae, as seen in most moulds. Yeast size can vary greatly depending on the species, typically measuring 3–4 μm in diameter, although some yeasts can reach over 40 μm.

The yeast species *Saccharomyces cerevisiae* has been used in baking and in fermenting alcoholic beverages for thousands of years. It is also extremely important as a model organism in modern cell biology research, and is one of the most thoroughly researched eukaryotic micro-organisms. Researchers have used it to gather information about the biology of the eukaryotic cell and ultimately human biology. Other species of yeast, such as *Candida albicans*, are opportunistic pathogens and can cause infections in humans. These infections can range from very mild to very severe in individuals. Yeasts have recently been used to generate electricity in microbial fuel cells, and produce ethanol for the biofuel industry.

Baker's Yeast

Baker's yeast is the common name for the strains of yeast commonly used as a leavening agent in baking bread and bakery products, where it converts the fermentable sugars present in the dough into carbon dioxide and ethanol. Baker's yeast is almost always of the species *Saccharomyces cerevisiae*, which is the same species commonly used in alcoholic fermentation, and so is also called brewer's yeast.

The use of steamed or boiled potatoes, water from potato boiling or sugar in a bread dough provides food for the growth of yeasts, however, too much sugar will dehydrate them. Yeast is inhibited by both salt and sugar, but more so with salt than sugar. Fats such as butter or eggs slow down yeast growth, however others say the effect of fat on dough remains unclear, presenting evidence that small amounts of fat are beneficial for baked bread volume.

Saccharomyces exiguus (also known as *S. minor*) is a wild yeast found on plants, fruits, and grains that is occasionally used for baking; it is not, however, generally used in a pure form, but comes from being propagated in a sourdough starter.

Types of baker's yeast

Baker's yeast is available in a number of different forms, the main differences being the moisture contents. Though each version has certain advantages over the others, the choice of which form to use is largely a question of the requirements of the recipe at hand and the training of the cook preparing it. Dry yeast forms are good choices for longer-term storage, often lasting several months at room temperatures without significant loss of viability. With occasional allowances for liquid content and temperature, the different forms of commercial yeast are generally considered interchangeable.

1. Cream yeast is the closest form to the yeast slurries of the 19th century, being essentially a suspension of yeast cells in liquid, siphoned off from the growth medium. Its primary use is in industrial bakeries with special high-volume dispensing and mixing equipment, and it is not readily available to small bakeries or home cooks.

2. Compressed yeast is essentially cream yeast with most of the liquid removed. It is a soft solid, beige in colour, and arguably best known in the consumer form as small, foil-wrapped cubes of cake yeast. It is also available in larger-block form for bulk usage. It is highly perishable; though formerly widely available for the consumer market, it has become less common in supermarkets in some countries due to its poor keeping properties, having been superseded in some such markets by active dry and instant yeast. It is still widely available for commercial use, and is somewhat more tolerant of low temperatures than other forms of commercial yeast; however, even there, instant yeast has made significant market inroads.

3. Active dry yeast is the form of yeast most commonly available to noncommercial bakers in the United States. It consists of coarse oblong granules of yeast, with live yeast cells encapsulated in a thick jacket of dry, dead cells with some growth medium. Under most conditions, active dry yeast must first be proofed or rehydrated. It can be stored at room temperature for a year or frozen for more than a decade, which means that it has better keeping qualities than other forms, but it is generally considered more sensitive than other forms to thermal shock when actually used in recipes.

4. Instant yeast appears similar to active dry yeast, but has smaller granules with substantially higher percentages of live cells per comparable unit volumes. It is more perishable than active dry yeast, but also does not require rehydration, and can usually be added directly to all but the driest doughs. Instant yeast generally has a small amount of ascorbic acid added as a preservative. Some producers provide two or more forms of instant yeast in their product portfolio; for example, LeSaffre's 'SAF Instant Gold' is designed specifically for doughs with high sugar contents.

5. Rapid-rise yeast is a variety of dried yeast (usually a form of instant yeast) that is of a smaller granular size, thus it dissolves faster in dough, and it provides greater carbon dioxide output to allow faster rising. There is considerable debate as to the value of such a product; while most

baking experts believe it reduces the flavour potential of the finished product, Cook's Illustrated magazine, among others, feels that at least for direct-rise recipes, it makes little difference. Rapid-rise yeast is often marketed specifically for use in bread machines.

MOULD CULTURES

Stock cultures of moulds usually are carried on slants of suitable agar medium, e.g. malt-extract agar, and may be preserved in the spore state for long periods by lyophilisation (freeze drying) or as soil stocks. There are a number of different ways of preparing spore or mycelial cultures for use on a plant scale. These include: (i) surface growth on a liquid or agar medium in a flask or similar container, (ii) surface growth on media in shallow layers in trays, (iii) growth on loose, moistened wheat bran which may be acidified or may have liquid nutrient added, e.g. corn-steep liquor, (iv) growth on previously sterilised and moistened bread or crackers, and (v) growth by the submerged method in an aerated liquid medium, usually resulting in pellets composed of mycelium, with or without spores. The mould spores are recovered in different ways, depending on the method of production. They may be washed or drawn from dry surfaces, may be left in dry material that is ground up or powdered, or for convenience in use may be incorporated in some dry powder, e.g. flour. The pellets, of course, are used as such.

Penicillium roqueforti

Penicillium roqueforti is a common saprotrophic fungus from the family *Trichocomaceae*. Widespread in nature, it can be isolated from soil, decaying organic matter, and plants. The major industrial use of this fungus is the production of blue cheeses, flavouring agents, antifungals, polysaccharides, proteases and other enzymes. The fungus has been a constituent of Roquefort, Stilton, Danish blue and other blue cheeses eaten by humans since about 50 AD.

As this fungus does not form visible fruiting bodies, descriptions are based on macromorphological characteristics of fungal colonies growing on various standard agar media, and on microscopic characteristics. When grown on Czapek yeast autolysate (CYA) agar or yeast-extract sucrose (YES) agar, *P. roqueforti* colonies are typically 40 mm in diameter, olive brown to dull green (dark green to black on the reverse side of the agar plate), with a velutinous texture. Grown on malt extract (MEA) agar, colonies are 50 mm in diameter, dull green in colour (beige to greyish green on the reverse side), with arachnoid (with many spider-web-like fibres) colony margins.

Penicillium camemberti

Penicillium camemberti is a species of fungus used in the production of Camembert and Brie cheeses, on which colonies of *P. camemberti* form a hard, white crust. It is responsible for giving these cheeses their distinctive taste.

Aspergillus oryzae

Aspergillus oryzae is a filamentous fungus (a mould). It is used in Chinese and Japanese cuisine to ferment soyabeans. It is also used to saccharify rice, other grains, and potatoes in the making of alcoholic beverages such as *huangjiu*, *sake*, and *shōchū*. The domestication of *A. oryzae* occurred at least two thousand years ago. *A. oryzae* is used for the production of rice vinegars.

Chapter 18

Fermented and Microbial Foods

INTRODUCTION

Fermentation in food processing typically is the conversion of carbohydrates to alcohols and carbon dioxide or organic acids using yeasts, bacteria or a combination thereof, under anaerobic conditions. A more restricted definition of fermentation is the chemical conversion of sugars into ethanol. The science of fermentation is known as zymurgy.

Fermentation usually implies that the action of micro-organisms is desirable, and the process is used to produce alcoholic beverages such as wine, beer, and cider. Fermentation is also employed in the leavening of bread, and for preservation techniques to create lactic acid in sour foods such as sauerkraut, dry sausages, kimchi and yogurt or vinegar (acetic acid) for use in pickling foods.

YEAST BREAD INGREDIENTS

There are only four ingredients you need to make yeast bread: flour, yeast, water, and salt. All other ingredients are there to add flavour, nutrition, colour, and to change the characteristics of the crumb. Here's what yeast bread ingredients do.

Flour

Flour provides the structure for the product. The gluten or protein in flour, combines to form a web that traps air bubbles and sets. Starch in flour sets as it heats to add to and support the structure. In yeast breads, we want a lot of gluten formation, since it forms a stretchy web that traps carbon dioxide and steam during baking, to give bread its texture (also known as crumb). Fats and sugars help prevent gluten formation. There is some simple sugar available in flour, which feeds the yeast. So if you have a bread recipe with no sugar source, that's okay—the yeast will have enough to 'eat' from the flour. The rising times will just be longer.

Bread flour is high protein flour, and produces bread that has a higher volume because it contains more stretchy gluten. Loaves made with bread flour rest for 10–15 minutes after rising before shaping the loaves so the gluten relaxes a bit and the dough is easier to work. All-purpose flour works just fine for most breads.

Whole grain flours do not have as much gluten because there are other ingredients like the bran and germ which get between the gluten molecules. Whole grain flours are usually combined with bread or all-purpose flour to make a better crumb.

Fat

Fat coats gluten molecules so they can't combine as easily, contributing to the finished product's tenderness. Yeast breads that have a high proportion of fat to flour are much more tender, don't rise as high, and have a very tender mouth-feel. Fat also contributes flavour to the bread, and helps the bread brown while baking.

Sugar

Sugar adds sweetness, as well as contributing to the product's browning. The main role for sugar in yeast breads is to provide food for the yeast. As the yeast grows and multiplies, it uses the sugar, forming by-products of carbon dioxide and alcohol, which give bread its characteristic flavour. Sugar tenderises bread by preventing the gluten from forming. Sugar also holds moisture in the finished product.

Eggs

Eggs are a leavening agent and the yolks add fat for a tender and light texture. The yolks also act as an emulsifier for a smooth and even texture in the finished product. When lots of eggs are used, they contribute to the flavour of the finished product.

Liquid

Liquid helps carry flavourings throughout the product, forms gluten bonds, and reacts with the starch in the protein for a strong but light structure. Liquids also act as steam during baking, contributing to the tenderness of the product. Yeast needs liquid in order to develop, reproduce, multiply, and form by-products which make the bread rise.

Salt

Salt strengthens gluten, and adds flavour. Salt enhances flavours. In yeast breads, salt helps moderate the effect of the yeast so the bread doesn't rise too quickly.

Yeast

Yeast is a one-celled plant, available in dried form, instant blend, and live cakes. In yeast bread, yeast multiplies and grows by using available sugars and water, giving off carbon dioxide and ethyl alcohol (fermentation). As long as air is available, the yeast multiplies. In bread recipes where the bread rises for a second time, you are told to 'punch down' the dough. This breaks up small clusters or colonies of yeast cells so they can get in contact with more air and food, which is why the second rise is usually shorter than the first rise.

Sourdough breads depend on yeast and bacteria starter (mixture of flour, yeast, liquid, bacteria) to provide the special sour flavour. The bacteria lowers the pH of the bread mixture, which adds to the flavour. Since the bread is more acidic (lower pH), this bread keeps longer than ordinary yeast bread. You can make starter in your own kitchen without adding any yeast if you do a lot of yeast bread baking, because the yeast cells are present in your kitchen. If you are new to working with yeast, however, add yeast to your starter. And here's an interesting point: San Francisco Sourdough bread can only be made in San Francisco! Scientists discovered that the bacteria in the bread was original to the area, and a wild yeast native to San Francisco was the only type that would grow with the special bacteria. Mixes are now made in that city and shipped to other parts of the country so you can make San Francisco sourdough in your home, but that special bacteria and yeast will not grow in your home kitchen, as they do for ordinary sourdough starters.

Leavening Agent

A leavening agent is any one of a number of substances used in doughs and batters that cause a foaming action which lightens and softens the finished product. The leavening agent incorporates gas bubbles into the dough—this may be air incorporated by mechanical means, but usually it is carbon dioxide produced by biological agents, or by chemical agents reacting with moisture, heat, acidity or other triggers. When a dough or batter is mixed, the starch in the flour mixes with the water in the dough to form a matrix (often supported further by proteins like gluten or other polysaccharides like pentosans or xanthan gum), then gelatinises and 'sets'; the holes left by the gas bubbles remain.

Biological leaveners

Micro-organisms that release carbon dioxide as part of their life cycle can be used to leaven products. Varieties of yeast are most often used, particularly *Saccharomyces* species (such as baker's yeast, *Saccharomyces cerevisiae*), though some recipes also rely on certain bacteria. Yeast leaves behind waste by-products (particularly ethanol and some autolysis products) that contribute to the distinctive flavour of yeast breads. In the naturally leavened sourdough breads, the flavour is further enhanced by various lactic acid bacteria (*Lactobacilli*) or acetic acid bacteria (*Acetobacter*).

Leavening with yeast is a process based on fermentation, biologically changing the chemistry of the dough or batter as the yeast works. Unlike chemical leavening, which usually activates as soon as the water combines the acid and base chemicals, yeast leavening requires proofing, which allows the yeast time to reproduce and consume carbohydrates in the flour.

Yeast can also be used to make alcoholic beverages like beer or wine. The resulting cast-off yeast, known as barm, can be used as a leavener and was probably ancestral to the use of modern pure-cultured yeast. Non-European cultures have used other by-products of making alcoholic beverages as leaveners, as in Ecuador: 'In olden times when the sediment of chicha called *concho* was used as a ferment, we had good bread; and now with better mills good quality bread has disappeared entirely.'

While not as widely known, bacterial fermentation is sometimes used, occasionally providing a drastically changed flavour profile from a yeast fermentation; a well-known example is salt rising bread, which uses a culture of the *Clostridium perfringens* bacterium.

Some typical biological leaveners are:
1. Beer (unpasteurised—live yeast).
2. Buttermilk.
3. Hinger beer.
4. Kefir.
5. Sourdough starter.
6. Yeast.
7. Yogurt.

Chemical leaveners

Chemical leaveners are chemical mixtures or compounds that release gases (usually carbon dioxide) when they react with moisture and heat; they are almost always based on a combination of acid (usually a low molecular weight organic acid) and an alkali; these leave behind a chemical salt. Chemical leaveners are used in quick breads and cakes, as well as cookies and numerous other applications where a long biological fermentation is impractical or undesirable. Chemical leavening was first publicised by Amelia Simmons in her American Cookery, published in 1796, wherein she mentions the use of pearl ash as a leavening agent. Since chemical expertise is required to create a functional chemical leaven without leaving behind off-flavours from the chemical precursors involved, such substances are often mixed into premeasured combinations for maximum results. These are generally referred to as baking powders.

Chemical leavening agents include: (i) baking powder, (ii) baking soda (sodium bicarbonate), (iii) monocalcium phosphate, (iv) sodium aluminium phosphate (SALP), (v) sodium acid pyrophosphate (SAPP), (vi) other phosphates, (vii) ammonium bicarbonate (hartshorn, horn salt, bakers ammonia), (viii) potassium bicarbonate (potash), (ix) potassium bitartrate (cream of tartar), (x) potassium carbonate (pearlash), and (xi) hydrogen peroxide.

Leavening by Bread Yeast

Many breads are leavened by yeast. The yeast used for leavening bread is *Saccharomyces cerevisiae*, the same species used for brewing alcoholic beverages. This yeast ferments carbohydrates in the flour, including any sugar, producing carbon dioxide. Most bakers in the US leaven their dough with commercially produced baker's yeast. Baker's yeast has the advantage of producing uniform, quick, and reliable results, because it is obtained from a pure culture. Many artisan bakers produce their own yeast by preparing a 'growth culture' which they then use in the making of bread. When this culture is kept in the right conditions, it will continue to grow and provide leavening for many years.

Both the baker's yeast and the sourdough method of baking bread follow the same pattern. Water is mixed with flour, salt and the leavening agent (baker's yeast or sourdough starter). Other additions (spices, herbs, fats, seeds, fruit, etc.) are not needed to bake bread, but are often used. The mixed dough is then allowed to rise one or more times (a longer rising time results in more flavour, so baker's often punch down the dough and let it rise again), then loaves are formed, and (after an optional final rising time) the bread is baked in an oven.

Many breads are made from a straight dough, which means that all of the ingredients are combined in one step, and the dough is baked after the rising time. Alternatively, dough can be made using a preferment, when some of the flour, water, and the leavening are combined a day or so ahead of baking, and allowed to ferment overnight. On the day of the baking, the rest of the ingredients are added, and the rest of the process is the same as that for straight dough. This produces a more flavourful bread with better texture. Many bakers see the starter method as a compromise between the highly reliable results of baker's yeast, and the flavour/complexity of a longer fermentation. It also allows the baker to use only a minimal amount of baker's yeast, which was scarce and expensive when it first became available. Most yeasted preferments fall into one of three categories: *poolish* or *pouliche*, a loose-textured mixture composed of roughly equal amounts of flour and water (by weight); *biga*, a stiff mixture with a higher proportion of flour; and pâte fermentée, which is simply a portion of dough reserved from a previous batch. Sourdough (also known as *levain* or 'natural leaven') takes it a step further, creating a preferment with flour and water that propagates naturally occurring yeast and bacteria (usually *Saccharomyces exiguus*, which is more acid-tolerant than *S. cerevisiae*, and various species of *Lactobacillus*).

Sourdough

The sour taste of sourdoughs actually comes not from the yeast, but from a *Lactobacillus*, with which the yeast lives in symbiosis. The *Lactobacillus* feeds on the by-products of the yeast fermentation, and in turn makes the culture go sour by excreting lactic acid, which protects it from spoiling (since most microbes are unable to survive in an acid environment).

Sourdough breads are most often made with a sourdough starter (not to be confused with the starter method discussed above). A sourdough starter is a culture of yeast and lactobacillus. It is essentially a dough-like or pancake batter-like flour/water mixture in which the yeast and lactobacilli live. A starter can be maintained indefinitely by periodically discarding a part of it and refreshing it by adding fresh flour and water. (When refrigerated, a starter can last weeks without needing to be fed.) There are starters owned by bakeries and families that are several human generations old, much revered for creating a special taste or texture. Starters can be obtained by taking a piece of another starter and growing it, or they can be made from scratch. There are hobbyist groups on the web who will send their starter for a stamped, self-addressed envelope, and there are even mailorder companies that sell different starters from all over the world. An acquired starter has the advantage of being more proven and established (stable and reliable, resisting spoiling and behaving predictably) than from-scratch starters.

Steam

The rapid expansion of steam produced during baking leavens the bread, which is as simple as it is unpredictable. The best known steam-leavened bread is the popover. Steam-leavening is unpredictable since the steam is not produced until the bread is baked.

Steam leavening happens regardless of the rising agents (baking soda, yeast, baking powder, sour dough, beaten egg whites, etc.).

1. The leavening agent either contains air bubbles or generates carbon dioxide.
2. The heat vapourises the water from the inner surface of the bubbles within the dough.
3. The steam expands and makes the bread rise.

It is actually the main factor in the rise of bread once it has been put in the oven. CO_2 generation, on its own, is too small to account for the rise. Heat kills bacteria or yeast at an early stage, so the CO_2 generation is stopped.

Bacteria

Salt rising bread employs a form of bacterial leavening that does not require yeast. Although the leavening action is not always consistent, and requires close attention to the incubating conditions, this bread is making a comeback due to its unique cheese-like flavour and fine texture.

Aeration

Aerated bread is leavened by carbon dioxide being forced into dough under pressure. The technique is no longer in common use, but from the mid-19th to 20th centuries bread made this way was somewhat popular in the United Kingdom, made by the Aerated Bread Company and sold in its high-street tearooms.

Fats or shortenings

Fats such as butter, vegetable oils, lard or that contained in eggs affects the development of gluten in breads by coating and lubricating the individual strands of protein and also helping hold the structure together. If too much fat is included in a bread dough, the lubrication effect will cause the protein structures to divide. A fat content of approximately 3 per cent by weight is the concentration that will produce the greatest leavening action. In addition to their effects on leavening, fats also serve to tenderise the breads they are used in and also help to keep the bread fresh longer after baking.

Bread improvers

Bread improvers are often used in producing commercial breads to reduce the time needed for rising, and to improve texture and volume. Chemical substances commonly used as bread improvers include ascorbic acid, hydrogenchloride, sodium metabisulphate, ammonium chloride, various phosphates, amylase, and protease. Sodium/salt is one of the most common additives used in production. In addition to enhancing flavour and restricting yeast activity, salt affects the crumb and the overall texture by stabilising and strengthening the gluten. Some artisan bakers are foregoing early addition of salt to the dough, and are waiting until after a 20 minute 'rest'. This is known as an autolyse, and is done with both refined and with whole grain flours.

Chemistry of Bread Flavour

The compounds responsible for bread flavour sensation appear to be unstable. More than 70 different organic compounds have been identified in preferments, dough, oven vapours, and bread. Those compounds, which include several organic acids, alcohols, carbonyls, and esters, arise through a complex series of reactions during fermentation and baking. Both fermentation and baking of dough are essential to develop an acceptable bread flavour. Many of the compounds formed during fermentation are volatilised during baking. Evidence suggests that reactions between free amino groups and reducing sugars predominate in crust browning and in producing bread flavour stimuli. Bread crust contains larger amounts of carbonyl compounds than the crumb. A gradual loss of carbonyl compounds from the crust parallels the staling of bread.

How yeast bread is made

Both commercial bakers and home bakers make bread from a dough that consists of at least four ingredients—flour, water or milk, salt, and yeast. The dough may also contain eggs, shortening, sugar or other foods. Most commercial bakers in the United States and many other countries use enriched dough for white bread.

They enrich their dough by adding vitamins and minerals, or they use already enriched flour. Most commercial dough also contains substances called dough conditioners and shelf-life improvers. Dough conditioners, such as chlorine dioxide and potassium bromate, help give bread a smooth, even texture. Shelf-life improvers include monoglycerides, which help keep bread from becoming stale, and calcium propionate, which reduces the growth of mould and bacteria.

Dough is made into bread by one of two processes, conventional bread making or continuous bread making. Conventional bread making is used by most bakeries. Home bakers also use variations of conventional bread making. Continuous bread making is used by only the largest bakeries.

In conventional bread making, the ingredients are mixed by one of two chief methods, the sponge-and-dough method or the straight dough method. In the sponge-and-dough method, the ingredients are combined in two stages. The first stage mixes all the yeast and about two-thirds of the flour and water or milk. This mixture is called a sponge. Bakers let the sponge ferment (rise) at about 85°F (29°C) for up to 16 hours. Then they add the rest of the ingredients, and the mixture ferments again for a short time. In the straight dough method, all the ingredients are combined at once and fermented for about 3 hours at 85°F (29°C). After either of these fermenting processes, the dough is divided into pieces and shaped. It is then fermented again for a short time in a process called proofing and baked in an oven at about 450°F (232°C).

Continuous bread

Continuous bread making uses highly specialised equipment to mix the ingredients and prepare the dough for baking. In the most common method, all the ingredients except the flour are first combined to form a mixture called a broth. After fermenting in a tank, the broth is pumped to a mixer and the flour is added. In the mixer, the ingredients are combined under pressure to form dough. The dough is then divided, shaped, and sent to an oven for baking. This process produces bread of uniform shape, texture, and quality. After bread has been baked, it is removed from the oven to cool. In commercial bakeries, the loaves are placed in cooling machines where their temperature is reduced to about 100°F (38°C). The bread may then be sliced and wrapped in paper or plastic film.

The food value of bread: Enriched white bread provides important amounts of protein, starch, iron, and three B vitamins—niacin, riboflavin, and thiamine. Milling removes from wheat most of these substances, which are naturally present in the grain. Whole-wheat bread provides almost all the natural vitamins and minerals of wheat, including niacin, riboflavin, thiamine, vitamin E, and iron and calcium. Whole-wheat bread also contains bran, an important source of fibre. White bread has little fibre.

Components of bread flavour originate from fermentative and thermal reactions. Enzymes provide precursors for both processes, and their influence should be controlled. Enzymes are now replacing other improving additives in breadmaking, indirectly affecting bread flavour. Amylases produce reducing sugars, which are: (i) fermentable substrates for fermentative microflora leading to numerous aromatic compounds, those of lower volatility remaining in bread, and (ii) precursors of many components (mainly carbonyls) after reacting with amino acids in nonenzymatic browning reactions. Proteases produce peptides and amino acids, which, like sugars, participate in metabolic and thermal reactions and can occasionally be a source of bitter peptides. Lipoxygenase from soya or faba flour, used in some breadmaking processes, gives unstable products decomposing to carbonyl compounds generating off flavours in bread.

In addition, the ingredients, the breadmaking process, and the baking conditions modify enzymatic activity and bread flavour.

Rye Bread

Rye bread is a type of bread made with various percentages of flour from rye grain. It can be light or dark in colour, depending on the type of flour used and the addition of colouring agents, and is typically denser than bread made from wheat flour. It is higher in fibre than many common types of bread and is often darker in colour and stronger in flavour.

While rye and wheat are genetically close enough to interbreed (the resulting hybrids are known as triticale), there are some substantial differences in the biochemistry of wheat and rye that can drastically affect the breadmaking process. A key issue is amylases—while wheat amylases are generally not heat stable and have no effect on the stronger wheat gluten, rye amylase remains active at substantially higher temperatures. Since rye gluten is not particularly strong, the main structure of the bread is based on complex polysaccharides, including rye starch and pentosans, and the amylases in the flour can break down the resulting structure, inhibiting the rise of the dough.

There are two common solutions: The traditional manner, acidification, uses *Lactobacillus* cultures in a naturally-derived sourdough starter to inactivate the rye amylases, which cannot function in an acidic environment, and to help gelatinise the starches in the dough matrix. In areas where obtaining wheat has traditionally been impractical because of marginal growing conditions or supply difficulties, this has been the most important technique to creating lighter breads.

Pure rye bread: Pure rye bread contains only rye flour, without any wheat. German-style pumpernickel, a dark, dense, and close-textured loaf, is made from crushed or ground whole rye grains, usually without wheat flour, baked for long periods at low temperature in a covered tin. Rye and wheat flours are often used to produce a rye bread which has a lighter texture, colour and flavour than pumpernickel. Light or dark rye flour can be used to make rye bread; the flour is classified according to the amount of bran left in the flour after milling.

Straight rye breads: A simple, all-rye bread can be made using a sourdough starter and rye meal; it will not rise as high as a wheat bread, but will be more moist with a substantially longer keeping time. Such breads are often known as black breads, partly from their darker colour than wheat breads (enhanced by long baking times, creating Maillard reactions in the crumb), and partly from their perceived lower social status than the lighter, more expensive wheat breads.

Multigrain rye breads: It is fairly common to combine rye with other grains and seeds. In southern Germany and Switzerland, for example, it is not uncommon to find a variant of Vollkornbrot with sunflower seeds instead of the rye seeds, and some traditional recipes also substitute whole wheat grains for the rye grains.

Crisp rye flatbreads: There are three different types of rye crisp bread: yeast fermented, sourdough fermented and cold bread crisp bread. Most of the crisp bread produced in Scandinavia is baked following three to four hours of fermentation. Sourdough crisp breads are used in Finland, Estonia, Latvia, Lithuania, Poland, Germany and India. The third type of crisp bread is the so-called cold bread crisp bread, essentially a type of hardtack (known in Sweden particularly as knäckebröd), which is baked without the addition of any leavening. The dough gets the right texture from a foaming process, where air is incorporated into the cooled dough, which also leads to the almost white colour of the finished bread. Crisp bread owes its long shelf-life to its very low water content (5–7 per cent).

Rye quick breads: Rye flour is sometimes used in chemically-leavened quick bread recipes as well, either batter-type or dough-type (similar to Irish soda bread). In such cases, it can be used in similar applications as whole wheat flour, since an egg matrix often provides the bread structure rather than the grain's gluten.

Health benefits: Rye bread contains a large amount of fibre and only a little fat. Rye bread does not create high spikes in blood sugar as white bread and other breads do.

MALT BEVERAGE

Malt beverage is an American term for both alcoholic and non-alcoholic fermented beverages, in which the primary ingredient is barley, which has been allowed to sprout (malt) slightly before it is processed. By far, the most predominant malt beverage is beer, of which there are two main styles: ale and lager. A non-alcoholic beverage brewed in this fashion is technically identical to 'non-alcoholic beer'. Such a beverage may be prepared by using a slightly altered brewing process which yields very little alcohol (technically less than 0.5 per cent by volume).

The term 'malt beverage' is often used by trade associations of groups of beer wholesalers (e.g. Tennessee Malt Beverage Association) to avoid any negative connotations associated with beer. Additionally, the term is applied to many other flavoured beverages prepared from malted grains to which natural or artificial flavours have been added to make them taste similar to wines, fruits, colas, ciders or other beverages.

This subcategory has been called 'malternative', as in Smirnoff Ice (US and French version) or 'maltini', as in 3SUM, which also has energy components like caffeine. Marketing of such products in the United States has increased rapidly in recent years.

In most jurisdictions, these products are regulated in a way identical to beer, which allows a retailer with a beer license to sell a seemingly wider product line. This also generally avoids the steeper taxes and stricter regulations associated with distilled spirits.

Microbiology of Beer

Beer is the world's most widely consumed and probably oldest of alcoholic beverages; it is the third most popular drink overall, after water and tea. It is produced by the brewing and fermentation of starches, mainly derived from cereal grains—most commonly malted barley, although wheat, maize (corn), and rice are widely used. Most beer is flavoured with hops, which add bitterness and act as a natural preservative, though other flavourings such as herbs or fruit may occasionally be included.

Barley is the source of the fermentable sugars in modern beer. Malt is formed by germinating or malting, barley seeds. The plant cells convert starch in the endosperm to fermentable sugars. Additionally, plant proteases reduce the total protein and make amino acids available for the yeast. The malt is then dried (~50°C) and roasted (~75°C).

Fermentation

The alcohol in beer is produced by yeast fermentation. The final alcohol content is determined by comparing the initial and final specific gravities. The final alcohol content in commercial beer is controlled by tax laws rather than by the yeast. Normal mixing and transferring the wort to a fermentation vessel will aerate the wort. Initially, the yeast will grow quickly as they use aerobic respiration. When the oxygen is depleted the yeast will switch to fermentation and produce ethyl alcohol.

Carbonation is added to beer by bubbling in CO_2 or by a secondary fermentation in which sugar or unfermented wort is added to the bottled beer. Commercial beer is aged several weeks and pasteurised in the bottle. Some beers are filtered rather than pasteurised to remove contaminating microbes.

Spoilage

Chlorophenols form when phenols in the wort combine with chlorine in water to give a plasticlike taste to the beer. Visible light (400–520 nm) causes the production of the skunk-smelling mercaptan from humulone. After the initial transfer of wort, aeration can result in oxidation of a variety of chemicals in the beer resulting in off-tastes.

Off-tastes and odours are produced most often by wild yeast and lactic acid bacteria (*Lactobacillus* and *Pediococcus*). *Micrococcus kristinae* is the only aerobic bacterium reported in beer spoilage. During the 1990s, gram-negative strictly anaerobic bacteria including *Pectinatus*, *Selenomonas lacticifex*, *Zymophilus*, and *Megasphaera* were isolated from spoiled beer.

Some yeast strains produce acetaldehyde which gives a rotten-apple taste to beer. Diacetyl, dimethyl sulphide, *cis*-3-hexanal, and organic acids are the most frequent products of contaminating bacteria. Table 18.1 shows various types of beer.

Table 18.1. Types of beer.

Type	Yeast	Method of preparation	Function of yeast
Lager	Saccharomyces cerevisiae (Bottom strain)	Fermented barley releases starches and amylase enzymes (malting). Enzymes in malt hydrolyse starch to fermentable sugars (mashing). Liquid (wort) is sterilised. Hops added for flavour. Yeast added; incubated at 3°–10°C. (Steam beer is incubated at 10°–21°C.) Wort is added to beer for secondary fermentation.	Converts sugar into alcohol and CO_2; can produce >6 per cent alcohol. Yeast grows on the bottom of fermentation vessel.
Ale	S. cerevisiae (Top strain)	As in lager; incubated at 10°–21°C. Sugar added to the beer for secondary fermentation.	Converts sugar into alcohol and CO_2; produces <4 per cent alcohol. Yeast grows at the top of fermentation vessel.
Lambic	Not inoculated; wild yeast include Kloeckera apiculata, Brettanomyces lambicus, S. cerevisiae	As in lager using 30 per cent wheat mixed with barley malt. Incubated at 10°–12°C.	Convert sugar into alcohol, CO_2, organic acids, and esters; produces <4 per cent alcohol.
Sake	S. cerevisiae	Aspergillus oryzae converts start in steamed rice into sugar; yeast added; incubated at 20°C.	Converts sugar into alcohol; 14–16 per cent alcohol.

Beer Defects and Diseases

Recently the Innsbruck Medical University team behind this revelation has shown—in layman's terms —is that beer offers a resultant anti-inflammatory effect which may have a 'beneficial impact on coronary heart diseases'. More specifically, *in vitro* tests on peripheral mononuclear blood cells demonstrated that beer extracts blocked the effects of said interferon-gamma—'one of the most important messengers in inflammatory response and mainly produced as part of the cellular immune response'.

To cut right to the chase: 'Beer extracts inhibit, among other things, the production of neopterin and the degradation of tryptophan by suppressing T-cell response.'

The team notes that 'this suppression might be connected with the calming effect of beer since its normalising effect on the tryptophan balance improves the availability of the happiness hormone serotonin'. Agreeably, the alcohol content of the beer is irrelevant, although lead boffin Professor Dietmar Fuchs inevitably cautioned that the potentially beneficial effects discovered 'must of course be weighed against the negative effects and dangers of drinking alcohol'.

Fuchs added: 'The effects could indeed be observed on extracts of alcohol-free beers. Our findings must, therefore, not be understood as an encouragement to drink alcohol.'

The term defects will be applied here to undesirable characteristics with causes that are not microbial, such as (i) turbidity due to unstable protein, protein-tannin complexes, starch, and resin, (ii) off-flavours caused by poor ingredients or contact with metals, and (iii) poor physical characteristics. This discussion will be limited to the troubles caused by micro-organisms and therefore termed beer infections or beer diseases. The mash in the brewhouse may undergo butyric acid fermentation by *Clostridium* spp. or lactic acid fermentation by lactics if the mash is held too long at temperatures favouring these bacteria.

Off-flavours so produced may carry over into the beer. The pitching yeast ordinarily is contaminated with bacteria and wild yeasts may be a source of spoilage organisms. Yeasts and bacteria produce turbidity when they grow in beer, and beer yeasts carried over from the fermentation may be responsible for cloudiness. Likewise, wild yeasts, e.g. *Saccharomyces pastorianus,* can cause Cloudiness in beer. Yeasts can be inhibited or excluded by keeping out air, fermenting most of the sugar in the wort to produce a 'dry' beer, using good cultures of beer yeasts, and sanitising the plant adequately. Yeasts also may be responsible for off-tastes and off-odours. Thus, for example, bitterness may be caused by *S. pastorianus*, and an esterlike taste by *Hansenula anomala.* Most yeasts produce fruity odours, and some produce hydrogen sulphide from the hop extract in the beer. Yeasts able to utilise the dextrins in beer (e.g. *Saccharomyces diastaticus)* are potential spoilage organisms.

The bacteria causing beer diseases are mostly from the genera *Pediococcus, Lactobacillus, Flavobacterium,* and *Acetobacter.*

'Sarcina sickness', characterised by sourness, turbidity, and ropiness of beer, is caused by *Pediococcus cerevisiae.* Because the cocci often aggregate in fours or tetrads, they were first thought to be sarcinae.

Some lactobacilli, being tolerant to acid and hop antiseptics, can grow in beer. *Lactobacillus pastorianus* and *L. diastaticus* cause sourness and a silky turbidity. These bacteria produce lactic, acetic, and formic acids and alcohol and carbon dioxide from sugars, and are especially bad in top fermentations such as are used for ales.

Zymomonas anaerobium, when growing in beer, causes a silky turbidity and produces an odour reminiscent of hydrogen sulphide and apples. It forms carbon dioxide and alcohol. It is easily killed by heat and rarely occurs in pasteurised beer.

Obesumbacterium proteus is responsible for a parsniplike odour and taste in wort and in beer. It produces alcohol and acid and is not tolerant of a pH as low as 4.2. It has been found as a common contaminant of pitching yeast.

Species of *Acetobacter* and *Gluconobacter*, which are tolerant of acid and hop antiseptics, can cause sourness of wort or beer under aerobic conditions. Exposure to oxygen can occur in worts that are stored too long, in empty beer barrels, and in pitching yeast. A number of species can cause sourness; *Gluconobacter oxydans* subsp. *suboxydans* and *G. oxydans* subsp. *industrius* may produce ropiness; and *A. pasteurianus* has been blamed for turbidity and sourness.

Other incompletely described, unidentified bacteria have been blamed for beer diseases. *Micrococcus, Streptococcus*, and *Bacillus* species have been accused of causing trouble but in some instances probably merely were present. *Streptococcus mucilaginosus*, which probably is a pediococcus, has been reported to cause ropiness.

It should be re-emphasised that all the yeasts and bacteria that cause infection or diseases in wort and beer are killed by boiling the wort and hops and must enter thereafter from equipment, the air, the water or the pitching yeast and that aseptic and sanitary precautions will help prevent these troubles.

Other Malt Beverages and Beer Types

Variations in malt beverages or beer types are usually related to: (i) alcohol content, (ii) concentration of malt and hops used, (iii) length of ageing, (iv) initial total solids (related to fermentable carbohydrate present and remaining after fermentation), and (v) temperature of fermentation.

Malt liquor is a North American term referring to a type of beer with high alcohol content. In legal statutes, the term often includes any alcoholic beverage above or equal to 5 per cent alcohol by volume made with malted barley. In common parlance, however, it is used for high-alcohol beers made with ingredients and processes resembling those in American-style lager. Malt liquor is distinguished from other beers of high alcohol content in that the brewing process is seen by many critics as targeting high alcohol content and economy rather than quality. However, this label is subject to the viewpoint of the brewer, as there are indeed examples of brews containing high-quality, expensive ingredients that brewers have chosen to label as 'malt liquors'.

Pilsener also has the unique claim to being 'the world's first golden beer'. A modern pilsener has a very light, clear colour from pale to golden yellow, and a distinct hop aroma and flavour. Pilseners are identified by their participation in categories like 'European-Style Pilsener' at the World Beer Cup or other similar competitions. A pilsener is generally regarded as different from other pale lagers by a more prominent hop character, particularly from the use of Saaz noble hops and spring (soft) water. While pilsener is best defined in terms of its characteristics and heritage, the term is also used by some brewers (particularly in North America) to indicate their 'premium' beer, whether or not it has a particular hop character.

Low-calorie, **light** or **no-carbohydrate** beers are made from prehydrolysed wort. Fungal enzymes (glucoamylases and amylases) are used to hydrolyse the dextrin to maltose and glucose, which can be completely fermented to alcohol; the net result is a lower concentration of remaining carbohydrate.

Bock is originally a dark beer, a modern bock can range from light copper to brown in colour. The style is very popular, with many examples brewed internationally.

Ale is a type of beer brewed from malted barley using a warm fermentation with a strain of brewer's yeast. The yeast will ferment the beer quickly, giving it a sweet, full bodied and fruity taste. Most ales contain hops, which help preserve the beer and impart a bitter herbal flavour that balances the sweetness of the malt.

Weiss beer, porter, and **stout** are ales in that top yeasts are employed in their manufacture. Weiss beer is a light, tart ale made chiefly from wheat. Porter and stout are dark, heavy, sweet ales.

Related Beverages

Sake is a rice-based alcoholic beverage of Japanese origin. It is sometimes spelled saké to show the pronunciation more clearly. To make beer or sake, the sugar needed to produce alcohol must first be converted from starch. However, the brewing process for sake differs from beer brewing as well, notably in that for beer, the conversion of starch to sugar and sugar to alcohol occurs in two discrete steps, but with sake they occur simultaneously. Additionally, alcohol content also differs between sake, wine, and beer. Wine generally contains 9–16 per cent alcohol and most beer is 3–9 per cent, whereas undiluted sake is 18–20 per cent alcohol, although this is often lowered to around 15 per cent by diluting the sake with water prior to bottling.

Pulque or *octli*, is a milk-coloured, somewhat viscous alcoholic beverage made from the fermented sap of the maguey plant, and is a traditional native beverage of Mexico.

Ginger beer is a carbonated drink that is flavoured primarily with ginger and sweetened with sugar or artificial sweeteners. Most ginger beer produced commercially is a manufactured soft drink.

The original recipe requires only ginger, sugar, water, lemon zest and yeast. Fermentation over a few days turns the mixture into ginger beer.

Wines

Wine is an alcoholic beverage, made of fermented fruit juice, usually from grapes. The natural chemical balance of grapes lets them ferment without the addition of sugars, acids, enzymes or other nutrients.

Grape wine is produced by fermenting crushed grapes using various types of yeast. Yeast consumes the sugars in the grapes and converts them into alcohol. Different varieties of grapes and strains of yeasts produce different types of wine.

Wines made from other fruits, such as apples and berries, are normally named after the fruit from which they are produced (for example, apple wine or elderberry wine) and are generically called fruit wine or country wine (not to be confused with the French term *vin de pays*). Others, such as barley wine and rice wine (i.e. sake), are made from starch-based materials and resemble beer and spirit more than wine, while ginger wine is fortified with brandy. In these cases, the term 'wine' refers to the higher alcohol content rather than production process.

Production of Fruit Alcohol

Alcohol and acids are two primary products of fermentation, both used to good effect in the preservation of foods. Several alcohol-fermented foods are preceded by an acid fermentation and in the presence of oxygen and *acetobacter*, alcohol can be fermented to produce acetic acid. Most food spoilage organisms cannot survive in either alcoholic or acidic environments. Therefore, the production of both these end products can prevent a food from undergoing spoilage and extend its shelf-life.

Primitive wines and beers have been produced, with the aid of yeasts, for thousands of years, although it was not until about four hundred years ago that micro-organisms associated with the fermentation were observed and identified. It was not until the 1850's that Louis Pasteur demonstrated unequivocally the involvement of yeasts in the production of wines and beers. Since then, the knowledge of yeasts and the conditions necessary for fermentation of wine and beer has increased to the point where pure culture fermentations are now used to ensure consistent product quality. Originally, alcoholic fermentations would have been spontaneous events that resulted from the activity of micro-organisms naturally present. These non-scientific methods are still used today for the home preparation of many of the world's traditional beers and wines.

Alcoholic drinks fall into two broad categories: wines and beers. Wines are made from the juice of fruits and beers from cereal grains. The principal carbohydrates in fruit juices are soluble sugars; the principal carbohydrate in grains is starch, an insoluble polysaccharide. The yeasts that bring about alcoholic fermentation can attack soluble sugars but do not produce starch-splitting enzymes. Wines can therefore be made by the direct fermentation of the raw material, while the production of beer requires the hydrolysis of starch to yield sugars fermentable by yeast, as a preliminary step.

Raw fruit juice is usually a strongly acidic solution, containing from 10 to 25 per cent soluble sugars. Its acidity and high sugar concentration make it an unfavourable medium for the growth of bacteria but highly suitable for yeasts and moulds. Raw fruit juice naturally contains many yeasts, moulds, and bacteria, derived from the surface of the fruit. Normally the yeast used in alcoholic fermentation is a strain of the species *Saccharomyces cerevisiae*.

The fermentation may be allowed to proceed spontaneously or can be 'started' by inoculation with a must that has been previously successfully fermented by *S. cerevisiae* var. *ellipsoideus*. Many modern wineries eliminate the original microbial population of the must by pasteurisation or by treatment with sulphur dioxide. The must is then inoculated with a starter culture derived from a pure culture of a suitable strain of wine yeast. This procedure eliminates many of the uncertainties and difficulties of older methods. At the start of the fermentation, the must is aerated slightly to build up a large and vigorous yeast population; once fermentation sets in, the rapid production of carbon dioxide maintains anaerobic conditions, which prevent the growth of undesirable aerobic organisms, such as bacteria and moulds. The temperature of fermentation is usually from 25° to 30°C, and the duration of the fermentation process may extend from a few days to two weeks. As soon as the desired degree of sugar disappearance and alcohol production has been attained, the microbiological phase of wine making is over. Thereafter, the quality and stability of the wine depend very largely on preventing further microbial activity, both during the 'ageing' in wooden casks and after bottling.

At all stages during its manufacture, fruit juice alcohol is subject to spoilage by undesirable microorganisms. Pasteur, whose descriptions of the organisms responsible and recommendations for overcoming them are still valid today, first scientifically explored the problem of the 'diseases' of wines. The most serious aerobic spoilage processes are brought about by film-forming yeasts and acetic acid bacteria, both of which grow at the expense of the alcohol, converting it to acetic acid or to carbon dioxide and water. The chief danger from these organisms arises when access of air is not carefully regulated during ageing. Much more serious are the diseases caused by fermentative bacteria, particularly rod-shaped lactic acid bacteria, which utilise any residual sugar and impart a mousy taste to the wine. Such wines are known as turned wines. Since oxygen is unnecessary for the growth of lactic acid bacteria, wine spoilage of this kind can occur even after bottling. These risks of spoilage can be minimised by pasteurisation after bottling.

Grape wine

Grape wine is perhaps the most common fruit juice alcohol. Because of the commercialisation of the product for industry, the process has received most research attention and is documented in detail. The production of grape wine involves the following basic steps: crushing the grapes to extract the juice; alcoholic fermentation; maltolactic fermentation if desired; bulk storage and maturation of the wine in a cellar; clarification and packaging. Although the process is fairly simple, quality control demands that the fermentation is carried out under controlled conditions to ensure a high quality product.

The distinctive flavour of grape wine originates from the grapes as raw material and subsequent processing operations. The grapes contribute trace elements of many volatile substances (mainly terpenes) which give the final product the distinctive fruity character. In addition, they contribute nonvolatile compounds (tartaric and malic acids) which impact on flavour and tannins which give bitterness and astringency. The latter are more prominent in red wines as the tannin components are located in the grape skins. Although yeasts are the principal organisms involved, filamentous fungi, lactic acid bacteria, acetic acid bacteria and other bacterial groups all play a role in the production of alcoholic fruit products.

Normal grapes harbour a diverse micro-flora, of which the principal yeasts (*Saccharomyces cerevisiae*) involved in desirable fermentation are in the minority. Lactic acid bacteria and acetic acid bacteria are also present. The proportions of each and total numbers present are dependent upon a number of external environmental factors including the temperature, humidity, stage of maturity, damage at harvest and application of fungicides. It is essential to ensure proliferation of the desired species at the expense of the non-desired ones. This is achieved through ensuring fermentation conditions are such to encourage *Saccharomyces* species.

The fermentation may be initiated using a starter culture of *Saccharomyces cerevisiae*—in which case the juice is inoculated with populations of yeast of 10^6 to 10^7 cfu/ml juice. This approach produces a wine of generally expected taste and quality. If the fermentation is allowed to proceed naturally, utilising the yeasts present on the surface of the fruits, the end result is less controllable, but produces wines with a range of flavour characteristics. It is likely that natural fermentations are practiced widely around the world, especially for home production of wine.

During alcoholic fermentation, yeasts are the prominent species. The composition of fruit juice—its acid and sugar level and low pH favour the growth of yeasts and production of ethanol that restricts the growth of bacteria and fungi. In natural fermentations, there is a progressive pattern of yeast growth. Several species of yeast, including *Kloeckera, Hanseniaspora, Candida* and *Metschnikowia*, are active for the first two to three days of fermentation. The build up of end products (ethanol) is toxic to these yeasts and they die off, leaving *Saccharomyces cerevisiae* to continue the fermentation to the end. *S. cerevisiae* can tolerate much higher levels of ethanol (up to 15 per cent v/v or more) than the other species who only tolerate up to 5 or 8 per cent alcohol. Because of its tolerance of alcohol, *S. cerevisiae* dominates wine fermentation and is the species that has been commercialised for starter cultures.

Traditionally, fermentation was carried out in large wooden barrels or concrete tanks. Modern wineries now use stainless steel tanks as these are more hygienic and provide better temperature control. White wines are fermented at 10° to 18°C for about seven to fourteen days. The low temperature and slow fermentation favours the retention of volatile compounds. Red wines are fermented at 20° to 30°C for about seven days. This higher temperature is necessary to extract the pigment from the grape skins.

Factors affecting wine fermentation

There are several variables which can affect the fermentation process and final quality of wine. Factors which are most important to control are:

1. The clarification and pretreatment of juice.
2. Chemical composition of the juice.
3. Temperature of the fermentation.
4. The influences of other micro-organisms.

Clarification and pretreatment of juice

Excessive clarification removes many of the natural yeasts and flora. This is beneficial if a tightly controlled induced fermentation is desired, but less so if the fermentation is a natural one. Long periods of settling out however, encourage the growth of natural flora, which can contribute to the fermentation.

Chemical composition of juice

The main constituents of grape juice are glucose (75 to 150 g/l), fructose (75 to 150 g/l), tartaric acid (2 to 10 g/l), malic acid (1 to 8 g/l) and free amino acids (0.2 to 2.5 g/l). The main reaction is the fermentation of glucose and fructose to ethanol and carbon dioxide. However, the presence of nitrogenous and sulphurous products also contributes to the fermentation. The addition of sulphur dioxide to the juice delays the growth of yeast, but does not necessarily inhibit growth of the non-Saccharomyces strains. Fruits generally contain sufficient substrates—soluble sugars—for the yeast to ferment and convert into an acceptable concentration of alcohol. Sugar can be added to fruit juices with a low sugar content, to increase the amount of fermentable substrate.

Temperature

Temperature has an impact on the growth and activity of different strains of yeast. At temperatures of 10° to 15°C, the non-Saccharomyces species have an increased tolerance to alcohol and therefore have the potential to contribute to the fermentation.

Influence of other micro-organisms

Other micro-organisms have the potential to influence wine production at all stages of the process. Prior to harvest, yeasts grow on the surface of grapes. Fungicides are used in an attempt to control their growth, but these disturb the natural balance of flora, thus making it difficult to carry out a 'natural' fermentation. Overuse of fungicides can lead to the development of resistant strains of yeast which have the potential to produce toxins which destroy the desirable yeast species. These yeasts are known as 'killer' strains. Other microbes have further chances to influence the fermentation during the clarification process, after fermentation and during maturation and bottling when *acetobacter* species can oxidise the alcohol and produce acetic acid.

About two to three weeks after the alcoholic fermentation is finished wines often undergo a malolactic fermentation. This occurs naturally and lasts for about four weeks. It is a lactic acid fermentation, initiated by lactic acid bacteria resident in the wine. Inoculating the fermented wine with cultures of *Leuconostoc oenos* can start the process if it is desired. The main reaction of these bacteria is the decarboxylation of L-malic acid to L-lactic acid, which decreases the acidity of the wine and increases its pH by about 0.3 to 0.5 units. Wines produced from grapes grown in colder climates tend to have a higher concentration of malic acid and a lower pH (3.0 to 3.5) and the taste benefits from this slight decrease in acidity. The benefits of this process are that it imparts a more mellow flavour to the wine. The growth of malolactic bacteria also contributes to the taste of the wine. Wines that have undergone a malolactic fermentation appear to be less susceptible to any further damage from other bacteria. This could be because *L. oenos* has used up all available substrate, or it may have secreted bacteriocins which prevent the growth of other species. Although the malolactic fermentation seems to be a useful process, not all wines benefit from it. Wines produced from grapes in warmer climates tend to be less acidic (pH > 3.5) and a further reduction in acidity may have adverse effects on the quality of the wine. Decreasing the acidity also increases the pH to values which can allow spoilage organisms to multiply. It is difficult to prevent the malolactic fermentation from taking place naturally, especially later on after the wine has been bottled. In low acid wines, the acidity may be adjusted after this fermentation has taken place. The malolactic fermentation can be prevented by controlling several factors: the wine pH (<3.2); ethanol content (>14 per cent) and levels of sulphur dioxide (>50 mg/l). The bacteriocin nisin can also be used to control the growth of malolactic bacteria. However, the subtle blend of aromas and flavours that contribute to the final taste may be lost by such stringent control.

The conversion of malic acid to lactic acid is one of the main reactions carried out by wine lactic acid bacteria. *L. oenos* needs to be present in significant numbers (greater than 10^6 cfu/ml) for the reaction to take place at a suitable pace. The bacteria use residual pentose and hexose sugars in the wine as a substrate for growth. The main reaction is the deacidification (or decarboxylation) of malic acid. In addition to this, the by-products of the reaction impart flavours and aromas to the wine.

During storage, wines are prone to non-desirable microbial changes. Yeasts, lactic acid bacteria, acetic acid bacteria and fungi can all spoil or taint wines after the fermentation process is completed. The changes that occur are increased acidification through the formation of acetic and other acids from alcohol; increased carbonation through a secondary fermentation of residual sugars and flavour changes through the metabolism of numerous compounds.

PRODUCTS OF YEAST FERMENTATION

The major products of yeast fermentation are alcoholic drinks and bread. With respect to fruits and vegetables, the most important products are fermented fruit juices and fermented plant saps. Virtually any fruit or sugary plant sap can be processed into an alcoholic beverage. The process is well known being essentially an alcoholic fermentation of sugars to yield alcohol and carbon dioxide. It should be noted that alcohol production requires special licences or is prohibited in many countries.

Fermented Fruit Juices

There are many fermented drinks made from fruit in Africa, Asia and Latin America. These include drinks made from bananas, grapes and other fruit. Grape wine is perhaps the most economically important fruit juice alcohol. It is of major economic importance in Chile, Argentina, South Africa, Georgia, Morocco and Algeria. Because of the commercialisation of the product for industry, the process has received most research attention and is documented in detail. Banana beer is probably the most wide spread alcoholic fruit drink in Africa and is of cultural importance in certain areas. Alcoholic fruit drinks are made from many other fruits including dates in North Africa, pineapples in Latin America and jack fruits in Asia.

Red grape wine

Red grape wines are made in many African, Asian and Latin American countries including Algeria, Morocco and South Africa. Red grape wine is an alcoholic fruit drink of between 10 and 14 per cent alcoholic strength. The colour ranges from a light red to a deep dark red. It is made from the fruit of the grape plant (*Vitis vinifera*). There are many varieties of grape used including Cabernet Sauvignon, Grenache, Nebbiolo, Pinot Noir, and Torrontes.

The skins of the grape are allowed to be fermented in red wine production, to allow for the extraction of colour and tannins, which contribute to the flavour. The grapes contribute trace elements of many volatile substances, which give the final product the distinctive fruity character. In addition, they contribute nonvolatile compounds (tartaric and malic acids) which impact on flavour and tannins, which give bitterness and astringency.

Raw material preparation

Ripe and undamaged grapes should be used. Red grapes are crushed to yield the juice plus skins, which is known as must.

Processing

The crushed grapes are transferred to fermentation vessels. The ethanol formed during this fermentation assists with the extraction of pigments from the skins. This takes between 24 hours and three weeks depending on the colour of the final product required.

The skins are then removed and the partially fermented wine is transferred to a separate tank to complete the fermentation. The fermentation can be from naturally occurring yeasts on the skin of the grape or using a starter culture of *Saccharomyces cerevisiae*—in which case the juice is inoculated with populations of yeast. This approach produces a wine of generally expected taste and quality. If the fermentation is allowed to proceed naturally, utilising the yeasts present on the surface of the fruits, the end result is less controllable, but produces wines with a range of flavour characteristics.

Traditionally, fermentation was carried out in large wooden barrels or concrete tanks. Modern wineries now use stainless steel tanks as these are more hygienic and provide better temperature control. Fermentation stops naturally when all the fermentable sugars have been converted to alcohol or when the alcoholic strength reaches the limit of tolerance of the strain of yeast involved. Fermentation can be stopped artificially by adding alcohol, by sterile filtration or centrifugation.

Some wines can be drunk immediately. However, most wines develop distinctive favours and aromas by ageing in wooden casks. Process of fermented red grape wine is shown in Fig. 18.1.

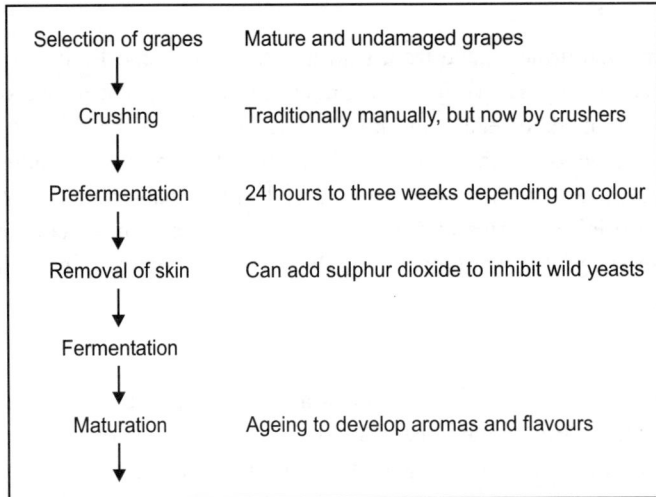

Selection of grapes — Mature and undamaged grapes

Crushing — Traditionally manually, but now by crushers

Prefermentation — 24 hours to three weeks depending on colour

Removal of skin — Can add sulphur dioxide to inhibit wild yeasts

Fermentation

Maturation — Ageing to develop aromas and flavours

Fig. 18.1. Process of fermented red grape wine.

Packaging and storage

Traditionally wine was delivered to the point of sale in casks. The product is traditionally packaged in glass bottles with corks, made from the bark of the cork oak (*Quercus suber*). The bottles should be kept out of direct sunlight. During storage, wines are prone to non-desirable microbial changes. Yeasts, lactic acid bacteria, acetic acid bacteria and fungi can all spoil or taint wines after the fermentation process is completed.

White grape wine

White grape wines are made in many African, Asian and Latin American countries including Algeria, Morocco and South Africa. White grape wine is an alcoholic fruit drink of between 10 and 14 per cent alcoholic strength. It is prepared from the fruit of the grape plant (*Vitis vinifera*), and is pale yellow in colour. There are many varieties used including Airen, Chardonnay, Palomino, Sauvignon Blanc and Ugni Blanc. The main difference between red and white wines is the early removal of grape skins in white wine production.

The distinctive flavour of grape wine originates from the grapes as raw material and subsequent processing operations. The grapes contribute trace elements of many volatile substances (mainly terpenes) which give the final product the distinctive fruity character.

Preparation of raw materials

Ripe and undamaged grapes should be used. The grapes are crushed to yield the juice and the skins are removed and separated out. Sometimes the juice is clarified by allowing it to stand for 24 to 48 hours at 5° to 10°C, by filtering or centrifugation. Pectolytic enzymes may be added to accelerate the breakdown of cell wall tissue and to improve the clarity of juice. Excessive clarification removes many of the natural yeasts and flora. This is beneficial if a tightly controlled induced fermentation is desired, but less so if the fermentation is a natural one. Long periods of settling out however, encourage the growth of natural flora, which can contribute to the fermentation.

Processing

The clarified juice is transferred to a fermentation tank where fermentation either begins spontaneously or is induced by the addition of a starter culture. Traditionally, fermentation was carried out in large wooden barrels or concrete tanks. Modern wineries now use stainless steel tanks as these are more hygienic and provide better temperature control. White wines are fermented at 10° to 18°C for about seven to fourteen days. The low temperature and slow fermentation favours the retention of volatile compounds. The fermentation can be from naturally occurring yeasts on the skin of the grape or using a starter culture of *Saccharomyces cerevisiae*.

This approach produces a wine of generally expected taste and quality. If the fermentation is allowed to proceed naturally, utilising the yeasts present on the surface of the fruits, the end result is less controllable, but produces wines having a range of flavour characteristics. It is likely that natural fermentations are practised widely around the world, especially for home production of wine. During storage, wines are prone to non-desirable microbial changes. Yeasts, lactic acid bacteria, acetic acid bacteria and fungi can all spoil or taint wines after the fermentation process is completed. Process of fermented white grape wine is shown in Fig. 18.2.

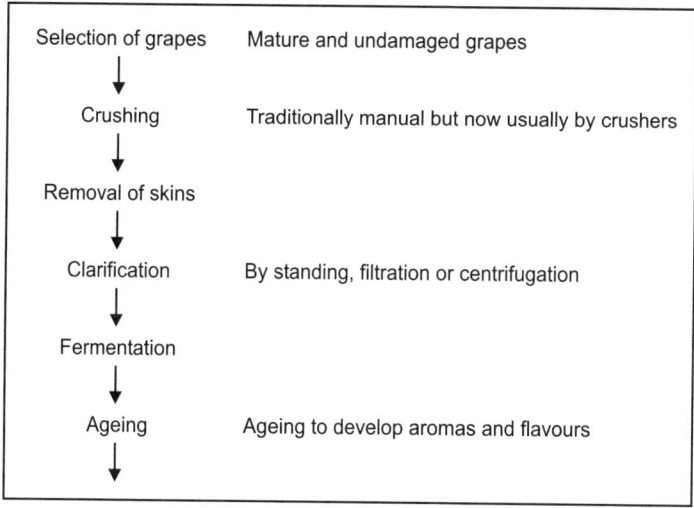

Fig. 18.2. Process of fermented white grape wine.

Packaging and storage

Traditionally wine was delivered to the point of sale in casks. The product is traditionally packaged in glass bottles with corks, made from the bark of the cork oak (*Quercus suber*). The bottles should be kept out of direct sunlight. During storage, wines are prone to non-desirable microbial changes. Yeasts, lactic acid bacteria, acetic acid bacteria and fungi can all spoil or taint wines after the fermentation process is completed.

Banana beer

Banana beer is made from bananas, mixed with a cereal flour (often sorghum flour) and fermented to an orange, alcoholic beverage. It is sweet and slightly hazy with a shelf-life of several days under correct storage conditions. There are many variations in how the beer is made. For instance *Urwaga* banana beer in Kenya is made from bananas and sorghum or millet and *Lubisi* is made from bananas and sorghum.

Preparation of raw materials

Ripe bananas (*Musa* spp.) are selected. The bananas should be peeled. If the peels cannot be removed by hand then the bananas are not sufficiently ripe.

Processing

The first step of the process is the extraction of banana juice. Extraction of a high yield of banana juice without excessive browning or contamination by spoilage micro-organisms and proper filtration to produce a clear product is of great importance. Grass is used as an aid in obtaining clarified juice.

One volume of water is added to every three volumes of banana juice. This makes the total soluble solids low enough for the yeast to act. Cereals are ground and roasted and added to improve the colour and flavour of the final product. The mixture is placed in a container, which is covered in polythene to ferment for 18 to 24 hours. The raw materials are not sterilised by boiling and therefore provide an excellent substrate for microbial growth.

It is essential that proper hygienic procedures are followed and that all equipment is thoroughly sterilised to prevent contaminating bacteria from competing with the yeast and producing acid instead of alcohol. This can be done by cleaning with boiling water or with chlorine solution. Care is necessary to wash the equipment free of residual chlorine as this would interfere with the actions of the yeast. Strict personal hygiene is also essential.

For many traditional fermented products, the micro-organisms responsible for the fermentation are unknown to scientists. However there has been research to identify the micro-organisms involved in banana beer production. The main micro-organism involved, is *Saccharomyces cerevisiae* which is the same organism involved in the production of grape wine. However many other micro-organisms associated with the fermentation have been identified. These varied according to the region of production. After fermentation the product is filtered through cotton cloth. Process of fermented banana beer is shown in Fig. 18.3.

Packaging and storage

Packaging is usually only required to keep the product for its relatively short shelf-life. Clean glass or plastic bottles are used. The product is kept in a cool place away from direct sunlight.

Cashew wine

Cashew wine is made in many countries in Asia and Latin America. Cashew wine is a light yellow alcoholic drink prepared from the fruit of the cashew tree (*Ancardium occidentale*). It contains an alcohol content of between 6 and 12 per cent alcohol.

Preparation of raw materials

In gathering the fruits and transporting them to the workshop, the prime purpose should be to have the fruit arrive in the very best condition possible. Cashew apples are sorted and only mature undamaged cashew apples should be selected. These should be washed in clean water.

Processing

The cashew apples are cut into slices to ensure a rapid rate of juice extraction when crushed in a juice press. The fruit juice is sterilised in stainless steel pans at a temperature of 85°C in order to eliminate wild yeast. The juice is filtered and treated with either sodium or potassium metabisulphite to destroy or inhibit the growth of any undesirable types of micro-organisms—acetic acid bacteria, wild yeasts and moulds. Wine yeast (*Saccharomyces cerevisiae* var *ellipsoideus*) are added. Once the yeast is added, the contents are stirred well and allowed to ferment for about two weeks. The wine is separated from the sediment. It is clarified by using fining agents such as gelatine, pectin or casein which are mixed with the wine. Filtration is carried out with filter-aids such as fullers earth. The filtered wine is transferred to wooden vats.

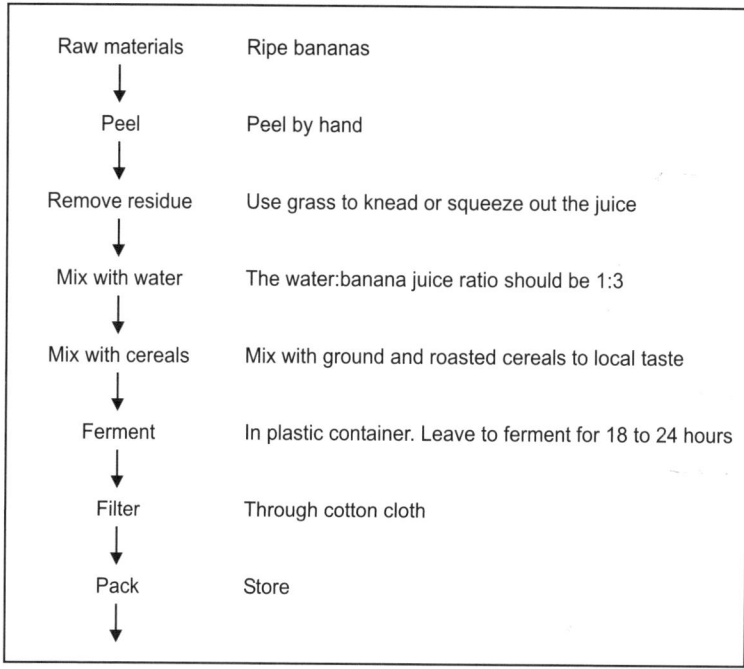

Fig. 18.3. Process of fermented banana beer.

The wine is then pasteurised at 50°–60°C. Temperature should be controlled, so as not to heat it to about 70°C, since its alcohol content would vapourise at a temperature of 75°–78°C. It is then stored in wooden vats and subjected to ageing. At least six months should be allowed for ageing.

If necessary, wine is again clarified prior to bottling. During ageing, and subsequent maturing in bottles many reactions, including oxidation, occur with the formation of traces of esters and aldehydes, which together with the tannin and acids already present enhance the taste, aroma and preservative properties of the wine. Process of fermented cashew wine is shown in Fig. 18.4.

Packaging and storage

The product is packaged in glass bottles with corks. The bottles should be kept out of direct sunlight.

Tepache

Tepache is a light, refreshing beverage prepared and consumed throughout Mexico. In the past, *tepache* was prepared from maize, but nowadays various fruits such as pineapple, apple and orange are used. The pulp and juice of the fruit are allowed to ferment for one or two days in water with some added brown sugar. The mixture is contained in a lidless wooden barrel called a 'tepachera', which is covered with cheese cloth. After a day or two, the *tepache* is a sweet and refreshing beverage. If fermentation is allowed to proceed longer, it turns into an alcoholic beverage and later into vinegar. The micro-organisms associated with the product include *Bacillus subtilis*, *B. graveolus* and the yeasts, *Torulopsis insconspicna*, *Saccharomyces cerevisiae* and *Candida queretana*.

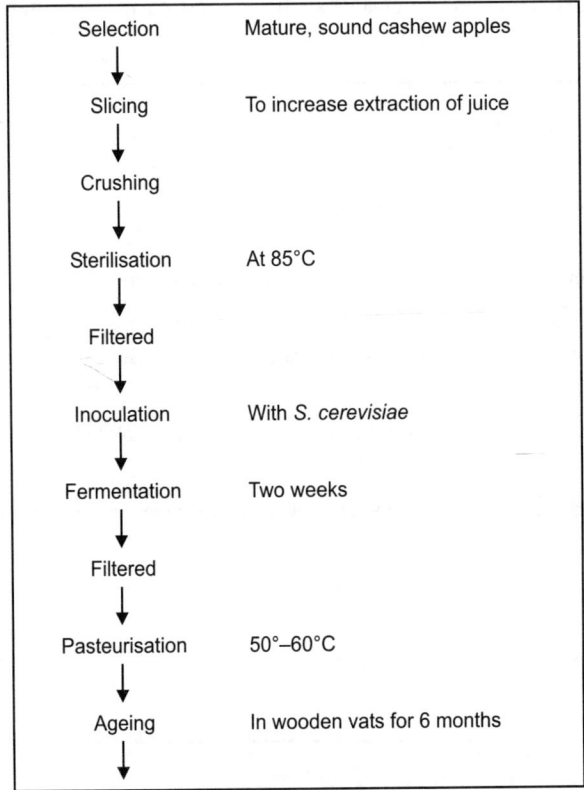

Fig. 18.4. Process of fermented cashew wine.

Colonche

Colonche is a sweet, fizzy beverage produced in Mexico by fermenting the juice of the fruits of the prickly pear cacti—mainly *Opuntia* species. The procedure for preparing *colonche* is essentially the same as has been followed for centuries. The cactus fruits are peeled and crushed to obtain the juice, which is boiled for 2–3 hours. After cooling, the juice is allowed to ferment for a few days. Sometimes old *colonche* or *tibicos* may be added as a starter. *Tibicos* are gelatinous masses of yeasts and bacteria, grown in water with brown sugar. They are also used in the preparation of *tepache*.

Fortified grape wines

Fortified wines are made in the Republic of South Africa and North Africa. Fortified wines are made by adding spirits to wines, either during or after fermentation, with the result that the alcohol content of the wines is raised to around 20 per cent, i.e. approximately double that of table wines.

Date wine

Date wines are popular in Sudan and North Africa. They are made using a variety of methodologies. *Dakhai* is produced by placing dates in a clean earthenware pot. For every one volume of dates between two and four volumes of boiling water are added. This is allowed to cool and is then sealed for three days. More warm water is then added and the container sealed again for seven to ten days. Many variations of date wine exist: *El madfuna* is produced by burying the earthenware pots underground. *Benti merse* is produced from a mixture of sorghum and dates. *Nebit* is produced from date syrup.

Sparkling grape wine

Sparkling grape wines are made in the Republic of South Africa. Sparkling wines can be made in one of three ways. The cheapest method is to carbonate wines under pressure. Unfortunately, the sparkle of these wines quickly disappears, and the product is considered inferior to the sparkling wines produced by the traditional method of secondary fermentation. This involves adding a special strain of wine yeast (*S. cerevisiae* var. *ellipsoideus*)—a champagne yeast—to wine that has been artificially sweetened. Carbon dioxide produced by fermentation of the added sugar gives the wine its sparkle. In the original champagne method, which is still widely used today, this secondary fermentation is carried out in strong bottles, capable of withstanding pressure but early in the nineteenth century a method of fermenting the wine in closed tanks was devised, this being considerably cheaper than using bottles.

Jack-fruit wine

Jack-fruit wine is an alcoholic beverage made by ethnic groups in the eastern hilly areas of India. As its name suggests, it is produced from the pulp of jack-fruit (*Artocarpus heterophyllus*). Ripe fruit is peeled and the skin discarded. The seeds are removed and the pulp soaked in water. Using bamboo baskets, the pulp is ground to extract the juice, which is collected in earthenware pots. A little water is added to the pots along with fermented wine inoculum from a previous fermentation. The pots are covered with banana leaves and allowed to ferment at 18° to 30°C for about one week. The liquid is then decanted and drunk. During fermentation, the pH of the wine reaches a value of 3.5 to 3.8, suggesting that an acidic fermentation takes place at the same time as the alcoholic fermentation. Final alcohol content is about 7 to 8 per cent within a fortnight.

Fermented Plant Saps

Virtually any sugary plant sap can be processed into an alcoholic beverage. The process is well known being essentially an alcoholic fermentation of sugars to yield alcohol and carbon dioxide. Many alcoholic drinks are made from the juices of plants including coconut palm, oil palm, wild date palm, nipa palm, raphia palm and kithul palm.

Palm wine

Palm 'wine' is an important alcoholic beverage in West Africa where it is consumed by more than 10 million people.

Palm wine can be consumed in a variety of flavours varying from sweet unfermented to sour fermented and vinegary alcoholic drinks. There are many variations and names including *emu* and *ogogoro* in Nigeria and *nsafufuo* in Ghana. It is produced from sugary palm saps. The most frequently tapped palms are raphia palms (*Raphia hookeri* or *R. vinifera*) and the oil palm (*Elaeis guineense*). Palm wine has been found to be nutritious. The fermentation process increases the levels of thiamin, riboflavin, pyridoxin and vitamin B_{12}. Like many African alcoholic beverages, palm wine has a very short shelf-life. The product is not preserved for more than one day. After this time accumulation of an excessive amount of acetic acid makes it unacceptable to consumers. The bark of a tree (*Saccoglottis gabonensis*) may be added as a preservative. The alkaloid and phenolic compounds which are extracted into the wine have antimicrobial effect.

Preparation of raw materials

Sap is collected by tapping the palm. Tapping is achieved by making an incision between the kernels and a gourd is tied around to collect the sap which is collected a day or two later. The fresh palm juice is a sweet, clear, colourless juice containing 10–12 per cent sugar and is neutral. The quality of the final wines is determined mostly by the conditions used in the collection of the sap. Often the collecting gourd is not washed between collections and residual yeasts in the gourd quickly begin the fermentation.

Processing

The sap is not heated and the wine is an excellent substrate for microbial growth. It is, therefore, essential that proper hygienic collection procedures are followed to prevent contaminating bacteria from competing with the yeast and producing acid instead of alcohol. Fermentation starts soon after the sap is collected and within an hour or two, the sap becomes reasonably high in alcohol (up to 4 per cent). If allowed to continue to ferment for more than a day, the sap begins turning into vinegar, although the vinegary flavour is preferred by some.

Organisms responsible include *S. cerevisiae*, and *Schizosaccharomyces pombe*, and the bacteria *Lactobacillus plantarum* and *L. mesenteroides*. There are reports that the yeasts and bacteria originate from the gourd, palm tree, and tapping implements. However the high sugar content of the juice would seem to selectively favour the growth of yeasts which might originate from the air. This is supported by the fact that fermentation also takes place in plastic containers.

Within 24 hours the initial pH is reduced from 7.4–6.8 to 5.5 and the alcohol content ranges from 1.5 to 2.1 per cent. Within 72 hours the alcohol levels increase from 4.5 to 5.2 per cent and the pH is 4.0. Organic acids present are lactic acid, acetic acid and tartaric acid.

The main control points are extraction of a high yield of palm sap without excessive contamination by spoilage micro-organisms, and proper storage to allow natural fermentation to take place. Process of fermented palm wine is shown in Fig. 18.5.

Packaging and storage

Packaging is usually only required to keep the product for its relatively short shelf-life. Clean glass or plastic bottles should be used. The product should be kept in a cool place away from direct sunlight.

Toddy

Throughout Asia, particularly India and Sri Lanka. Toddy is an alcoholic drink made by the fermentation of the sap from a coconut palm. It is white and sweet with a characteristic flavour. It is between 4 and 6 per cent alcohol and has a shelf-life of about 24 hours.

Preparation of raw materials

The sap is collected by slicing off the tip of an unopened flower. The sap oozes out and can be collected in a small pot tied underneath the flower.

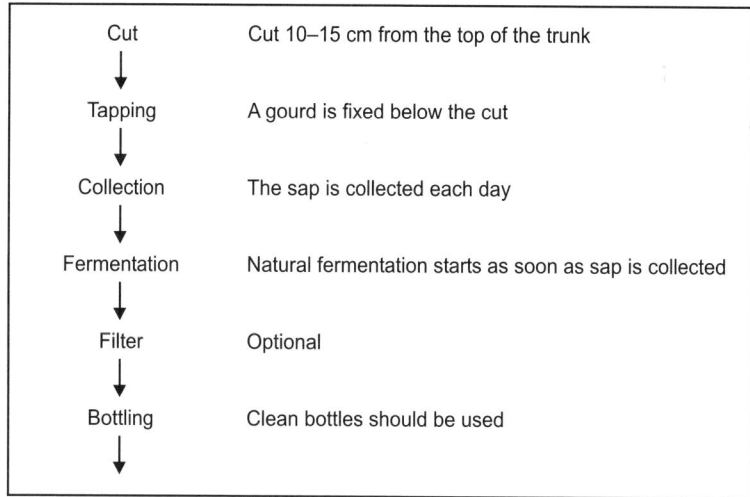

Fig. 18.5. Process of fermented palm wine.

Processing

The fermentation starts as soon as the sap collects in the pots on the palms, particularly if a small amount of toddy is left in the pots. The toddy is fully fermented in six to eight hours. The product is usually sold immediately due to its short shelf-life. Process of fermented toddy is shown in Fig. 18.6.

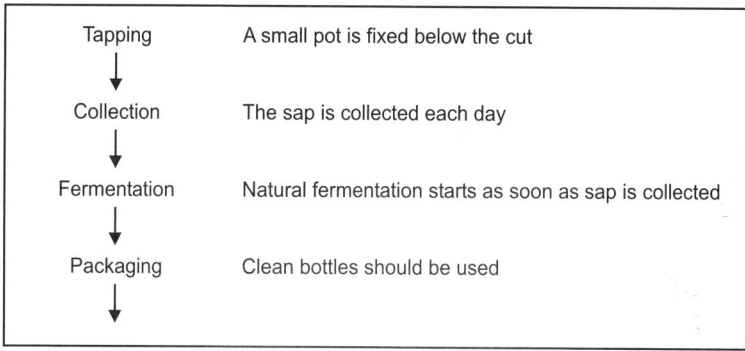

Fig. 18.6. Process of fermented toddy.

Packaging and storage

Packaging is usually only required to keep the product for its relatively short shelf-life. This is usually clean glass or plastic bottles. The product should be kept in a cool place away from direct sunlight.

Pulque

Pulque is the national drink in Mexico, where, it is claimed, it originated with the early Aztecs. Pulque is a traditional beverage that now forms the basis of a national industry, together with the spirits mezcal and tequila that are obtained from it. Pulque plays an important role in the nutrition of low income people in Mexico with B vitamins being present in nutritionally important levels.

Pulque is a milky, slightly foamy, acidic and somewhat viscous beverage. It is obtained by fermentation of aguamiel, which is the name given to the juices of various cacti, notably *Agave atrovirens* and *A. americana* which are often called the 'Century plant' in English. The alcohol content on pulque varies between six and seven per cent.

The beverage obtained upon distilling pulque is called 'Mezcal', and if manufactured in the Tequila region from a numbered distillery, it is referred to as 'Tequila'. The drink is often considered an aphrodisiac. The name Ticyaol is given to a good strain that makes one particularly virile. Pulque is frequently the potion of choice used by women during menstruation.

Preparation of raw materials

The juices are extracted from the plants when they are eight to ten years old and fermentation takes place spontaneously, although occasionally the juices are inoculated with a starter from previous fermentations.

Processing

The juice is allowed to ferment naturally through a mixed fermentation although yeast (*Saccharomyces carbajali*) is the main actor. *Lactobacillus plantarum* produces lactic acid and the viscosity of pulque is caused by the activity of two species of *Leuconostoc* which produce dextrans. During fermentation of the juices of the plant, the soluble solids are reduced from between 25–30 per cent to 6 per cent; the pH falls from 7.4 to between 3.5 and 4.0; the sucrose content falls from 15 to 1 per cent and vitamin levels are increased.

For instance the vitamin content (milligrams of vitamins per 100 g of product) increases from 5 to 29 for thiamine, 54 to 55 for niacin and 18 to 33 for riboflavin.

Packaging and storage

Packaging is only required to keep the product for its relatively short shelf-life. Clean glass or plastic bottles should be used. The product should be kept in a cool place away from direct sunlight.

Ulanzi (Bamboo wine)

Ulanzi is a fermented bamboo sap obtained by tapping young bamboo shoots during the rainy season. It is a clear, whitish drink with a sweet and alcoholic flavour.

Preparation of raw materials

The bamboo shoots should be young in order to obtain a high yield of sap. The growing tip is removed and a container fixed in place to collect the sap. The container should be clean in order to prevent contamination of the fresh sap.

Processing

The raw material is an excellent substrate for microbial growth and fermentation begins immediately after collection. Fermentation takes between five and twelve hours depending on the strength of the final product desired.

Packaging and storage

Packaging is usually only required to keep the product for its relatively short shelf-life.

Basi (sugar cane wine)

Basi is a sugar cane wine made in the Philipppines by fermenting boiled, freshly extracted, sugar cane juice. A dried powdered starter is used to initiate the fermentation. The mixture is allowed to ferment for up to three months, and to age for up to one year. The final product is light brown in colour and has a sweet and a sour flavour. A similar product called *shoto sake* is made in Japan.

Muratina

Muratina is an alcoholic drink made from sugar cane and *muratina* fruit in Kenya. The fruit is cut in half, sun dried and boiled in water. The water is removed and the fruit is again sun dried. The fruit is added to a small amount of sugar cane juice and incubated in a warm place for 24 hours, after which it is removed and sun dried. The dried fruit is then added to a barrel of sugar cane juice which is allowed to ferment for between one and four days. The final product has a sour alcoholic taste.

Winemaking critical control points

1. Cold soak.
2. Mid-fermentation.
3. End of primary fermentation.
4. Mid-malolactic fermentation.
5. Completion of MLF.
6. Topping wine.
7. Barrel ageing.
8. Final bottling blend.
9. Bottled wine.

Wine defects caused by yeast and bacteria

1. Yeast:
   (a) Ethyl acetate.
   (b) Sulphides.
   (c) Aldehydes.
   (d) 4-ethyl phenol/4-ethyl guiaicol.
2. Bacteria:
   (a) Acetic acid (VA).
   (b) Biogenic amines.
   (c) Mousy.
   (d) Geranium.

Wine spoilage ecology

1. Yeast and bacteria live/work together.
   (a) Beneficial.
   (b) Spoilage.
2. Spoilage is typically caused by more than one organism (spoilage consortium).
   (a) Perceived spoilage is often a blend of metabolites from several organisms.
3. Some microbes can serve as 'indicators' of potential spoilage.

Spoilage microbes

1. *Acetobacter* sp./*Gluconobacter* sp.

2. *Pediococcus* spp.
3. *Lactobacillus* spp.
4. *Brettanomyces bruxellensis*.
5. *Zygosaccharomyces bailii*.
6. Wild (apiculate) yeast.
7. *Saccharomyces cerevisiae*.
8. *Oenococcus oeni*.

Example: Lactobacillus

Methods

1. Sense of smell.
2. Plating.
3. Tasting.
4. VA measure.

Benefits of microscopy

1. Rapid time to results.
2. Effective for cell counting.
3. Viability estimates.
4. Low cost per sample.
5. Easy to use methods.

LACTIC ACID BACTERIA AND WINE SPOILAGE

Lactic acid bacteria (LAB) are responsible for many fermented foods such as sauerkraut, pickles and yogurt. They have also been isolated from wines at various states of vinification. In wines they are responsible for malolactic fermentation (MLF) which can be beneficial in some cases and undesirable in others.

Besides conducting MLF, these bacteria under certain conditions can also cause undesirable changes in wine flavour which renders the wine undrinkable. Many species of LAB do not conduct MLF and their growth in wine can cause some serious wine spoilage.

Nature of Lactic Acid Bacteria

Lactic acid bacteria found in wine belong to three genera, namely:

1. *Leuconostoc*—Heterofermentative cocci, oval or spherical, occur in pairs or chains.
2. *Pediococcus*—Homofermentative cocci, often found in tetrads.
3. *Lactobacillus*—Homofermentative or heterofermentative rods, found singly or in chains.

These organisms are Gram-positive, catalase-negative, nonsporing cocci, coccobacilli or rods. They are microaerophilic that means they grow well under conditions of low oxygen content. Since they can grow under low oxygen conditions, they can grow throughout the wine (as opposed to on the surface of the wine) even though the container is kept full.

The bacteria can metabolise sugars, acids and other constituents in wine and produce several compounds. Some of these are undesirable and constitute spoilage.

Source of Lactic Acid Bacteria

The bacteria can be found on the surface of grapes and grape leaves. During the harvest, the bacteria gain entry into the winery with the grapes. Their population on the surface of the fruit is generally low and it depends on the level of maturity and the condition of the fruit. Another source of these organisms in a winery is the contamination equipment. These may include pumps, valves and storage containers. Wooden barrels which are often difficult to clean and sanitise can be a source of these bacteria if the barrels contain MLF wine and were not properly cleaned.

Occurrence of Lactic Acid Bacteria at Various Stages of Vinification

At crush the bacterial population is small, about 10^3 to 10^4 cells/ml. Species belonging to genera *Lactobacillus*, *Pediococcus* and *Leuconostoc* have been found to occur at this stage. In the next stage, i.e. alcoholic fermentation, the population of these bacteria declines. This may be due to the competition by yeast and formation of ethanol and sulphur dioxide by the yeast during the alcoholic fermentation.

Following the alcoholic fermentation, the surviving bacteria grow vigorously and conduct MLF. The cell population can reach as high as 10^6 to 10^8 cells/ml. Usually species of Leuconostoc grow and conduct MLF but in the case of high pH wines (pH 3.5 and above), species of Pediococcus and Lactobacillus could be involved in MLF. After MLF the fate of lactic acid bacteria depends on wine composition and how the wine is handled. If the wine pH is high (>3.5), and the SO_2 level is inadequate, then the spoilage causing species of LAB can grow and spoil the wine. For this reason special attention should paid to the wines during storage after MLF.

Nature of Spoilage by Lactic Acid Bacteria

The nature and the extent of wine spoilage by LAB depends on several factors such as the type of bacteria, composition of the wine and vinification practices. Based on the substrate used lactic spoilage has been classified as follows:

1. Fermentation of sugars: LAB, including those involved in MLF, metabolise sugars such as glucose and fructose, and produce lactic acid and acetic acid. The resulting wine acquires a sour vinegar-like aroma due to high VA levels. This is a serious spoilage and occurs in must with stuck fermentation or wines with higher residual sugars (sweet wines). A less serious form of lactic spoilage can occur in dry wines. In these wines the LAB utilises pentose sugars, trace amounts of glucose and fructose, and produces lactic and acetic acid as a by-product. When sugars are attacked by LAB, lactic and acetic acids are produced. Formation of these acids increases the titratable acidity and lowers the pH. The decrease in pH restricts the growth of those organisms.

2. Degradation of glycerol: Breakdown of glycerol by LAB results in the formation of lactic acid, acetic acid and acrolein. The wine smells acetic, butyric and acquires a bitter taste due to acrolein.

3. Fermentation of tartaric acid: In this kind of spoilage, the LAB ferments tartaric acid and forms lactic acid, acetic acid and carbon dioxide. Degradation of tartaric acid occurs especially in wines with low acidity and high pH (pH above 3.5). The titratable acidity is further reduced and the wine acquires an acetic aroma and disagreeable taste. In advanced cases the wine is sometimes referred to as mousy.

4. Fermentation of citric acid: Citric acid content of a wine can decrease during MLF. Depending on the species of bacteria and the wine pH. Citric acid degradation has been positively correlated with the formation of diacetyl and acetone as well as acetic acid.

5. Ropiness: Certain species of *Leuconostoc* have been found to produce dextran slime or mucilaginous substances in wine. The wine appears oily and may not necessarily have high volatile acidity. In general, the lactic acid bacteria (as a group) are involved in the fermentation of malic acid and other wine constituents. Their activity results in the formation of several components that impart off flavours to wine. Some of the terms used in describing the lactic spoilage in wine include: acetic or sour, buttery, cheesy, sauerkraut-like, bitter, pickle aroma, mousy and geranium.

6. Other off aromas: Very unpleasant odours associated with lactic spoilage include mousy and geranium-like aromas. The mousy aroma has been attributed to the formation of a compound called acetyltetrahydropyridine. Two species of lactobacillus have been shown to produce these mousy odour compounds.

Sometimes a wine can develop a geranium-like odour which makes it undrinkable. This odour is caused by a compound known as 2-ethoxyhexa-3,5-diene. This compound is produced from the decomposition of sorbic acid by the LAB. In sweet wines sorbic acid is often added to prevent the growth of unwanted yeast (yeast growth can cause refermentation).

When the sorbic acid is attacked by LAB, 2-ethoxyhexa-3,5-diene is formed which imparts the geranium-like odour to the wine. To prevent this odour the growth of LAB in sweet wines containing sorbic acid should be controlled.

Factors Influencing the Growth of Lactic Acid Bacteria (LAB) in Wine

We have discussed the nature and extent of wine spoilage by LAB. In order to prevent wine spoilage by these micro-organisms, it is important to know the various factors that influence the growth of these microbes in wine so that one can manipulate these factors to reduce the risk of spoilage. The three important factors that deserve some consideration include:

1. Must/wine composition.
2. Vinification practices.
3. Interrelationships with other organisms.

Must/Wine composition

Wine pH

Wine pH is one of the most important factors influencing the growth of LAB. It affects the initiation and duration of malolactic fermentation MLF, it influences the type of species of bacteria that may develop in wine and it also affects the metabolic behaviour of the organism and thereby determines the kind of by-products formed as a result of bacterial activity. In the wine pH range of 3.0 to 4.0, the time needed for the completion of MLF decreases with an increase in pH. Bousbouras and Kunkee reported that at pH 3.15 it took 23.4 weeks to complete MLF; whereas at pH 3.83, it was completed in just two weeks.

Many researchers have noted the effect of pH on the species of bacteria that can grow in wine. Generally at pH below 3.5, the MLF is often dominated by *Leuconostoc*, whereas, above pH 3.5, species of *Pediococcus* and *Lactobacillus* seem to flourish. It should be noted here that many strains of *Lactobacillus* are involved in wine spoilage.

Another important pH effect not commonly realised is the effect of pH on the metabolic behaviour of the organisms. For example at pH 3.5 and above, LAB are more likely to decompose sugars, tartaric acid and citric acid. As mentioned earlier, fermentation of sugar leads to higher volatile acidity (VA) levels in wine.

From the foregoing discussion it should be obvious that controlling wine pH is one of the keys to controlling wine spoilage by LAB.

Sulphur dioxide (SO₂)

Sulphur dioxide is an effective germicide commonly used by the winemakers to control the growth of harmful bacteria. The SO_2 in wine exists in free and bound forms. All these forms remain in an equilibrium which is influenced by pH. Concentration of the molecular SO_2 form of free SO_2 which is also the most toxic form increases with a decrease in wine pH. Therefore, maintaining low pH is helpful in making SO_2 the most effective tool to control LAB. The bound form of SO_2 has also been reported to have a detrimental effect on LAB. In wine, SO_2 is bound to certain carbonyl compounds such as acetaldehyde. When LAB attacks the carbonyl compound, the bound SO_2 is released. It is this liberated free SO_2 that prevents further growth of the bacteria. SO_2 is an effective germicide and concentrations of 0.8 ppm molecular SO_2 will be adequate to control the growth of LAB in wine.

Alcohol

Generally LAB can survive and grow in table wines. There is some variation between various species regarding alcohol tolerance. For example; Lactobacillus trichods has been found in wine containing 20 per cent alcohol. The alcohol tolerance is influenced by pH and storage temperature.

Oxygen and carbon dioxide

Although microaerophilic conditions are desirable for the growth of LAB, the evidence suggests that a small amount of O_2 may be necessary. It is however, widely recognised that the presence of CO_2 stimulates the growth of LAB. This may be a factor stimulating MLF in wines left on the lees which would contain a fair amount of dissolved CO_2. Kelly, Asmudson, and Hopcroft concluded that this was likely due to low levels of O_2 as they observed the same effect using N_2.

Nutrients

LAB require a source of energy such as carbohydrates and inorganic salts. In addition they also need other growth factors such as vitamins and amino acids. Yeast autolysis (which occur during prolonged lees contact) resulting in increased nutrient content can render a young wine prone to attack by LAB.

Vinification practices

Many vinification practices can influence growth of LAB in a winery. Some of the important practices include: fruit condition, must treatment (adjustment), clarification, fermentation conditions, skin contact time (in case of red wine), lees contact, wine clarification, storage and winery sanitation.

Sound fruit has a low population of LAB on the surface, therefore, using clean and healthy fruit is important in reducing the number of microbes that would enter the winery at harvest. Sulphur dioxide is often added at the crush. It is one of the most effective measures in controlling the growth of LAB. Winemakers not sulphiting the must at crush in order to reduce sulphites in wine are taking a bigger risk in exposing their wines to bacterial spoilage. High pH musts usually contain low acid levels. The acidity and pH of such a must should be adjusted with tartaric acid additions before fermentation. This will enable fermentation to occur at low pH, and thus reduce the chances of spoilage by LAB. Clarifying white must by settling or other means reduces the suspended solids in the must. This practice is suggested for discouraging MLF in white wine.

Fermentation conditions affect the growth of LAB. For example, in case of a stuck fermentation, LAB can attack sugar and increase volatile acidity (VA) levels in wine. Controlling the fermentation so that it proceeds rapidly, evenly, and reaches dryness, is a sound enological practice to prevent any damage from LAB. A young wine left on the lees for a long time will be prone to MLF. This is due to the availability of nutrients released by yeast autolysis and a reduced CO_2 environment. For controlling LAB, early racking is recommended.

Wine clarification, especially using tight filter pads or a 0.45 micron membrane filter will reduce the bacterial population and consequently the chance of spoilage. Of all the winery practices, cleaning and sanitisation of equipment and containers is one of the most important practices that a winemaker must employ to control the wine spoilage.

Interrelationships with other organisms

LAB does not seem to grow well in must during alcoholic fermentation. It seems that yeast has an inhibitory effect on the growth of LAB. This could be due to several reasons such as competition and depletion of nutrients by yeast, competition by natural yeast flora (e.g. *Pichia*), formation of ethanol, SO_2 and other inhibitory compounds by the yeast. Contrary to the antagonistic effects of the yeast, there are however, some reports that suggest that yeast may have stimulatory influences on the growth of LAB. For example, prolonged contact with the lees can result in enrichment of young wine by yeast autolysis. This in turn can stimulate the growth of LAB.

Other micro-organisms such as *Botrytis cineria* and acetic acid bacteria have been reported to have a stimulating effect on LAB. LAB are often found in association with acetic acid bacteria and there is some evidence indicating a symbiotic relationship between these organisms. Bacteriophages are known to destroy the LAB. These phages have been isolated from wine. Not much is known about the inhibitory impact of these phages on LAB in wine and its influence on wine quality.

Recommendations to winemakers

Since LAB are involved in MLF as well as wine spoilage, a winemaker needs to decide up front whether to encourage MLF. If the choice is to encourage MLF (and avoid spoilage), then the following recommendations should be followed and MLF must be conducted under controlled conditions.

1. Use clean, healthy and high acid fruit.
2. Add a small dose of SO_2 at crush. (About 25–30 ppm based on must pH.)
3. Adjust the must pH if necessary. A pH range of 3.3 to 3.5 is desirable for MLF. Since MLF causes an increase in pH, it is advisable to conduct MLF at the lowest must pH as practically possible.
4. Inoculate the must with a pure starter culture of ML bacteria. The preferred time of inoculation is the 2nd or 3rd day after the alcoholic fermentation has begun. Low ethanol, low SO_2 and warm fermentation conditions favour MLF.
5. Take precautions to avoid a stuck fermentation. This would include not using overripe or mouldy grapes, using a good dose of vigorously growing, pure culture of yeast, adding yeast nutrient and maintaining controlled temperature conditions. Do not allow fermentation temperature to exceed about 30°C or 86°F.
6. Monitor MLF and as soon as it is completed, treat the wine to prevent further growth of any LAB.

If the winemaker's choice is not to encourage MLF then the following recommendations should be followed as a guide to prevent MLF as well as spoilage due to LAB:

1. Use sound fruit for making wine.

2. Add SO_2 at crush, about 50 to 75 ppm based on must pH.
3. In a low acid and high pH must, add tartaric acid to bring the pH to 3.3 or lower.
4. In the case of white wine, clarify the must (reduce suspended solids) before fermentation.
5. Control fermentation temperature. Use well prepared, pure culture yeast starter. Use yeast nutrient if needed.
6. In the case of red wine, prevent must temperature from exceeding 85°F. Punching the cap and keeping the cap moist is important.
7. After the must is fermented dry, promptly rack the wine off the lees and add enough SO_2 to attain 0.8 ppm molecular SO_2 level.
8. Clarify and stabilise the wine and store in clean containers.
9. Clean and sanitise equipment and containers before processing the wine.
10. Sterile filter and store wine at cool cellar temperatures.

Chapter 19

Miscellaneous Fermented Food Products

INTRODUCTION

Generally, a significant increase in the soluble fraction of a food is observed during fermentation. The quantity as well as quality of the food proteins as expressed by biological value, and often the content of watersoluble vitamins is generally increased, while the antinutritional factors show a decline during fermentation. Fermentation results in a lower proportion of dry matter in the food and the concentrations of vitamins, minerals and protein appear to increase when measured on a dry weight basis. Single as well as mixed culture fermentation of pearl millet flour with yeast and lactobacilli significantly increased the total amount of soluble sugars, reducing and nonreducing sugar content, with a simultaneous decrease in its starch content. Combination of cooking and fermentation improved the nutrient quality of all tested sorghum seeds and reduced the content of antinutritional factors to a safe level in comparison with other methods of processing. Mixed culture fermentation of pearl millet flour with *Saccharomyces diastaticus*, *Saccharomyces cerevisiae*, *Lactobacillus brevis* and *Lactobacillus fermentum* was found to improve its biological utilisation in rats. Most traditional fermented food products are made by a complex interaction of different micro-organisms. This chapter deals with the products made when there is not a single dominant set of micro-organisms.

VINEGAR

Vinegar is the product of a mixed fermentation of yeast followed by acetic acid bacteria. Vinegar, literally translated as sour wine, is one of the oldest products of fermentation used by man. It is the acetic acid produced by the fermentation of alcohol (ethanol) which gives the characteristic flavour and aroma to vinegar.

It can be made from almost any fermentable carbohydrate source, for example fruits, vegetables, syrups and wine. The basic requirement for vinegar production is a raw material that will undergo an alcoholic fermentation. Apples, pears, grapes, honey, syrups, cereals, hydrolysed starches, beer and wine are all ideal substrates for the production of vinegar. To produce a high quality product it is essential that the raw material is mature, clean and in good condition.

Indigenous vinegars can be made quite simply by the spontaneous fermentation of a fruit or alcohol. All that is necessary is an alcoholic substrate, strains of acetic-acid forming bacteria (*acetobacter*) and oxygen to enable the oxidation of alcohol. However, this process is very slow and vinegars produced by this method tend to be of inferior quality. Controlled fermentation conditions produce a more acceptable product. A wide range of raw materials can be made into vinegar.

Coconut Water Vinegar

A clear liquid with a distinctive acetic acid taste with a hint of a coconut flavour.

Raw material preparation

Coconut water is a waste product, which is produced in appreciable quantities in the Philippines, Sri Lanka, Thailand and other countries. Its conversion into vinegar therefore presents an attractive option for decreasing wastage and producing a valuable product.

Processing

Coconut water is a good base for vinegar, but its sugar content is too low (only about 1 per cent). Sugar needs to be added to bring the level of sugar up to 15 per cent. After the addition of sugar, the coconut juice is allowed to ferment for about seven days, during which time the sugar is converted to alcohol. An alternative method is to pasteurise the coconut water and sugar mixture and add yeast.

After this initial fermentation, strong vinegar (10 per cent v/v) is added to stimulate the growth of acetic acid bacteria and discourage further yeast fermentation. The acetic acid fermentation takes approximately one month, yielding a vinegar with approximately 6 per cent acetic acid. The fermentation will take less time than this if a generator is used. After fermentation, the vinegar must be stored in anaerobic conditions to prevent spoilage by the oxidation of acetic acid.

Clarification can be achieved by stirring with a well beaten egg white, heating until the egg white coagulates and filtering.

Pineapple Peel Vinegar

This product enables the utilisation of pineapple peels, which are usually discarded during the processing or consumption of the fruit. The product has a distinct, very light pineapple flavour and has the same uses as any commercial vinegar.

Raw material preparation

The peels should be from very well washed ripe pineapples (damaged, rotten or infected fruits should not be used as a source of peels). Use only the peels, not the leaves or stems. The water used should be potable water, boiled if necessary. All the equipment should be well cleaned, as well as the bottles, which should also be steam-sterilised before use.

Processing

The peels should be cut into thin strips and put into clay or pewter pots. Aluminium or iron pots should not be used. Sugar and clean water are added. Each pot is then inoculated and covered with a clean cotton cloth, held around the pot with an adhesive tape, to prevent contamination by insects or dust. The inoculated pineapple is fermented at room temperature (about 20°–22°C) for about eight days. The acidity should be checked daily. The water level should be maintained during this period. The product should be increasingly acid and by the eighth day it should have the required concentration of 4 per cent acetic acid in vinegar.

If higher acidity is desired the product is left to ferment for another one or two days. The development of acidity should be checked by tasting the product during fermentation. The residual bacteria removed may be reused as a residue inoculum two or three times more.

The traditional process may be improved by a two-stage fermentation in which alcohol is first formed by yeast (*Saccharomyces cerevisiae*) and the 'must' is then inoculated with acetic acid bacteria

(*Acetobacter pasteurianus*). In outline, the process involves liquidising the peels and diluting with water (water:pulp is 4:1), adjusting the pH to 4.0 using sodium bicarbonate and adding yeast nutrient (ammonium phosphate) at 0.14 g per litre. A starter culture is added at 2.7 g per litre and the fermentation allowed to take place at 25°C for two days.

The 'must' is then filtered and inoculated with acetic acid bacteria and allowed to ferment for eleven days with aeration of the 'must'. Other parts of the process are similar. Additional equipment includes a pH meter, refractometer, liquidiser, fermentation locks and equipment for preparing the starter cultures. Process of fermented pineapple peel vinegar is shown in Fig. 19.1.

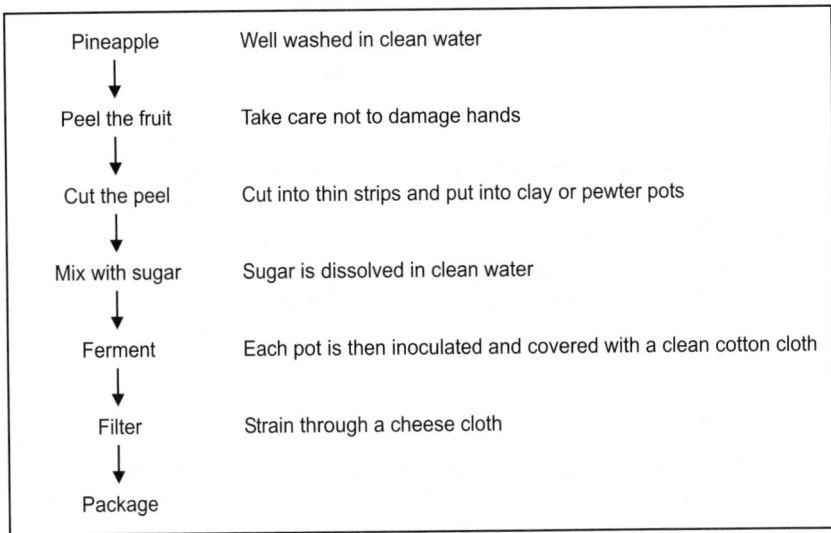

Fig. 19.1. Process of fermented pineapple peel vinegar.

Packaging and storage

The vinegar is bottled in clean glass bottles and stored in a cool dark place.

Palm Wine Vinegar

Palm wine vinegar is a produced across West Africa. It is a vinegar containing about 4 per cent acetic acid, produced from the oxidation of palm wine. It is mainly consumed by people in urban areas as a salad dressing and meat tenderiser, although it also has medicinal uses and is valued in certain rituals. Palm wine is fermented using the same process as for grape wine vinegar—the oxidation of alcohol to acetic acid. The spontaneous process takes about four days. The optimum fermentation temperature is 30°C.

Coconut Toddy Vinegar

Coconut toddy vinegar is produced throughout South Asia particularly Sri Lanka. It is a clear liquid with a strong acetic acid flavour and a hint of coconut flavour. The fresh toddy is strained, prior to allowing yeast fermentation to occur naturally for 48 to 72 hours. The yeast cells and debris are then removed by progressive sedimentation. After two to four weeks of settling the fermented toddy is placed in barrels. The alcohol is then converted into acetic acid by acetic acid bacteria which are naturally present. The process can be hastened by adding vinegar as a starter. The fermented toddy is converted into vinegar in about three months. Ageing for six months, results in a pleasantly flavoured final product.

Quick process pickles

Quick process pickles are easy to make but do not really constitute a fermented food product. For this technique, vegetables are soaked in a low salt solution for a few hours. They are then drained and placed in a container. The container is filled with a hot vinegar and spice mixture or a hot oil and spice mixture. There are hundreds of different recipes utilising locally available fruit and vegetables.

COCOA PRODUCTS

Cocoa Powder

A fine brown powder with the characteristic taste of cocoa. It is a major ingredient in the confectionery and bakery industries. The product has a short shelf-life. 'Drinking chocolate' is a mixture of cocoa powder and sugar.

Raw material preparation

Cocoa beans are the seeds of the cocoa plant (*Theobroma cacao*). Cocoa pods are cut from the cocoa tree. The pods are cut and the beans removed. Only fully ripe and undamaged beans should be selected. It is important that the beans are processed quickly.

Processing

It was formerly believed that cocoa beans were fermented to remove the adhering pulp. However a good flavour in the final cocoa or chocolate is dependent on good fermentation. Fermentation is carried out in a variety of ways but all depend on heaping a quantity of fresh beans with their pulp and allowing micro-organisms to produce heat. The majority of beans are fermented in heaps although better results are obtained using boxes, which result in a more even fermentation.

Fermentation lasts from five to six days. During the first day the adhering pulp is liquified and drains away with the temperature rising steadily. The initial alcoholic fermentation gives way to acetification. This and other chemical changes cause the temperature to rise in excess of 50°C. The beans die. It was thought in the past that death was mainly due to increasing temperature. It is now known that acetic acid at a concentration of 1 per cent in the bean is the cause of death and that it is only enhanced by heat, lactic acid and ethanol. The pH value of the cotyledon drops from 6.45 to 4.5 over 120 hours and that during the same period the acetic acid content increased from 0 to 1.36 per cent, while the lactic acid content increased from 0.005 to 0.12 per cent. When the bean dies maceration of the tissue takes place, allowing enzymes and substrate to mix freely. The possible substrates for enzymes are carbohydrates, lipids, phenolics and amino acids. In addition it is known that the bacteria can metabolise alcohols and organic acids of various kinds. The changing chemical picture is complex. Possible major substrates for micro-organisms are carbohydrates, lipids, phenolics and amino acids. Unlike some flavours and aromas, that of chocolate is not attributable to a single compound.

During fermentation the external appearance of the beans changes. At first they are pinkish with a covering of white mucilage. Gradually the colour darkens and the mucilage disappears. The beans on the surface are always darker than those deeper in the heap or box, indicating that the colour change is oxidative. As the beans are mixed, their colour becomes a more uniform orange-brown and they are only slightly sticky. At this stage they are ready for drying.

The beans need to be dried to a moisture content of less than 7.5 per cent. The beans are dried by either being spread out in the sun in layers a few centimetres thick or in artificial dryers. There are numerous types of dryers but it is important that any smoky products of combustion do not come in contact with the beans otherwise taints will appear in the final product. The beans are cleaned to remove the extraneous matter.

Cocoa beans consist of an outer skin that needs to be removed and inner 'nib'. The shell is sometimes removed before roasting and sometimes after roasting.

For cocoa powder roasting temperatures of 120° to 150°C are used. There are many designs of roasters: both batch and continuous systems. The operation is controlled so that the cocoa is heated to the required temperature without burning the shell or the cotyledon. The heat is applied evenly over a long period of up to 90 minutes to produce even roasting. The bean must not be contaminated with any combustion products from the fuel used and provision must be made for the escape of any volatile acids, water vapour and decomposition products of the bean. After roasting the beans are cooled quickly to prevent scorching. The roasted nibs are ground into a powder in a plate mill. The resulting powder is sieved through fine silk, nylon or wire mesh.

To produce cocoa powder, some of the cocoa butter needs to be removed. With low fat cocoa powder, more than 90 per cent of the cocoa butter is removed. With medium fat cocoa powder, more than 78 per cent of the cocoa butter has been removed. Finally high fat cocoa powder has less than 78 per cent of the cocoa butter removed. Extrusion, expeller or screw presses are used in the cocoa industry to remove the cocoa. The cake from the mill is ground in a hammer mill to produce the cocoa powder. Process of fermented cocoa powder is shown in Fig. 19.2.

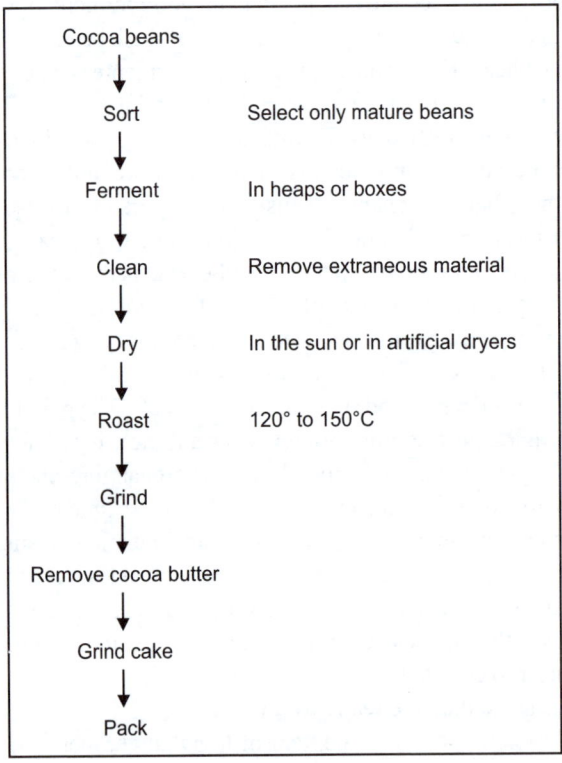

Fig. 19.2. Process of fermented cocoa powder.

Packaging and storage

Cocoa powder is hygroscopic (picks up moisture from the air) and should be protected, especially in humid climates. Lidded tins or sealed polythene bags should be used.

Chocolate

A brown solid oily product with the characteristic taste of chocolate. It is a major ingredient in the confectionery and bakery industries.

Preparation of raw materials

Cocoa beans are the seeds of the cocoa plant (*Theobroma cacao*). Cocoa pods are cut from the trees, and the beans are removed from the pods. Only fully ripe and undamaged beans should be selected. It is important that the beans are processed quickly.

Processing

Fermentation, drying and cleaning of the beans have been described already. For cocoa butter production the roasting temperatures are 100° to 104°C. There are many designs of roasters: both batch and continuous systems. The operation is controlled so that the cocoa is heated to the required temperature without burning the shell or the cotyledon. The heat is applied evenly over a long period of up to 90 minutes to produce even roasting; the nib must not be contaminated with any combustion products from the fuel used and provision must be made for the escape of any volatile acids, water vapour and decomposition products of the nib. After roasting the beans are cooled quickly to prevent scorching.

Roasting will have already loosened the shell. The beans are then lightly crushed with the object of preserving large pieces of shell and nib and avoiding the creation of small particles and dust. The cocoa bean without its shell is known as a 'cocoa nib'. The valuable part of the cocoa bean is the nib, the outer shell being a waste material of little value.

Alkalisation is a treatment that is sometimes used before and sometimes after grinding to modify the colour and flavour of the product. This was developed in the Netherlands in the last century and is sometimes known as 'Dutching'. This involves soaking the nib or the cocoa mass in potassium or sodium carbonate. By varying the ratio of alkali to nib, a wide range of colours of cocoa powder can be produced. Complete nib penetration may take an hour. After alkalisation the cocoa needs to be dried slowly. The cocoa nib is ground into 'cocoa liquor' (also known as 'unsweetened chocolate' or 'cocoa mass'). The grinding process generates heat and the dry granular consistency of the nib is turned into a liquid as the high amount of fat contained in the nib melts.

There are various pretreatments to develop the flavour of the cocoa mass with and without reaction solutions. These include the 'Luwa thin-layer evaporator', 'Petzomat thin-layer process', 'Cocovap process', 'Lehman KFA process' and 'Carle-Montanari process'.

Extrusion, expeller, or screw presses are used in the cocoa industry for the production of cocoa butter from whole beans, and mixtures of fine nib dusts, small nibs, and immature beans. Research in the Kerala Agricultural University has led to develop a suitable pressure device capable of separating cocoa butter from ground cocoa mass ideally suitable for small scale manufacturers. In Peru a simple screw press is used to extract cocoa butter from beans. The crude cocoa butter is filtered through cloth and allowed to solidify.

To produce plain chocolate, cocoa mass is mixed with sugar and sufficient cocoa butter to enable the chocolate to be moulded. The ratio of mass to sugar varies according to the national taste. The mixture is ground to such a degree that the chocolate is smooth to the palate. At one time this was done by a lengthy process in melengeurs—heavy granite rollers in a revolving granite bed—but nowadays grinding is done in a series of rolls. The chocolate is then 'Conched'. This may last for several hours. The chocolate is heated, this helps to drive off volatile acids, thereby reducing acidity when present in the raw bean, and the process finishes the development of flavour and makes the chocolate homogeneous. Similar processes are involved in the manufacture of milk chocolate. The milk is added in various ways either in powder form to the mixture of mass, sugar and cocoa butter or by condensing first with sugar, adding the mass and drying this mixture under vacuum. The product is called 'crumb' and this is ground and conched in a similar manner to plain chocolate. After conching the chocolate has to be tempered before it is used for moulding or for enrobing confectionery centres. Tempering involves cooling and reaching the right physical state for rapid setting after moulding or enrobing.

COFFEE

A fine dark brown powder made from roasted coffee beans. Brewed with boiling water and consumed as a drink.

Raw Material Preparation

Coffee beans are harvested from two plants *Coffea arabica* and *Coffea canephora* variety *robusta*. Only ripe berries should be used in coffee production. Berries can be placed in water so that immature berries which float can be identified and discarded.

Processing

Dry processing is the simpler of the two processing methods and is popular in Brazil for the processing of *Robusta* coffee and in Sri Lanka for processing *Arabica* coffee. The coffee cherries are dried immediately after harvest by sun drying on a clean dry floor or on mats. The dried berry is then hulled to remove the pericarp. This can be done by hand using a pestle and mortar or in a mechanical huller. The mechanical hullers usually consist of a steel screw, the pitch of which increases as it approaches the outlet so removing the pericarp. The hulled coffee is cleaned by winnowing.

Wet processing involves squeezing the berry in a pulping machine or pounding in a pestle and mortar to remove the outer fleshy material (mesocarp and exocarp) and leave the bean covered in mucilage. This mucilage is removed by fermentation. Fermentation involves placing the beans in plastic buckets or tanks and allowing them to sit, until the mucilage is broken down. Natural enzymes in the mucilage and yeasts and bacteria in the environment work together to break down the mucilage. The coffee should be stirred occasionally and ever so often a handful of beans should be tested by washing in water. If the mucilage can be washed off and the beans feel gritty rather than slippery, the beans are ready. There is much debate about the fermentation of coffee beans. Some researchers feel that the mucilage breakdown is caused by enzymatic breakdown. For instance Wellman has stated that enymatic fermentation starts immediately the beans have been squeezed from the fresh berries. If these 'pulped' beans are piled up or put in a container and protected from any bacterial or other contamination the fermentation will progress. After a number of hours the enzymes of the pulp will have acted on the torn tissues, gorged with starches, sugars and pectins, in such a manner that, without any microbial intervention, the remaining pulp will be easily detached from the beans and washed off in water. However most investigators acknowledge the necessity for the presence of micro-organisms for the depectinisation of the beans.

The following micro-organisms have been isolated: *Leuconostoc mesenteroides*; *Lactobacillus plantarum*; *Lactobacillus brevis*, *Streptococcus faecalis*, *Aerobacter* (*Enterobacter*) and *Escherichia*, pectinolytic species of *Bacillus*, *Saccharomyces marscianus*, *S. bayanus* and a *Flavobacterium* sp., *Erwinia dissolvens*, *Fusarium* spp., *Aspergillus* spp. and *Penicillium*.

The beans should then be washed immediately as 'off' flavours develop quickly. To prevent cracking the coffee beans should be dried slowly to 10 per cent moisture content (wet basis). Drying should take place immediately after to prevent 'off' flavours developing. The same drying methods can be used for this as for the dry processed coffee.

After drying the coffee should be rested for 8 hours in a well ventilated place. The thin parchment around the coffee is removed either by hand, in a pestle and mortar or in a small huller. The hulled coffee is cleaned by winnowing.

The final flavour of the coffee is heavily dependent on how the beans are roasted. Roasting is a time temperature dependent process. The roasting temperature needs to be about 200°C. The degree of roast is usually assessed visually. One method is to watch the thin white line between the two sides of the bean, when this starts to go brown the coffee is ready. As preferences vary considerably from region to region, a lot of research will need to be done to find the locally acceptable degree of roast. Coffee beans can be roasted in a saucepan as long as they are continually stirred. A small improvement is made by roasting the coffee in sand, as this provides a more even heat. A roaster will produce a higher quality product. Grinding is a means of adding value to a product. However, it is fraught with difficulties. It is easy to make an assessment of an intact bean, while a ground product presents some difficulty. The fear of adulteration and the use of low quality produce is justified. Because of this there is a great deal of market resistance to ground coffee.

This market resistance can only be overcome by consistently producing a good product. There are basically two types of grinders—manual grinders and motorised grinders. Process of fermented coffee is shown in Fig. 19.3.

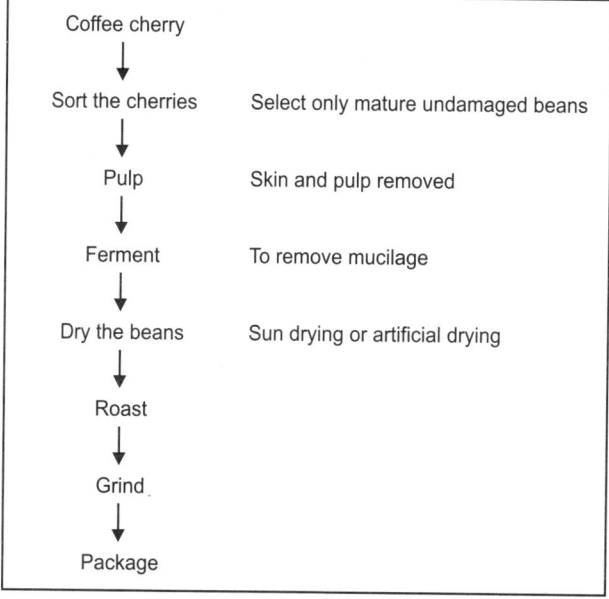

Fig. 19.3. Process of fermented coffee.

Packaging and storage

Roasted beans can be stored in sacks. Milled beans need to be packaged quickly to prevent the loss of volatile flavour components. The packaging material should be airtight. Polythene is not suitable as it is a low barrier to loss of aroma.

OTHER MIXED FERMENTATION PRODUCTS

Vanilla

Vanilla is produced in Madagascar, Indonesia and various South Pacific islands. It is a dark brown pod about 20 cm in length. Vanilla is produced by fermenting the pods of the orchids of the genus vanilla. The pods are first sun dried for 24 to 36 hours and then blanched in hot water (65°C) for two to three minutes. The pods are then fermented in boxes and dried again.

Tabasco

Tabasco sauce is made in Mexico and Guatemala. The chilli pods are harvested, ground into a paste and placed in a container with salt. The hot and fiery sauce develops.

Tea

In the production of tea, there is a process referred to as fermentation. However microbial activity is not involved in the so-called 'fermentation' of tea. The chemical changes are effected by enzymes alone. Fermentation rooms are used where moisture and temperature can be controlled. During fermentation even further darkening of the leaf occurs and the typical aroma develops. By subjective judgement of the aroma's intensity the period necessary for completion is gauged.

FERMENTED VEGETABLES

Fermented vegetables are made with lactic acid bacteria, which is a valuable technique humans have been using for thousands of years. This preservation method has numerous health advantages. Fermented vegetables are rich in nutrients, fibre and digestion-enhancing enzymes. They also help the intestinal tract maintain a healthy balance of flora by increasing beneficial bacteria. The simple and natural process of lactic acid fermentation now is being rediscovered, especially by those who are aware of the failures of the modern diet. One only has to observe health statistics briefly to become aware that the American diet must change if we are to live full and productive lives. The consumption of fermented vegetables addresses numerous dietary and health issues simultaneously. You're probably familiar with sauerkraut—its the most common fermented vegetable product. There are several reasons for sauerkraut's popularity; consider its unique taste, legendary nutritional and medicinal properties and the ease with which its made. Sauerkraut barely begins to tell the story of fermented foods—a story that repeats itself around the globe, from the pungent flavour of Korea's kimchi to Tanzania's fermented gruel, togwa.

Sauerkraut

Sauerkraut, directly translated from German: 'sour herb' or 'sour cabbage', is finely shredded cabbage that has been fermented by various lactic acid bacteria, including *Leuconostoc*, *Lactobacillus*, and *Pediococcus*. It has a long shelf-life and a distinctive sour flavour, both of which result from the lactic acid that forms when the bacteria ferment the sugars in the cabbage. It is, therefore, not to be confused with coleslaw, which receives its acidic taste from vinegar.

Producing sauerkraut

Sauerkraut is made by a process of pickling called lacto-fermentation that is analogous to how traditional (not heat-treated) pickled cucumbers and kimchi are made. Fully-cured sauerkraut keeps for several months in an airtight container stored at or below 15°C (59°F). Neither refrigeration nor pasteurisation is required, although these treatments prolong storage life.

Fermentation by lactobacilli is introduced naturally, as these airborne bacteria culture on raw cabbage leaves where they grow. Yeasts also are present, and may yield soft sauerkraut of poor flavour when the fermentation temperature is too high. The fermentation process has three phases. In the first phase, anaerobic bacteria such as *Klebsiella* and *Enterobacter* lead the fermentation, and begin producing an acidic environment that favours later bacteria. The second phase starts as the acid levels become too high for many bacteria, and *Leuconostoc mesenteroides* and other *Leuconostoc* spp. take dominance. In the third phase, various *Lactobacillus* species, including *L. brevis* and *L. plantarum*, ferment any remaining sugars, further lowering the pH. There are unpasteurised sauerkrauts on the market. Properly cured sauerkraut is sufficiently acidic to prevent a favourable environment for the growth of *Clostridium botulinum*, the toxins of which cause botulism.

Health benefits

Health benefits have been claimed for raw sauerkraut. It contains vitamin C, lactobacilli, and other nutrients. However, the low pH and abundance of lactobacilli may upset the intestines of people who are not used to eating acidic foods.

Before frozen foods and the importation of foods from the Southern Hemisphere became readily available in northern and central Europe, sauerkraut provided a source of nutrients during the winter. Captain James Cook always took a store of sauerkraut on his sea voyages, since experience had taught him it prevented scurvy. German sailors continued this practice even after the British Royal Navy had switched to limes, earning the British sailor the nickname 'Limey' while his German counterpart became known as a 'Kraut'. Sauerkraut is also a source of biogenic amines, such as tyramine, which may cause adverse reactions in sensitive people. It also provides various cancer-fighting compounds including isothiocyanate and sulphoraphane.

Similar foods

There are many other vegetables that are preserved by a similar process:
1. Korean *kimchi*.
2. Japanese *tsukemono*.
3. Chinese *suan cai*.
4. Filipino *atchara*.

Also a feed for cattle, silage, is made the same way.

Salt for Pickling

For pickling any variety of common salt is suitable as long as it is pure. Impurities or additives can cause problems. Salt with chemicals to reduce caking should not be used as they make the brine cloudy. Salt with lime impurities can reduce the acidity of the final product and reduce the shelf-life of the product. Salt with iron impurities can result in the blackening of the vegetables. Magnesium impurities impart a bitter taste. Carbonates can result in pickles with a soft texture.

Dry salted fermented vegetables

With dry salting, the vegetable is treated with dry salt. The salt extracts the juice from the vegetable and creates the brine. The vegetable is prepared, washed in potable cold water and drained. For every 100 kg of vegetables 3 kg of salt is needed. The vegetables are placed in a layer of about 2.5 cm depth in the fermenting container (a barrel or keg). Salt is sprinkled over the vegetables. Another layer of vegetables is added and more salt added. This is repeated until the container is three quarters full. A cloth is placed above the vegetables and a weight added to compress the vegetables and assist the formation of a brine which takes about 24 hours. As soon as the brine is formed, fermentation starts and bubbles of carbon dioxide begin to appear. Fermentation takes between one and four weeks depending on the ambient temperature. Fermentation is complete when no more bubbles appear, after which time the pickle can be packaged in a variety of mixtures. These can be vinegar and spices or oil and spices.

Sauerkraut process

Lactic acid bacteria are the primary group of organisms involved in sauerkraut fermentation. They can be divided into three groups according to their types and end products:

Leuconostoc mesenteroides	An acid and gas producing coccus.
Lactobacillus plantarum and	Bacilli that produce acid and a small amount of gas.
L. cucumeris	
Lactobacillus pentoaceticus	Acid and gas producing bacilli.
(*L. Brevis*)	

In addition to the desirable bacteria there are a range of undesirable micro-organisms present on cabbage (and other vegetable material) which can interfere with the sauerkraut process if allowed to multiply unchecked. The quality of the final product depends largely on how well the undesirable organisms are controlled during the fermentation process. Some of the typical spoilage organisms utilise the protein as an energy source, producing unpleasant odours and flavours.

Fermentation process

Shredded cabbage or other suitable vegetables are placed in a jar and salt is added. Mechanical pressure is applied to the cabbage to expel the juice, which contains fermentable sugars and other nutrients suitable for microbial activity. The first micro-organisms to start acting are the gas-producing cocci (*L. mesenteroides*). These microbes produce acids. When the acidity reaches 0.25 to 0.3 per cent (calculated as lactic acid), these bacteria slow down and begin to die off, although their enzymes continue to function. The activity initiated by the *L. mesenteroides* is continued by the lactobacilli (*L. plantarum* and *L. cucumeris*) until an acidity level of 1.5 to 2 per cent is attained. The high salt concentration and low temperature inhibit these bacteria to some extent. Finally, *L. pentoaceticus* continues the fermentation, bringing the acidity to 2 to 2.5 per cent thus completing the fermentation.

The end products of a normal kraut fermentation are lactic acid along with smaller amounts of acetic and propionic acids, a mixture of gases of which carbon dioxide is the principal gas, small amounts of alcohol and a mixture of aromatic esters. The acids, in combination with alcohol form esters, which contribute to the characteristic flavour of sauerkraut. The acidity helps to control the growth of spoilage and putrefactive organisms and contributes to the extended shelf-life of the product. Changes in the sequence of desirable bacteria or indeed the presence of undesirable bacteria, alter the taste and quality of the product.

Effects of temperature on sauerkraut process

The optimum temperature for sauerkraut fermentation is around 21°C. A variation of just a few degrees from this temperature alters the activity of the microbial process and affects the quality of the final product. Therefore, temperature control is one of the most important factors in the sauerkraut process. A temperature of 18° to 22°C is most desirable for initiating fermentation since this is the optimum temperature range for the growth and metabolism of *L. mesenteroides*. Temperatures above 22°C favour the growth of *Lactobacillus* species.

Effects of salt on the sauerkraut process

Salt plays an important role in initiating the sauerkraut process and affects the quality of the final product. The addition of too much salt may inhibit the desirable bacteria, although it may contribute to the firmness of the kraut. The principle function of salt is to withdraw juice from the cabbage (or other vegetable), thus making a more favourable environment for development of the desired bacteria.

Generally, salt is added to a final concentration of 2.0 to 2.5 per cent. At this concentration, lactobacilli are slightly inhibited, but cocci are not affected. Unfortunately, this concentration of salt has a greater inhibitory effect against the desirable organisms than against those responsible for spoilage.

The spoilage organisms can tolerate salt concentrations up to between 5 and 7 per cent, therefore it is the acidic environment created by the lactobacilli that keep the spoilage bacteria at bay, rather than the addition of salt. In the manufacture of sauerkraut, dry salt is added at the rate if 1 to 1.5 kg per 50 kg cabbage (2 to 3 per cent). The use of salt brines is not recommended in sauerkraut making, but is common in vegetables that have a low water content. It is essential to use pure salt since salts with added alkali may neutralise the acid.

Use of starter cultures

In order to produce sauerkraut of consistent quality, starter cultures (similar to those used in the dairy industry) have been recommended. Not only do starter cultures ensure consistency between batches, they speed up the fermentation process as there is no time lag while the relevant microflora colonise the sample. Because the starter cultures used are acidic, they also inhibit the undesirable micro-organisms. It is possible to add starters traditionally used for milk fermentation, such as *Streptococcus lactis*, without adverse effect on final quality. Because these organisms only survive for a short time (long enough to initiate the acidification process) in the kraut medium, they do not disturb the natural sequence of micro-organisms. On the other hand, if *Leuconostoc mesenteroides* is added in the early stages, it gives a good flavour to the final product, but alters the sequence of subsequent bacterial growth and results in a product that is incompletely fermented.

If gas producing rods (for example *L. pentoaceticus*) are added to the sauerkraut, this disturbs the balance between acetic and lactic acids—more acetic acid and less lactic acid are produced than normal—and the fermentation never reaches completion. If lactic acid, non-gas producing rods (*L. cucumeris*) are used as a starter, again the kraut is not completely fermented and the resulting product is bitter and more susceptible to spoilage by yeasts.

It is possible to use the juice from a previous kraut fermentation as a starter culture for subsequent fermentations. The efficacy of using old juice depends largely on the types of organisms present in the juice and its acidity. If the starter juice has an acidity of 0.3 per cent or more, it results in a poor quality kraut. This is because the cocci which would normally initiate fermentation are suppressed by the high acidity, leaving the bacilli with sole responsibility for fermentation.

If the starter juice has an acidity of 0.25 per cent or less, the kraut produced is normal, but there do not appear to be any beneficial effects of adding this juice. Often, the use of old juice produces a sauerkraut which has a softer texture than normal.

Spoilage and defects in the sauerkraut process

The majority of spoilage in sauerkraut is due to aerobic soil micro-organisms which break down the protein and produce undesirable flavour and texture changes. The growth of these aerobes can easily be inhibited by a normal fermentation.

Soft kraut can result from many conditions such as large amounts of air, poor salting procedure and varying temperatures. Whenever the normal sequence of bacterial growth is altered or disturbed, it usually results in a soft product. It is the lactobacilli, which seem to have a greater ability than the cocci to break down cabbage tissues, which are responsible for the softening. High temperatures and a reduced salt content favour the growth of lactobacilli, which are sensitive to higher concentrations of salt. The usual concentration of salt used in sauerkraut production slightly inhibits the lactobacilli, but has no effect on the cocci. If the salt content is too low initially, the lactobacilli grow too rapidly at the beginning and upset the normal sequence of fermentation. Another problem encountered is the production of dark coloured sauerkraut. This is caused by spoilage organisms during the fermentation process. Several conditions favour the growth of spoilage organisms. For example, an uneven distribution of salt tends to inhibit the desirable organisms while at the same time allowing the undesirable salt tolerant organisms to flourish. An insufficient level of juice to cover the kraut during the fermentation allows undesirable aerobic bacteria and yeasts to grow on the surface of the kraut, causing off flavours and discolouration. If the fermentation temperature is too high, this also encourages the growth of undesirable microflora, which results in a darkened colour. Pink kraut is a spoilage problem. It is caused by a group of yeasts which produce an intense red pigment in the juice and on the surface of the cabbage. It is caused by an uneven distribution of or an excessive concentration of salt, both of which allow the yeast to multiply. If conditions are optimal for normal fermentation, these spoilage yeasts are suppressed.

Brine salted fermented vegetables

Brine is used for vegetables which inherently contain less moisture. A brine solution is prepared by dissolving salt in water (a 15 to 20 per cent salt solution). Fermentation takes place well in a brine of about 20 salometer. As a general guide, a fresh egg floats in a 10 per cent brine solution. Properly brined vegetables will keep well in vinegar for a long time. The duration of brining is important for the overall keeping qualities. The vegetable is immersed in the brine and allowed to ferment. The strong brine solution draws sugar and water out of the vegetable, which decreases the salt concentration. It is crucial that the salt concentration does not fall below 12 per cent, otherwise conditions do not allow for fermentation. To achieve this, extra salt is added periodically to the brine mixture.

Once the vegetables have been brined and the container sealed, there is a rapid development of micro-organisms in the brine. The natural controls which affect the microbial populations of the fermenting vegetables include the concentration of salt and temperature of the brine, the availability of fermentable materials and the numbers and types of micro-organisms present at the start of fermentation. The rapidity of the fermentation is correlated with the concentration of salt in the brine and its temperature.

Most vegetables can be fermented at 12.5° to 20° salometer salt. If so, the microbial sequence of lactic acid bacteria generally follows the classical sauerkraut fermentation described by Pederson. At higher salt levels of up to about 40° salometer, the sequence is skewed towards the development of a homofermentation, dominated by *Lactobacillus plantarum*. At the highest concentrations of salt (about 60° salometer) the lactic fermentation ceases to function and if any acid is detected during brine storage it is acetic acid, presumably produced by acid-forming yeasts which are still active at this concentration of salt.

Brine salted fermentation of vegetables (pickles)

Pickled cucumbers are another fermented product that has been studied in detail and the process is known. The fermentation process is very similar to the sauerkraut process, only brine is used instead of dry salt. The washed cucumbers are placed in large tanks and salt brine (15 to 20 per cent) is added. The cucumbers are submerged in the brine, ensuring that none float on the surface—this is essential to prevent spoilage. The strong brine draws the sugar and water out of the cucumbers, which simultaneously reduces the salinity of the solution. In order to maintain a salt solution so that fermentation can take place, more salt has to be added to the brine solution. If the concentration of salt falls below 12 per cent, it will result in spoilage of the pickles through putrefaction and softening.

A few days after the cucumbers have been placed in the brine, the fermentation process begins. The process generates heat which causes the brine to boil rapidly. Acids are also produced as a result of the fermentation.

During fermentation, visible changes take place which are important in judging the progress of the process. The colour of the cucumber surface changes from bright green to a dark olive green as acids interact with the chlorophyll. The interior of the cucumber changes from white to a waxy translucent shade as air is forced out of the cells. The specific gravity of the cucumbers also increases as a result of the gradual absorption of salt and they begin to sink in the brine rather than floating on the surface.

Microbes involved in the fermentation process

As with the sauerkraut process, the gram positive coccus—*Leuconostoc mesenteroides* predominates in the first stages of pickle fermentation. This species is more resistant to temperature changes and tolerates higher salt concentration than the subsequent species. As fermentation proceeds and the acidity increases, lactobacilli start to take over from the cocci. The active stage of fermentation continues for between 10 to 30 days, depending upon the temperature of the fermentation. The optimum temperature for *L. cucumeris* is 29° to 32°C. During the fermentative period, the acidity increases to about 2 per cent and the strong acid producing types of bacteria reach their maximum growth. If sugar or acetic acid is added to the fermenting mixture during this time it increases the production of acid.

Problems in pickles

The production of excessive amounts of acid during the fermentation, results in shrivelling of the pickles, possibly due to over-activity of the *L. mesenteroides* species. If the brine is stirred, it may introduce air, which makes conditions more favourable for the growth of spoilage bacteria. In general, if the pickles are well covered with brine, the salt concentration is maintained and the temperature is at an optimum, it should be quite simple to produce good quality pickles.

Nonsalted, lactic acid fermented vegetables

Some vegetables are fermented by lactic acid bacteria, without the prior addition of salt or brine. Examples of non-salted products include *gundruk* (consumed in Nepal), *sinki* and other wilted fermented leaves. The detoxification of cassava through fermentation includes an acid fermentation, during which time the cyanogenic glycosides are hydrolysed to liberate the toxic cyanide gas.

The fermentation process relies on the rapid colonisation of the food by lactic acid producing bacteria, which lower the pH and make the environment unsuitable for the growth of spoilage organisms. Oxygen is also excluded as the *Lactobacilli* favour an anaerobic atmosphere. Restriction of oxygen ensures that yeasts do not grow. For the production of sinki, fresh radish roots are harvested, washed and wilted by sun-drying for one to two days. They are then shredded, re-washed and packed tightly into an earthenware or glass jar, which is sealed and left to ferment. The optimum fermentation time is twelve days at 30°C. Sinki fermentation is initiated by *L. fermentum* and *L. brevis*, followed by *L. plantarum*. During fermentation the pH drops from 6.7 to 3.3. After fermentation, the radish substrate is sun-dried to a moisture level of about 21 per cent. For consumption, sinki is rinsed in water for two minutes, squeezed to remove the excess water and fried with salt, tomato, onion and green chilli. The fried mixture is then boiled in rice water and served hot as soup along with the main meal.

Pit fermentations

South Pacific pit fermentations are an ancient method of preserving starchy vegetables without the addition of salt. The raw materials undergo an acid fermentation within the pit, to produce a paste with good keeping qualities. Pit fermentations are also used in other parts of the world—for example in Ethiopia, where the false banana (*Ensete ventricosum*) is fermented in a pit to produce a pulp known as kocho. Foods preserved in pits can last for years without deterioration, therefore pits provide a good, reliable cheap means of storage. Root crops and bananas are peeled before being placed in the pit, while breadfruit are scraped and pierced. Food is left to ferment for three to six weeks, after which time it becomes soft, has a strong odour and a paste-like consistency. During fermentation, carbon dioxide builds up in the pit, creating an anaerobic atmosphere. As a result of bacterial activity, the temperature rises much higher than the ambient temperature. The pH of the fruit within the pit decreases from 6.7 to 3.7 within about four weeks. Inoculation of the fruit in the pit with lactic acid bacteria greatly speeds up the process. The fermented paste can be left in the pit and removed as required. Usually, it is removed and replaced with a second batch of fresh food to ferment. The fermented food is washed and fibrous material removed. It is then dried in the sun for several hours to remove the volatile odours, and pounded into a paste. Grated coconut or coconut cream and sugar may be added and the mixture is wrapped in banana leaves and either baked or boiled.

PRINCIPLES OF ACETIC ACID FERMENTATION

The main desirable fermentation carried out by acetic acid bacteria is the production of vinegar. Vinegar, literally translated as sour wine, is one of the oldest products of fermentation used by man. It can be made from almost any fermentable carbohydrate source, for example fruits, vegetables, syrups and wine. Whatever the raw material used, the fermentation process follows a definite sequence.

The basic requirement for vinegar production is a raw material that will undergo an alcoholic fermentation. Apples, pears, grapes, honey, syrups, cereals, hydrolysed starches, beer and wine are all ideal substrates for the production of vinegar. The best raw materials are cider and wine, which are widely used in Europe and the United States. To produce a high quality product it is essential that the raw material is mature, clean and in good condition.

Microbes Involved in the Vinegar Process

The production of vinegar depends on a mixed fermentation, which involves both yeasts and bacteria. The fermentation is usually initiated by yeasts which break down glucose into ethyl alcohol with the liberation of carbon dioxide gas. Following on from the yeasts, *acetobacter* oxidise the alcohol to acetic acid and water.

Yeast reaction:

$$C_6H_{12}O_6 \quad \rightarrow \quad 2C_2H_5OH + 2CO_2$$

Glucose   yeast   ethyl alcohol + carbon dioxide

Bacterial reaction:

$$C_2H_5OH + O_2 \quad \rightarrow \quad CH_3COOH + H_2O$$

Alcohol   acetic acid   water

The yeasts and bacteria exist together in a form known as commensalism. The acetobacter are dependent upon the yeasts to produce an easily oxidisable substance (ethyl alcohol). It is not possible to produce vinegar by the action of one type of micro-organism alone.

For a good fermentation, it is essential to have an alcohol concentration of 10 to 13 per cent. If the alcohol content is much higher, the alcohol is incompletely oxidised to acetic acid. If it is lower than 13 per cent, there is a loss of vinegar because the esters and acetic acid are oxidised. In addition to acetic acid, other organic acids are formed during the fermentation which become esterified and contribute to the characteristic odour, flavour and colour of the vinegar. Acetaldehyde is an intermediate product in the transformation of the reducing sugar in fruit juice to acetic acid or vinegar. Oxygen is required for the conversion of acetaldehyde to acetic acid. In general, the yield of acetic acid from glucose is approximately 60 per cent. That is three parts of glucose yield two parts acetic acid.

Micro-organisms involved in the fermentation of vinegar

The organisms involved in vinegar production usually grow at the top of the substrate, forming a jelly like mass. This mass is known as 'mother of vinegar'. The mother is composed of both acetobacter and yeasts, which work together. The principal bacteria are *Acetobacter acetic, A. xylinum* and *A. ascendens.* The main yeasts are *Saccharomyces ellipsoideus* and *S. cerevisiae.* It is important to maintain an acidic environment to suppress the growth of undesirable organisms and to encourage the presence of desirable acetic acid producing bacteria. It is common practice to add 10 to 25 per cent by volume of strong vinegar to the alcoholic substrate in order to attain a desirable fermentation. The alcoholic fermentation of sugars should be completed before the solution is acidified because any remaining sugar will not be converted to alcohol after the acetic acid is added. Incomplete fermentation of the juice results in a 'weak' product. The acetic acid strength of good vinegar should be approximately 6 per cent.

Fermentation methods

Small scale production

Vinegar can be made at home at the small scale by introducing oxygen into barrels of wine or cider and allowing fermentation to occur spontaneously. This process is not very rigorously controlled and often results in a poor quality product.

The Orleans process

The Orleans process is one of the oldest and well known methods for the production of vinegar. It is a slow, continuous process, which originated in France. High grade vinegar is used as a starter culture, to which wine is added at weekly intervals. The vinegar is fermented in large (200 litres) capacity barrels. Approximately 65 to 70 litres of high grade vinegar is added to the barrel along with 15 litres of wine. After one week, a further 10 to 15 litres of wine are added and this is repeated at weekly intervals. After about four weeks, vinegar can be withdrawn from the barrel (10 to 15 litres per week) as more wine is added to replace the vinegar. One of the problems encountered with this method is that of how to add more liquid to the barrel without disturbing the floating bacterial mat. This can be overcome by using a glass tube which reaches to the bottom of the barrel. Additional liquid is poured in through the tube and therefore does not disturb the bacteria. Wood shavings are sometimes added to the fermenting barrel to help support the bacterial mat.

Quick vinegar method

Because the Orleans process is slow, other methods have been adapted to try and speed up the process. The German method is one such method. It uses a generator, which is an upright tank filled with beechwood shavings and fitted with devices which allow the alcoholic solution to trickle down through the shavings in which the acetic acid bacteria are living. The tank is not allowed to fill as that would exclude oxygen which is necessary for the fermentation. Near the bottom of the generator are holes which allow air to be drawn in the air rises through the generator and is used by the acetic acid bacteria to oxidise the alcohol. This oxidisation also releases considerable amounts of heat which must be controlled to avoid causing damage to the bacteria.

Problems in vinegar production

Many of the problems of vinegar production are concerned with the presence of nematodes, mites, flies and other insects. These pests can be controlled by adherence to good hygiene and pasteurisation of the vinegar. Problems associated with the fermentative process include the presence of a whitish film on the surface of the vinegar. This is sometimes called *Mycoderma vini* and is composed of yeast-like organisms, which grow aerobically and oxidise the carbon containing compounds to carbon dioxide and water. They also alter the flavour and alcohol content of the vinegar. This problem can, however, be controlled by adding one part vinegar to three parts of the alcoholic solution or by storing the alcoholic liquid in filled closed containers.

TYPICAL PRODUCTS OF BACTERIAL FERMENTATIONS

Many products are produced by bacterial fermentations. These include the fruit and vegetable pickles produced by lactic acid fermentation and the products of alkaline bacterial fermentations. Lactic acid bacteria pickling is still carried out at the domestic scale. However industrial scale processes have been developed for the production of most types of pickles. Pickles can be made by storing prepared vegetables in a weak brine solution, by dry salting or allowing the vegetables to ferment without salt.

Dry Salted Pickles

Dry salting is used for pickling many vegetables and fruits including limes, lemons and cucumbers. For dry salt pickling any variety of common salt is suitable as long as it is pure. Impurities or additives can cause problems:

1. Chemicals to reduce caking should not be used as they make the brine cloudy.
2. Lime impurities can reduce the acidity of the final product and reduce the shelf-life of the product.
3. Iron impurities can result in the blackening of the vegetables.
4. Magnesium impurities impart a bitter taste.
5. Carbonates can result in pickles with a soft texture.

Dry salted lime pickle

Dry salted lime pickles are produced in Asia and Africa. They are particularly popular in India, Pakistan and North Africa. With dry salting, the limes are treated with dry salt. The salt extracts and juice from the vegetable and create the brine. The final product is a sour lime pickle. Spices are added depending on local preference. In India and Pakistan, the pickle is usually very spicy and hot due to the addition of chilli. It is usually eaten as a condiment.

Preparation of raw materials

The limes need to be selected and prepared. Only fully ripe limes without bruising or damage should be used. All limes need to be washed in potable cold water, drained, and then cut into quarters. Spices should be of good quality and free of mould.

Processing

Limes are placed in a layer, approximately 2.5 cm deep, into the fermenting container (a barrel or keg). One kilogram of salt is added for every four kilograms of limes. The salt is sprinkled over the vegetables. Another layer of vegetables is added and more salt added. This is repeated until the container is three quarters full. A cloth is placed above the vegetables and a weight added to compress the vegetables and assist in the formation of a brine. The formation of a brine takes about 24 hours. The container is then placed in the sun for a week.

As soon as the brine is formed, fermentation starts. As fermentation starts bubbles of carbon dioxide appear. Fermentation takes between one and four weeks depending on the ambient temperature. Fermentation is complete when no more bubbles appear. Process of fermented dry salted lime pickle is shown in Fig. 19.4.

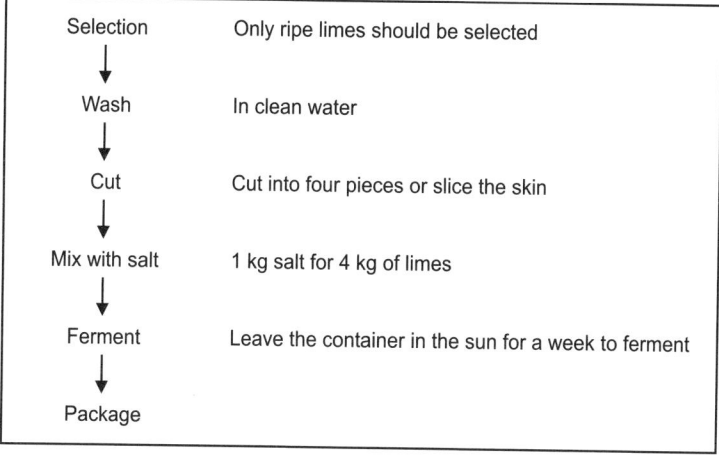

Fig. 19.4. Process of fermented dry salted lime pickle.

Packaging and storage

The vegetables can be removed from the brine and packaged in a variety of mixtures which may consist of vinegar and spices or oil and spices. Lime pickle can be packed in small polythene bags and sealed or in clean jars and capped. Lime pickles keep well if stored in a cool place. Due to the high acid level of the final product, the risk of food poisoning is low.

Pickled cucumbers

Pickled cucumbers are made in Africa, Asia and Latin America. Cucumbers undergo a typical lactic acid fermentation and change from a pale product to a darker green and more transparent product. *Khalpi* is a cucumber pickle popular during the summer months in Nepal.

Raw material preparation

Fully ripe cucumbers without bruising or damage are washed in potable cold water and drained. The cucumbers can be pickled whole or sliced. With *khalpi* the cucumbers are washed, sliced and cut into 5–8 cm pieces.

Processing

One kg of salt is added to every 20 kg of small cucumbers and 15 kg of large cucumbers. The brine should be formed within 24 hours by osmosis. If the brine formed by osmosis does not cover the cucumbers 40° Salometer brine is added to the desired level. A day or two after the tank is filled and closed the brine should be stirred in order to help equalise the concentration of salt throughout the mass. As soon as the brine is formed, fermentation starts and bubbles of carbon dioxide appear. Fermentation takes between one and four weeks depending on the ambient temperature. Fermentation is complete when no more bubbles appear. During fermentation the brine becomes cloudy for the first few days due to the growth of bacteria. Later if the brine is not covered, a filmy yeast growth will often occur on the surface. Process of fermented dry pickled cucumbers is shown in Fig. 19.5.

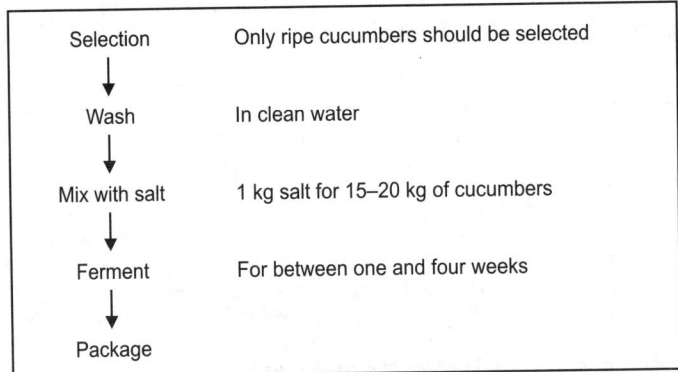

Fig. 19.5. Process of fermented dry pickled cucumbers.

Packaging and storage

Cucumber pickle is usually stored in clean capped jars. They keep well if stored in a cool place. Due to the high acid level of the final product, the risk of food poisoning is low. With *khalpi* in Nepal, oil is added.

Pak-Gard-Dong (pickled leafy vegetable)

Pak-Gard-Dong is a fermented mustard leaf (*Brassica juncea*) product made in Thailand. The mustard leaves are washed, wilted in the sun, mixed with salt, packed into containers for 12 hours. The water is then drained and a 3 per cent sugar solution added. They are again allowed to ferment for three to five days at room temperature. Micro-organisms associated with the fermentation include *Lactobacillus brevis*, *Pediococcus cerevisiae* and *Lactobacillus plantarum*.

A similar product (*Hum choy*) is made in the South of China. This is produced by fermenting a local leafy vegetable. The leaves are washed and drained. They are then covered in salt and hung on racks to dry in the sun. The wilted leaves are placed in earthenware pots and covered with rice water, obtained after washing rice grains. The pots are sealed and the leaves allowed to ferment for four days. The product can be stored for up to two months if the seal is not broken.

Tempoyak (pickled durian)

Tempoyak is the fermented pulp of a durian fruit (*Durio zibethinus*) from Malaysia. It has the distinctive durian smell and a creamy yellow colour. It is made by mixing durian pulp with salt and placing in a sealed container. Fermentation takes about seven days.

Pickled beetroots

In Russia beetroot is pickled by cleaning, slicing and placing in a container with salt. Due to the high sucrose level, dextrans are produced giving the product a slimy texture.

Lamoun makbous (pickled lemons)

Pickled lemons are popular in Asia. In west Asia and north Africa they are known as *lamoun makbous* and *msir*. Lemons are washed in clean water, sliced and covered in salt. After at least 24 hours, they are drained and mixed with oil and spices.

Brined Fruit and Vegetable Pickles

For brine pickling any variety of common salt is suitable as long as it is pure. Impurities or additives can cause problems:

1. Chemicals to reduce caking should not be used as they make the brine cloudy.
2. Lime impurities can reduce the acidity of the final product and reduce the shelf-life of the product.
3. Iron impurities can result in the blackening of the vegetables.
4. Magnesium impurities impart a bitter taste.
5. Carbonates can result in pickles with a soft texture.

Green mango pickle

Mango pickle is a very popular pickle in many Asian, African and Latin American countries. It is a major product of India, Pakistan and Bangladesh and it is estimated that the annual production of mango pickle in South Africa is over 10,000 tons.

Green mango pickle is a hot, spicy pickle with a sour taste. It is eaten as a condiment. Preservation is caused by a combination of salt, increased acidity and to a small extent the spices. It is known as *burong mangga* and *dalok* in the Philippines.

Preparation of the raw material

The fresh, fully mature, firm but unripe mangoes must be carefully selected to ensure a good quality product. The best pickles are obtained from fruit at early maturity when the fruit has reached almost maximum size. Riper fruit results in pickles with a fruity odour and lacking the characteristic and predominant green mango flavour.

The green mangoes need to be inspected and any damaged fruit rejected. The fruit is washed in clean water and drained. After draining, the fruit is cut. Sharp knives with preferably stainless blades should be used. Iron or copper equipment should be avoided. A single stroke should be used during the cutting process to ensure minimum damage and avoiding mushiness in the final product.

Processing

The sliced mangoes are soaked in brine solution. Sodium metabisulphite (1000 ppm) and 1 per cent calcium chloride are added. The containers are stored until the mangoes are pickled. The brine is then drained off and spices are mixed with the mango slices. Process of fermented green mango pickle is shown in Fig. 19.6.

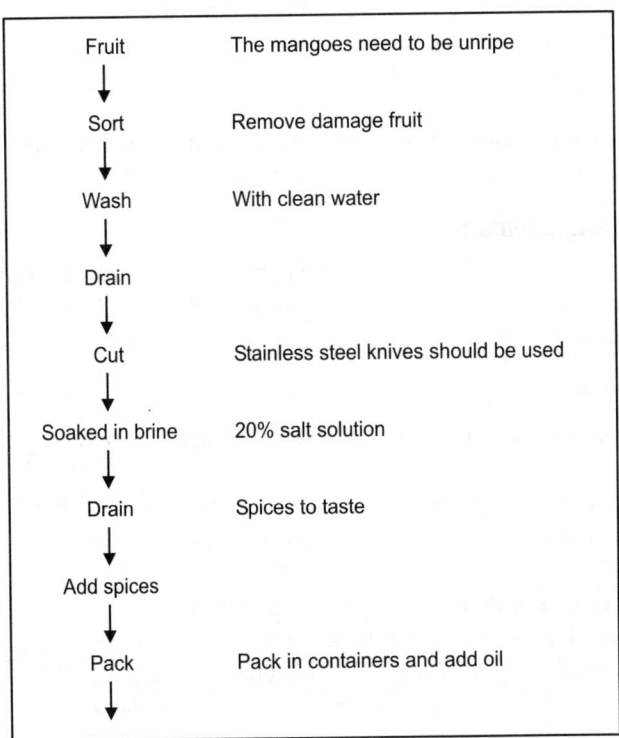

Fig. 19.6. Process of fermented green mango pickle.

Packaging and storage

The mixture is then packed and oil added onto the surface of the mixture. The mangoes should be firmly pressed down in the container. Good quality vegetable oil such as sunflower oil should be used and finely ground chilli powder can be added to the oil for flavour and colour. Mango pickle can be packed in small polythene bags and sealed or in clean jars and capped. Mango pickle keeps well if stored in a cool place. If it is processed well, it can be kept for several months. Due to the high acid level of the final product, the risk of food poisoning is low.

Lime pickle (brined)

Lime pickles are produced in Asia, Latin America and Africa. They are particularly popular in India, Pakistan and North Africa. Lime pickle is made from salted pieces of lime packed in a salty, spicy liquor, like a semisolid gravy. It is brownish red and the lime peels are yellow or pale green with a sour and salty taste. It is eaten as a condiment with curries or other main meals. If processed well, the product can be kept for several months.

Preparation of raw materials

The limes need to be selected and prepared. Only fully ripe limes without bruising or damage should be used. All the limes need to be washed in potable cold water and drained. The limes are dipped in hot water (60°–65°C) for about five minutes. They are then cut into pieces in order to expose the interior and allow salt to be absorbed more quickly. All spices should be of good quality and free of mould.

Processing

The prepared limes are covered with a brine solution. This causes water to be drawn out of the pieces by osmosis. It is important to ensure that the surface is covered with juice, and leave for 24 hours. If necessary, the fruits should be pressed down to hold them below the liquid. Once the limes have been placed in the brine, there is a rapid development of micro-organisms and fermentation begins. After fermentation the limes are dried in the sun until the skin becomes brown. Process of fermented lime pickle is shown in Fig. 19.7.

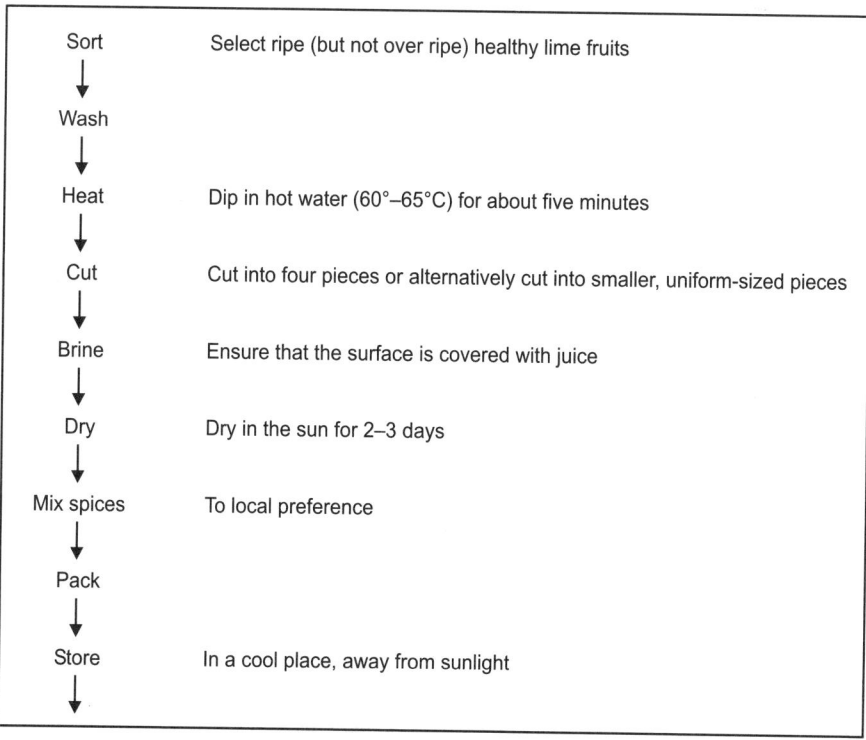

Fig. 19.7. Process of fermented lime pickle.

Packaging and storage

The limes are mixed with spices and oils according to local taste and tradition. Lime pickle can be packed in small polythene bags and sealed or in clean jars and capped. Lime pickle keeps well if stored in a cool place. Due to the high acid level of the final product, the risk of food poisoning is low.

Kimchi (pickled cabbage)

Kimchi is probably the most important processed food product in Korea. It is an essential dish, eaten at most mealtimes. Production is estimated at over one million tons, mainly at household level. Daily consumption is estimated at 150 to 250 grams per person. *Kimchi* is a general name for a range of closely related fermented products. It is similar to Sauerkraut in Europe and the United States. There are numerous variations of *kimchi* depending on the production technique. The main pickled cabbage *kimchis* are *tongbaechu-kimchi*, *tongkimchi* and *bossam-kimchi*. This section refers to *kimchi* produced from cabbage, the following section deals with pickled radish products.

Preparation of raw materials

Appropriate cultivars of Chinese cabbage, with light-green coloured soft leaves and compact structures with no defects, are required for production of *kimchi*. After removing outer leaves and roots from the cabbage, it is cut into small pieces.

Processing

The prepared cabbage is placed in a salt solution (8–15 per cent) for two to seven hours in order to increase the salt content of the cabbage to between 2.0–4.0 per cent (w/w). It is then rinsed several times with freshwater and drained to remove extra water by centrifugation or by allowing to stand. *Kimchi* fermentation is carried out by various micro-organisms present in the raw materials and ingredients used in the preparation of kimchi. Among the two hundred bacteria isolated form kimchi, the important micro-organisms in kimchi fermentation are known to be *Lactobacillus plantarum*, *L. brevis*, *Streptococcus faecalis*, *Leuconostoc mesenteroides* and *Pediococcus pentosaceus*. After fermentation, the product can be left to mature for several weeks if refrigeration is available. If stored under warm conditions, the *kimchi* deteriorates rapidly. Process of fermented *kimchi* (pickled cabbage) is shown in Fig. 19.8.

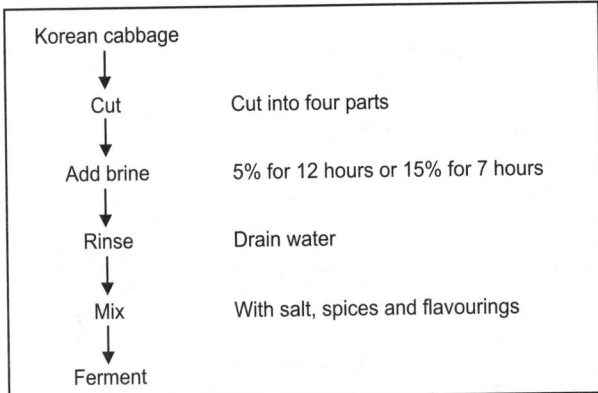

Fig. 19.8. Process of fermented *kimchi* (pickled cabbage).

Green olives

Olives are a brine fermented product which undergo an essential pretreatment with lye to remove substances which are toxic to bacteria and would, if left in the olives, prevent fermentation. Green olives are placed in a 2 per cent sodium hydroxide (lye) solution at 21° to 24°C until the lye penetrates the flesh. Cold water is added to the solution, which, dilutes the mixture until the lye is completely removed. The lye treatment is necessary to remove a bitter glucoside compound (oleuropein) from the outer tissues of the olive. Oleuropein is highly toxic to bacteria and therefore needs to be removed in order for a fermentation to take place. After the glucoside has been removed, the olives are placed in barrels with a 1 to 10 per cent brine solution and allowed to undergo a spontaneous fermentation. The optimum fermentation temperature is 24°C. The fermentation period usually takes between two and three months. Once fermentation is complete, the olives are packed in airtight jars and sterilised which produces a good quality product with a long storage life.

Black olives

When ripe olives are used, they are placed in a 5 to 7 per cent brine solution to soften the outer tissue before lye is added. This pretreatment allows the lye to penetrate the fruit more easily. In ripe fruit, the glucoside is situated more deeply within the tissue. After soaking in brine, the lye solution (0.7 to 2.0 per cent) is added and, after soaking, the olives are washed clean. They are then packed in barrels with a 2 to 5 per cent brine solution and allowed to undergo fermentation for two to six weeks, depending on the external temperature. Unlike immature olives, the ripe one are exposed to air during fermentation. This is to oxidise the polyphenols in the tissue to a black colour, which is dependent upon oxygen and the small amounts of sodium hydroxide which are left on the olives. The finished product is packed in a 3 to 5 per cent brine solution and then sterilised. *Bacillus subtilis* may produce pectolytic enzymes which result in a soft product. If the wash water used for removing the lye is below 60°C, many species of undesirable bacteria can survive which result in a low quality product.

Jack-fruit pickle

Young green jack fruit is pickled in India and Sri Lanka. Young green jack fruit are peeled and cut into 1.2 to 1.8 cm thick slices. The slices are placed in a container and covered in an 8 per cent common salt solution. They are weighed down to keep them submerged in the brine. The brine solution is increased by 2 per cent each day until it reaches 15 per cent. The slices are then left for 8–10 days in the brine. Vinegar and spices are added prior to packaging.

Pickled radish

A number of pickled radish products are produced in Korea. These include: *kaktugi, tongchimi, chonggak-kimchi, seokbakji, yolmu-kimchi dan moogi kach doo ki gactuki* and *mootsanji*.

Pickled cucumber

A variety of brine pickled cucumber products are made around the world. *Oi sobagi* and *oiji* are made in Korea. In Egypt cucumbers are pickled by soaking in brine to produce *torshi khiar*.

Pickled leafy vegetables

There are many other brine pickled leafy vegetables around the world.
For instance:
1. *Pak-sian-dong*: This is a popular pickled leafy vegetable *Pak Sian* (*Gynadropsis pentaphylla*) in Thailand. The fresh vegetable is cleaned and wilted in the sun for one to two hours. It is then placed in brine and fermented for two to three days at room temperature.
2. *Sayur asin* fermented wilted mustard cabbage (*Brassica juncea*) from Indonesia. It is also known as *kiam chai* in Thailand and *kiam chaye* in Malaysia.

Other pickled vegetables and fruits

1. *Naw-mai-dong*: pickled bamboo shoots (*Bambusa glaucescens*) from Thailand.
2. *Hom-dong*: pickled red onions from Thailand.
3. *Jeruk*: pickled vegetables including ginger and papaya from Malaysia.
4. Pickled carrots and turnips are produced in Asia and Africa. They are known as *hua-chai po* in Thailand and *tai tan tsoi* in China.
5. *Nukamiso-zuke*: Vegetables fermented in rice bran, salt and water in Japan.
6. Bananas are pickled in the West Indies.
7. Fermented sweet peppers (*torshi felfel*) are produced in west Asia and Africa.
8. Cauliflower stalks are fermented to produce achar *tandal* in India.
9. Aubergines (*torshi betingen*) are pickled in west Asia.

NONSALTED LACTIC ACID BACTERIA PRODUCTS

Gundruk (Pickled Leafy Vegetable)

Gundruk is particularly popular in Nepal. The annual production of *gundruk* in Nepal is estimated at 2000 tons and most of the production is carried out at the household level. *Gundruk* is obtained from the fermentation of leafy vegetables in Nepal. It is served as a side dish with the main meal and is also used as an appetiser. Gundruk is an important source of minerals particularly during the off-season when the diet consists of mostly starchy tubers and maize which tend to be low in minerals.

Preparation of raw materials

In the months of October and November, during the harvest of the first broad mustard, radish and cauliflower leaves, large quantities of leaves accumulate—much more than can be consumed fresh. These leaves are allowed to wilt for one or two days and then shredded with a knife or sickle.

Processing

Shredded leaves are tightly packed in an earthenware pot and warm water (at about 30°C) is added to cover all the leaves. The pot is then kept in a warm place. After five to seven days, a mild acidic taste indicates the end of fermentation and the *gundruk* is removed and sun-dried. This process is similar to sauerkraut production except that no salt is added to the shredded leaves prior to *gundruk* fermentation. The ambient temperature at the time of fermentation is about 18°C. *Pediococcus* and *Lactobacillus* species are the predominant micro-organisms during gundruk fermentation. The fermentation is initiated by *L. cellobiosus* and *L. plantarum*, and other homolactics make a vigorous growth from the third day onwards. Pediococcus pentosaceus increases in number on the fifth day and thereafter declines. During fermentation, the pH drops slowly to a final value of 4.0 and the amount of acid (as lactic) increases to about 1 per cent on the sixth day. It has been found that a disadvantage with the traditional process of gundruk fermentation is the loss of 90 per cent of the carotenoids, probably during sun-drying. Improved methods of drying might reduce the vitamin loss. Process of fermented *gundruk* (pickled leafy vegetable) is shown in Fig. 19.9.

Kocho (Pickled False Banana)

False banana (*Ensete ventricosum*) is fermented in a pit to produce a pulp known as *kocho*. Foods preserved in pits can last for years without deterioration. Pits therefore provide a good, reliable cheap means of storage.

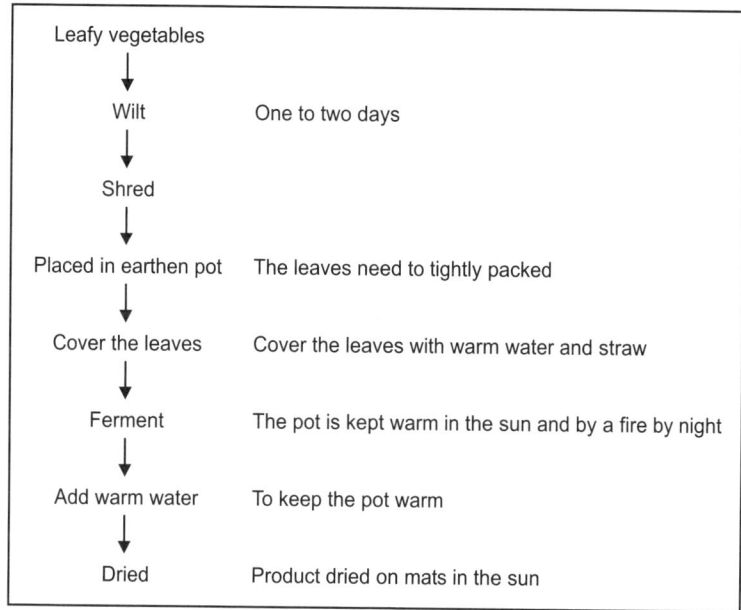

Leafy vegetables

Wilt — One to two days

Shred

Placed in earthen pot — The leaves need to tightly packed

Cover the leaves — Cover the leaves with warm water and straw

Ferment — The pot is kept warm in the sun and by a fire by night

Add warm water — To keep the pot warm

Dried — Product dried on mats in the sun

Fig. 19.9. Process of fermented *gundruk* (pickled leafy vegetable).

Processing

The type of soil and its drainage are important in the selection of a pit site. Pits are often lined with stones to prevent the soil from the side walls falling into the bottom. A family pit may be 0.6 to 1.5 metres deep and 1.2 to 2 metres wide with a capacity of about fifty breadfruits. A community pit is usually much larger, with the capacity to hold up to 1000 breadfruit.

A family pit requires at least 1000 green banana leaves and four sacks of dried banana leaves for lining the walls and top. It is essential that proper attention is given to hygiene of the pit and the fruit to be stored in it.

The central stems are removed from fresh banana leaves and they are wilted in the sun until they become soft and pliable. The pit is lined with dry leaves, then green leave are folded and arranged, overlapping each other, around the sides of the pit and extending over the top. At least two or three layers of banana leaves are used to seal the pit and prevent contamination by the soil. Washed, peeled food is placed in the pit, green banana leaves are folded over the top of the food and heavy stones are placed on top to weigh down the leaves.

Root crops and bananas are peeled before placing in the pit, breadfruit are scraped and pierced. Food is left to ferment for three to six weeks, after which time it becomes soft, has a strong odour and a paste-like consistency. The fermented paste can be left in the pit and removed as required. Usually, it is removed and replaced with a second batch of fresh food to ferment. The fermented food is washed and fibrous material removed.

It is then dried in the sun for several hours to remove the volatile odours. It is then pounded into a paste. Grated coconut or coconut cream and sugar added and the mixture is wrapped in banana leaves and either baked or boiled. During fermentation, carbon dioxide builds up in the pit, creating an anaerobic atmosphere. As a result of bacterial activity, the temperature rises much higher than the ambient temperature. The pH of the fruit within the pit decreases from 6.7 to 3.7 within about four weeks. Inoculation of the fruit in the pit with lactic acid bacteria greatly speeds up the process.

In the South Pacific pit fermentations are an ancient method of preserving starchy vegetables such as banana, plantain, breadfruit, cassava, taro, sweet potato, arrowroot and yams. The products undergo an acid fermentation, to produce a paste with good keeping qualities. It is usually pounded with a little sugar, coconut cream or fresh coconut and boiled or baked to make a type of pudding.

Sinki (Pickled Radish)

Sinki is a sour pickle prepared from radish tap roots. It is consumed traditionally in India, Nepal and parts of Bhutan, where it is used as a base for soup or eaten as a pickle. It is one of the most popular pickles in Nepal. Fresh radish roots are harvested, washed and wilted by sun-drying for one to two days. They are then shredded, re-washed and packed tightly into an earthenware or glass jar, which is sealed and left to ferment. The optimum fermentation time is twelve days at 30°C. Sinki fermentation is initiated by *L. fermentum* and *L. brevis*, followed by *L. plantarum*. During fermentation the pH drops from 6.7 to 3.3. After fermentation, the radish substrate is sun-dried to a moisture level of about 21 per cent. There is a second processing method involving fermentation in a clay lined pit for two to three months. For consumption, sinki is rinsed in water for two minutes, squeezed to remove the excess water and fried with salt, tomato, onion and green chilli. The fried mixture is then boiled in rice water and served hot as soup along with the main meal.

Sunki

Sunki is a non-salted and fermented vegetable product prepared from the leaves of 'Otaki-turnip' in Kiso district, Nagano prefecture, Japan. Sunki is eaten with rice and in miso soup. The Otaki-turnip is boiled, inoculated with '*Zumi*' (a wild small apple) dried Sunki from the previous year and allowed to ferment for one to two months. *Sunki* is produced under low temperature (in winter season). Micro-organisms involved include *Lactobacillus plantarum*, *L. Brevis*, *Bacillus coagulans* and *Pediococcus pentosaceus*.

Kanji

In Northern India and Pakistan carrots, especially a variety that is deep purple in colour, are fermented to make a traditional ready to serve drink known as *kanji*. *Kanji* is very popular and considered to have cooling and soothing properties and to be of high nutritional value. After thorough washing the carrots are finely grated. Each kilogram of grated carrot is mixed with 7 litres of water, 200 g of salt, 40 g of crushed mustard seed and 8 g of hot chilli powder. The mixture is then placed in a glazed earthenware vessel, which is almost entirely sealed, leaving only a tiny hole for gases released during fermentation to escape. The mixture is then allowed to ferment for seven to ten days. The type of fermentation that takes place is known as a lactic fermentation, which must be carried out in the absence of air. Lactic acid bacteria produce lactic acid which reduces the pH (i.e. increases the acidity) to a level that prevents the growth of food poisoning organisms. The final product is slightly acidic in taste and has an attractive purple-red colour. After fermentation the drink is strained through fine muslin and has to be consumed within 3 or 4 days after which it goes bad. Each kg of grated carrot yields just over 7 litres of *kanji*.

Fermented Tea Leaves

In South East Asia, tea leaves (*Camellia sinensis*) are fermented to make a sour-tasting snack. In Myanmar the product is called *leppet-so*, in Thailand it is known as *miang*.

ALKALINE BACTERIAL PRODUCTS

Kawal

Kawal is a strong smelling Sudanese, protein-rich food prepared by fermenting the leaves of a wild African legume, *Cassia obtusifolia* and is usually cooked in stews and soups. It is used as a meat replacer or a meat extender. Its protein is of high quality, rich in sulphur amino acids which are usually obtained from either fish or meat.

Raw material preparation

The *Sickle Pod* plant (*Cassia obtusifolia*) is a wild legume that grows in Sudan. The leaves are collected late in the rainy season when the plant is fully grown. All the stems, pods and flowers are removed. The leaves are not washed, since it is thought that natural micro-organisms on the leaves are important for the correct fermentation.

Process and principles of preservation

The leaves of the leguminous plant are pounded into paste without releasing the juice. The paste is placed in an earthenware jar and covered with sorghum leaves. The whole jar is sealed with mud and buried in the ground up to the neck in a cool place. Every three days the contents are mixed by hand.

The fermentation takes about fourteen days. The fermentation is extremely complex. The main micro-organisms are *Bacillus subtilis* and *Propionibacterium* spp. Lactic acid bacteria including *Lactobacillus plantarum*; yeasts including *Candida krusei* and *Saccharomyces* spp. and moulds including *Rhizopus* spp. are also involved.

After about fourteen days, the strongly smelling black fermented paste is made into small balls and sun-dried for five days. Process of fermented kawal is shown in Fig. 19.10.

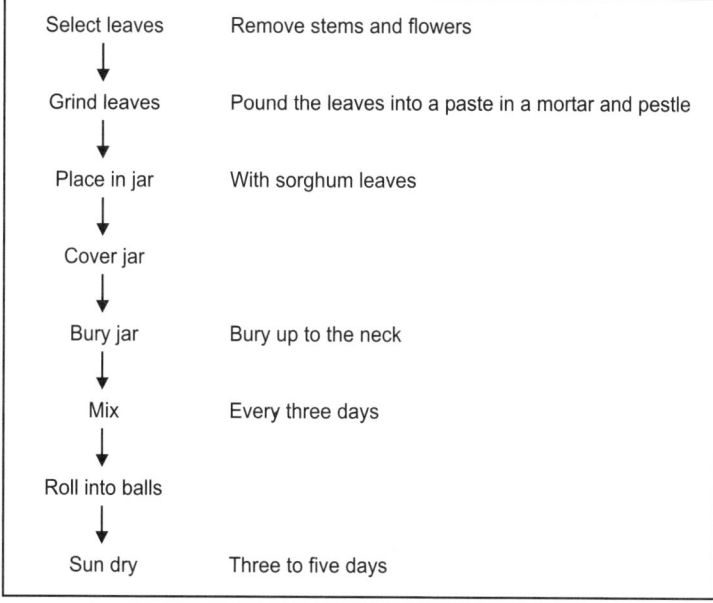

Fig. 19.10. Process of fermented kawal.

Ombolo wa koba

In Zaire cassava leaves are fermented to produce *ombolo wa koba* which is traditionally eaten with boiled cassava and plantain bananas. Cassava leaves are allowed to wilt and turn black. This takes about three to four days. The cassava leaves are then chopped up and placed in a pot of boiling water for about one hour. During this processing stage, a water soluble extract of ash is produced by placing the ash of burnt dried banana skins and palm tree flowers in a strainer and pouring water through it. The extract is then added to the boiled cassava leaves.

The extract is alkaline and neutralises the cyanhydric acid liberated when the leaves are chopped up. Salt and dried fish or meat is also added. After allowing the cassava leaf mixture to cool a little, acid palm oil is then added. This reacts with the excess alkali and neutralises it. The product is now ready to be eaten.

TEA PROCESSING

Tea processing is the method in which the leaves from the tea plant *Camellia sinensis* are transformed into the dried leaves for brewing tea. The categories of tea are distinguished by the processing they undergo. In its most general form, tea processing involves different manners and degree of oxidation of the leaves, stopping the oxidation, forming the tea and drying it. The innate flavour of the tealeaves is determined by the type of cultivar of the tea bush, the quality of the plucked tea leaves, and the manner and quality of the production processing they undergo (Fig. 19.11).

Although each type of tea has different taste, smell, and visual appearance, tea processing for all tea types consists of a very similar set of methods with only minor variations:

1. Picking: Tea leaves and flushes, which includes a terminal bud and two young leaves, are plucked from *Camellia sinensis* bushes typically twice a year during early spring and early summer or late spring. Autumn or winter pickings of tea flushes are much less common, though they occur when climate permits. Picking is done by hand when a higher quality tea is needed, or where labour costs are not prohibitive. Hand-picking is done by pulling the flush with a snap of the wrist and does not involve twisting or pinching the flush, since doing the latter reduces the quality of the leaves. Tea flushes and leaves can also be picked by machine, though there will be more broken leaves and partial flushes. It is also more difficult to harvest by machine on mountain slopes where tea is often grown.

2. Withering/Wilting: The tea leaves will begin to wilt soon after picking, with a gradual onset of enzymatic oxidation. Wilting is used to remove excess water from the leaves and allows a very slight amount of oxidation. The leaves can be either put under the sun or left in a cool breezy room to pull moisture out from the leaves. The leaves sometimes lose more than a quarter of their weight in water during wilting. The process is also important in promoting the breakdown of leaf proteins into free amino acid and increases the availability of freed caffeine both of which changes the taste of the tea.

3. Bruising: In order to promote and quicken oxidation, the leaves may be bruised by shaking and tossing in a bamboo tray, tumbling in baskets or by being kneaded or rolled-over by heavy wheels. The bruising breaks down the structures within and outside of the leaf cells and allows from the commingling of oxidative enzymes with various substrates, which allows for the beginning of oxidation. This also releases some of the leaf juices, which may aid in oxidation and change the taste profile of the tea.

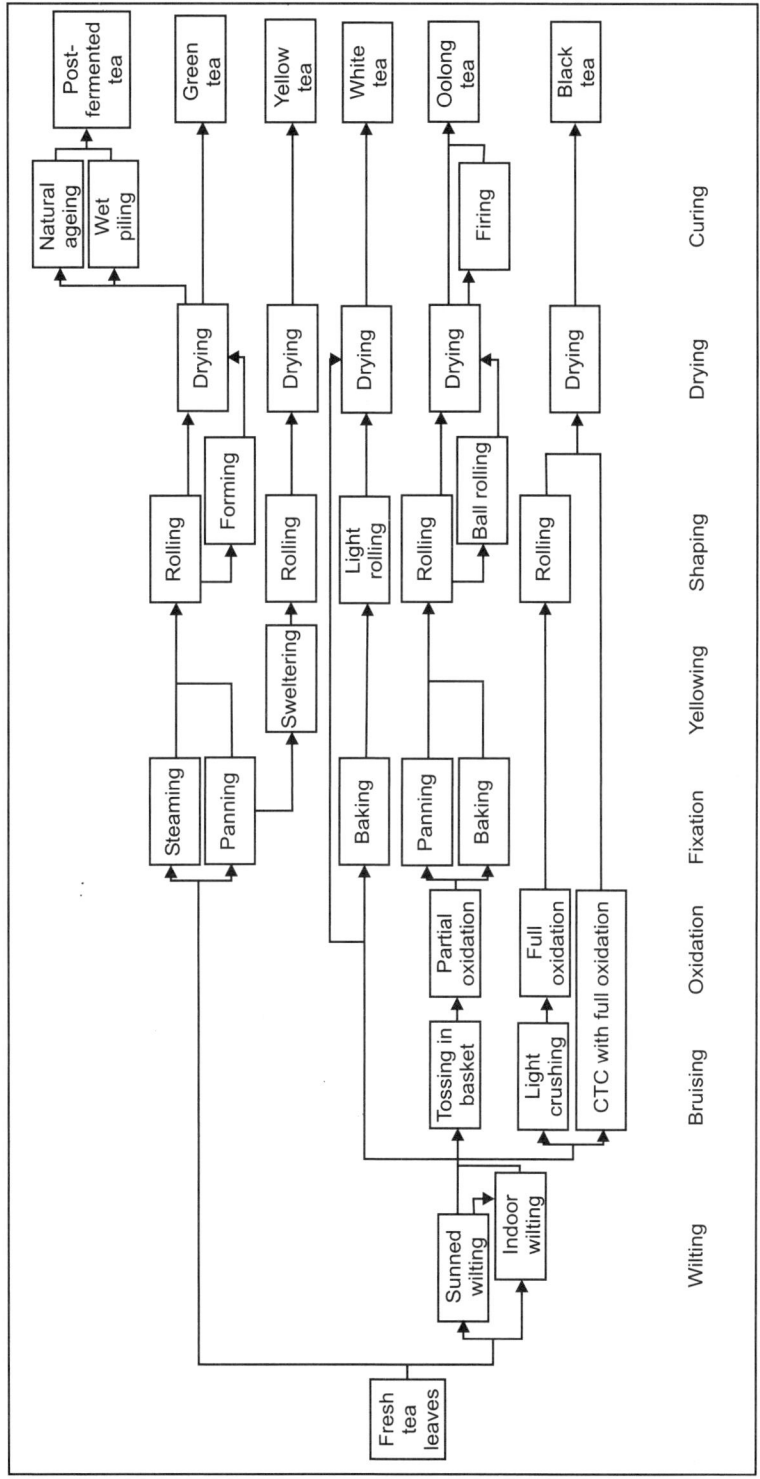

Fig. 19.11. Tea leaf processing methods for the six most common types of tea.

4. Oxidation/Fermentation: For teas that require oxidation, the leaves are left on their own in a climate-controlled room where they turn progressively darker. This is accompanied by agitation in some cases. In this process the chlorophyll in the leaves is enzymatically broken down, and its tannins are released or transformed. This process is sometimes referred to as 'fermentation' in the tea industry. The tea producer may choose when the oxidation should be stopped, which depends on the desired qualities in the final tea as well as the weather conditions (heat and humidity). For light oolong teas this may be anywhere from 5–40 per cent oxidation, in darker oolong teas 60–70 per cent, and in black teas 100 per cent oxidation. Oxidation is highly important in the formation of many taste and aroma compounds, which give a tea its liquor colour, strength, and briskness. Depending on the type of tea desired, under or over-oxidation/fermentation can result in grassy flavours, or overly thick winey flavours.

5. Fixation/Kill-green: Kill-green or *shaqing* is done to stop the tea leaf oxidation at a desired level. This process is accomplished by moderately heating tea leaves, thus deactivating their oxidative enzymes and removing unwanted scents in the leaves, without damaging the flavour of the tea. Traditionally, the tea leaves are panned in a wok or steamed, but with advancements in technology, kill-green is sometimes done by baking or 'panning' in a rolling drum. In some white teas and some black teas such as CTC blacks, kill-green is done simultaneously with drying.

6. Sweltering/Yellowing: Unique to yellow teas, warm and damp tea leaves from after kill-green are allowed to be lightly heated in a closed container, which causes the previously green leaves to yellow. The resulting leaves produce a beverage that has a distinctive yellowish-green hue due to transformations of the leaf chlorophyll. Through being sweltered for 6–8 hours at close to human body temperatures, the amino acids and polyphenols in the processed tea leaves undergo chemical changes to give this tea its distinct briskness and mellow taste.

7. Rolling/Shaping: The damp tea leaves are then rolled to be formed into wrinkled strips, by hand or using a rolling machine which causes the tea to wrap around itself. This rolling action also causes some of the sap, essential oils, and juices inside the leaves to ooze out, which further enhances the taste of the tea. The strips of tea can then be formed into other shapes, such as being rolled into spirals, kneaded and rolled into pellets or tied into balls, cones and other elaborate shapes. In many type of oolong, the rolled strips of tea leaf are then rolled to spheres or half spheres and is typically done by placing the damp leaves in large cloth bags, which are then kneaded by hand or machine in a specific manner.

8. Drying: Drying is done to 'finish' the tea for sale. This can be done in a myriad of ways including panning, sunning, air drying or baking. However, baking is usually the most common. Great care must be taken to not over-cook the leaves. The drying of the produced tea are responsible for many new flavour compounds particularly important in green teas.

9. Ageing/Curing: While not always required, some teas required additional ageing, secondary-fermentation or baking to reach their drinking potential. For instance, a green tea pu-erh, prior to curing into a post-fermented tea, is often bitter and harsh in taste, but becomes sweet and mellow through fermentation by age or dampness. As well, oolong can benefit from ageing if fired over charcoal. Flavoured teas are manufactured in this stage by spraying the tea with aromas and flavours or by storing them with their flavourants.

Without careful moisture and temperature control during its manufacture and life thereafter, fungi will grow on tea. This form of fungus causes real fermentation that will contaminate the tea and may render the tea unfit for consumption.

Specific Processing of Tea

Tea is traditionally classified based on the degree or period of 'fermentation' the leaves have undergone:

1. White tea: Young leaves or new growth buds that have undergone minimal oxidation through a slight amount of wilting before halting the oxidation with heat. Though the young leaves may be shaped before drying, leaf buds processed into white tea are usually dried immediately after wilting. The buds may be shielded from sunlight to prevent formation of chlorophyll. White tea is produced in lesser quantities than most other styles, and can be correspondingly more expensive than tea from the same plant processed by other methods. It is less well-known in countries outside of China, though this is changing with increased western interest in organic or premium teas.

2. Green tea: This tea has undergone the least amount of oxidation. The oxidation process is halted through quick application of heat after tea picking, either with steam the Japanese method or by dry cooking in hot pans, the traditional Chinese method. Tea leaves may be left to dry as separate leaves or they may be rolled into small pellets to make Gunpowder tea. This process is time consuming and is typically done with pekoes of higher quality. The tea is processed within one to two days of harvesting, and if done correctly retains most of the chemical composition of the fresh leaves from which it was produced.

3. Oolong (Wulong): Oxidation is stopped somewhere between the standards for green tea and black tea. The processing typically takes two to three days from wilting to drying with a relatively short oxidation period of several hours. In Chinese, semi-oxidised teas are collectively grouped as blue tea, while the term 'oolong' is used specifically as a name for certain semi-oxidised teas. Common wisdom about lightly oxidised teas in Taiwan (a large producer of Oolong) is that too little oxidation upsets the stomach of some consumers. Even so, some producers attempt to minimise oxidation in order to produce a specific taste.

4. Black tea/Red tea: The tea leaves are allowed to completely oxidise. Black tea is the most common form of tea in southern Asia (Sri Lanka, India, Pakistan, Bangladesh, etc.) and in the last century many African countries including Kenya, Burundi, Rwanda, Malawi and Zimbabwe. The literal translation of the Chinese word is red tea, which is used by some tea lovers. The Chinese call it red tea because the actual tea liquid is red. Westerners call it black tea because the tea leaves used to brew it are usually black. However, red tea may also refer to rooibos, an increasingly popular South African tisane. Black tea is first withered to induce protein breakdown and reduce water content (68–77 per cent of original), heavily rolled or torn to bruise and disrupt the leaf cell structures and activate oxidation. The oxidation process takes between 45–90 minutes to 3 hours and is done at high humidity between 20°–30°C, transforming much of the catechins of the leaves into complex tannin.

5. Black tea produced through CTC processing: Black tea is further classified as either orthodox or as Crush, Tear, Curl (CTC), a production method developed around 1932. Unblended black teas are also identified by the estate they come from, their year and the flush (first, second or autumn). Orthodox processed black teas are further graded according to the post-production leaf quality by the Orange Pekoe system, while CTC teas use a different grading system.

6. Post-fermented tea: Teas that undergo a second oxidation, such as Pu-erh, Liu'an, and Liubao, are collectively referred to as secondary or post-fermentation teas in English. In Chinese they are categorised as Dark tea or black tea. This is not to be confused with the English term Black tea, known in Chinese as red tea. Pu-erh, also known as Póu léi (Polee) in Cantonese is the most common type of post-fermetation tea in the market.

7. Yellow tea: This tea is processed in a similar manner to green tea but instead of immediate drying after fixation is stacked, covered, and gently heated in a humid environment. This initiates oxidation in the chlorophyll of the leaves through nonenzymatic and non-microbial means, which results in a yellowish or greenish-yellow colour. This tea is popular in Japanese tea ceremonies due to its appearance, but the flavour as well is distinctive. The name derives from this 'yellowing' process, and possibly includes a reference to the colour yellow which indicates the emperor, as this was a tea popular at court ceremonies for its bright colour and smooth pouring before the Imperial court.

GREEN TEA

Green Tea Fermentation

For the production of green tea, the fresh leaves are withered in hot pans at a temperature of 160°F (Chinese method) or steamed (Japanese method); then rolled to break them up and liberate their juices; then 'fired'.

It will be observed that the chief difference between black and green tea is that the former is fermented, while the latter is not; and one of the main results of fermentation seems to be to render the tannic acid less soluble, so that, as we shall shortly see, an infusion of green tea contains more tannin than an infusion of black. In former days a good deal of so-called green tea was really made in the same way as black, and subsequently 'faced' with Prussian blue or indigo to give it the proper colour.

We have seen that the quality of teas varies with the age of the leaf from which they are prepared, the younger leaves yielding the finest tea. Apart from this cause of variation, teas show marked differences according to the country and district in which they are produced.

Chinese teas have the most delicate flavour of any, but are rather lacking in 'body'; they are also devoid of any marked astringency. Indian teas, and especially those produced in Assam, have the greatest degree of 'body' and astringency. This makes them powerful teas, suited rather for blending with milder varieties than for drinking alone.

Ceylon teas have plenty of body, and a rich and peculiar flavour, but have not so much strength or pungency as the Indian varieties. According to the district in which they are produced, Chinese black teas may be divided into:

1. Monings, from North China, with a small and delicate leaf and a peculiar malty flavour.
2. Kaisows, from South China, the so-called red-leaf teas, because the original teas grown in this district had a reddish leaf.
3. Oolongs, from Formosa, pungent and slightly bitter, yielding a pale infusion, and chiefly used for purposes of blending.
4. Scented orange Pekoe and scented Caper come from the Canton district, and yield a pale, strong infusion with an aromatic flavour, for which reason they are used to give bouquet to blends. Caper is really an unfermented tea, highly fired, and standing intermediate between the black and green varieties.

CACAO

Fermentation of Cacao

The cacao fruits are opened and the pulp and seeds are transferred to larger containers. This is either performed by farmers, plantation workers or in large cocoa factories where it can be done by machines.

The cacao beans are later transferred to wooden crates or baskets with banana leaves in between and on top to enable an optimal fermentation. The duration of the fermentation depends on the variety and is from 2 to more than 7 days. The length of the fermentation also affects the aroma, so if well-developed aroma is wanted the beans are fermentation for a longer time.

Extracting, fermenting and drying cacao beans

Following the growing and harvesting period, the cacao pods are processed and prepared for their distribution.

Extraction: To extract the cacao bean, cacao pods are split open with measured force. It is important to protect the cacao bean when opening the pods so as not to damage them or compromise their juice.

Fermenting: The beans and pulp are moulded into a conical heap. The heap is then rolled in banana leaves, making sure that it's entirely shut. In this closed environment, the cacao beans ferment for a given period of time (usually not more than a week). Fermentation results in the beans' colour change from purple to brown, and the emergence of a cacao butter aroma reminiscent to that of chocolate. An optional part of cacao bean cultivation, fermenting is only performed by certain growers. It still remains a debate amongst growers and chocolate manufacturers, many of which skip the fermentation process altogether.

Drying: Following either harvesting or fermentation, the beans must be dried before being distributed or processed into cacao butter. They are scattered over bamboo mats that allow for ventilation and are left to dry for two to four weeks. As the dehydration process progresses, the beans are regularly turned to prevent the formation of mould and bacteria.

In industrialised cacao processing plants, drying is done in special ventilated chambers that protect the cacao beans from high levels of humidity. Nevertheless, their flavour is not comparable to those dried naturally under the sun of the tropics, nor is the quality of the butter they produce.

More hubs

Tempering chocolate

If you are looking to master the art of handling chocolate, learning to temper chocolate should be high up on your to-do list. Tempering is important to chocolate-making, as it preserves the chocolate's original characteristics. Cool down your chocolate too quickly, and it will form sugar crystals that give it a rough, grainy texture. Cool it down too slowly, and it will retain a gummy, elastic quality.

Tempering stabilises the relationship between the butter fat and the cocoa solids present in chocolate. This process (also known as emulsification) enables chocolate to be handled effortlessly when using moulds and chocolate fondant. Tempering also aids in preserving the chocolate's flavour, quality, and appearance for longer periods of time, as well as preserving its flavour and appearance.

When a chocolate is manufactured, it is tempered before being moulded and finished. But once a tempered chocolate is melted, it must be tempered again before it cools down into a solid piece.

It's easy to recognise untempered chocolate, because it blooms, acquiring a dull, brittle appearance, and sometimes looks cloudy and white on the surface. To temper chocolate, you will need a plastic or silicon dough scraper and a cold, flat surface that will easily lower the temperature of your chocolate.

Professional chocolatiers prefer to use a slab of marble. If this isn't an option, use an baking sheet placed upside-down on the counter. If you wish to cool your chocolate faster, put a plate with ice beneath the baking sheet to accelerate the process.

Melt your chocolate and make sure that its smooth and homogeneous before you start tempering. Pour more than half of the chocolate over your tempering surface. Using your plastic dough scraper, spread the chocolate in a circular motion, thinning it gently. Scrape the chocolate up and spread it thinly in a circle once again. Repeat this process for about five minutes or until temperature reaches 82°F. Once the temperature is right, return the tempered chocolate into the bowl and mix it into the remaining melted chocolate. Once combined, the chocolate cannot exceed a temperature of 90°F. Your chocolate is now tempered and ready for use.

Growing and harvesting cacao beans

If you are located in a region surrounding the Equator or if your climatic conditions will allow for their growth, harvesting cacao beans can be a profitable hobby. Whether you simply wish to know about the cultivation of cacao beans or you are researching a business plan, these basics of cacao bean cultivation and processing should give you a good idea of how cacao beans are treated in the making of chocolate.

Tropical areas within 20 degrees of the equator are the best places to grow the Theobroma cacao tree. An exacting tree specimen, cacao trees can only grow under specific temperatures, altitudes, and other atmospheric conditions, such as humidity, wind, and sun.

Cacao trees grow best when a protective canopy lies over them, much like is the case in their natural jungle habitats. However, they can also be grown entirely without protection, as they do in the islands of the Caribbean, Jamaica, and Trinidad.

Part 1-Growing as a cacao tree begins to grow, it takes the size of a small to medium tree. After 36 months, the cacao tree starts to bear fruit and continues to be productive for decades to come. Usually active for 10–50 years, cacao trees eventually lose fruit-bearing capabilities.

Four easy ways to melt chocolate

As is the case in many chocolate recipes, chocolate must be melted in order to be incorporated into a dessert. But melting chocolate to perfection, let alone baking it, isn't easy to master. It takes a combination of experience and instinct to melt chocolate without burning it or altering its unique composition.

Below we have compiled four different chocolate-melting techniques that you can implement in your everyday cooking.
1. Caramel brownies: 1 cup all-purpose flour, pre-sifted 1/4 tsp., iodised salt 1/2 tsp., double acting baking powder 1 1/4 cup, white granulated sugar 1/3 cup, unsweetened baking cocoa powder 3 tbsp., chocolate cook and serve.
2. Recipe for home-made hot chocolate: On a cold winter's day or evening, one of the most commonly consumed beverages is hot chocolate. Hot chocolate is a delectable treat, no matter if it is ordered pre-made from a coffee shop, made from a mix or made from scratch. However, using your own recipe for home-made hot chocolate produces a beverage with so much more meaning.
3. Chocolate chip cookie recipe: This is a contest for the best chocolate chip cookie recipe on the planet. Many people have tried to recreate this age old classic of gooey chocolate and scrumptious cookie but only a few have actually gotten it right. Every single cookbook you look into will

have a version of this popular American favourite. A contest is now being held to find the absolute best chocolate chip cookie recipe on the planet.

4. Chocolate cake recipe: For many people, when you ask them what their favourite cake flavour is, the answer is likely to be chocolate. In fact, some people love chocolate so much that they would probably worship at an altar to ensure a steady supply! So how do you decide which chocolate cake recipe you will bake for that special occasion or those just because moments when you need a chocolate fix?

SOYA SAUCE

Soya sauce is a condiment produced by fermenting soyabeans with *Aspergillus oryzae* or *Aspergillus sojae* moulds, along with water and salt. After the fermentation, which yields moromi, the moromi is pressed, and two substances are obtained: a liquid, which is the soya sauce, and a cake of (wheat and) soya residue, the latter being usually reused as animal feed. Most commonly, a grain is used together with the soyabeans in the fermentation process, but not always. Also, some varieties use roasted grain. Soya sauce is a traditional ingredient in East and Southeast Asian cuisines, where it is used in cooking and as a condiment. In more recent times, it is also being used in Western cuisine and prepared foods.

Soya sauce may be made either by fermentation or by hydrolysis; some commercial sauces contain a mixture of fermented and chemical sauces. Traditional soya sauces are made by mixing soyabeans and grain with cultures such as *Aspergillus oryzae* and other related micro-organisms and yeasts. The resulting substance is called 'koji' (note that the term 'koji' is used both for the mixture of soyabeans, wheat, and mould; as well as for only the mould).

In older times, the koji was then fermented naturally in giant urns and under the sun, which was believed to contribute additional flavours. Today, the koji is generally placed in a 'muro' which is a temperature and humidity controlled incubation chamber. Some soya sauces made in the Japanese way or styled after them contain about fifty per cent wheat.

Some brands of soya sauce are often made from acid-hydrolysed soya protein instead of brewed with a traditional culture. This process may take only three days. Although they have a different flavour, aroma, and texture when compared to brewed soya sauces, they have a longer shelf-life and are more commonly produced for this reason. Some people feel the hydrolysed sauces taste better, but some prefer the naturally brewed varieties.

The clear plastic packets of dark sauce common with Chinese-style take out food typically use a hydrolysed vegetable protein formula. Some higher-quality hydrolysed vegetable protein products with no added salt, sugar or colourings are sold as low-sodium soya sauce alternatives called 'liquid aminos' in health food stores, similar to the way salt substitutes are used. Carcinogens may form during the manufacture of chemical sauce.

Types of Soya Sauce

Soya sauce has been integrated into the traditional cuisines of many East Asian and Southeast Asian cultures. Soya sauce is widely used as a particularly important flavouring in Japanese, Thai, Korean, and Chinese cuisine. Despite their rather similar appearance, soya sauces produced in different cultures and regions are different in taste, consistency, fragrance and saltiness. Soya sauce retains its quality longer when kept away from direct sunlight.

Chinese soya sauce

Chinese soya sauce is primarily made from soyabeans, with relatively low amounts of other grains. There are two main varieties:

1. Light or fresh soya sauce is a thin (low viscosity), opaque, lighter brown soya sauce. It is the main soya sauce used for seasoning, since it is saltier, has less noticeable colour, and also adds a distinct flavour. The light soya sauce made from the first pressing of the soyabeans is called tóuchōu, which can be loosely translated as first soya sauce or referred to as premium light soya sauce. Tóuchōu is sold at a premium because, like extra virgin olive oil, the flavour of the first pressing is considered superior. An additional classification of light soya sauce, shua-nghuáng, is double-fermented to add further complexity to the flavour. These last two more delicate types are used primarily for dipping.
2. Dark and old soya sauce, a darker and slightly thicker soya sauce, is aged longer and contains added molasses to give it its distinctive appearance. This variety is mainly used during cooking, since its flavour develops during heating. It has a richer, slightly sweeter, and less salty flavour than light soya sauce. Dark soya sauce is partly used to add colour and flavour to a dish after cooking, but, as stated above, is more often used during the cooking process, rather than after.

In traditional Chinese cooking, these soya sauces were employed in strategic ways to achieve a flavour and colour for the dish.

Another type, thick soya sauce, is a dark soya sauce that has been thickened with starch and sugar. It is occasionally flavoured with MSG. This sauce is not usually used directly in cooking, but more often as a dipping sauce or poured on food as a flavourful addition.

Japanese soya sauce

Buddhist monks introduced soya sauce into Japan in the 7th century, where it is known as shōyu. The Japanese word tamari is derived from the verb tamaru that signifies 'to accumulate', referring to the fact that tamari was traditionally a liquid by-product produced during the fermentation of miso. Japan is the leading producer of tamari.

Shōyu is traditionally divided into five main categories depending on differences in their ingredients and method of production. Most, but not all Japanese soya sauces include wheat as a primary ingredient, which tends to give them a slightly sweeter taste than their Chinese counterparts. They also tend towards an alcoholic sherry-like flavour, sometimes enhanced by the addition of small amounts of alcohol as a natural preservative. The widely varying flavours of these soya sauces are not always interchangeable, some recipes only call for one type or the other, much like a white wine cannot replace a red's flavour or beef stock does not produce the same results as fish stock.

Production process

The explanation of Honjozo (genuine fermented) type is explained as follows. First, put soyabeans and one without lipid in water, pressure and boil them. Roast wheat and smash them up. Following sentence is the main process.

1. Mix an equal amount of boiled soyabeans and roasted wheat. Add a little spore of the mould (only for making soya sauce). Mix again for a few days. After this, they changed into enough amount of the mould.
2. Put saline solution into that culture of the mould.

3. They are fermented by the mould. On this time, wild nature lactic acid bacteria make lactic acid in them. After this, wild nature yeasts make alcohol. Most of soya sauce's smell are chemicals produced in this process by the moulds. In the moulds, an amino-glycosidic reaction takes place.
4. Fold them in nylon cloth and squeeze it. Then they are divided into the liquid and other. This liquid is nearly soya sauce.
5. Heat the liquid, and filter out the contamination in the liquid.
6. Finally, pour the liquid into a container.

Related micro-organisms

Koji: Koji is a fungus of genus Aspergillus that is used for fermenting many ingredients in Japanese cuisine. Three species are used for brewing soya sauce:
1. *Aspergillus oryzae*: Strains with high proteolytic capacity are used for brewing soya sauce. This fungus is also used for saccharification of steamed rice for brewing sake.
2. *Aspergillus sojae*: This fungus also has a high proteolytic capacity.
3. *Aspergillus tamari*: This fungus is used for brewing tamari.

Microbes contained in Koji:
1. *Bacillus* spp. (genus): This organism is likely to grow soya sauce ingredients, bring to generate odours and ammonia.
2. *Lactobacillus* species: This organism produces a lactic acid increases the acidity in the feed.

Soya sauce varieties

1. *Koikuchi* (dark colour): Originating in the Kantō region, its usage eventually spread all over Japan. Over 80 per cent of the Japanese domestic soya sauce production is of *koikuchi*, and can be considered the typical Japanese soya sauce. It is produced from roughly equal quantities of soyabean and wheat. This variety is also called *kijōyu* or *namashōyu* when it is not pasteurised.
2. *Usukuchi* (light colour): Particularly popular in the Kansai region of Japan, it is both saltier and lighter in colour than *koikuchi*. The lighter colour arises from the use of amazake, a sweet liquid made from fermented rice, that is used in its production.
3. *Tamari*: Produced mainly in the Chūbu region of Japan, *tamari* is darker in appearance and richer in flavour than *koikuchi*. It contains little or no wheat; wheat-free *tamari* can be used by people with gluten intolerance. It is the 'original' Japanese soya sauce, as its recipe is closest to the soya sauce originally introduced to Japan from China. Technically, this variety is known as misōdamari, as this is the liquid that runs off miso as it matures.
4. *Shiro* (white): In contrast to *tamari* soya sauce, *shiro* soya sauce uses mostly wheat and very little soyabean, lending it a light appearance and sweet taste. It is more commonly used in the Kansai region to highlight the appearances of food, for example *sashimi*.
5. *Saishikomi* (twice-brewed): This variety substitutes previously-made *koikuchi* for the brine normally used in the process. Consequently, it is much darker and more strongly flavoured. This type is also known as *kanro shōyu* or 'sweet shōyu'.

Newer varieties of Japanese soya sauce include:
1. *Gen'en* (reduced salt): This version contains 50 per cent less salt than regular shōyu for health conscious consumers.
2. *Usujio* (light salt): This version contains 20 per cent less salt than regular shōyu.

All of these varieties are sold in the marketplace in three different grades according to how they were produced:

1. *Honjōzō* (genuine fermented): Contains 100 per cent genuine fermented product.
2. *Kongō-jōzō* (mixed fermented): Contains genuine fermented shōyu mash mixed with 30–50 per cent of chemical or enzymatic hydrolysate of plant protein.
3. *Kongō* (mixed): Contains *Honjōzō* or *Kongōj-ōzō shōyu* mixed with 30–50 per cent of chemical or enzymatic hydrolysate of plant protein.

All the varieties and grades may be sold according to three official levels of quality:

1. *Hyōjun*: Standard grade, contains more than 1.2 per cent total nitrogen.
2. *Jōkyū*: Upper grade, contains more than 1.35 per cent of total nitrogen.
3. *Tokkyū*: Special grade, contains more than 1.5 per cent of total nitrogen.

Soya sauce is also commonly known as *shōyu* in Hawaii.

MISO

Miso is a traditional Japanese seasoning produced by fermenting rice, barley and/or soyabeans, with salt and the fungus *kōjikin*, the most typical miso being made with soya. The result is a thick paste used for sauces and spreads, pickling vegetables or meats, and mixing with dashi soup stock to serve as miso soup called *misoshiru*, a Japanese culinary staple. High in protein and rich in vitamins and minerals, miso played an important nutritional role in feudal Japan. Miso is still very widely used in Japan, both in traditional and modern cooking, and has been gaining worldwide interest. Miso is typically salty, but its flavour and aroma depend on various factors in the ingredients and fermentation process. There is a very wide variety of miso available. Different varieties of miso have been described as salty, sweet, earthy, fruity, and savoury.

The earliest form of miso is known as 'Hishio'. Hishio is a kind of salty seasoning which is made from grain. The origin of the miso of Japan is not completely clear.

1. Grain and fish misos had been manufactured in Japan since the Neolithic era (Jōmon period). These are called 'Jōmon miso'.
2. This miso predecessor originated in China during the 3rd century BC or earlier. It is likely that Hishio, and other fermented soya-based foods, were introduced to Japan at the same time as Buddhism in the 6th century AD. This fermented food was called 'Shi'.

Until the Muromachi era, miso was made without grinding the soyabeans, somewhat like natto. In the Kamakura era, a common meal was made up of a bowl of rice, some dried fish, a serving of miso, and a fresh vegetable.

In the Muromachi era, Buddhist monks discovered that soyabeans could be ground into a paste, spawning new cooking methods using miso to flavour other foods. In medieval times, the word 'Temaemiso', meaning home-made miso, appeared. Miso production is a relatively simple process and so home-made versions spread throughout Japan. Miso was used as military provisions during the Sengoku era and making miso was an important economic activity for daimyos of that era.

During the Edo period miso was also called *hishio* and *kuki* and various type of miso that fit with each climate and culture was formed throughout Japan.

These days miso is produced industrially in large quantities and traditional home-made miso has become a rarity. In recent years, many new types of miso have appeared. For example, there are ones with added soup stocks or calcium or reduced salt for health, etc.

Flavour

The taste, aroma, texture, and appearance of miso all vary by region and season. Other important variables that contribute to the flavour of a particular miso include temperature, duration of fermentation, salt content, variety of kōji, and fermenting vessel. The most common flavour categories of miso are:
1. *Shiromiso*, 'white miso'.
2. *Akamiso*, 'red miso'.
3. *Awasemiso*, 'mixed miso'.
4. *Hatchomiso*.

Although white and red (*shiromiso* and *akamiso*) are the most common types of misos available, different varieties may be preferred in particular regions of Japan. In the eastern Kantō region that includes Tokyo, the darker brownish *akamiso* is popular while the western Kansai region encompassing Osaka, Kyoto, and Kobe prefer the lighter *shiromiso*. *Hatchomiso* is favoured in the Tokai area.

Ingredients

The ingredients used to produce miso may include any mix of soyabeans, barley, rice, buckwheat, millet, rye, wheat, hemp seed, and cycad, among others. Lately, producers in other countries have also begun selling miso made from chickpeas, corn, azuki beans, amaranth, and quinoa. Fermentation time ranges from as little as five days to several years. The wide variety of Japanese miso is difficult to classify, but is commonly done by grain type, colour, taste, and background.
1. *Mugi*: Barley.
2. *Tsubu*: Whole wheat/barley.
3. *Genmai*: Brown rice.
4. *Moromi*: Chunky, healthy (kōji is unblended).
5. *Nanban*: Mixed with hot chili pepper for dipping sauce.
6. *Taima*: Hemp seed.
7. *Sobamugi*: Buckwheat.
8. *Hadakamugi*: Rye.
9. *Nari*: Made from cycad pulp, Buddhist temple diet.
10. *Gokoku*: '5 grain': soya, wheat, barley, proso millet, and foxtail millet.

Many regions have their own specific variation on the miso standard. For example, the soyabeans used in Sendai miso are much more coarsely mashed than in normal soya miso.

Miso made with rice such as *shinshu* and *shiro* are called kome miso. Types of miso are divided by main ingredients.
1. *Kome* miso, 'rice miso': Colour is yellow, yellowish white or red, etc. Whitish miso is made from boiled soyabean, but reddish miso is made from steamed soyabean. Much of *Kome* miso is consumed in Eastern Japan, *Hokuriku* and *Kinki* areas.
2. *Mugi* miso, 'barley miso': Whitish miso is produced in *Kyusyu*, Whestern *Chugoku* area in Japan, *Shikoku* areas. *Mugi* miso has a peculiar smell. Northern *Kanto* area produces reddish miso.
3. *Mame* miso, 'soyabean miso': Miso is a darker, more reddish brown than *kome* miso. This is not so sweet, but has some astringency and good *umami*. This miso requires a long maturing term. *Mame* miso is consumed in mostly *Aichi* prefecture, part of *Gifu* prefecture and part of *Mie* prefecture.

4. *Tyougou* miso, 'mixed miso': This comes in various types, because it consists of other varieties of miso mixed together. This may improve the weak points of each type of miso. For example, *Mame* miso is very salty. But when combined with *Kome* miso, the finished product has a mild taste.

5. Red miso: This is aged for a long time, such as over one year. Therefore, due to Maillard reaction, the colour of this miso changes gradually from white to red or black, thus giving it the name red miso. Features of the taste are saltiness, and some astringency with *umami*. Factors in the depth of colour are the formula of the soyabeans themselves and the quantity of soyabeans used. Generally, steamed soyabeans are more deeply coloured than boiled soyabeans.

6. White miso: The most widely produced miso, made in many regions of the country. Its main ingredients are rice, barley, and a small quantity of soyabeans. If you added a greater quantity of soyabeans, the miso would be red or brown. Compared with red miso, white miso has a very short brewing time. The taste is sweet, but the *umami* is soft (compared to red miso).

Storage and Preparation

Miso typically comes as a paste in a sealed container requiring refrigeration after opening. Natural miso is a living food containing many beneficial micro-organisms such as *Tetragenococcus halophilus* which can be killed by overcooking. For this reason, it is recommended that the miso be added to soups or other foods being prepared just before they are removed from the heat. Using miso without any cooking may be even better. Outside of Japan, a popular practice is to only add miso to foods that have cooled in order to preserve *kōjikin* cultures in miso. Nonetheless miso and soya foods play a large role in the Japanese diet and many cooked miso dishes are popularly consumed.

Usage

Miso is a part of many Japanese-style meals. It most commonly appears as the main ingredient of miso soup, which is eaten daily by much of the Japanese population. The pairing of plain rice and miso soup is considered a fundamental unit of Japanese cuisine. This pairing is the basis of a traditional Japanese breakfast. Miso is used in many other types of soup and souplike dishes, including some kinds of ramen, udon, nabe, and imoni. Generally, such dishes have the title *miso* prefixed to their name (for example, *miso-udon*), and have a heavier, earthier flavour and aroma compared to other Japanese soups that are not miso-based.

Many traditional confections use a sweet, thick miso glaze, such as mochidango. Miso glazed treats are strongly associated with Japanese festivals, although they are available year-round at supermarkets. The consistency of miso glaze ranges from thick and taffy-like to thin and drippy.

Soya miso is used to make a type of pickle called 'misozuke'. These pickles are typically made from cucumber, daikon, hakusai or eggplant, and are sweeter and less salty than the standard Japanese salt pickle. Other foods with miso as an ingredient include:

1. Dengaku (sweetened miso used for grilling).
2. Yakimochi (charcoal-grilled miso covered mochi).
3. Miso braised vegetables or mushrooms.
4. Marinades: Fish or chicken can be marinated in miso and sake overnight to be grilled.
5. Corn on the cob in Japan is often coated with shiro miso, wrapped in foil and grilled.
6. Sauces: Sauces like misoyaki (a variant on teriyaki) are common.

7. Dips: Used as a dip to eat with vegetables (e.g. cucumbers, daikon, carrots, etc.).
8. Side dish: Miso is often eaten not only as a condiment but also as a side dish. Mixed or cooked miso with spices/ vegetables are called 'okazu-miso', which are often eaten along with hot rice, or spread over onigiri.

Nutrition and Health

The nutritional benefits of miso have been widely touted by commercial enterprises and home cooks alike. Claims that miso is high in vitamin B_{12} have been contradicted in some studies. Part of the confusion may stem from the fact that some soya products are high in B vitamins (though not necessarily B_{12}) and some, such as soya milk, may be fortified with vitamin B_{12}. Some, especially proponents of healthful eating, suggest that miso can help treat radiation sickness, citing cases in Japan and Russia where people have been fed miso after the Chernobyl nuclear disaster and the atomic bombings of Hiroshima and Nagasaki. Notably, Japanese doctor Shinichiro Akizuki, director of Saint Francis Hospital in Nagasaki during World War II, theorised that miso helps protect against radiation sickness.

Some experts suggest that miso is a source of *Lactobacillus acidophilus*. Lecithin, a kind of phospholipid caused by fermentation, which is effective in the prevention of high blood pressure. However, miso is also relatively high in salt which can contribute to increased blood pressure in the small percentage of the population with sodium-sensitive pre-hypertension or hypertension. Based on the other results of double-blind controlled studies of sodium and hypertension, there is no definitive evidence that high sodium intake leads to negative clinical conditions such as hypertension in healthy persons. Clinical evidence indicates wide-population heterogeneity in response to sodium.

TEMPEH

Tempeh or tempe (Indonesian), is a traditional soya product originally from Indonesia. It is made by a natural culturing and controlled fermentation process that binds soyabeans into a cake form, similar to a very firm vegetarian burger patty. Tempeh is unique among major traditional soya-foods in that it is the only one that did not originate in the Sinosphere.

It originated in today's Indonesia, and is especially popular on the island of Java, where it is a staple source of protein. Like tofu, tempeh is made from soyabeans, but tempeh is a whole soyabean product with different nutritional characteristics and textural qualities. Tempeh's fermentation process and its retention of the whole bean give it a higher content of protein, dietary fibre, and vitamins. It has a firm texture and strong flavour. Because of its nutritional value, tempeh is used worldwide in vegetarian cuisine; some consider it to be a meat analogue.

Production of Tempeh

Tempeh begins with whole soyabeans, which are softened by soaking and dehulled, then partly cooked. Speciality tempehs may be made from other types of beans, wheat or may include a mixture of beans and whole grains. A mild acidulent, usually vinegar, may be added in order to lower the pH and create a selective environment that favours the growth of the tempeh mould over competitors. A fermentation starter containing the spores of fungus *Rhizopus oligosporus* is mixed in. The beans are spread into a thin layer and are allowed to ferment for 24 to 36 hours at a temperature around 30°C (86°F). In good tempeh, the beans are knitted together by a mat of white mycelia.

Under conditions of lower temperature or higher ventilation, gray or black patches of spores may form on the surface—this is not harmful, and should not affect the flavour or quality of the tempeh.

This sporulation is normal on fully mature tempeh. A mild ammonia smell may accompany good tempeh as it ferments, but it should not be overpowering. In Indonesia, ripe tempeh (two or more days old) is considered a delicacy.

Nutrition

The soya protein in tempeh becomes more digestible as a result of the fermentation process. In particular, the oligosaccharides that are associated with gas and indigestion are greatly reduced by the *Rhizopus* culture. In traditional tempeh making shops, the starter culture often contains beneficial bacteria that produce vitamins such as B_{12} (though it is uncertain whether this B_{12} is always present and bioavailable). In western countries, it is more common to use a pure culture containing only *Rhizopus oligosporus* which makes very little B_{12} and could be missing *Klebsiella pneumoniae* which has been shown to produce significant levels of B_{12} analogues in tempeh when present. Whether these analogues are true, bioavailable B_{12}, hasn't been thoroughly studied yet.

Preparation

In the kitchen, tempeh is often prepared by cutting it into pieces, soaking in brine or salty sauce, and then frying. Cooked tempeh can be eaten alone, or used in chili, stir frys, soups, salads, sandwiches, and stews. Tempeh has a complex flavour that has been described as nutty, meaty, and mushroom-like. Tempeh freezes well, and is now commonly available in many western supermarkets as well as in ethnic markets and health food stores. Tempeh performs well in a cheese grater, after which it may be used in the place of ground beef (as in tacos). When thin sliced and deep fried in oil, tempeh obtains a crispy golden crust while maintaining a soft interior—its sponge-like consistency make it suitable for marinades. Dried tempeh (whether cooked or raw) provides an excellent stew base for backpackers.

Types of tempeh

Types of tempeh are listed in Table 19.1.

Table 19.1. Types of tempeh.

Name	Description
Tempe bacem	Tempeh boiled with spices and palm sugar, and then fried for a few minutes to enhance the taste. The result is damp, spicy, sweet and dark-coloured tempeh.
Tempe bongkrèk	Made from or with coconut press cake.
Tempe bosok (*busuk*)	Rotten tempeh, used in small amounts as a flavouring.
Tempe gembus	Made from okara.
Tempe gódhóng	Tempeh wrapped in banana leaves.
Tempe goreng	Deep-fried tempeh.
Tempe mendoan	Thinly sliced tempeh, battered and deep fried quickly resulting in limp texture.
Tempe kedelai	Simply tempeh, made from soyabeans.
Tempe kering	Raw tempeh cut into little sticks, deep fried then mixed with spices and sugar, often mixed with separately fried peanuts and anchovies (ikan teri), this can be stored up to a month if cooked properly.
Tempe murni	Tempeh made in plastic wrap without any additives such as grated raw papaya (lit. pure soyabean cake).
Tempe oncom	Also onchom; made from peanut press cake; orange colour; *Neurospora sitophila*.

A new form of tempeh based on barley and oats instead of soya was developed by scientists at the Swedish Department of Food Science in 2008. It can be produced in climate regions where it is not possible to grow soya beans.

ANG-KHAK

Ang-khak, also known *äs anka*, angquac, beni-koji, aga-koji, red rice or Chinese red rice, is manufactured by solid state fermentation (SSF) of rice using various strains of *Monascus purpureus* and other related strains. During fermentation, the rice becomes pigmented, its colour varying from a bright yellow to orange red and deep purple. When fermentation is accomplished, Ang-khak is dried, milled and brought to the market, the shelf life being about one year. Ang-khak is being used in China, Taiwan, the Philippines, Thailand, and presumably in many other countries in the Orient. It is a commercial product in the southern provinces of China, in the Philippines, and in Indonesia. In Addition to providing colour, red rice is used to add flavour to foods and to inhibit undesirable bacteria that might cause food spoilage. The outstanding features of Ang-khak are:
1. Agricultural raw materials are easily available.
2. Yields are high.
3. High pigment stability (pH, sunlight, temperature).
4. No signs of toxicity (acute, chronical, mutagenicity) or cancerogenicity.
5. Effective in curing urinal incontinence of infants and Asthma.
6. Contains Monacolin a hypocholesterinemic agent.
7. Thrombolytic.

NATTO

Natto is a traditional Japanese food made from soyabeans fermented with *Bacillus subtilis*. It is popular especially as a breakfast food. As a rich source of protein and good bacteria, natto and the soyabean paste miso formed a vital source of nutrition in feudal Japan. Natto can be an acquired taste because of its powerful smell, strong flavour, and slippery texture. In Japan natto is most popular in the eastern regions, including Kanto, Tohoku, and Hokkaido.

Natto is most commonly eaten at breakfast to accompany rice, possibly with some other ingredients, for example soya sauce, tsuyu broth, mustard, scallions, grated daikon, okra, or a raw quail egg. In Hokkaido and northern Tohoku region, some people dust natto with sugar. Natto is also commonly used in other foods, such as natto- sushi, natto toast, in miso soup, tamagoyaki, salad, as an ingredient in okonomiyaki, or even with spaghetti or as fried natto. A dried form of natto, having little odour or sliminess, can be eaten as a nutritious snack. There is even natto ice cream. Soyabeans are sometimes crushed and fermented. This is called Hikiwarinatto. It is a food that is easy to digest, so Hikiwarinatto is very healthy.

The perceived flavour of natto- can differ greatly between people; some find it tastes very strong and cheesy and may use it in small amounts to flavour rice or noodles, while others find it tastes bland and unremarkable.

SOYABEAN CHEESE

Soyabean cheese, tou-fu-ju or tofu, is a Chinese fermented food made by soaking soyabeans, grinding them to a paste, and then filtering them through linen. The protein in the filtrate is curdled by means of a magnesium or calcium salt, after which the curd is pressed into blocks. The blocks, arranged on trays, are held in a fermentation chamber for a month at about 14°C, during which period white moulds, probably *Mucor* spp., develop. Final ripening takes place in brine or in a special wine.

MINCHIN

Fermented minchin is made from wheat gluten from which the starch has been removed. The moist, raw gluten is placed in a closed jar and allowed to ferment for 2 to 3 weeks, after which it is slated. A typical specimen was found to contain seven species of moulds, nine of bacteria, and three of yeasts. The final product is cut into strips to be boiled, backed or fried.

IDLI

Idli is a south Indian savoury cake popular throughout India. The cakes are usually two to three inches in diameter and are made by steaming a batter consisting of fermented black lentils (de-husked) and rice. The fermentation process breaks down the starches so that they are more readily metabolised by the body. Steamed idli in India may have been an imported idea from Indonesia. The earliest mention of idli in India occurs in Kannada writing of Shivakotiacharya in 920 CE.

Idli, a fermented food of India, is made from rice and black gram mungo in equal parts. The ingredients are washed and soaked separately, ground, mixed, and finally allowed to ferment overnight. When the batter has risen enough, it is cooked by steaming and served hot. *Leuconostoc mesenteroides* grows first in the batter, leavening it, and is followed by *Streptococcus faecalis* and finally *Pediococcus cerevisiae*, all of which contribute to the acidity.

Most often eaten at breakfast or as a snack, idlis are usually served in pairs with chutney, sambar or other accompaniments. Mixtures of crushed dry spices such as milagai podi are the preferred condiment for idlis eaten on the go.

POI

Poi is a Hawaiian word for the primary Polynesian staple food made from the corm of the taro plant (known in Hawaiian as *kalo*). Poi is produced by mashing the cooked corm (baked or steamed) until it is a highly viscous fluid. Water is added during mashing and again just before eating, to achieve a desired consistency, which can range from liquid to dough-like (poi can be known as two-finger or three-finger, alluding to how many fingers you would have to use to eat it, depending on its consistency).

Poi made from Taro should not be confused with:

1. Samoan poi, which is a creamy dessert created by mashing ripe bananas with coconut cream.
2. Tahitian po'e, which is a sweet, pudding-like dish made with bananas, papaya or mangoes cooked with manioc and coconut cream.

Poi has a paste-like texture and a delicate flavour. The flavour changes distinctly once the poi has been made. Fresh poi is sweet and edible all by itself. Each day thereafter the poi loses sweetness and turns slightly sour. Because of this, some people find poi more palatable when it is mixed with milk and/or sugar. The speed of this fermentation process depends upon the bacteria level in the poi. To slow the souring process, poi should be stored in a cool, dark location (such as a kitchen cupboard). Poi stored in the refrigerator should be squeezed out of the bag into a bowl, and a thin layer of water drizzled over the top to keep a crust from forming. Sour poi is still quite edible with salted fish or lomi salmon on the side. Sourness is prevented by freezing or dehydrating, although the resulting poi tends to be bland in comparison with the fresh product. For best thawing results place in a microwave with a layer of tap water over the surface of the frozen poi. Sour poi is also used as a cooking ingredient, usually in breads and rolls. It has a smooth, creamy mouthfeel.

Other Uses

Poi has been used as a milk substitute for babies born with an allergy to dairy products because of its nutritional value. It is also used as a baby food for babies with severe food allergies.

THE WAY AHEAD

Fermentation is one of the oldest forms of food preservation technology in the world. Indigenous fermented foods such as bread, cheese and wine, have been prepared and consumed for thousands of years and are strongly linked to culture and tradition, especially in rural households and village communities. Fermented foods are popular throughout the world and in some regions make a significant contribution to the diet of millions of individuals. For instance Soya sauce is consumed throughout the world and is a fundamental ingredient in diets from Indonesia to Japan. Over one billion litres of soya sauce are produced each year in Japan alone. In Africa fermented cassava products (like *gari* and *fufu*) are a major component of the diet of more than 800 million people and in some areas these products constitute over 50 per cent of the diet. Fermentation is a relatively efficient, low energy preservation process, which increases the shelf life and decreases the need for refrigeration or other forms of food preservation technology. It is, therefore, a highly appropriate technique for use in developing countries and remote areas where access to sophisticated equipment is limited. There is tremendous scope and potential for the use of micro-organisms towards meeting the growing world demand for food, through efficient utilisation of available natural food and feed stocks and the transformation of waste materials.

There is a danger that the introduction of 'western foods' with their glamorous image will displace these traditional fermented foods. Although fermentation of foods has been in use for thousands of years for the preservation and improvement of a range of foods, the microbial and enzymatic processes responsible for the transformations were, and still are, largely unknown. Because of the tremendously important role indigenous fermented fruits and vegetables play in food preservation and their potential to contribute to the growing food needs of the world, it is essential that the knowledge of their production is not lost. Moreover, it is essential to increase the knowledge and understanding of the methods of preparation, in order to improve the efficiency of fermentation, especially the traditional processes as the yields of traditional fermentation processes are often low and sometimes the products are unsafe. This section discusses potential areas for improvement of indigenous fermented fruit and vegetable products. It can be divided into four main areas:

1. Improve the understanding of the fermented products.
2. Refine the processes.
3. Disseminate the improvements.
4. Create a supportive policy environment.

Improving the Understanding of Fermented Products

For fermented products such as cheese, bread, beer and wine, which are produced on a commercial scale, a good understanding of the microbial processes has been developed. However, with many of the fermented products in Africa, Asia and Latin America, knowledge of the processes involved is poor. It is likely that the basic principles apply across the board, but production conditions vary enormously from region to region, giving rise to numerous variations of the basic fermented product. It is not the intention or the desire to standardise the process and thereby lose this huge diversity, rather it is to harness the tremendous potential these methods have to contribute to increasing not only the quantity, but quality of food available to the world's population.

There are two main reasons for gaining a better understanding of indigenous fermented products:

1. Documenting the traditional knowledge to ensure that the huge diversity is not lost.
2. Developing a scientific understanding of the microbial processes, with a view to improving the efficiency of the process.

Documenting the traditional knowledge

Fermentation is one of the oldest food processing technologies in the world. The knowledge of how to make these products has often been passed down from parent to child (usually mother to daughter) and belongs to that undervalued body of 'indigenous knowledge'. Most of this knowledge has not been documented and is in danger of being lost as technologies evolve and families move away from traditional food preservation practices. The collection and preservation of indigenous knowledge is of interest to governments, historians, anthropologists and scientists, to name but a few. Several individuals and organisations are actively involved in research in this area.

Several research institutes and scientists in Africa, Asia and Latin America are recording information on traditional fermented foods.

Intermediate Technology has been collecting information about traditional food products from Africa, Asia and Latin America. This included the following fermented food products: *kenkey*, *ogi*, *injera*, fermented sweet bread, sorghum beer, palm wine, banana beer, pineapple peel vinegar, lime pickle, tamarind pickle, mango pickle, *gari*, vegetable pickle, coconut toddy, yoghurt, *ayib* and *dawdawa*.

The Special Program on Biotechnology and Development Cooperation for the Netherlands Government was established in 1992 to improve the access of developing countries to biotechnological expertise and innovation with a focus on using biotechnology for the benefit of small-scale farmers and producers. Part of the program involved a competition to identify farmers' existing biotechnology practises. This program resulted in the collection of valuable information about traditional fermented food products. Finally, the Food and Agriculture Organisation of the United Nations sees the value in collecting and preserving this source of knowledge.

Developing a scientific understanding of the microbial processes

Most traditional fermented products are made by natural fermentations carried out in a non-sterile environment. The specific environmental conditions cause a gradual selection of micro-organisms responsible for the desired final product. This is appropriate for small-scale production for home consumption. However, the method is difficult to control and there are risks of accompanying microflora causing spoilage and unsafe products.

If the processes are to be refined, with a view to production on a larger scale, it is essential to have a scientific understanding of the fermentation processes. This can be developed by:

1. The isolation and characterisation of the essential micro-organisms involved.
2. The determination of the role of external factors in fermentations and the effects of these on the metabolism of micro-organisms.
3. The investigation of the effects of pre-treatments of raw materials on the fermentation process.
4. The identification of the options for further processing and how these affect the taste and texture of the product.

This research is capital intensive and usually requires scarce foreign exchange. It requires the use of sophisticated equipment and reagents backed with a consistent energy and water supply which are not always available in developing countries. To meet the current and future challenges in developing countries, it is important that these countries develop the capabilities to benefit from improvements in fermentation methodologies. Biotechnologies need to be developed which are affordable by the poor, since it is they who are likely to benefit most by improvements to the traditional processes.

Refining the Process

The art of traditional processes needs to be refined to incorporate objective methods of process control and to standardise quality of the final product without losing their desirable attributes such as improved keeping quality, taste and nutritional qualities. Science based fermentation research has often focused mainly on improving the metabolic properties of the micro-organisms used as a starter culture, using the techniques of selection, mutation and genetic modification. To achieve this a full understanding of the fermentation process is needed. The properties of the starter culture must be known and culture conditions must be controllable. This means that science based fermentation research currently has little to offer traditional food processing.

Process control

Once the details of the fermentation process and the microbes involved are known and understood, it is possible to begin to refine and improve the process. The commercially produced products, such as bread, wine, soya sauce and pickles are all examples of processes which have been studied and optimised. Recently traditional fermented products in Africa have been industrialised. In Nigeria, Dadwa (a fermented legume product) is now made by Cadburys and in Zimbabwe, traditional fermented milk is made industrially and sold as 'Lacto'. The areas where the efficiency and yield of food fermentation processes can be increased are:

1. The selection or development of more productive microbial strains.
2. The control and manipulation of culture conditions.
3. The improvement of product purification and concentration.

Techniques to control the fermentation processes could include the development of pure starter cultures. Developing these by laboratory selection or genetic engineering is not viable. A more feasible approach would be to exploit the ecological principle of inoculum enrichment by natural selection. Another approach to stabilise fermentation under nonsterile conditions is the use of multi-strain dehydrated starters which can be stored at ambient temperature. These are already used for the manufacture of tempeh.

Quality control

The aim of quality control is to ensure that every batch of food produced has a satisfactory and uniform quality. This does not necessarily mean that it is the highest quality possible but that it reaches the standard the customers are willing to pay for. Inadequate quality control can have an adverse effect on local demand for the product. This is particularly a problem for small-scale traditional production. In modern industrial applications, the fermentation equipment and processes are controlled using expensive technology, resulting in a consistent product of a known quality. Traditional practises take place in a less predictable environment. This can result in mistakes including sour beer and mouldy pickles.

It is often felt that traditional products made at the small scale are unhygienic and unsafe. This is sometimes true. However, the case is often overstated. Many fermented foods are inherently safe due to low moisture contents or high acidity. Lime pickle from India and Gundruk from Nepal are good examples. Several of the steps in traditional processing are designed to reduce contamination. These include boiling, adding salt and sun drying.

Quality control procedures are essential for the production of safe products and contribute to the success of small food processing businesses. Appropriate quality control procedures need to be developed and implemented. These procedures need to be developed with the processors who must understand and apply them. The quality of food is highly subjective. What is acceptable to one customer is not acceptable to another. It is important to carry out participative research to identify ways to improve the quality control procedures for fermented food products.

The sort of areas that should be investigated include:

1. Selecting good quality raw materials.
2. Processing under correct conditions.
3. Ensuring high standards of personal hygiene by the food processors.
4. Ensuring the processing area is sufficiently clean.
5. Using correct packaging.

Disseminating Improvements

Documentation of the traditional methods of food fermentation and research to identify improved methods of production are meaningless if the results are not disseminated to those who are likely to put them into practice. There is a danger of mystifying the fermentation process by enrobing it in scientific theory. What was once a simple process carried out by any family member, in the confines of the household, using locally available equipment and materials, could become a process to be feared. It is important to be realistic and to ensure that the improvements recommended are ones which can easily be put into practice. The aim is not to deter the production of fermented foods at the small scale, but to encourage their production and consumption on a larger scale.

Fermented foods often have a stigma attached to them—they are considered as poor man's food. As soon as a family can afford to buy processed foods, they move away from carrying out home fermentation. This is a pity, because as we have seen earlier, fermented food products have many nutritional advantages which surpass western-style fast foods and processed foods. Where cultural values attached to the fermented food are strong, it is unlikely that there will be an image problem. For example, kimchi is considered part of the national heritage in Korea. It is a vital ingredient of all meals and as such is a highly valued food. This is reflected in the amount of research carried out on the product and the detailed understanding of the process, which already exists.

It is not difficult to gain access to village people, both to collect the traditional information and to disseminate improved practices. Numerous organisations are involved in field projects. They can be used to organise training sessions and group meetings for the dissemination of new methods, for example, for the use of pure starter cultures.

One of the problems likely to be encountered is gaining access to starter cultures and other improved methods. Agricultural extension services should take a responsibility for the promotion and the supply of starter cultures at a price which is affordable.

Creating a Supportive Environment for Production of Fermented Food Products

Developing countries need to build their resources of trained, knowledgeable individuals, who are able to apply the basic microbiological principles to the production of fermented foods. Extra support should be made available to train professionals in this discipline.

Fermented foods should be recognised as part of each countries heritage and culture and efforts made to preserve the methods of production. A recognised body (government or non-government) should take the responsibility for the collection of details and the promotion of fermented food products. Consumers need to be made aware of the numerous benefits of fermented foods and their prejudices against fermented foods, especially those traditionally produced at the home scale, dispelled.

Many traditional fermented foods are produced from minor or wild fruits and vegetables, many of which are being lost through deforestation and loss of biodiversity.

Chapter 20

Food and Enzymes from Micro-organisms

INTRODUCTION

Enzymes are commonly used in food processing and in the production of food ingredients. Enzymes traditionally isolated from culturable micro-organisms, plants, and mammalian tissues are often not well-adapted to the conditions used in modern food production methods. The use of recombinant DNA technology has made it possible to manufacture novel enzymes suitable for specific food-processing conditions. Such enzymes may be discovered by screening micro-organisms samples from diverse environments or developed by modification of known enzymes using modern methods of protein engineering or molecular evolution.

As a result, several important food-processing enzymes such as amylases and lipases with properties tailored to particular food applications have become available. Another important achievement is improvement of microbial production strains. For example, several microbial strains recently developed for enzyme production have been engineered to increase enzyme yield by deleting native genes encoding extracellular proteases.

Moreover, certain fungal production strains have been modified to reduce or eliminate their potential for production of toxic secondary metabolites. In this chapter, we will discuss the safety of micro-organisms used as hosts for enzyme-encoding genes, the construction of recombinant production strains, and methods of improving enzyme properties.

MICRO-ORGANISMS AS FOOD: SINGLE CELL PROTEIN (SCP)

Commonly referred to as SCP, these products are dried cells of micro-organisms such as algae, actinomycetes, bacteria, yeasts, moulds and higher fungi which are grown in large fermentors. The product at present is largely used as animal feed. One of the earliest known use of SCP as a natural source of food comes from Africa: Spirulina, a blue-green alga growing in the lake Chad region of Africa develops into a mat which is scooped out periodically by the natives and dried in sun to be eaten as food. During the world war, baker's yeast (*Saccharomyces cerevisiae*) and Torula yeast (*Candida utilis*) were grown on a large scale using molasses and sulphite waste liquor from pulp and paper industry as media to produce a protein supplement for animals and human beings.

There have been several candidates for SCP production from time to time and the substrate used for the cultivation of these micro-organisms are also variable. The most advanced process for SCP production on a methanol substrate was developed by the then Imperial Chemical Industries of UK by growing *Methylophilus* (*Pseudomonas*) methylotrophus in large fermentors.

There are several limitations in the use of SCP for human consumption and they are due to: (i) high nucleic acid contents of many micro-organisms that would result in kidney stone formation or gout, (ii) poor digestibility, gastrointestinal problems and skin reactions, and (iii) the possible presence of toxic or carcinogenic compounds from residues of substrates. However, dried food-grade yeasts and their autolysates have been used for many years.

Dried mycelia of mushrooms, by virtue of their pleasant flavour can be used in soups, sauces or gravy formulations. The high capital costs and the need for sterility controls render SCP expensive in developing countries where food shortages are common. As animal feed, SCP grown on agricultural residues should certainly find a place in the future economy of developing nations. It is, however, noteworthy that Dabur in India is manufacturing and selling spirulina for human consumption. Many groups of micro-organisms are used as sources of proteins. Some of the micro-organisms with their carbon and energy sources are given in Table 20.1.

Table 20.1. Single cell protein (SCP) and mycoprotein produced on the selected substrates.

Microgial micro-organisms groups		Protein (%/100 g, on dry weight basis)	Substrates
Algae	Chlorella pyrenoidosa (36)[a]	–	CO_2 (10%), light
	Scenedesmus acutus (20)[b]	–	CO_2 sunlight
	Spirulina maxima (15)[b]	53	CO_2 (5%), combustion gases, bicarbonate, sunlight (in pond)
Bacteria	Achromobacter delvacvate	–	Diesel oil in fermenter
	Bacillus megaterium	–	Collagen meat packing waste in fermenter
	Cellumonas sp. (0.45)[c]	87	Bagasse
	Methylomonas clara (0.5)[c]	13	Methanol
	Pseudomonas sp. (1.0)[c]	–	n-alkanes fuel oil
Actinomycetes	Nocardia sp. (0.98)[c]	–	n-alkanes
	Thermomonpspora fusca (0.4)[c]	5.6	Cellulose pulp
Fungi			
Yeasts	Candida lipolytica (0.88)[c]	65–69	n-alkanes
	C. utilis (0.39)[c]	–	Potato starch waste
	B. utilis	54	Sulphite liquor
	Saccharomyces cerevisiae (0.5)[c]	53	Molasses
	Saccharomyces cerevisiae (0.5)[c]	45	Beer
	S. fragilis	54	Milk whey
	Rhodotorula glutinis	–	Domestic sewage
	Torulopsis sp.	–	Methanol
Moulds	Aspergillus niger	50	Molasses
	Trichoderma viride	64	Straw, starch
	Paecilomyces varioti	55	Sulphite waste liquor
Mushrooms	Agaricus campestris	36–45	Glucose
	Morchella crassipes	31	Glucose, cheese whey, sulphite, liquor.

[a]Yield g/day (on dry weight basis); [b]yield g/m²/day (on dry weight basis); [c]yield dry weight basis (g/g substrate used). Values in parantheses—denote yield of biomass.

Substrates Used for Production of Content SCP

A variety of substrates are used for SCP production. However, availability of necessary substrates is of considerable biological and economic importance for the production of SCP. Algae which contain chlorophylls, do not require organic wastes. They use free energy from sunlight and carbon dioxide from air, while bacteria (except photoautotrops) and fungi require organic wastes, as they do not contain chlorophylls. The major components of substrates are the raw materials which contain sugars (sugarcane, sugarbeet and their processed products), starch (grains, tapioca, potato, and their by-products), lignocelluloses from woody plants and herbs having residues with nitrogen and phosphorous contents and other raw materials (whey and refuses from processed food). Organic wastes are also generated by certain industries and are rich in aromatic compounds or hydrocarbons. Recent price-increase in petroleum and refined petroleum products has made hydrocarbons and chemicals derived from them (such as methanol and ethanol) less attractive as raw materials for SCP production that renewable sources such as agricultural wastes or by-products.

Commercial Production of SCP

The raw materials that can be used for single-cell protein manufacture include whey, sulphate waste liquors, hydrocarbon waste from the petroleum industry, and the vats used to produce alcoholic beverages. The production process involves growth of the organisms in large fermenting tanks with forced aeration for vigorous cell-growth manufacture process used by British Petroleum Industry for single-cell protein from hydrocarbons is represented in Fig. 20.1.

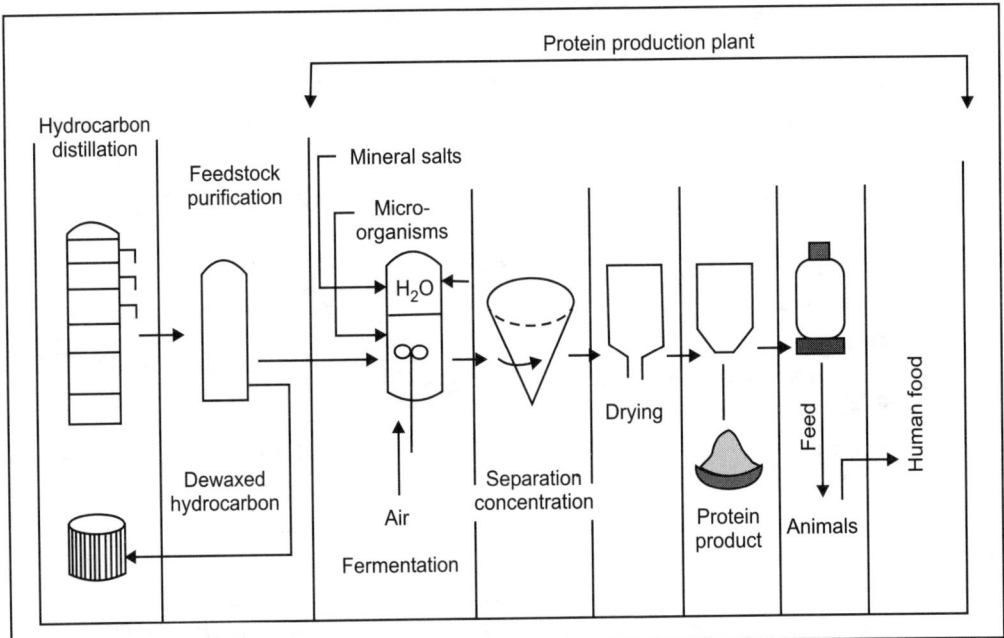

Fig. 20.1. Diagrammatic representation of commercial production of single cell from hydrocarbons.

Micro-organisms and their raw material used in the production of single-cell protein are listed in Table 20.2.

Table 20.2. Micro-organisms and their raw material used in the production of single-cell protein.

Micro-organisms	Raw materials	
Bacteria	*Hygrogenomonas, Cellulomonas, Pseudomonas*, etc.	Hydrocarbon wastes from petroleum industry.
Fungi		
Yeasts	*Candida* spp., *Saccharomyces fragilis, Torula* sp., *Rhodotorula* spp.	Whey, ethyl alcohol, starches, *n*-paraffins, sulphite waste, etc.
Moulds	*Aspergillus terreus, Trichoderma reesei, Penicillium* spp.	Paper-pulp, starches, coffee wastes, straw, bassage, etc.
Algae	*Scenedesmus acutues, Scenedesmus acutues, Spirulina, Chlorella*	In culture ponds.

Advantages of single-cell protein manufacture

1. Micro-organisms grow very vigorously and produce a high yield. It has been calculated that 100 lbs of yeast produces about 250 tons of protein within 24 hours. Algae grown in ponds produce 20 tons (dry weight) of protein per acre/year. The yield of protein is 10–15 times higher than soyabeans and 20–50 times higher than corn.
2. Industrial wastes or by-products are utilised as raw materials for micro-organisms.
3. The protein content in the cells of micro-organisms is reported to be very high 60 per cent protein in dried cells of *Pseudomonas* spp; 40–50 per cent in yeast cells and 20–40 per cent in algal cells have been calculated.
4. Yeasts grown in this process possess high vitamin content.
5. All essential amino acids are contained by single-cell proteins.

Disadvantages of single-cell protein manufacture

1. Yeasts show lower growth rates, lower protein and lower methionine content.
2. Moulds also have their limitations due to lower growth rates and lower protein content.
3. Algae have cellulose in their cell walls which are not digestible. They also accumulate heavy metals which may prove harmful to living beings.
4. Since the bacterial cells are small in size and have low density, their harvesting from the fermented medium becomes difficult and costly.
5. Bacterial cells possess high nucleic acid content which may prove detrimental to human beings by increasing the uric acid level in blood. Additional steps to overcome this problem make the production costly.

Primary and secondary micro-organisms

Micro-organisms may be termed 'primary' when grown directly for the purpose in mind and 'secondary' when they are recovered as a by-product of a fermentation.

Nutritional Value of SCP

Nowadays, considerable information is available on the composition of microbial cells, e.g. protein, amino acid, vitamin, and minerals. Commercial value of SCP depends on their nutritional performance and nevertheless, it has to be evaluated to the prevalent feed protein. SCPs either from alkanes or methanols, are characterised by good content and balance in essential amino acids.

Composition of growth medium governs the protein and lipid contents of micro-organisms. Yeasts, moulds and higher fungi have higher cellular lipid content and lower nitrogen and protein contents, when grown in media having high amount of available carbon as energy source and low nitrogen.

Ignoring a few extreme values, the mean crude protein in dry matter of algae and yeasts, on conventional substrates, lies between 50 and 60 per cent, for alkane yeasts between 55 and 65 per cent, and for bacteria about 80 per cent. A high content of nucleic acid free protein is extremely important for the economic efficiency of the procedure in SCP production. Because of high protein and fat contents, the contribution of carbohydrates to the nutritional value of SCP is not of prime importance. The crude ash content is determined in particular by the nutrient salts of the fermentation medium. Estimation of crude protein is based on total nitrogen which is multiplied by the factor 6.25. The protein content of micro-organisms computed in this manner does not give the exact figure of protein content, as in the estimation of total nitrogen, the value of nucleic acid is also included which is somewhat erroneous.

The most important measure of nutritional value is the actual performance of SCP products as determined in feeding studies. The determinants of the utility of SCP product for application as food for human beings and feed for animals differ. For human beings, protein digestibility and protein efficiency ratio (PER), biological value or net protein utilisation (NPU), determined in rats, are the parameters for food application, whereas for animals, metabolisable energy, protein digestibility and feed conversion ratio (weight of ration consumer/weight gain) are the measures or performance in broiler, chickens, swine and calves (and egg laying in hens).

Digestibility (D) is the percentage of total nitrogen consumed, which is absorbed through the alimentary tract. It is calculated as below:

$$D = \frac{Ni - Fn}{Ni}$$

where,

Ni = nitrogen ingested from SCP.

Fn = nitrogen content in faeces after feeding SCP.

Biological value (B) is the percentage of total nitrogen assimilated which is retained by the body, taking into account the simultaneous loss of endogenous nitrogen through excretion in urine. This is expressed by the following formula:

$$B = \frac{Ni - (Fn + Un)}{(Ni - Fn)} \times 100$$

where,

Un = nitrogen content in urine after feeding SCP.

Protein efficiency is the proportion of nitrogen retained when protein under test is fed compared with that retained when a reference protein (e.g. egg albumin) is fed.

Nutritional values of SCP product are given in Table 20.3 which indicates that protein digestibility range from good to very good and is true for bacteria and yeasts growth on unconventional substrates.

However, there are certain problems which warrant the use of SCP products as human foods such as: (i) high content of nucleic acid leading to development of kidney stone and gout if consumed in high quantity, (ii) possibility for the presence of toxic secondary metabolites, and (iii) poor digestibility and stimulation of gastrointestinal and skin reactions.

Table 20.3. Nutritional value of food protein.

Food protein	Analytical composition (%)		Essential amino acids (g/100 g crude protein)		Biological coefficient (%)		Digestibility of crude protein (%)*	Metabolisable energy for (Kcal/kg)
	Total nitrogen	Crude protein (N × 6.25)	Lysine	Threonine	NPU	NPV		
Algae	8.0	45–71	5.7	5.2	–	–	82	–
Dried skimmed milk	5.7	35.9	8.0	–	87	31.2	–	2510
Soyabean meal	7.0	44	6.4	4.0	64	65	–	2240
Alkane yeast (toprina – LBP)	11.2	7.0	7.4	4.2	91	96	92	2540
Bacteria from methanol	11.5	72	6.2	4.6	84	88.4	91	3468

*Digestibility determined by pig feeding; NPU = Net protein utilisation; NPV = Net protein value.

FATS FROM MICRO-ORGANISMS

Fats (more properly lipids) are synthesised in appreciable amounts by certain yeasts, yeast like organisms, and moulds, but production in this manner has been employed only during periods of emergency, e.g. a state of war, when cheaper and more easily available animal and plant lipids were not available in sufficient quantity.

Organisms Used

Among the yeasts, *Candida pulcherrima, Torulopsis lipofera, Saccharomyces cerevisiae*, and *Rhodotorula glutinis* have been studied for their fat production, and the first was used for this purpose in Germany and Sweden during World War II. The yeast like *Trichosporon pullulans* was used by the Germans during World War I, as were special strains of the mould *Geotrichum candidum*.

Raw Materials

Media for fat production should in general have a high carbon-to-nitrogen ratio, a good supply of phosphates, and for most organisms a pH on the acid side. In fat production by *Trichosporon pullulans*, good growth first is obtained in a mash with a high ratio of nitrogen to carbon, and fat production is carried out in a medium with a high ratio of carbon to nitrogen. Molasses, cellulose waste, hydrolysed wood, and spent sulphite liquor are among the sources of carbohydrate employed. Nitrogen can be in the form of ammonium salts, urea, urine, yeast water, molasses slop or extracts of grains. Salts to be added include potassium chloride, monopotassium phosphate, and magnesium sulphate. Addition of small amounts of alcohol or sodium acetate increases yields of lipids.

The choice of a yeast will depend on its ability to utilise both pentoses and hexoses or only the latter. *Geotrichum candidum* is able to utilise the lactose in whey, to which some additional nitrogenous food and salts may be added.

Production of Fat

Since all the previously mentioned organisms grow best under aerobic conditions, their growth for fat production has been in thin layers on trays or other flat areas when *Trichosporon pullulans* or a mould was employed and in well-aerated tanks when yeasts were grown submerged. The optimal temperature varies with the organism employed, ranging from 15° to 20°C for *T. pullulans* to 25° to 30°C or slightly higher for moulds and yeasts. A fairly long period is required for maximal fat production by most of the organisms mentioned. *T. pullulans*, for example, requires 2 to 3 days to attain growth and 6 to 8 days more for maximal yields of lipids. Fields of lipids vary widely with the organisms and with methods of production. Recovery of lipids is by extraction with solvents, with or without autolysis.

PRODUCTION OF AMINO ACIDS

Currently, the amino acids used in amino acid products are mainly manufactured by the fermentation method using natural materials, similar to yogurt, beer, vinegar, miso(bean paste), soyasauce, etc.

Fermentation Method is a Natural Mechanism

The amino acid fermentation method is a method for the production of amino acids utilising the phenomenon that micro-organisms convert nutrients to various vital components necessary to themselves.

With the fermentation method, raw materials such as syrups are added to micro-organism culture media, and the proliferating micro-organisms are allowed to produce amino acids. It is enzymes that play an important role here. Enzymes, which are proteins to catalyse chemical reactions in the living body, are indispensable to degrade and synthesise substances. Consecutive reactions by 10 to 30 kinds of enzymes are involved in the process of fermentation, and various amino acids are produced as a result of these reactions.

Screen a Superior Micro-organism First

In order to produce amino acids using micro-organisms, it is important to find a micro-organism with a high potential for producing amino acids. One gram of natural soil contains about 100 million micro-organisms. From these a useful one can be picked out.

Once a micro-organism suitable for the fermentation method has been selected, it is necessary to enhance its potential, that is, to make improvements to take full advantage of the potential of the organism.

Generally, micro-organisms produce the 20 kinds of amino acids only in the amounts necessary to themselves. They have a mechanism for regulating the quantities and qualities of enzymes to yield amino acids only in the needed amounts. Therefore, it is necessary to release this regulatory mechanism in order to manufacture the target amino acid in large amounts.

The yield of an amino acid depends on the quantities and qualities of the enzymes. The yield increases if the enzymes involved in the production of the target amino acid are present in large quantities under workable conditions, while it decreases if the enzymes are present in small quantities. Suppose that a micro-organism has a metabolic pathway $A \rightarrow (a) \rightarrow B \rightarrow (b) \rightarrow C \rightarrow (c) \rightarrow D$ (a, b, and c are enzymes). In order to produce only amino acid C in large amounts, you have to enhance the actions only of enzymes a and b and to get rid of the action of enzyme c. Strains are improved using various techniques to make this process possible. A fermentation tank is filled with syrups/sugars derived from sugar cane, corn, and cassava, and then fermentation conditions are set so that the stirring conditions, air supply, temperature, and pH are optimum. Finally, only the target amino acid is obtained from this fermented broth in high purity (Fig. 20.2).

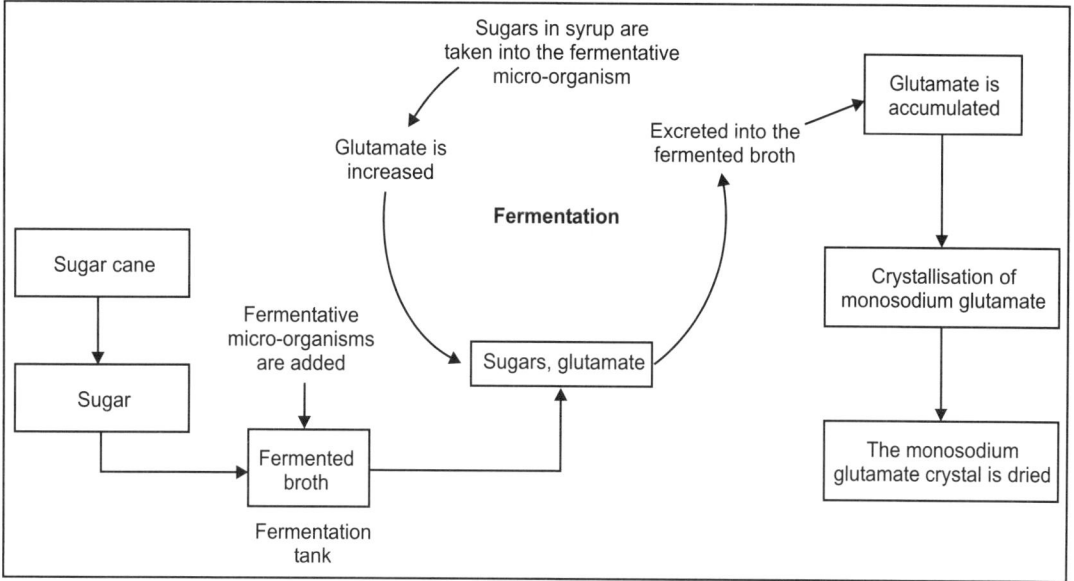

Fig. 20.2. Production of mono sodium glutamate by fermentation.

Other Production Methods of Amino Acids

In addition to the fermentation method, the enzymatic reaction and extraction methods are used for producing amino acids. With the enzymatic reaction method, an amino acid precursor is converted to the target amino acid using 1 or 2 enzymes.

This enzyme method allows the conversion to a specific amino acid without microbial growth, thus eliminating the long process from glucose. This method comes into its own when the amino acid precursor is supplied at low prices.

With the extraction method, natural proteins are degraded to various amino acids, but the amount of each amino acid contained in the raw material proteins naturally restricts the yield.

The fermentation method has the advantage of mass production at low cost, which was the great impetus for expanding the amino acid market. The manufacturing method of glutamate shifted from the extraction method to the fermentation method in the 1960s. Subsequently, a similar shift to the fermentation method took place for the other amino acids in rapid succession.

Generally, amino acids cannot be manufactured in quantities without deactivating the regulatory mechanism that micro-organisms possess. However, the glutamate-producing micro-organism has such a rare characteristic that glutamate can be produced solely by setting special fermentation conditions without improving the strain.

A fermentation tank is fed with raw materials such as syrup derived from sugarcane, and glutamate-producing micro-organisms are fermented under the appropriate conditions. During this fermentation process, glutamate is excreted from the micro-organisms into the fermented broth. This is how glutamate is obtained in large amounts.

PRODUCTION OF OTHER SUBSTANCES ADDED TO FOOD

Dextran is an extracellular bacterial polymer of D-glucopyranose with predominantly α- (1→6) linkage in the main chain and a variable amount of α-(1→2), α-(1→3), α-(1→4) branched linkages. Other workers have also reported formation of dextran from different strains of bacteria that were primarily *Leuconostoc* strains. The specificity of the synthesised linkages in the dextran is strain dependent. Among many dextran producing species the dextran produced by *L. mesenteroides* NRRL B512F and *L. mesenteroides* NRRL B1299 have been well characterised and classified. Dextran from *L. mesenteroides* B512F contains 95 per cent of α-(1→6) linkages and 5 per cent of α-(1→3) branch linkages; whereas insoluble dextran from *L. mesenteroides* 1299 contains 63 per cent α-(1→6), 27 per cent of α-(1→2) and 8 per cent of α-(1→3) linkages.

Dextran and Xanthan

Dextran is a bacterial polysaccharide, which is commercially available, and it is used as drugs, especially as blood plasma volume expander. Dextran has found industrial applications in food, pharmaceutical and chemical industries as adjuvant, emulsifier, carrier and stabiliser. Cross-linked dextran is known as Sephadex, which is widely used for the separation and purification of protein. In food industry dextran is currently used as thickener for jam and ice cream. It prevents crystallisation of sugar, improves moisture retention, and maintains flavour and appearance of various food items.

Dextran is produced at the industrial level by the fermentation of sucrose-rich media. Several research workers have optimised fermentation conditions for maximum dextran production. It has been reported earlier that molecular weight and yield of dextran production depends on the process variables such as temperature, sucrose and the acceptor concentration. It was also mentioned that medium containing nitrogen source supplemented with different salts increased dextran production. Xanthan is a polyionic hydropolysaccharide made by *Xanthomonas campestris* when grown in a glucose-based medium. Xanthan has many possible uses in the food industry, particularly as a stabiliser. Xanthan differs from dextran in that it is not hydrolysed or degraded by human beings or animals and is excreted intact.

Lactic Acid Fermentation

Lactic acid fermentation is a biological process by which sugars such as glucose, fructose, and sucrose, are converted into cellular energy and the metabolic by-product lactate. It is an anaerobic fermentation reaction that occurs in some bacteria and animal cells, such as muscle cells, in the absence of oxygen. If oxygen is present in the cell, many organisms will by-pass fermentation and undergo cellular respiration; however, facultative anaerobic organisms will both ferment and undergo respiration in the presence of oxygen. In homofermentative fermentation, one molecule of glucose is ultimately converted to two molecules of lactic acid. Heterofermentative fermentation, in contrast, yields carbon dioxide and ethanol in addition to lactic acid, in a process called the phosphoketolase pathway.

Chemical process

The process of lactic acid fermentation using glucose is summarised below. In homolactic fermentation, one molecule of glucose is converted to two molecules of lactic acid:

$$C_6H_{12}O_6 \rightarrow 2CH_3CHOHCOOH$$

In heterolactic fermentation, the reaction proceeds as follows, with one molecule of glucose converted to one molecule of lactic acid, one molecule of ethanol, and one molecule of carbon dioxide:

$$C_6H_{12}O_6 \rightarrow CH_3CHOHCOOH + C_2H_5OH + CO_2$$

Before lactic acid fermentation can occur, the molecule of glucose must be split into two molecules of pyruvate. This process is called glycolysis.

Glycolysis

To extract chemical energy from glucose, the glucose molecule must be split up into two molecules of pyruvate. This process also generates two molecules of adenosine triphosphate as an immediate energy yield and two molecules of NADH.

$$C_6H_{12}O_6 + 2ADP + 2P_i + 2NAD^+ \rightarrow 2CH_3COCOO^- + 2ATP + 2NADH + 2H_2O + 2H^+$$

In aerobic respiration, the pyruvate is further oxidised completely, generating additional ATP and NADH in the citric acid cycle and by oxidative phosphorylation. However, this can occur only in the presence of oxygen. Oxygen is toxic to organisms that are obligate anaerobes, and is not required by facultative anaerobic organisms. In the absence of oxygen, one of the fermentation pathways occurs in order to regenerate NAD^+; lactic acid fermentation is one of these pathways.

Fermentation

Lactic acid fermentation is the simplest type of fermentation. In essence, it is a redox reaction. In anaerobic conditions, the cell's primary mechanism of ATP production is glycolysis. Glycolysis reduces—that is, transfers electrons to—NAD^+, forming NADH. However, there is only a limited supply of NAD^+ available in a cell. For glycolysis to continue, NADH must be oxidised—that is, have electrons taken away—to regenerate the NAD^+. This is usually done through an electron transport chain in a process called oxidative phosphorylation; however, this mechanism is not available without oxygen.

Instead, the NADH donates its extra electrons to the pyruvate molecules formed during glycolysis. Since the NADH has lost electrons, NAD^+ regenerates and is again available for glycolysis. Lactic acid, for which this process is named, is formed by the reduction of pyruvate.

In homolactic acid fermentation, both molecules of pyruvate are converted to lactate. In heterolactic acid fermentation, one molecule of pyruvate is converted to lactate; the other is converted to ethanol and carbon dioxide. Homolactic acid fermentation is unique in that it is one of the only respiration processes that do not produce a gas as a by-product.

Purpose

Some bacteria and yeasts organisms are unable to cope with the presence of oxygen. These organisms use fermentation as a method of obtaining energy in the form of ATP. Because the production of lactic acid frees up NAD^+, the process of glycolysis can continue.

Lactic acid fermentation also occurs in animal muscle cells under conditions when oxygen is low. Extreme exercise would be an example of this. In this situation, the lactate is carried away by the circulatory system to the liver, where it is converted back to pyruvate through the Cori cycle.

Fermentation, however, is far less effective than cellular respiration, producing only two ATP molecules per glucose molecule consumed. The typical yield from cellular respiration is anywhere from 34–38 molecules of ATP. Thus, it is typically seen only in small organisms, such as bacteria and yeast, that can survive on this low energy yield.

Applications

Lactic acid fermentation is used in many areas of the world to produce foods that cannot be produced through other methods. The most commercially important genus of lactic acid-fermenting bacteria is

Lactobacillus, though other bacteria and even yeast are sometimes used. Two of the most common applications of lactic acid fermentation are in the production of yogurt and sauerkraut.

Yogurt production

The main method of producing yogurt is through the lactic acid fermentation of milk with harmless bacteria. The primary bacteria used are typically *Lactobacillus bulgaricus* and *Streptococcus thermophilus*, and US law requires all yogurts to contain these two cultures (though others may be added as probiotic cultures). These bacteria produce lactic acid in the milk culture, decreasing its pH and causing it to congeal. The bacteria also produce compounds that give yogurt its distinctive flavour. An additional effect of the lowered pH is the incompatibility of the acidic environment with many other types of harmful bacteria.

For a probiotic yogurt, additional types of bacteria such as *Lactobacillus acidophilus* are also added to the culture.

Sauerkraut

Lactic acid fermentation is also used in the production of sauerkraut. The main type of bacteria used in the production of sauerkraut is of the genus *Leuconostoc*.

As in yogurt, when the acidity rises due to lactic acid-fermenting organisms, many other pathogenic micro-organisms are killed. The bacteria produce lactic acid, as well as simple alcohols and other hydrocarbons. These may then combine to form esters, contributing to the unique flavour of sauerkraut.

Kimchi

Kimchi also uses lactic acid fermentation.

Citric Acid

Citric acid is a commercially important product that has been obtained by submerged fermentation of glucose or sucrose by *Aspergillus niger*. This work was undertaken to determine the potential of food processing solid residues as a substrate for citric acid production by solid state fermentation using *Aspergillus niger*. Yields of citric acid varied considerably and were found to depend significantly on the strain of *Aspergillus niger* used and the following factors: the type of raw material fermented, the initial moisture content of the substrate, the amount of methyl alcohol present, and the fermentation time and temperature. Under favourable conditions, yields from more than 50 to nearly 90 per cent were obtained on the basis of the amount of carbohydrate consumed. The results of this study indicate that food processing solid residues can serve as a low-cost substrate for citric acid production by solid state fermentation using *Aspergillus niger*.

Citric acid fermentation is one of the rare examples of industrial fermentation technology where academic discoveries have worked in tandem with industrial know-how, in spite of an apparent lack of collaboration, to give rise to an efficient fermentation process. The current world market estimates suggest that upwards of 4.0×10^5 tons citric acid per year may be produced. Citric acid is a major product but the upward trend in its use seen over many years is an annual 2–3 per cent increase. The demand for this particular metabolite is increasing day by day which requires a much more efficient fermentation process for higher yield product. When applied to appropriate mass balances, it is possible to predict the utilisation of substrates and the yield of individual products. Fermentation media for citric acid biosynthesis should consist of substrates necessary for the growth of micro-organism, primarily the carbon, nitrogen and phosphorus sources. Moreover, water and air can be included as fermentation substrates.

The basic substrates for citric acid fermentation using submerged technique of fermentation are beet or cane-molasses. The present investigation deals with the kinetic study of citric acid fermentation. Cane-molasses was employed as the basal fermentation media in the stirred fermentor under the submerged fermentation conditions. The study revealed the nutritional status of the organism and basic fermentation parameters.

PRODUCTION OF ENZYMES

The protein biocatalysts, called enzymes, used by living cells are responsible for numerous metabolic processes of the cell. The use of microbial enzymes, although only recently understood, has been going on for centuries. Since micro-organisms are responsible for the fermentations of beer, wine, bread, cheese, and various vegetables, all these processes are examples of cell-mediated conversions or applications of enzymes.

Amylase

Amylase is an enzyme that catalyses the breakdown of starch into sugar. Amylase is present in human saliva, where it begins the chemical process of digestion. Foods that contain much starch but little sugar, such as rice and potato, taste slightly sweet as they are chewed because amylase turns some of their starch into sugar in the mouth.

The pancreas also makes amylase (alpha amylase) to hydrolyse dietary starch into disaccharides and trisaccharides which are converted by other enzymes to glucose to supply the body with energy. Plants and some bacteria also produce amylase. Specific amylase proteins are designated by different Greek letters. All amylases are glycoside hydrolases and act on α-1,4-glycosidic bonds.

Classification of amylases

α-Amylase

(EC 3.2.1.1) (alternate names: 1,4-α-D-glucan glucanohydrolase; glycogenase) The α-amylases are calcium metalloenzymes, completely unable to function in the absence of calcium. By acting at random locations along the starch chain, α-amylase breaks down long-chain carbohydrates, ultimately yielding maltotriose and maltose from amylose or maltose, glucose and 'limit dextrin' from amylopectin. Because it can act anywhere on the substrate, α-amylase tends to be faster-acting than β-amylase. In animals, it is a major digestive enzyme and its optimum pH is 6.7–7.0.

In human physiology, both the salivary and pancreatic amylases are α-amylases. They are discussed in much more detail at α-amylase. Also found in plants (adequately), fungi (ascomycetes and basidiomycetes) and bacteria (*Bacillus*).

β-Amylase

(EC 3.2.1.2) (alternate names: 1,4-α-D-glucan maltohydrolase; glycogenase; saccharogen amylase) Another form of amylase, β-amylase is also synthesised by bacteria, fungi, and plants. Working from the non-reducing end, β-amylase catalyses the hydrolysis of the second α-1,4-glycosidic bond, cleaving off two glucose units (maltose) at a time. During the ripening of fruit, β-amylase breaks starch into maltose, resulting in the sweet flavour of ripe fruit.

Both α-amylase and β-amylase are present in seeds; β-amylase is present in an inactive form prior to germination, whereas α-amylase and proteases appear once germination has begun. Cereal grain amylase is key to the production of malt. Many microbes also produce amylase to degrade extracellular starches. Animal tissues do not contain β-amylase, although it may be present in micro-organisms contained within the digestive tract.

γ-Amylase

(EC 3.2.1.3) (alternative names: Glucan 1,4-α-glucosidase; amyloglucosidase; Exo-1,4-α-glucosidase; glucoamylase; lysosomal α-glucosidase; 1,4-α-D-glucan glucohydrolase) In addition to cleaving the last α(1-4)glycosidic linkages at the nonreducing end of amylose and amylopectin, yielding glucose, γ-amylase will cleave α(1–6) glycosidic linkages. Unlike the other forms of amylase, γ-amylase is most efficient in acidic environments and has an optimum pH of 3.

Production of Amylase

From moulds

Moulds are used as sources of amylases as well as of other hydrolytic enzymes, the species and strain of mould being selected especially for the purpose. *Rhizopus delemar*, *Mucor rouxii*, and related species have been employed in the Amylo process, in which a starchy grain mash is saccharified by amylases produced by the mould growing on it. This process has been applied principally to the preparation of mashes for alcoholic fermentation by yeasts. For the production of preparations rich in amylases, *Aspergillus oryzae* has been used most, although *A. niger* has been recommended for submerged methods of production. The preparation of koji, the *A. oryzae* starter for soyasauce that is rich in amylases as well as other hydrolytic enzymes.

Moistened, steamed wheat or rice bran is used for the production of amylases from *A. oryzae* by the tray method, in which the mould is grown on thin layers of the medium in trays, or the drum method, in which the bran is tossed loosely in a rotating drum. A maximal yield is obtained by the tray method in 40 to 48 hr at about 30°C in an atmosphere with a high humidity and adequate ventilation. The amylases are extracted from the mycelium and may be purified by precipitation and washing or may be concentrated as desired. Other hydrolytic enzymes also are present in such preparations.

From bacteria

Bacillus subtilis has been the principal bacterium used for the production of amylases, although other species of bacteria are known to yield these enzymes. Most bacteria produce more α-amylase than β-amylase. Production may be by the surface-growth method on shallow layers of mash in trays or by the submerged method. Bacterial amylase may be purified and concentrated by dialysis, condensation, and fractional precipitation.

Uses

Amylase enzymes find use in bread making and to break down complex sugars such as starch (found in flour) into simple sugars. Yeast then feeds on these simple sugars and converts it into the waste products of alcohol and CO_2. This imparts flavour and causes the bread to rise. While amylase enzymes are found naturally in yeast cells, it takes time for the yeast to produce enough of these enzymes to break down significant quantities of starch in the bread. This is the reason for long fermented doughs such as sour dough. Modern bread making techniques have included amylase enzymes (often in the form of malted barley) into bread improver thereby making the bread making process faster and more practical for commercial use.

When used as a food additive Amylase has E number E1100, and may be derived from swine pancreas or mould mushroom. Bacilliary amylase is also used in clothing and dishwasher detergents to dissolve starches from fabrics and dishes. Workers in factories that work with amylase for any of the above uses are at increased risk of occupational asthma.

Invertase

Invertase catalyses the hydrolysis of sucrose to glucose and fructose. The invertase of yeasts is a fructosidase in that it attacks the fructose end of the sucrose molecule, in contrast to the glucosidase of moulds, which attacks the glucose end. Industrially, invertase is produced mainly by growth of special strains of *Saccharomyces cerevisiae* (bottom type) in a medium that contains sucrose, an ammonium salt, and phosphate buffer and other minerals and is adjusted to about pH 4.5. Incubation is for about 8 hr at 28° to 30°C. For recovery of the invertase the yeast cells are filtered off, compressed, plasmolysed, and autolysed. The invertase extracted from the cells may be dried with sugar or held in a sucrose sirup, or the enzyme may be purified by dialysis, ultrafiltration, adsorption, and elution. Most commercial preparations of invertase are not highly purified.

Uses

Invertase is used in the confectionery industry to make invert sugar for the preparation of liqueurs and ice creams in which the crystallisation of sugars from high concentrations is to be avoided. In soft-center, chocolate-coated candies, e.g. Maraschino cherries, invertase incorporated in the centers softens the fondant after it has been coated with chocolate. Invertase is added to sucrose sirups to hydrolyse that sugar and in this way to prevent crystallisation on standing. It also has been used in the manufacture of artificial honey.

Pectolytic Enzymes

Pectin, which is methylated polygalacturonic acid, is important in food industries because of its ability to form gels with sugar and acid. In jellies this characteristic is desirable, but it is not desirable in fruit juices. Most authorities agree that chiefly two enzymes are involved in the hydrolysis of pectin: pectinesterase, to hydrolyse the pectin to methanol and polygalacturonic acid (pectic acid), and polygalacturonase, to hydrolyse the polygalacturonic acid to monogalacturonic acid. Further hydrolysis would yield sugars and other products.

The mixture of pectolytic enzymes sometimes is called pectinase (pectase, pectinols, or filtragols), a term which will be used here for a mixture of pectolytic enzymes such as is produced by micro-organisms. Pectinase is yielded by a number of moulds and by various bacteria, including the clostridia involved in retting. Only the fungal type of pectinase is produced industrially to any extent, and this from moulds such as species of *Aspergillus*, *Penicillium*, and other genera. The mycelium is developed on a medium containing pectin or a pectinlike compound; a nitrogen source, such as plant, yeast or malt extract, ammonia, peptone, etc. and mineral salts. The mycelium is harvested, macerated, and extracted, and the crude enzyme mixture thus obtained may be precipitated and concentrated.

Uses

Pectinases from extracts of plant materials or from fungi are used in the food industries for the clarification of fruit juices, wines, vinegars, sirups, and jellies that may contain suspended pectic material. Treatment of fruit juices with pectinase helps prevent jelling of the juices upon concentration. The addition of pectinase to crushed fruit, e.g. grapes, aids in the expression of the juice and results in wines that clarify readily. Partial deesterification by means of pectinesterase to yield modified pectins which set slowly is employed in the manufacture of candy jellies of high sugar content.

Proteolytic Enzymes

The proteolytic enzymes or proteases, include the proteinases, which catalyse the hydrolysis of the protein molecule into large fragments, and the peptidases, which hydrolyse these polypeptide fragments as far down as amino acids. The proteolytic enzyme preparations from micro-organisms are proteases, i.e. mixtures of proteinases and peptidases. Proteases also are prepared from plant or animal sources. Papain, for example, from the papaya fruit, is injected into meat animals before slaughter, so that the meat will be tenderised by the enzyme during cooking.

From bacteria

For the most part, bacterial protease is prepared from cultures of *Bacillus subtilis*, although many other bacteria yield proteases. A high-yielding strain is selected, special culture media are employed, and temperature and degree of aeration are adjusted to favour the production of protease over that of amylase. The medium or mash has a fairly high content of carbohydrate (2 to 6 per cent), as well as of protein, and also contains mineral salts. Incubation is for 3 to 5 days at about 37°C with adequate ventilation. The filtrate from the culture is concentrated, and the enzymes are used in this form, purified further, or absorbed onto some inert material, such as, sawdust. The enzyme mixture also contains varying amounts of amylases.

From moulds

Protease preparations from moulds also contain other enzymes. Thus the koji for soya sauce or the Taka-Diastase for pharmaceutical purposes contains a variety of enzymes. It is possible, however, to select strains of moulds that give high yields of proteases and comparatively low yields of other enzymes. The mould also can be chosen for its ability to produce proteases which are active under acid conditions or active under alkaline conditions. The methods of preparation of mould proteases are similar to those for the production of amylases. *Aspergillus oryzae* is a good source of proteases, although other moulds have been recommended. Many different media have been suggested, including those containing wheat bran, soyabean cake, alfalfa meal, middlings, yeast, and other materials. Recovery of the enzyme is by extraction, concentration, and precipitation, as for other hydrolytic enzymes.

Uses

The proteases from micro-organisms are used primarily for their proteinase activity. Bacterial proteases have been applied to the digestion of fish livers to liberate fish oil, to the tenderisation of meat, and to the clarification and maturing of malt beverages. Fungal proteases are active in the manufacture of soya sauce and other Oriental mould-fermented foods and may be added to bread dough, where, along with amylase, they help improve the consistency of the dough. They also may be used for chill-proofing beer and ale by removal of protein haze (the fungal tannase present also may be helpful), for the tenderisation of meats, for thinning egg white so that it can be filtered before drying, and for the hydrolysis of the gelatinous protein material in fish waste and press water to facilitate concentration and drying.

Glucose Oxidase

Glucose oxidase is produced by the submerged growth of *Aspergillus niger* or another mould. It is used to remove glucose from egg white or whole eggs to facilitate drying, prevent deterioration, and improve the whipping properties (of the reconstituted dried whites). It has been employed also to extend the shelf-life of canned soft drinks by retarding the pick-up of iron and the fading of colour. Oxidation of the glucose by glucose oxidase forms gluconic acid and hydrogen peroxide, the latter then being decomposed by the catalase in the same preparation. A combination of glucose oxidase and catalase is used to remove small residues of oxygen in packaged foods.

Other Enzymes

Cellulase, catalysing the hydrolysis of cellulose to cellulodextrins and glucose, has been recommended for producing more fermentable sugar in brewer's mashes, clarifying orange and lemon juices and concentrates, and tenderising green beans. Microbial lipase removes fat from yolk residues in dried egg albumen, assists mould spores in production of blue-cheese flavour in spreads, and adds to the flavour of milk chocolate. Dextransucrase increases viscosity by production of dextran in sucrose-containing foods. Flavour-producing enzymes, both from raw foods and from micro-organisms, are receiving special attention. Lactase from *Saccharomyces fragilis* may find use in hydrolysis of the lactose in whey to glucose and galactose, which are less laxative sugars. Catalase, the enzyme that converts hydrogen peroxide to water and oxygen is commercially prepared from *Aspergillus niger*, *Penicillium vitale*, and *Micrococcus lysodelilaticus*. Catalase is used in many applications where the removal of hydrogen peroxide is desired, for example, in cake baking, irradiated foods, and hydrogen peroxide sterilisation. Glucose isomerase converts glucose to fructose and is used in the corn milling industry. Commercially, *Streptomyces* or *Bacillus coagulans* is used. Undoubtedly more kinds of enzymes could be added to those mentioned.

SECTION V

Foods in Relation to Disease

Chapter 21

Bacterial Agents of Foodborne Illness

INTRODUCTION

Throughout our lifetimes we are subjected to risks and hazards of all kinds. Foods should be safer today than in the 'good old days', due to the knowledge we have gained of bacteria and sanitation, as well as to increased regulations. However, due to large-scale, high-speed food processing, alteration of traditional processing methods resulting in less control of micro-organisms, proliferation of heat-and-eat convenience foods, and nationwide distribution with increased potential for mishandling, it is possible for outbreaks of foodborne illness to occur that involve many people. The agents that cause human illness and can be transmitted by foods are bacteria, viruses, fungi, parasites, chemicals, and toxins naturally present in plants and animals. A foodborne disease outbreak is defined by the centres for disease control (CDC) as an incident in which two or more persons experience a similar illness, usually gastrointestinal, after ingesting a common food, and epidemiological analysis implicates the food as the source of the illness. For botulism or chemical poisoning, one case constitutes on outbreak (Fig. 21.1). A microbial foodborne illness may result from ingesting a food containing either pathogenic micro-organisms or a toxin or poison. When a pathogenic micro-organism is the etiologic agent, the illness is called an infection. If a toxin or poison is the causative agent, the illness is called a food intoxication or food poisoning.

AEROMONAS HYDROPHILA

Aeromonas hydrophila are Gram-negative, nonspore-forming, rod-shaped, facultative anaerobic bacilli belonging to the family Aeromonadaceae. Although *A. hydrophila* is the focus of this section, other aeromonads, such as *A. caviae* and *A. sobria*, have also been isolated from human faeces and from water sources.

Morphologically, aeromonads are indistinguishable from members of the Enterobacteriaceae family, such as *E. coli*. They also share many biochemical characteristics, with the differentiation being that aeromonads are oxidase positive and Enterobacteriaceae are oxidase negative.

Sources

Previous work has firmly established that *Aeromonas* species, including *A. hydrophila*, are ubiquitous in the environment. These organisms have been found in lakes, rivers, marine waters, sewage effluents, and drinking waters, among other places. The concentration of Aeromonas species varies with the environment being investigated. In clean rivers, lakes, and storage reservoirs, concentrations of *Aeromonas* spp. have been found to typically be around 10^2 CFU/ml.

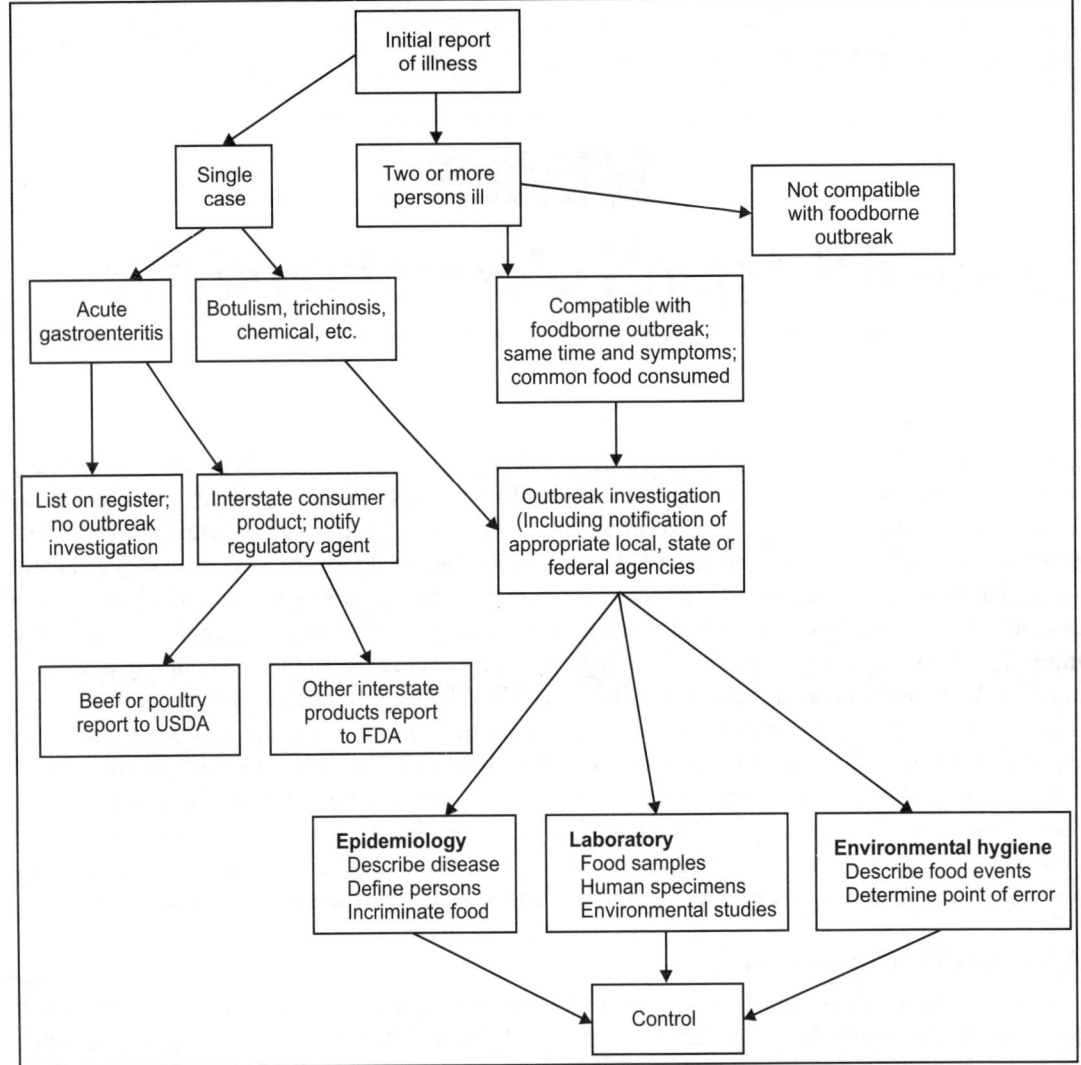

Fig. 21.1. A scheme for handling foodborne disease complaints, to be implemented by state and local health departments.

Groundwaters generally contain less, with fewer than 1 CFU/ml. Additionally, drinking water immediately leaving the treatment plant has been found to contain between 0 and 10^2 CFU/ml, with potentially higher concentrations in drinking water distribution systems, attributed to growth in biofilms. Depending on the study, *A. hydrophila* comprised 20–60 per cent of the aeromonads isolated. *Aeromonas* spp. have been found to grow between 5° and 45°C. Water temperature is a significant factor for *Aeromonas* growth.

Coinciding with the optimal growth range of Aeromonas, seasonal variation has been reported for public water systems, with *Aeromonas* more often recovered during the warmer months. The same trend has been observed with stool samples.

Health Effects

In recent years, *A. hydrophila* has gained public health recognition as an opportunistic pathogen. It has been implicated as a potential agent of gastroenteritis, septicaemia, cellulitis, colitis, and meningitis, and is frequently isolated from wound infections sustained in aquatic environments. It has also recently been implicated in respiratory infections. Treatment for infection with *Aeromonas* is generally not necessary for gastrointestinal illness. However, for other presentations of infection, antibiotic therapy is usually implemented. Individuals at the greatest risk of infection are children, the elderly, and the immunocompromised.

Exposure

The common routes of infection suggested for *Aeromonas* are the ingestion of contaminated water or food or contact of the organism with a break in the skin. No person-to-person transmission has been reported. It should be noted that although *A. hydrophila* is water based, waterborne outbreaks have not been reported, and waterborne transmission has not been well established. For example, various studies have been unsuccessful in linking patient isolates of *A. hydrophila* with isolates recovered from the water supply. As mentioned above, the growth of *A. hydrophila* is temperature dependent. Therefore, the risk of infection is highest in the summer months, when these micro-organisms are multiplying more rapidly.

The dose necessary to cause infections in humans has not been established. In the limited number of studies done, the dose was quite high, and only a limited number of participants were infected. The virulence of the strain is one factor that can influence the infectious dose needed. For *A. hydrophila*, the virulence of the organism is, at least in part, thought to result from the production of specific enterotoxins. The primary toxins are haemolysins. In addition, some aeromonads produce a range of cell surface and secreted proteases that may enhance their virulence. It has been demonstrated that a significant proportion of the *A. hydrophila* isolated from water (chlorinated and unchlorinated supplies) contained genes responsible for enterotoxigenic or cytotoxic activity. Expression of virulence factors has been shown to be influenced by environmental temperature. *A. hydrophila* isolated from the environment produced significantly less enterotoxins when grown at 37°C compared with 28°C, whereas the clinical isolates tested produced more enterotoxins at 37°C than at 28°C. The temperature of the human body is approximately 37°C; therefore, strains that produce virulence factors at this temperature are likely to be more important as pathogens.

Treatment Technology

As mentioned previously, aeromonads are ubiquitous in many water environments. Consequently, they will be present in most source waters used for drinking water production. The methods currently used for treatment and disinfection are effective in minimising the level of aeromonads in the finished drinking water. For example, it has been shown that *A. hydrophila* is generally more susceptible to chlorine and monochloramine than coliforms. Chlorine dioxide has also been shown to be an effective disinfectant. In the distribution system, there is the potential for *Aeromonas* to regrow. Maintaining chlorine at or above 0.2 mg/l should provide adequate control of *A. hydrophila* in the water. However, it is difficult to control its growth in biofilms.

The most effective approach for controlling *Aeromonas* growth is to limit the *Aeromonas* spp. entering the distribution system through effective treatment and maintenance, to maintain temperatures below 14°C, to provide free chlorine residuals above 0.1–0.2 mg/l, and to limit the levels of organic carbon compounds. If there are significant increases in *Aeromonas* concentrations in a drinking water supply, this indicates a general deterioration of bacteriological quality.

Assessment

Some studies have been undertaken to determine if the indicators currently used in the drinking water industry, including *E. coli*, total coliforms, and HPC, can be used as surrogates for the presence of *Aeromonas*. Several studies, including a large study in England, showed no relationship between *Aeromonas* incidence and coliforms, *E. coli* or HPCs. Although all the studies had similar findings, not all could draw definite conclusions, because of limited sample sizes, minimal occurrences of coliforms, and/or the absence of *E. coli* in the water.

When looking at the overall public health significance of *A. hydrophila* in drinking water, further epidemiological studies are needed to ascertain the relationship between *Aeromonas* illness and the presence of these organisms in drinking water. The European Community has established a drinking water standard for *A. hydrophila* of no more than 20 CFU/100 ml in water leaving the treatment plant and 200 CFU/100 ml in distribution system water. These values are based on an assessment of achievability, motivated by a precautionary approach, and not on the public health significance of their occurrence in drinking-water. Based on what is currently known, treated drinking water probably represents a very low risk. However, it is advisable to minimise the concentration of *A. hydrophila*, as well as other aeromonads, in drinking water supplies until their public health significance has been fully investigated.

BACILLUS CEREUS

Bacillus cereus is a spore-forming bacterium that can be frequently isolated from soil and some food. *B. cereus* spores are more resistant to heat and chemical treatments than vegetative pathogens such as *Salmonella*, *E. coli*, *Campylobacter*, and *Listeria monocytogenes*. If *B. cereus* grows in food, it can cause two different types of foodborne illness in humans—vomiting very shortly after eating contaminated food or diarrhea after a longer incubation.

Symptoms and Disease Process

Two different toxins are involved in these foodborne illnesses. The emetic (vomiting) form of *B. cereus* has an onset time of 0.5 to 6 hours after consumption, with primary symptoms of vomiting and nausea and occasionally diarrhea. Recovery occurs in less than 24 hours. The diarrheal illness has a mean onset time of between 6 and 15 hours, with symptoms of watery diarrhea, pain and nausea persisting for 24 hours. The diarrheal toxin is released in the body after ingestion of high numbers of cells (e.g. $>10^5$/g). It is the action of the toxin in the small intestine that causes diarrhea. In a small percentage of cases, both vomiting and diarrheal symptoms can occur if both types of toxins are produced.

Primary Routes of Transmission

Spores of *B. cereus* can be found widely in nature, including samples of dust, dirt, cereal crops, water, etc. so it is a common contaminant of raw agricultural commodities. Normal contamination levels are generally <100/g.

Starchy foods, such as rice or potatoes, are commonly associated with *B. cereus* emetic (vomiting) toxin outbreaks. Due to its preparation process, one of the most common food vehicles for transmission of emetic *B. cereus* illness is fried rice, and there have been several reported outbreaks. The spores of

B. cereus are activated in the initial preparation of the rice, which if stored at abusive temperatures (approximately 59° to 104°F or 15° to 40°C) for an extended time, will outgrow and produce a toxin that is heat stable and will not be inactivated during subsequent cooking.

The diarrhea-causing strains have been found in a wider selection of foods. Common sources include meat and vegetable items, soups and milk products. Unlike the emetic toxin, the diarrheal toxin is destroyed in cooking. If the spores experience conditions that permit growth, they can grow to levels where toxins are produced.

The types of *B. cereus* illness reported appear to differ significantly by geography. In Japan, the emetic form is found about 10 times more frequently than the diarrheal type. In Europe and North America, the diarrheal type is more frequently reported. These differences may be due to variations in diet among the world's regions.

Control

Heating can activate spores, which allows them to germinate and grow under favourable conditions. Time and temperature abuse of cooked food permits the activated spores to grow and produce toxins. Control relies on prompt refrigeration and cooling of foods quickly to less than 41°F (5°C) to minimise growth and toxin formation. Many of the emetic illnesses are due to improper holding of cooked rice at warm room temperatures, offering conditions where the activated spores in the rice are able to produce toxin. Foods should be promptly refrigerated or held above 140°F (60°C) to prevent growth of the cells.

Heating of a food after potential temperature abuse is not a foolproof control technique for *B. cereus*, since the emetic toxin is heat stable. The diarrheal toxin will, however, be destroyed by heating.

An additional concern regarding *B. cereus* is the resistance of the spores to peracetic acid treatments that may be used as an alternative to hydrogen peroxide for treatment of aseptic packaging materials. *B. cereus* spores are more resistant to some peracid products than other sporeformers. If the food product to be produced supports the growth of *B. cereus*, it is important to evaluate effectiveness of the treatment against *B. cereus* spores to ensure product safety.

BRUCELLA

Brucella is a genus of Gram-negative bacteria. They are small (0.5 to 0.7 by 0.6 to 1.5 μm), nonmotile, nonencapsulated coccobacilli, which function as facultative intracellular parasites (Fig. 21.2).

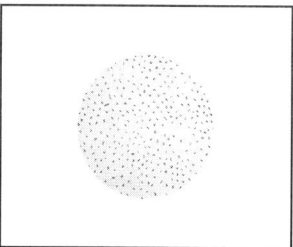

Fig. 21.2. *Brucella.*

Brucella is the cause of brucellosis, which is a zoonosis. It is transmitted by ingesting infected food, direct contact with an infected animal, or inhalation of aerosols. Transmission from human to human, for example through sexual intercourse or from mother to child, is exceedingly rare, but possible. Minimum infectious exposure is between 10–100 organisms. Brucellosis primarily occurs through occupational exposure (e.g. exposure to cattle, sheep, pigs), but also by consumption of unpasteurised milk products. There are a few different species of *Brucella*, each with slightly different host specificity. *B. melitensis* which infects goats and sheep, *B. abortus* which infects cattle, *B. suis* infects pigs, *B. ovis* infects sheep and *B. neotomae*. Recently new species were discovered, in marine mammals (*B. pinnipedialis* and s*B. ceti*), in the common vole *Microtus arvalis* (*B. microti*), and even in a breast implant (*B. inopinata*).

However, the new NCBI taxonomy has named all Brucella species *Brucella melitensis*. They include *Brucella melitensis* 16M and 5 other biovars: *abortus*, *canis*, *neotomae*, *ovis*, and *suis*.

Diagnosis

Brucella is isolated from a blood culture on Castaneda medium. Prolonged incubation (up to 6 weeks) may be required as they are slow-growing, but on modern automated machines the cultures often show positive results within seven days. On Gram-stain they appear as dense clumps of Gram-negative coccobacilli and are exceedingly difficult to see.

It is crucial to be able to differentiate *Brucella* from *Salmonella* which could also be isolated from blood cultures and are Gram-negative. Testing for urease would successfully accomplish the task; as it is positive for the *Brucella* and negative for the *Salmonella*. *Brucella* could also be seen in bone marrow.

Laboratory acquired brucellosis is common. This most often happens when the disease is not thought of until cultures become positive, by which time the specimens have already been handled by a number of laboratory staff. The idea of preventive treatment is to stop people who have been exposed to *Brucella* from becoming ill with the disease.

There are no clinical trials to be relied on as a guide for optimal treatment, but a three week course of rifampicin and doxycycline twice daily is the combination most often used, and appears to be efficacious; the advantage of this regimen is that it is oral medication and there are no injections; however, a high rate of side effects (nausea, vomiting, loss of appetite) has also been reported.

Human Brucellosis

The disease is characterised by acute undulating fever, headache, night sweats, fatigue and anorexia. Human brucellosis is not considered a contagious disease and people become infected by contact with fluids from infected animals (sheep, cattle or pigs) or derived food products like unpasteurised milk and cheese. Brucellosis is also considered an occupational disease because of a higher incidence in people working with animals (slaughterhouse cases). The real worldwide incidence of brucellosis is unknown because there is a low level of surveillance and reporting in *Brucella* endemic areas.

Blue light study

In a study published in *Science* in August 2007, it was revealed that *Brucella* reacts strongly to the presence of the blue spectrum in natural light, reproducing at a great rate and becoming infectious. Conversely, depriving *Brucella* of the blue wavelengths dropped its reproductive rate by 90 per cent, a result one of the co-authors called 'spectacular'.

CAMPYLOBACTER

Campylobacters are bacteria that are a major cause of diarrhoeal illness in humans and are generally regarded as the most common bacterial cause of gastroenteritis worldwide. In developed and developing countries, they cause more cases of diarrhoea than, for example, foodborne *Salmonella* bacteria. In developing countries, Campylobacter infections in children under the age of two years are especially frequent, sometimes resulting in death. In almost all developed countries, the incidence of human campylobacter infections has been steadily increasing for several years. The reasons for this are unknown.

Campylobacters are mainly spiral-shaped, S-shaped or curved, rod-shaped bacteria. There are 16 species and six subspecies assigned to the genus Campylobacter, of which the most frequently reported in human disease are *C. jejuni* (subspecies jejuni) and *C. coli*.

C. laridis and *C. upsaliensis* are also regarded as primary pathogens, but are generally reported far less frequently in cases of human disease. Most species prefer a micro-aerobic (containing 3–10 per cent oxygen) atmosphere for growth. A few species tend to favour an anaerobic environment, although they will grow under micro-aerobic conditions also.

The Disease

1. Campylobacteriosis is the disease caused by the presence of campylobacters. The onset of disease symptoms usually occurs two to five days after infection, but can range from one to ten days.
2. The most common clinical symptoms of campylobacter infections include diarrhoea (frequently with blood in the faeces), abdominal pain, fever, headache, nausea, and/or vomiting. The symptoms typically last three to six days.
3. A fatal outcome is rare and is usually confined to very young or elderly patients or to those already suffering from another serious disease such as AIDS.
4. Complications such as bacteremia, hepatitis, pancreatitis (infections of the blood, liver and pancreas respectively), and abortion have all been reported with various degrees of frequency. Post-infection complications may include reactive arthritis (painful inflammation of the joints which can last for several months) and neurological disorders such as Guillain-Barré syndrome, a polio-like form of paralysis that can result in respiratory and severe neurological dysfunction or death in a small, but significant, number of cases.
5. The high incidence of campylobacter diarrhoea, as well as its duration and possible sequelae, makes it highly important from a socio-economic perspective.

Sources and Transmission

1. Campylobacters are widely distributed and occur in most warm-blooded domestic, production and wild animals. They are prevalent in food animals such as poultry, cattle, pigs, sheep, ostriches and shell-fish; and in pets, including cats and dogs.
2. The main route of transmission is generally believed to be foodborne, via undercooked meats and meat products, as well as raw or contaminated milk. The ingestion of contaminated water or ice is also a recognised source of infection.
3. Campylobacteriosis is considered to be a zoonosis, a disease transmitted to humans from animals or animal products. In animals, campylobacters seldom cause disease.
4. One of the major gaps in our knowledge at present is the relative contribution of each of the above sources to the overall burden of disease. Since common-source outbreaks account for a rather small proportion of cases, the vast majority of reports are made sporadically, with no easily discernible pattern. Estimation of the importance of all known sources is therefore extremely difficult. In addition, the wide occurrence of campylobacters also hinders the development of strategies to control campylobacters in the food supply 'from farm to fork'.

Control and Prevention Methods

1. Treatment is not generally indicated, except electrolyte replacement and rehydration. Antimicrobial treatment (erythromycin, tetracycline, quinolones) is indicated in invasive cases or to eliminate the carrier state.
2. The prevention of infection requires control measures at all stages of the food chain, from agricultural production on the farm, to processing, manufacturing and preparation of foods in both commercial establishments and the domestic environment.
3. Specific intervention methods on the farm have been shown to reduce the incidence of campylobacter in poultry. Measures include enhanced biosecurity to avoid horizontal transmission of campylobacter from the environment to the flock of birds. This control option is feasible only where birds are kept in closed housing conditions.
4. There are no proven intervention methods to reduce campylobacter in cattle farms. Prevention of the contamination of raw milk on the farm is not consistently possible; therefore, consumption of raw milk should be avoided.
5. Good hygienic slaughtering practices will reduce contamination of carcasses by faeces, but will not guarantee the absence of campylobacter from meat and meat products. Education in hygienic handling of foods for abattoir workers and those involved in the production of raw meat is essential to keep microbiological contamination to a minimum.
6. The only effective method of eliminating campylobacter from contaminated foods is to introduce a bactericidal treatment, such as heating (e.g. cooking or pasteurisation) or irradiation.
7. Preventive measures for campylobacter infection in the household kitchen are similar to those used against other foodborne bacterial diseases.
8. In countries without adequate sewage disposal systems, faeces and articles soiled with faeces may need to be disinfected before disposal.

Recommendations for the Public and Travellers

1. Make sure your food is properly cooked and still hot when served.
2. Avoid raw milk and products made from raw milk. Drink only pasteurised or boiled milk.
3. Avoid ice unless you are sure it is made from safe water.
4. When the safety of drinking water is doubtful, boil it or if this is not possible, disinfect it with a reliable, slow-release disinfectant agent. These are usually available at pharmacies.
5. Wash hands thoroughly and frequently using soap, in particular after contact with pets or farm animals, or after having been to the toilet.
6. Wash fruits and vegetables carefully, particularly if they are eaten raw. If possible, vegetables and fruits should be peeled.
7. WHO's brochure A Guide on Safe Food for Travellers gives practical advice for safeguarding health when travelling.

Recommendations for Food Handlers

1. Both professional and domestic food handlers should be vigilant during the preparation of food and should observe hygienic rules of food preparation.
2. Professional food handlers who suffer from fever, diarrhoea, vomiting or visible infected skin lesions should report to their employer immediately.
3. More information for food handlers is given in the WHO Guide on Hygiene in Food Service and Mass Catering Establishments (Document code: WHO/FNU/FOS/94.5).

CLOSTRIDIUM BOTULINUM

Clostridium botulinum is a gram-positive, rod-shaped bacterium that produces neurotoxins, known as botulinum neurotoxins types A-G, that cause the flaccid muscular paralysis seen in botulism. It is also the main paralytic agent in botox. *C. botulinum* is an anaerobic spore-former, which produces oval, subterminal endospores and is commonly found in soil.

Clostridium botulinum is a rod-shaped micro-organism. It is an obligate anaerobe, meaning that oxygen is poisonous to the cells. However, *C. botulinum* tolerates traces of oxygen due to the enzyme called superoxide dismutase (SOD) which is an important antioxidant defense in nearly all cells exposed to oxygen. *C. botulinum* is only able to produce the neurotoxin during sporulation, which can only happen in an anaerobic environment. Other bacterial species produce spores in an unfavourable growth environment to preserve the organism's viability and permit survival in a dormant state until the spores are exposed to favourable conditions.

In the laboratory *Clostridium botulinum* is usually isolated in tryptose sulphite cycloserine (TSC) growth media in an anaerobic environment with less than 2 per cent of oxygen. This can be achieved by several commercial kits that use a chemical reaction to replace O_2 with CO_2. *C. botulinum* is a lipase negative micro-organism that grows between pH of 4.8 and 7 and it can't use lactose as a primary carbon source, characteristics important during a biochemical identification.

Symptoms of Botulism

Botulism neurotoxins prevent neurotransmitters from functioning properly. This means that they inhibit motor control. As botulism progresses, the patient experiences paralysis from top to bottom, starting with the eyes and face and moving to the throat, chest, and extremities. When paralysis reaches the chest, death from inability to breathe results unless the patient is ventilated. Symptoms of botulism generally appear 12 to 72 hours after eating contaminated food. With treatment, illness lasts from 1 to 10 days. Full recovery from botulism poisoning can take weeks to months. Some people never fully recover. In general, symptoms of botulism poisoning include the following: (i) nausea, (ii) vomiting, (iii) fatigue, (iv) dizziness, (v) double vision, (vi) dry skin, mouth and throat, (vii) drooping eyelids, (viii) difficulty swallowing, (ix) slurred speech, (x) muscle weakness, (xi) body aches, (xii) paralysis, and (xiii) lack of fever.

Infant botulism takes on a different form. Symptoms in an infant include lethargy, poor appetite, constipation, drooling, drooping eyelids, a weak cry, and paralysis.

Long-term effects of botulism

The majority of botulism patients never fully recover their pre-illness health. After three months to a year of recovery, persisting side-effects are most likely permanent. These long-term effects most often include fatigue, weakness, dizziness, dry mouth, and difficulty performing strenuous tasks. Patients also report a generally less happy and peaceful psychological state than before their illness.

Botulism diagnosis

If a patient displays symptoms of botulism, a doctor will most likely take a blood, stool, or gastric secretion sample. The most common test for botulism is injecting the patient's blood into a mouse to see whether the mouse displays signs of botulism, since other testing methods take up to a week.

Sometimes botulism can be difficult to diagnose, since symptoms can be mild or confused with those of Guillan-Barre Syndrome.

Treatment of botulism

If found early, botulism can be treated with an antitoxin that blocks circulation of the toxin in the bloodstream. This prevents the patient's case from worsening, but recovery still takes several weeks.

Prevention of botulism

Since botulism poisoning most commonly comes from foods improperly canned at home, the most important step in preventing botulism is to follow proper canning procedure. Ohio State University's Extension Service provides a useful guide to sanitary canning techniques. Further botulism prevention techniques include:

1. Not eating canned food if the container is bulging or if it smells bad, although not all strains on *Clostridium Botulinum* smell.
2. Storing garlic or herb-infused oil in the refrigerator.
3. Not storing baked potatoes at room temperature.

To prevent infant botulism, do not give even a small amount of honey to an infant, as honey is one source of infant botulism.

Phenotypes

The current nomenclature for *C. botulinum* recognises four physiological groups (I–IV). The classification is based on the ability of the organism to digest complex proteins. Studies at the DNA and rRNA level support the subdivision of the species into groups I–IV. Most outbreaks of human botulism are caused by group I (proteolytic) or II (non-proteolytic) *C. botulinum*. Group III organisms mainly cause diseases in animals.

There has been no record of Group IV *C. botulinum* causing human or animal disease (Table 21.1). Botulism poisoning can occur due to improperly preserved or home-canned, low-acid food that was not processed using correct preservation times and/or pressure.

Table 21.1. Phenotypic groups of *Clostridium botulinum*.

Properties	Group I	Group II	Group III	Group IV
Toxin Types	A, B, F	B, E, F	C, D	G
Proteolysis	+	–	Weak	–
Saccharolysis	–	+	–	–
Disease host	Human	Human	Animal	–
Toxin gene	Chromosome	Chromosome	Bacteriophage	Plasmid
Close relatives	*C. sporogenes,* *C. putrificum*	*C. butyricum,* *C. beijerinickii*	*C. haemolyticum,* *C. novyi* type A	*C. subterminale,* *C. haemolyticum*

Neurotoxin Types

Neurotoxin production is the unifying feature of the species *C. botulinum*. Seven types of toxins have been identified and allocated a letter (A-G). Most strains produce one type of neurotoxin but strains producing multiple toxins have been described. *Clostridium botulinum* producing B and F toxin types have been isolated from human botulism cases in New Mexico and California. The toxin type has been designated Bf as the type B toxin was found in excess to the type F. Similarly, strains producing Ab and Af toxins have been reported. There is evidence that the neurotoxin genes have been the subject of horizontal gene transfer, possibly from a viral source. This theory is supported by the presence of integration sites flanking the toxin in some strains of *C. botulinum*. However, these integrations sites are degraded indicating that the *C. botulinum* acquired the toxin genes quite far into the evolutionary past. Only types A, B, E, and F cause disease in humans while types C and D cause disease in cows, birds, and other animals but not in humans. The 'gold standard' for determining toxin type is a mouse bioassay, but the genes for types A, B, E, and F can now be readily differentiated using Real-time polymerase chain reaction (PCR).

Organisms genetically as they identified as other *Clostridium* species have caused human botulism; *Clostridium butyricum* producing type E toxin and *Clostridium baratii* producing type F toxin. The ability of *C. botulinum* to naturally transfer neurotoxin genes to other clostridia is concerning, especially in the food industry where preservation systems are designed to destroy or inhibit only *C. botulinum* but not other *Clostridium* species.

Clostridium Botulinum in Different Geographical Locations

A number of quantitative surveys for *C. botulinum* spores in the environment have suggested a prevalence of specific toxin types in given geographic areas, which remain unexplained.

North America

Type A *C. botulinum* predominates the soil samples from the western regions while type B is the major type found in eastern areas. The type B organisms were of the proteolytic type I. Sediments from the Great Lake regions were surveyed after outbreaks of botulism among commercially reared fish and only type E spores were detected. It has been noted in a survey that type A strains were isolated from soils that were neutral to alkaline (average pH 7.5) while type B strains were isolated from slightly acidic soils (average pH 6.25).

Europe

Clostridium botulinum type E is prevalent in aquatic sediments in Norway and Sweden, Denmark, the Netherlands, the Baltic coast of Poland and Russia. It was then suggested that the type E *C. botulinum* is a true aquatic organism, which was indicated by the correlation between the level of type E contamination and flooding of the land with seawater. As the land dried, the level of type E decreased and type B became dominant. In soil and sediment from the United Kingdom, *C. botulinum* type B predominates. In general, the incidence is usually lower in soil than in sediment. In Italy, a survey was conducted in the vicinity of Rome, and a low level of contamination was found; all strains were proteolytic *C. botulinum* type A or B.

Australia

Clostridium botulinum type A was found to be present in soil samples from mountain areas of Victoria. Type B organisms were detected in marine mud from Tasmania. Type A *C. botulinum* have been found in Sydney suburbs and types A and B were isolated from urban areas. In a well-defined area of the Darling-Downs region of Queensland, a study showed the prevalence and persistence of *C. botulinum* type B after many cases of botulism in horses.

Other

A 'mouse protection' or 'mouse bioassay' test determines the type of *C. botulinum* present using monoclonal antibodies. This can now also be accomplished using real-time PCR.

Clostridium botulinum is also used to prepare the medicaments Botox, Dysport, Xeomin, and Neurobloc used to selectively paralyse muscles to temporarily relieve muscle function. It has other 'off-label' medical purposes, such as treating severe facial pain, such as that caused by trigeminal neuralgia.

Botulin toxin produced by *C. botulinum* is often believed to be a potential bioweapon as it is so potent that it takes about 75 nanograms to kill a person (LD_{50} of 1 ng/kg, assuming an average person weighs ~75 kg); 500 grams of it would be enough to kill half of the entire human population.

Clostridium botulinum is a soil bacterium. The spores can survive in most environments and are very hard to kill. They can survive the temperature of boiling water at sea level, thus many foods are canned with a pressurised boil that achieves an even higher temperature, sufficient to kill the spores.

Growth of the bacterium can be prevented by high acidity, high ratio of dissolved sugar, high levels of oxygen, very low levels of moisture or storage at temperatures below 3°C (38°F) for type A. For example in a low acid, canned vegetable such as green beans that are not heated hot enough to kill the spores (i.e. a pressurised environment) may provide an oxygen free medium for the spores to grow and produce the toxin. On the other hand, pickles are sufficiently acidic to prevent growth; even if the spores are present, they pose no danger to the consumer. Honey, corn syrup, and other sweeteners may contain spores but the spores cannot grow in a highly concentrated sugar solution; however, when a sweetener is diluted in the low oxygen, low acid digestive system of an infant, the spores can grow and produce toxin. As soon as infants begin eating solid food, the digestive juices become too acidic for the bacterium to grow.

CLOSTRIDIUM PERFRINGENS

Clostridium perfringens (formerly known as *C. welchii*) is a Gram-positive, rod-shaped, anaerobic, spore-forming bacterium of the genus *Clostridium*. *C. perfringens* is ever present in nature and can be found as a normal component of decaying vegetation, marine sediment, the intestinal tract of humans and other vertebrates, insects, and soil. *C. perfringens* is a human pathogen sometimes, and other times it can be ingested and not cause any harm.

Clostridium perfringens is commonly encountered in infections as a component of the normal flora. In this case, its role in disease is minor.

Infections due to *C. perfringens* this disease shows evidence of tissue necrosis, bacteremia, emphysematous cholecystitis, and gas gangrene, which is also known as clostridial myonecrosis. The toxin involved in gas gangrene is known as α-toxin, which inserts into the plasma membrane of cells, producing gaps in the membrane that disrupt normal cellular function. *C. perfringens* can participate in polymicrobial anaerobic infections. After ingestion, bacteria multiply and lead to colic, diarrhea, and sometimes nausea.

The action of *C. perfringens* on dead bodies is known to mortuary workers as tissue gas and can be halted only by embalming.

Food Poisoning

In the United Kingdom and United States, *C. perfringens* bacteria are the third-most-common cause of foodborne illness, with poorly prepared meat and poultry the main culprits in harbouring the bacterium.

The *Clostridium perfringens* enterotoxin (CPE) mediating the disease is heat-labile (dies at 74°C) and can be detected in contaminated food, if not heated properly, and feces.

Incubation time is between 6 and 24 (commonly 10–12) hours after ingestion of contaminated food. Often, meat is well prepared but too far in advance of consumption. Since *C. perfringens* forms spores that can withstand cooking temperatures, if let stand for long enough, germination ensues and infective bacterial colonies develop. Symptoms typically include abdominal cramping and diarrhea; vomiting and fever are unusual. The whole course usually resolves within 24 hours. Very rare, fatal cases of clostridial necrotising enteritis (also known as Pig-Bel) have been known to involve 'Type C' strains of the organism, which produce a potently ulcerative β-toxin. This strain is most frequently encountered in Papua New Guinea.

It is likely that many cases of *C. perfringens* food poisoning remain subclinical, as antibodies to the toxin are common among the population. This has led to the conclusion that most of the population has experienced food poisoning due to *C. perfringens*.

Despite its potential dangers, *Clostridium perfringens* is used as the leavening agent in salt rising bread. The baking process is thought to reduce the bacterial contamination, precluding negative effects.

Gas Gangrene

Clostridium perfringens is the most common bacterial agent for Gas gangrene.

1. Gangrene is necrosis and putrefaction of tissues. Gas production forms bubbles of gas in muscle (crepitus) and smell in decomposing tissue.
2. After rapid and destructive local spread (which can take hours), systemic spread of bacteria and bacterial toxins may result in death. This is a problem in major trauma and in military contexts.
3. Gram-positive spore can form anaerobic bacilli.
4. It is a saprophyte, meaning it occurs in soil, H_2O, decomposing plant, human and animal feces.
5. Under appropriate conditions, spores can reactivate into a vegetative cell.
6. Can grow in anaerobic dead tissue or dirt. Produces cytotoxin that can lyse cells.
7. Traumatic wounds should be cleaned. Wounds that cannot be cleaned should not be stitched shut.
8. Spores can withstand boiling water. Autoclaving is necessary to ensure sterility.
9. Penicillin prophylaxis kills clostridia, and is thus useful for dirty wounds and lower leg amputations.
10. If detected on clinical grounds, should not wait for lab results.
11. If adrenaline used for injection is contaminated with spores, catastrophic reactions can result.
12. Prompt and adequate surgical attention is of paramount importance.
13. Grows readily on blood agar plate in anaerobic conditions and often produces a zone of haemolysis.
14. Growth in food can produce toxins causing acute, self-limiting diarrhea.
15. High infectious dose is required; carrier state persists for several days.

Colony Characteristics

On blood agar plates, *C. perfringens* grown anaerobically produces β-haemolytic, flat, spreading, rough, translucent colonies with irregular margins. A distinguishing characteristic of *C. perfringens* is a zone of double Beta Haemolysis. On a Nagler agar plate, containing 5–10 per cent egg yolk, is used to identify strains that produce α-toxin, a diffusible lecithinase that interacts with the lipids in egg yolk to produce a characteristic precipitate around the colonies. One-half of the plate is inoculated with antitoxin to act as a control in the identification.

ESCHERICHIA COLI

Escherichia coli (commonly abbreviated *E. coli*) is a Gram-negative rod-shaped bacterium that is commonly found in the lower intestine of warm-blooded organisms (endotherms). Most *E. coli* strains are harmless, but some, such as serotype O157:H7, can cause serious food poisoning in humans, and are occasionally responsible for product recalls. The harmless strains are part of the normal flora of the gut, and can benefit their hosts by producing vitamin K_2, and by preventing the establishment of pathogenic bacteria within the intestine. *E. coli* are not always confined to the intestine, and their ability to survive for brief periods outside the body makes them an ideal indicator organism to test environmental samples for fecal contamination. The bacteria can also be grown easily and its genetics are comparatively simple and easily manipulated or duplicated through a process of metagenics, making it one of the best-studied prokaryotic model organisms, and an important species in biotechnology and microbiology.

E. coli was discovered by German paediatrician and bacteriologist Theodor Escherich in 1885, and is now classified as part of the Enterobacteriaceae family of gamma-proteobacteria.

E. coli is Gram-negative, facultative anaerobic and non-sporulating. Cells are typically rod-shaped and are about 2 micrometres (μm) long and 0.5 μm in diameter, with a cell volume of 0.6–0.7 (μm)^3. It can live on a wide variety of substrates. *E. coli* uses mixed-acid fermentation in anaerobic conditions, producing lactate, succinate, ethanol, acetate and carbon dioxide. Since many pathways in mixed-acid fermentation produce hydrogen gas, these pathways require the levels of hydrogen to be low, as is the case when *E. coli* lives together with hydrogen-consuming organisms such as methanogens or sulphate-reducing bacteria.

Optimal growth of *E. coli* occurs at 37°C (98.6°F) but some laboratory strains can multiply at temperatures of up to 49°C (120.2°F). Growth can be driven by aerobic or anaerobic respiration, using a large variety of redox pairs, including the oxidation of pyruvic acid, formic acid, hydrogen and amino acids, and the reduction of substrates such as oxygen, nitrate, dimethyl sulphoxide and trimethylamine N-oxide. Strains that possess flagella can swim and are motile. The flagella have a peritrichous arrangement.

E. coli and related bacteria possess the ability to transfer DNA via bacterial conjugation, transduction or transformation, which allows genetic material to spread horizontally through an existing population. This process led to the spread of the gene encoding shiga toxin from Shigella to *E. coli* O157:H7, carried by a bacteriophage.

Diversity

As more is known about certain organisms, such as genetic information, the taxonomic classification of species is changed to reflect the advance in knowledge, however in the case of *Escherichia coli* due to its medical importance, this has not occurred (namely split into several genera/species) and remains one of the most diverse bacterial species: only 20 per cent of the genome is common to all strains. In fact, from the evolutionary point of view, the members of genus Shigella (*dysenteriae, flexneri, boydii, sonnei*) are actually *E. coli* strains 'in disguise' (i.e. *E. coli* is paraphyletic to the genus).

A strain of *E. coli* is a subgroup within the species that has unique characteristics that distinguish it from other *E. coli* strains. These differences are often detectable only at the molecular level; however, they may result in changes to the physiology or life-cycle of the bacterium. For example, a strain may gain pathogenic capacity, the ability to use a unique carbon source, the ability to take upon a particular ecological niche or the ability to resist antimicrobial agents. Different strains of *E. coli* are often host-specific, making it possible to determine the source of faecal contamination in environmental samples. For example, knowing which *E. coli* strains are present in a water sample allows researchers to make assumptions about whether the contamination originated from a human, another mammal or a bird.

New strains of *E. coli* evolve through the natural biological process of mutation and through horizontal gene transfer. Some strains develop traits that can be harmful to a host animal. These virulent strains typically cause a bout of diarrhoea that is unpleasant in healthy adults and is often lethal to children in the developing world. More virulent strains, such as O157:H7 cause serious illness or death in the elderly, the very young or the immunocompromised. *E. coli* is the type species of the genus and the type strain is ATCC 11775.

A common subdivison system of *E. coli*, but not based on evolutionary relatedness, is by serotype, which is based on major surface antigens (O antigen: part of lipopolysaccharide layer; H: flagellin; K antigen: capsule), e.g. O157:H7 (NB: K-12, the common laboratory strain is not a serotype).

Role as Normal Microbiota

E. coli normally colonises an infant's gastrointestinal tract within 40 hours of birth, arriving with food or water or with the individuals handling the child. In the bowel, it adheres to the mucus of the large intestine. It is the primary facultative anaerobe of the human gastrointestinal tract. (Facultative anaerobes are organisms that can grow in either the presence or absence of oxygen.) As long as these bacteria do not acquire genetic elements encoding for virulence factors, they remain benign commensals.

Role in Disease

Virulent strains of *E. coli* can cause gastroenteritis, urinary tract infections, and neonatal meningitis. In rarer cases, virulent strains are also responsible for haemolytic-uremic syndrome, peritonitis, mastitis, septicaemia and Gram-negative pneumonia.

Gastrointestinal infection

Certain strains of *E. coli*, such as O157:H7, O121 and O104:H21, produce potentially lethal toxins. Food poisoning caused by *E. coli* is usually caused by eating unwashed vegetables or undercooked meat. But it is not limited to these—as outbreaks in the United States have occurred even when eating shelled nuts, including Hazelnuts. O157:H7 is also notorious for causing serious and even life-threatening complications such as Haemolytic-uremic syndrome. This particular strain is linked to the 2006 United States *E. coli* outbreak due to fresh spinach. Severity of the illness varies considerably; it can be fatal, particularly to young children, the elderly or the immunocompromised, but is more often mild. Earlier, poor hygienic methods of preparing meat in Scotland killed seven people in 1996 due to *E. coli* poisoning, and left hundreds more infected. *E. coli* can harbour both heat-stable and heat-labile enterotoxins. The latter, termed LT, contains one A subunit and five B subunits arranged into one holotoxin, and is highly similar in structure and function to cholera toxins. The B subunits assist in adherence and entry of the toxin into host intestinal cells, while the A subunit is cleaved and prevents cells from absorbing water, causing diarrhea. LT is secreted by the Type 2 secretion pathway.

If *E. coli* bacteria escape the intestinal tract through a perforation (for example from an ulcer, a ruptured appendix or due to a surgical error) and enter the abdomen, they usually cause peritonitis that can be fatal without prompt treatment. However, *E. coli* are extremely sensitive to such antibiotics as streptomycin or gentamicin. This could change since, as noted below, *E. coli* quickly acquires drug resistance. Recent research suggests that treatment with antibiotics does not improve the outcome of the disease, and may in fact significantly increase the chance of developing haemolytic-uremic syndrome.

Intestinal mucosa-associated *E. coli* are observed in increased numbers in the inflammatory bowel diseases, Crohn's disease and ulcerative colitis. Invasive strains of *E. coli* exist in high numbers in the inflamed tissue, and the number of bacteria in the inflamed regions correlates to the severity of the bowel inflammation.

Epidemiology of gastrointestinal infection

Transmission of pathogenic *E. coli* often occurs via faecal-oral transmission. Common routes of transmission include: unhygienic food preparation, farm contamination due to manure fertilisation, irrigation of crops with contaminated greywater or raw sewage, feral pigs on cropland, or direct consumption of sewage-contaminated water. Dairy and beef cattle are primary reservoirs of *E. coli* O157:H7, and they can carry it asymptomatically and shed it in their faeces. Food products associated with *E. coli* outbreaks include raw ground beef, raw seed sprouts or spinach, raw milk, unpasteurised juice, unpasteurised cheese and foods contaminated by infected food workers via faecal-oral route.

According to the US Food and Drug Administration, the faecal-oral cycle of transmission can be disrupted by cooking food properly, preventing cross-contamination, instituting barriers such as gloves for food workers, instituting health care policies so food industry employees seek treatment when they are ill, pasteurisation of juice or dairy products and proper hand washing requirements.

Shiga toxin-producing *E. coli* (STEC), specifically serotype O157:H7, have also been transmitted by flies, as well as direct contact with farm animals, petting zoo animals, and airborne particles found in animal-rearing environments.

Urinary tract infection

Uropathogenic *E. coli* (UPEC) is responsible for approximately 90 per cent of urinary tract infections (UTI) seen in individuals with ordinary anatomy. In ascending infections, fecal bacteria colonise the urethra and spread up the urinary tract to the bladder as well as to the kidneys (causing pyelonephritis), or the prostate in males. Because women have a shorter urethra than men, they are 14-times more likely to suffer from an ascending UTI (Fig. 21.3).

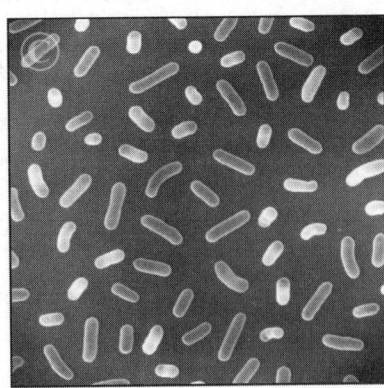

Fig. 21.3. *E. coli* bacteria, the most prevalent Gram-negative flora in the intestine.

Uropathogenic *E. coli* utilise P fimbriae (pyelonephritis-associated pili) to bind urinary tract endothelial cells and colonise the bladder. These adhesins specifically bind D-galactose-D-galactose moieties on the P blood-group antigen of erythrocytes and uroepithelial cells. Approximately 1 per cent of the human population lacks this receptor, and its presence or absence dictates an individual's susceptibility to *E. coli* urinary tract infections. Uropathogenic *E. coli* produce alpha- and beta-haemolysins, which cause lysis of urinary tract cells.

UPEC can evade the body's innate immune defences (e.g. the complement system) by invading superficial umbrella cells to form intracellular bacterial communities (IBCs). They also have the ability to form K antigen, capsular polysaccharides that contribute to biofilm formation. Biofilm-producing *E. coli* are recalcitrant to immune factors and antibiotic therapy and are often responsible for chronic urinary tract infections.

K antigen-producing *E. coli* infections are commonly found in the upper urinary tract. Descending infections, though relatively rare, occur when *E. coli* cells enter the upper urinary tract organs (kidneys, bladder or ureters) from the blood stream.

Neonatal meningitis

It is produced by a serotype of *Escherichia coli* that contains a capsular antigen called K1. The colonisation of the newborn's intestines with these stems, that are present in the mother's vagina, lead to bacteraemia, which leads to meningitis. And because of the absence of the IgM antibodies from the mother (these do not cross the placenta because FcRn only mediates the transfer of IgG), plus the fact that the body recognises as self the K1 antigen, as it resembles the cerebral glicopeptides, this leads to a severe meningitis in the neonates.

Laboratory Diagnosis

Typically diagnosis has been done by culturing on sorbitol-MacConkey medium and then using typing antiserum. However, current latex assays and some typing antisera have shown cross reactions with non-*E. coli* O157 colonies. Furthermore, not all *E. coli* O157 strains associated with HUS are nonsorbitol fermentors.

Other methods for detecting *E. coli* O157 in stool include ELISA tests, colony immunoblots, direct immunofluorescence microscopy of filters, as well as immunocapture techniques using magnetic beads. These assays are designed as screening tool to allow rapid testing for the presence of *E. coli* O157 without prior culturing of the stool specimen.

Antibiotic Therapy and Resistance

Bacterial infections are usually treated with antibiotics. However, the antibiotic sensitivities of different strains of *E. coli* vary widely. As Gram-negative organisms, *E. coli* are resistant to many antibiotics that are effective against Gram-positive organisms. Antibiotics which may be used to treat *E. coli* infection include amoxicillin as well as other semisynthetic penicillins, many cephalosporins, carbapenems, aztreonam, trimethoprim-sulphamethoxazole, ciprofloxacin, nitrofurantoin and the aminoglycosides.

Antibiotic-resistant *E. coli* may also pass on the genes responsible for antibiotic resistance to other species of bacteria, such as *Staphylococcus aureus*, through a process called horizontal gene transfer. *E. coli* often carry multidrug resistant plasmids and under stress readily transfer those plasmids to other species. Indeed, *E. coli* is a frequent member of biofilms where many species of bacteria exist in close proximity to each other. This mixing of species allows *E. coli* strains that are piliated to accept and transfer plasmids from and to other bacteria. Thus *E. coli* and the other enterobacteria are important reservoirs of transferable antibiotic resistance.

Beta-lactamase strains

Resistance to beta-lactam antibiotics has become a particular problem in recent decades, as strains of bacteria that produce extended-spectrum beta-lactamases have become more common. These beta-lactamase enzymes make many, if not all, of the penicillins and cephalosporins ineffective as therapy. Extended-spectrum beta-lactamase–producing *E. coli* are highly resistant to an array of antibiotics and infections by these strains are difficult to treat. In many instances, only two oral antibiotics and a very limited group of intravenous antibiotics remain effective.

Phage Therapy

Phage therapy—viruses that specifically target pathogenic bacteria—has been developed over the last 80 years, primarily in the former Soviet Union, where it was used to prevent diarrhoea caused by *E. coli*. Presently, phage therapy for humans is available only at the Phage Therapy Centre in the Republic of Georgia and in Poland. However, on January 2, 2007, the United States FDA gave Omnilytics approval to apply its *E. coli* O157:H7 killing phage in a mist, spray or wash on live animals that will be slaughtered for human consumption. The Bacteriophage T4 is a highly studied phage that targets *E. coli* for infection.

Vaccination

Researchers have actively been working to develop safe, effective vaccines to lower the worldwide incidence of *E. coli* infection. In March 2006, a vaccine eliciting an immune response against the *E. coli* O157:H7 O-specific polysaccharide conjugated to recombinant exotoxin A of *Pseudomonas aeruginosa* (O157-rEPA) was reported to be safe in children two to five years old. Previous work had already indicated that it was safe for adults. A phase III clinical trial to verify the large-scale efficacy of the treatment is planned.

In 2006 Fort Dodge Animal Health (Wyeth) introduced an effective live attenuated vaccine to control airsacculitis and peritonitis in chickens. The vaccine is a genetically modified avirulent vaccine that has demonstrated protection against O78 and untypeable strains.

In January 2007 the Canadian biopharmaceutical company bioniche announced it has developed a cattle vaccine which reduces the number of O157:H7 shed in manure by a factor of 1000, to about 1000 pathogenic bacteria per gram of manure.

In April 2009 a Michigan State University researcher announced that he has developed a working vaccine for a strain of *E. coli*. Mahdi Saeed, professor of epidemiology and infectious disease in MSU's colleges of Veterinary Medicine and Human Medicine, has applied for a patent for his discovery and has made contact with pharmaceutical companies for commercial production.

Model Organism in Life Science Research

Role in biotechnology

Because of its long history of laboratory culture and ease of manipulation, *E. coli* also plays an important role in modern biological engineering and industrial microbiology. The work of Stanley Norman Cohen and Herbert Boyer in *E. coli*, using plasmids and restriction enzymes to create recombinant DNA, became a foundation of biotechnology. Considered a very versatile host for the production of heterologous proteins, researchers can introduce genes into the microbes using plasmids, allowing for the mass production of proteins in industrial fermentation processes. Genetic systems have also been developed which allow the production of recombinant proteins using *E. coli*. One of the first useful applications of recombinant DNA technology was the manipulation of *E. coli* to produce human insulin. Modified *E. coli* have been used in vaccine development, bioremediation, and production of immobilised enzymes. *E. coli* cannot, however, be used to produce some of the more large, complex proteins which contain multiple disulphide bonds and, in particular, unpaired thiols, or proteins that also require post-translational modification for activity. Studies are also being performed into programming *E. coli* to potentially solve complicated mathematics problems such as the Hamiltonian path problem.

Model organism

E. coli is frequently used as a model organism in microbiology studies. Cultivated strains (e.g. *E. coli* K12) are well-adapted to the laboratory environment, and, unlike wild type strains, have lost their ability to thrive in the intestine. Many lab strains lose their ability to form biofilms. These features protect wild type strains from antibodies and other chemical attacks, but require a large expenditure of energy and material resources.

In 1946, Joshua Lederberg and Edward Tatum first described the phenomenon known as bacterial conjugation using *E. coli* as a model bacterium, and it remains the primary model to study conjugation. *E. coli* was an integral part of the first experiments to understand phage genetics, and early researchers, such as Seymour Benzer, used *E. coli* and phage T4 to understand the topography of gene structure. Prior to Benzer's research, it was not known whether the gene was a linear structure or if it had a branching pattern.

E. coli was one of the first organisms to have its genome sequenced; the complete genome of *E. coli* K12 was published by Science in 1997.

The long-term evolution experiments using *E. coli*, begun by Richard Lenski in 1988, have allowed direct observation of major evolutionary shifts in the laboratory. In this experiment, one population of *E. coli* unexpectedly evolved the ability to aerobically metabolise citrate. This capacity is extremely rare in *E. coli*. As the inability to grow aerobically is normally used as a diagnostic criterion with which to differentiate *E. coli* from other, closely related bacteria such as Salmonella, this innovation may mark a speciation event observed in the lab. By combining nanotechnologies with landscape ecology complex habitat landscapes can be generated with details at the nanoscale. On such synthetic ecosystems evolutionary experiments with *E. coli* have been performed in order to study the spatial biophysics of adaptation in an island biogeography on-chip.

Environmental Quality

E. coli bacteria have been commonly found in recreational waters and their presence is used to indicate the presence of recent faecal contamination, but *E. coli* presence may not be indicative of human waste. *E. coli* are harboured in all warm-blooded animals: birds and mammals alike. *E. coli* bacteria have also been found in fish and turtles. Sand and soil also harbour *E. coli* bacteria and some strains of *E. coli* have become naturalised. Some geographic areas may support unique populations of *E. coli* and conversely, some *E. coli* strains are cosmopolitan.

LISTERIA MONOCYTOGENES

Listeria monocytogenes, commonly referred to as *Listeria*, is a pathogen that causes listeriosis, a serious human illness. It is unlike most other foodborne pathogens because it can grow at proper refrigeration temperatures. In addition, *Listeria* is widely distributed in nature, and the organism has been recovered from farm fields, vegetables, animals and other environments such as food processing facilities, retail stores and home kitchens and ready-to-eat foods.

Symptoms and Disease Process

L. monocytogenes causes listeriosis, a serious infection with high hospitalisation rates for those who become ill. People at highest risk for a severe case include the elderly, the fetuses of pregnant women, and the immunosuppressed. It is unique among foodborne pathogens since its incubation time (time from ingestion of cells to illness) is at least seven days. Listeriosis is a rare disease with a high mortality rate, causing about 43 per cent of the food poisoning deaths in the United States. *L. monocytogenes* can also cause mild, flu-like symptoms in healthy individuals when consumed at very high levels.

A person with listeriosis has fever, muscle aches and occasional gastrointestinal symptoms such as nausea or diarrhea. If infection spreads to the nervous system, symptoms such as headache, stiff neck, confusion, loss of balance or convulsions can occur. Infected pregnant women may experience only a mild, flu-like illness; however, infections during pregnancy can lead to miscarriage or stillbirth, premature delivery or infection of the newborn.

Primary Routes of Transmission

Foods can become contaminated with *L. monocytogenes* along the continuum from farm to fork, in the produce growing environment, during processing or during handling and preparation in retail establishments and consumers' kitchens.

The primary route of transmission is through the ingestion of contaminated food. The International Life Sciences Institute in 2005 described high-risk foods for causing listeriosis as those with the following properties:
1. Have the potential for contamination with *L. monocytogenes*.
2. Support the growth of *L. monocytogenes* to high numbers.
3. Are ready-to-eat.
4. Require refrigeration.
5. Are stored for an extended period of time.

Because *Listeria* is abundant in nature and can be found almost anywhere, there can be a constant reintroduction of the organism into the food plant, retail setting, foodservice establishment and home. It is difficult to totally eliminate this contaminant from the food-handling environment, but the goal is to control it as effectively as possible, especially where it can contaminate ready-to-eat, refrigerated foods.

Although *L. monocytogenes* is the only member of the *Listeria* family that causes human illness, the presence of any member of the *Listeria* family in a food processing environment may indicate that conditions are favourable for *L. monocytogenes*.

Control

Effective control of *L. monocytogenes* requires prevention of contamination (to the extent possible) and prevention of growth through time/temperature or formulation control. Knowledge of potential harbourage sites is important, as contamination is more likely to occur when the organism has become established in a niche. Food processing plant surveys have found *Listeria* in the following locations (listed approximately in the order of prevalence): (i) floors, (ii) drains, (iii) coolers, (iv) cleaning aids such as brushes, sponges, etc., (v) product and/or equipment wash areas, (vi) food contact surfaces,

(vii) condensate, (viii) walls and ceilings, and (ix) compressed air. Control of *Listeria* relies on detecting and managing harbourage sites with thorough and frequent cleaning. This includes daily cleaning of floors and drains, and adequate attention to less frequently cleaned areas such as HVAC systems, walls, coolers and freezers. Also, damaged equipment, cracks, crevices and hollow areas must be part of sanitation and inspection schedules. It is essential to avoid creation of aerosols during cleaning, especially of floors and drains, to avoid spread of contaminants.

The organism is killed by normal food pasteurisation and cooking processes, and is typically sensitive to most sanitisers at recommended rates. Contamination may occur after the cooking process in the processing environment, at retail locations and in the home. For example, post-pasteurisation contamination of food products can occur when the organism is dispersed via an aerosol. Prevention of growth is essential to avoid the potential for illness, because *L. monocytogenes* can grow at refrigerated temperatures, defeating one of the traditional food safety measures.

L. monocytogenes can survive on cold surfaces and can also multiply slowly at 34°F. It has also been shown to grow to a water activity as low as 0.92 and over a pH range of 4.4–9.43. Because the organism can grow under refrigeration, effective labelling to ensure product rotation in retail settings is an important control measure for ready-to-eat products.

Since this organism continues to elicit concern among consumers, regulators, processors and retailers, studies need to be carefully designed to ensure validity.

Background on Challenges to the Zero Tolerance Initiative

The FDA/Food Safety and Inspection Service risk assessment reinforces epidemiological conclusions that foodborne listeriosis is a moderately rare, although severe, disease. A study by the Food Products Association showed it is likely that low levels of *L. monocytogenes* are consumed routinely with limited effect. It is believed that 5 per cent of the general population may be asymptomatic carriers of *Listeria*, but the percentage may be higher in particular groups, such as slaughterhouse workers.

Extensive risk assessments and analyses have been conducted by the Food Safety and Inspection Service (FSIS), US Food and Drug Administration/FSIS7, World Health Organisation/Food and Agriculture Organisation, and International Life Sciences Institute to identify factors that contribute to risk of illness. This research is important because the prevalence in the food supply does not match the rate of illness in the population, and because the outcome of illness in susceptible individuals is very severe. These assessments have generally concluded that the ability of a food to support growth of *Listeria* enhances risk.

Because of this, US FDA issued draft Compliance Policy Guidelines in February, 2008 based on the ability of a product to support growth of *L. monocytogenes*. The USDA retains a zero tolerance policy for RTE foods, while other countries allow up to 100 cfu/g in certain foods.

MYCOBACTERIUM

Mycobacterium is a genus of Actinobacteria, given its own family, the Mycobacteriaceae. The genus includes pathogens known to cause serious diseases in mammals, including tuberculosis (*Mycobacterium tuberculosis*) and leprosy (*Mycobacterium leprae*).

Microbiological Characteristics

Mycobacteria are aerobic and nonmotile bacteria (except for the species *Mycobacterium marinum*, which has been shown to be motile within macrophages) that are characteristically acid-alcohol fast. Mycobacteria do not contain endospores or capsules and are usually considered Gram-positive. A recent paper in PNAS showed sporulation in *Mycobacterium marinum* and perhaps in *M. bovis*. However, this has been strongly argued by other scientists. While mycobacteria do not seem to fit the Gram-positive category from an empirical standpoint (i.e. they generally do not retain the crystal violet stain well), they are classified as an acid-fast Gram-positive bacterium due to their lack of an outer cell membrane. All *Mycobacterium* species share a characteristic cell wall, thicker than in many other bacteria, which is hydrophobic, waxy, and rich in mycolic acids/mycolates. The cell wall consists of the hydrophobic mycolate layer and a peptidoglycan layer held together by a polysaccharide, arabinogalactan. The cell wall makes a substantial contribution to the hardiness of this genus. The biosynthetic pathways of cell wall components are potential targets for new drugs for tuberculosis.

Many *Mycobacterium* species adapt readily to growth on very simple substrates, using ammonia or amino acids as nitrogen sources and glycerol as a carbon source in the presence of mineral salts. Optimum growth temperatures vary widely according to the species and range from 25°C to over 50°C.

Some species can be very difficult to culture (i.e. they are fastidious), sometimes taking over two years to develop in culture. Further, some species also have extremely long reproductive cycles— *M. leprae*, may take more than 20 days to proceed through one division cycle (for comparison, some *E. coli* strains take only 20 minutes), making laboratory culture a slow process. In addition, the availability of genetic manipulation techniques still lags far behind that of other bacterial species.

A natural division occurs between slowly and rapidly growing species. Mycobacteria that form colonies clearly visible to the naked eye within seven days on subculture are termed rapid growers, while those requiring longer periods are termed slow growers. Mycobacteria cells are straight or slightly curved rods between 0.2–0.6 µm wide by 1.0–10 µm long.

Pigmentation

Some mycobacteria produce carotenoid pigments without light. Others require photoactivation for pigment production.

1. Photochromogens (Group I): Produce nonpigmented colonies when grown in the dark and pigmented colonies only after exposure to light and reincubation, e.g. *M. kansasii*, *M. marinum*, *M. simiae*.
2. Scotochromogens (Group II): Produce deep yellow to orange colonies when grown in the presence of either the light or dark, e.g. *M. scrofulaceum*, *M. gordonae*, *M. xenopi*, *M. szulgai*.
3. Non-chromogens (Groups III and IV): Nonpigmented in the light and dark or have only a pale yellow, buff or tan pigment that does not intensify after light exposure, e.g. *M. tuberculosis*, *M. avium-intra-cellulare*, *M. bovis*, *M. ulcerans*, *M. fortuitum*, and *M. chelonae*.

Staining characteristics

Mycobacteria are classical acid-fast organisms. Stains used in evaluation of tissue specimens or microbiological specimens include Fite's stain, Ziehl-Neelsen stain, and Kinyoun stain. Mycobacteria appear phenotypically most closely related to members of *Nocardia*, *Rhodococcus* and *Corynebacterium*.

Ecological Characteristics

Mycobacteria are widespread organisms, typically living in water (including tap water treated with chlorine) and food sources. Some, however, including the tuberculosis and the leprosy organisms, appear to be obligate parasites and are not found as free-living members of the genus.

Pathogenicity

Mycobacteria can colonise their hosts without the hosts showing any adverse signs. For example, billions of people around the world have asymptomatic infections of *M. tuberculosis*. Mycobacterial infections are notoriously difficult to treat. The organisms are hardy due to their cell wall, which is neither truly Gram-negative nor positive. Additionally, they are naturally resistant to a number of antibiotics that disrupt cell-wall biosynthesis, such as penicillin. Due to their unique cell wall, they can survive long exposure to acids, alkalis, detergents, oxidative bursts, lysis by complement, and many antibiotics. Most mycobacteria are susceptible to the antibiotics clarithromycin and rifamycin, but antibiotic-resistant strains have emerged. As with other bacterial pathogens, surface and secreted proteins of *M. tuberculosis* contribute significantly to the virulence of this organism. There is an increasing list of extracytoplasmic proteins proven to have a function in the virulence of *M. tuberculosis*.

Medical classification

Mycobacteria can be classified into several major groups for purpose of diagnosis and treatment: *M. tuberculosis* complex, which can cause tuberculosis: *M. tuberculosis*, *M. bovis*, *M. africanum*, and *M. microti*; *M. leprae*, which causes Hansen's disease or leprosy; nontuberculous mycobacteria (NTM) are all the other mycobacteria, which can cause pulmonary disease resembling tuberculosis, lymphadenitis, skin disease or disseminated disease.

Phenotypic testing

Various phenotypic tests can be used to identify and distinguish different Mycobacteria species and strains. Phenotypic testing of Mycobacteria.

Mycosides

Mycosides are phenolic alcohols (such as phenolphthiocerol) that were shown to be components of mycobacterium glycolipids that are termed glycosides of phenolphthiocerol dimycocerosate. There are 18 and 20 carbon atoms in mycosides A, and B, respectively.

Species

In older systems, mycobacteria are grouped based upon their appearance and rate of growth. However, these are symplesiomorphies, and more recent classification is based upon cladistics (Fig. 21.4).

Slowly growing

Mycobacterium tuberculosis complex

Mycobacterium tuberculosis complex (MTBC) members are causative agents of human and animal tuberculosis. Species in this complex include:

1. *M. tuberculosis*, the major cause of human tuberculosis.
2. *M. bovis*.
3. *M. bovis* BCG.
4. *M. africanum*.
5. *M. canetti*.
6. *M. caprae*.
7. *M. microti*.
8. *M. pinnipedii*.

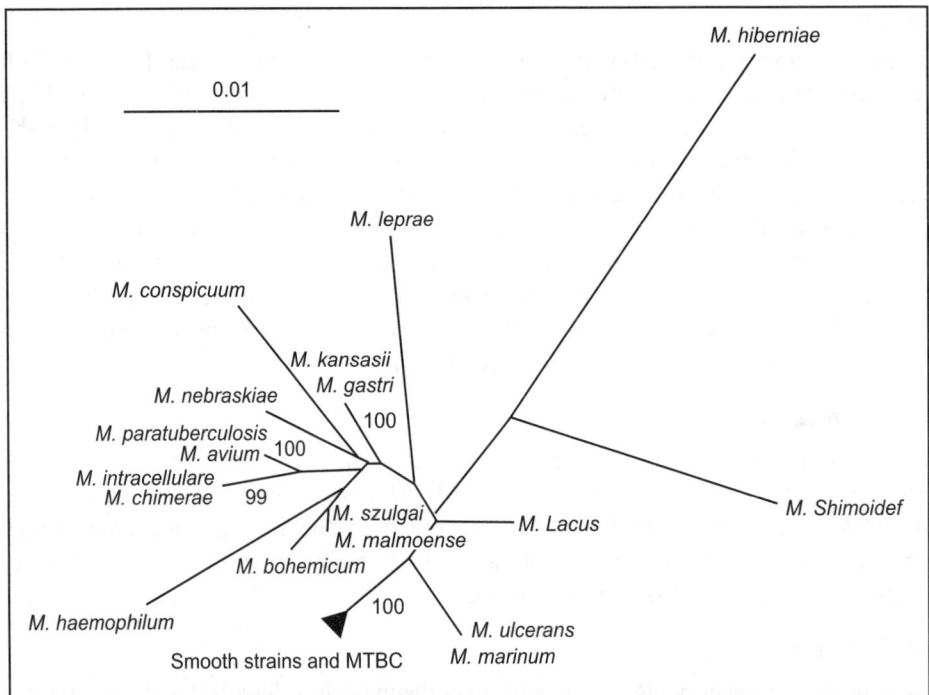

Fig. 21.4. Phylogenetic position of the Tubercle *Bacilli* within the Genus Mycobacterium. The black triangle corresponds to tubercle bacilli sequences that are identical or differing by a single nucleotide. The sequences of the genus Mycobacterium that matched most closely to those of *M. tuberculosis* were retrieved from the BIBI database (http://pbil.univ-lyon.fr/bibi/) and aligned with those obtained for 17 smooth and MTBC strains. The unrooted neighbour-joining tree is based on 1,325 aligned nucleotide positions of the 16S rRNA gene. The scale gives the pairwise distances after Jukes-Cantor correction. Bootstrap support values higher than 90 per cent are indicated at the nodes.

SHIGELLA

Shigella is a genus of Gram-negative, non-spore forming rod-shaped bacteria closely related to *Escherichia coli* and *Salmonella*. The causative agent of human shigellosis, *Shigella* causes disease in primates, but not in other mammals. It is only naturally found in humans and apes. During infection, it typically causes dysentery. The genus is named after Kiyoshi Shiga, who first discovered it in 1898.

Classification

Shigella species are classified by four serogroups:
1. Serogroup A: *S. dysenteriae* (12 serotypes).
2. Serogroup B: *S. flexneri* (6 serotypes).
3. Serogroup C: *S. boydii* (23 serotypes).
4. Serogroup D: *S. sonnei* (1 serotype).

Group A–C are physiologically similar; *S. sonnei* (group D) can be differentiated on the basis of biochemical metabolism assays. Three *Shigella* groups are the major disease-causing species: *S. flexneri* is the most frequently isolated species worldwide and accounts for 60 per cent of cases in the developing world; *S. sonnei* causes 77 per cent of cases in the developed world, compared to only 15 per cent of cases in the developing world; and *S. dysenteriae* is usually the cause of epidemics of dysentery, particularly in confined populations such as refugee camps.

Pathogenesis

Shigella infection is typically via ingestion (fecal–oral contamination); depending on age and condition of the host as few as 100 bacterial cells can be enough to cause an infection. *Shigella* causes dysentery that results in the destruction of the epithelial cells of the intestinal mucosa in the cecum and rectum. Some strains produce enterotoxin and Shiga toxin, similar to the verotoxin of *E. coli* O157:H7. Both Shiga toxin and verotoxin are associated with causing hemolytic uremic syndrome. *Shigella* invade the host through the M-cells in the gut epithelia of the large intestine, as they cannot enter directly through the epithelial cells. Using a Type III secretion system acting as a biological syringe, the bacterium injects IpaD protein into cell, triggering bacterial invasion and the subsequent lysis of vacuolar membranes using IpaB and IpaC proteins.

It utilises a mechanism for its motility by which its IcsA protein triggers actin polymerisation in the host cell (via N-WASP recruitment of Arp2/3 complexes) in a 'rocket' propulsion fashion for cell-to-cell spread. The most common symptoms are diarrhea, fever, nausea, vomiting, stomach cramps and flatulence. The stool may contain blood, mucus or pus. In rare cases, young children may have seizures. Symptoms can take as long as a week to show up, but most often begin two to four days after ingestion. Symptoms usually last for several days but can last for weeks. *Shigella* is implicated as one of the pathogenic causes of reactive arthritis worldwide.

Severe dysentery can be treated with ampicillin, TMP-SMX, or fluoroquinolones such as ciprofloxacin and of course rehydration. Medical treatment should only be utilised in severe cases. Antibiotics are usually avoided in mild cases because some *Shigella* are resistant to antibiotics, and usage of them may make the germ even more resistant.

Antidiarrheal agents may also worsen the sickness. Each of the *Shigella* genomes includes a virulence plasmid that encodes conserved primary virulence determinants. The *Shigella* chromosomes share most of their genes with that of *E. coli* K12 strain MG1655.

Identification

Shigella species are negative for motility and are nonlactose fermenters. (However, *S. sonnei* can ferment lactose). They typically do not produce gas from carbohydrates (with the exception of certain strains of *S. flexneri*) and tend to be overall biochemically inert. *Shigella* should also be urea hydrolysis negative. When inoculated to a triple sugar iron slant they react as follows: K/A, gas, H_2S. Indole reactions are mixed, positive and negative, with the exception of *S. sonnei* which is always indole negative.

STAPHYLOCOCCUS

Staphylococcus is a genus of Gram-positive bacteria. Under the microscope they appear round (cocci), and form in grape-like clusters. The *Staphylococcus* genus includes at least forty species. Of these, nine have two subspecies and one has three subspecies. Most are harmless and reside normally on the skin and mucous membranes of humans and other organisms. Found worldwide, they are a small component of soil microbial flora.

Biochemical Identification

Assignment of a strain to the genus *Staphylococcus* requires that it is a Gram-positive coccus that forms clusters, produces catalase, has an appropriate cell wall structure (including peptidoglycan type and teichoic acid presence) and G + C content of DNA in a range of 30–40 mol%. *Staphylococcus* species can be differentiated from other aerobic and facultative anaerobic Gram-positive cocci by several simple tests. *Staphylococcus* spp. are facultative anaerobes (capable of growth both aerobically and anaerobically). All species grow in the presence of bile salts and all are catalase positive. Growth also occurs in a 6.5 per cent NaCl solution. On Baird Parker Medium *Staphylococcus* spp. grow fermentatively, except for *S. saprophyticus* which grows oxidatively.

Staphylococcus spp. are resistant to bacitracin (0.04 U disc: resistance = <10 mm zone of inhibition) and susceptible to furazolidone (100 µg disc: resistance = <15 mm zone of inhibition). Further biochemical testing is needed to identify down to the species level. One of the most important phenotypical features used in the classification of staphylococci is their ability to produce coagulase, an enzyme that causes blood clot formation.

Coagulase-positive

Six species are currently recognised as being coagulase positive: *S. aureus*, *S. delphini*, *S. hyicus*, *S. intermedius*, *S. lutrae*, *S. pseudintermedius* and *S. schleiferi* subsp. coagulans. These species belong to two separate groups—the *S. aureus* (*S. aureus* alone) group and the *S. hyicus*-intermedius group (the remaining five).

A seventh species has also been described—*Staphylococcus leei*—from patients with gastritis.

1. *S. aureus* (formerly also called *Staphylococcus pyogenes*) is coagulase-positive, meaning that it produces coagulase. However, while the majority of *S. aureus* are coagulase-positive, some may be atypical in that they do not produce coagulase. *S. aureus* is also catalase-positive (meaning that it can produce the enzyme catalase) and able to convert hydrogen peroxide (H_2O_2) to water and oxygen, which makes the catalase test useful to distinguish *Staphylococci* from *Enterococci* and *Streptococci*.

2. *S. pseudintermedius* inhabits and sometimes infects the skin of domestic dogs and cats. This organism, too, can carry the genetic material that imparts multiple bacterial resistance. It is rarely implicated in infections in humans, as a zoonosis.

Coagulase-negative

1. *S. epidermidis*, a coagulase-negative staphylococcus species, is a commensal of the skin, but can cause severe infections in immune-suppressed patients and those with central venous catheters.

2. *S. saprophyticus*, another coagulase-negative species that is part of the normal vaginal flora, is predominantly implicated in genitourinary tract infections in sexually-active young women.

3. In recent years, several other *Staphylococcus* species have been implicated in human infections, notably *S. lugdunensis*, *S. schleiferi*, and *S. caprae*.

Common abbreviations for coagulase-negative staphylococcus species are CoNS and CNS.

Genomics and Molecular Biology

The first *S. aureus* genomes to be sequenced were those of N315 and Mu50 in 2001. Many more complete *S. aureus* genomes have been submitted to the public databases, making *S. aureus* one of the most extensively sequenced bacteria. The use of genomic data is now widespread and provides a valuable resource for researchers working with *S. aureus*. Whole genome technologies such as sequencing projects and microarrays have shown there is an enormous variety of *S. aureus* strains. Each contains different combinations of surface proteins and different toxins. Relating this information to pathogenic behaviour is one of the major areas of staphylococcal research. The development of molecular typing methods has enabled the tracking of different strains of *S. aureus*. This may lead to better control of outbreak strains. A greater understanding of how the staphylococci evolve, especially due to the acquisition of mobile genetic elements encoding resistance and virulence genes is helping to identify new outbreak strains and may even prevent their emergence.

PLESIOMONAS SHIGELLOIDES

Plesiomonas shigelloides is a species of bacteria. It is a Gram-negative, rod-shaped bacterium which has been isolated from freshwater, freshwater fish, and shellfish and from many types of animals including cattle, goats, swine, cats, dogs, monkeys, vultures, snakes, and toads.

Infections from this organism cause gastroenteritis, followed by septicemia in immune deficient patients. It is placed among the Enterobacteriaceae. Some *Plesiomonas* strains share antigens with *Shigella sonnei*, and cross-reactions with *Shigella* antisera occur. *Plesiomonas* can be distinguished from *Shigella* in diarrheal stools by an oxidase test. *Plesiomonas* is oxidase positive and *Shigella* is oxidase negative. *Plesiomonas* is negative for DNAse; this and other biochemical tests distinguish it from *Aeromonas* sp.

VIBRIO

Vibrio species account for a significant number of foodborne infections from the consumption of raw or undercooked shellfish. They require salt to grow, and are thus associated with ocean-sourced seafood. There are four *Vibrio* species of primary public health concern: *Vibrio vulnificus*, *Vibrio parahaemolyticus*, *Vibrio cholerae* O1 and *Vibrio cholerae* non-O1.

Vibrio vulnificus is found in most coastal waters, primarily in estuaries where the tide flows into a river causing fresh and salt water to mix. It is associated with plankton, shellfish and finfish. It is considered the most serious pathogenic *Vibrio* in industrialised nations. *Vibrio* parahaemolyticus is also found in coastal water estuarine environments. It is associated with marine fish and shellfish.

Vibrio cholerae O1 causes Asiatic or epidemic cholera. This organism may be found in the temperate estuarine and marine coastal areas. Cholera occurs in developing nations; periodically, epidemics can spread quickly in developing countries around the world. Sporadic cases occur periodically in industrialised nations.

Vibrio cholerae non-O1 infects only humans and other primates and has genetic differences from the 'O1' strain. Non-O1 strains cause a less severe disease. Pathogenic and nonpathogenic strains of the organism are found in marine and estuarine environments.

Symptoms and Disease Process

If immunocompromised people or those with impaired liver function consume seafood contaminated with even low levels of *Vibrio vulnificus*, a severe blood infection (septicemia) can occur. The microorganism enters the blood stream, causing septic shock, which is rapidly followed by death in many cases (about 50 per cent). More than 70 per cent of infected individuals have distinctive bulbous skin lesions. Consumption of contaminated seafood by healthy people can result in vomiting, diarrhea and abdominal pain. Symptoms begin around 38 hours after consumption of contaminated food, and the disease progresses rapidly.

Vibrio parahaemolyticus causes mild or moderate gastroenteritis with symptoms of diarrhea, abdominal cramps, nausea, vomiting, headache, fever and chills. The illness persists for about 2.5 days after an incubation period of four to 96 hours after ingestion. A Food and Drug Administration risk assessment determined that 15 per cent of oyster associated illnesses are caused by servings at or above 10,000/g at the time of harvest.

Vibrio cholerae O1 causes a mild or acute watery diarrhea. Onset is usually sudden, with incubation periods varying from six hours to five days. Symptoms include abdominal cramps, nausea, vomiting, dehydration and shock. Death may occur after severe fluid and electrolyte loss. Illness is caused when viable bacteria attach to the small intestine and produce cholera toxin. It is believed that the infectious dose is likely greater than one million organisms.

Vibrio cholerae non-O1 causes a gastroenteritis by the same name. Symptoms include diarrhea, abdominal cramps and fever, with vomiting and nausea occurring in approximately 25 per cent of infected individuals. Approximately 25 per cent of infected individuals will have blood and mucus in their stools. Diarrhea may last six to seven days and will usually occur within 48 hours after ingestion of the organism.

The infective dose is suspected to be more than one million organisms. Although rare, septicemia, as has been reported with *V. vulnificus*, has been reported and deaths have resulted.

Primary Routes of Transmission

Vibrio vulnificus has been isolated from oysters, clams and crabs. Consumption of these raw or recontaminated products may result in illness. Wound infections may result either from *Vibrio*-containing seawater contamination of an open wound or by cutting part of the body on an underwater sharp object (coral, fish, etc.), followed by contamination with the organism. There is no evidence of person-to-person transmission of *V. vulnificus*.

Vibrio parahaemolyticus has been associated with consumption of raw, improperly cooked or cooked and re-contaminated fish and shellfish.

Vibrio cholerae O1 is generally spread through contaminated water supplies by poor sanitation. Sporadic cases occur due to the consumption of raw or improperly cooked shellfish harvested from contaminated coastal waters. *Vibrio cholera* is part of the indigenous microflora of these waters.

Vibrio cholerae non-O1 is transmitted by consuming raw, improperly cooked or cooked and recontaminated shellfish.

Control

The primary control for *Vibrio* is harvesting seafood from safe waters. Many countries test coastal waters for safe harvesting. Raw oyster-related outbreaks are more frequent in the summer months and are more prevalent in Gulf Coast waters than in other areas of the United States. Thus, limiting the time of harvest may also be an effective control strategy.

After harvest, seafood should be chilled to less than 5°C (41°F) to prevent growth of *Vibrio*. Cooking seafood to at least 65°C (149°F) will destroy *Vibrio*; however, this is not a control strategy for those who choose to consume it raw.

Protection from post-process contamination with raw products is important for cooked products. Cooked seafood should be eaten within two hours or promptly chilled to less than 5°C (41°F). Growth parameters vary among the three *Vibrio* species (Table 21.2).

Table 21.2. Growth parameters vary among the three *Vibrio*.

	Temperature (°C)	pH	Water activity	Salt (per cent)
V. cholerae	10–43	5 – 9.6	0.97 – 0.998	0.1 – 4
V. parahaemolyticus	5–43	4.8–11	0.94–0.996	0.5–10
V. vulnificus	8–43	5–10	0.96–0.997	0.5–5

Research at the University of Delaware has shown that the use of high hydrostatic pressure inactivates pathogenic strains of *Vibrio*. High-pressure processing may be advantageous over thermal treatments since pathogens such as *Vibrio* can be inactivated while virtually all flavour, colour and nutritional constituents are maintained.

Chapter 22

Nonbacterial Agents of Foodborne Illness

INTRODUCTION

Some foodborne disease outbreaks are not caused by bacteria or their toxins but result from mycotoxins, viruses, rickettsias, parasitic worms or protozoa or from the consumption of food contaminated with toxic substances. The implication in human health is not clearly understood for the mycotoxins or for many of the viruses, but their incidence and the nature of their action in animals justify their discussion.

HELMINTHS

The helminths are worm-like parasites. The clinically relevant groups are separated according to their general external shape and the host organ they inhabit. There are both hermaphroditic and bisexual species. The definitive classification is based on the external and internal morphology of egg, larval, and adult stages.

Helminth is a general term meaning worm. The helminths are invertebrates characterised by elongated, flat or round bodies. In medically oriented schemes the flatworms or platyhelminths (platy from the Greek root meaning 'flat') include flukes and tapeworms. Roundworms are nematodes (nemato from the Greek root meaning 'thread'). These groups are subdivided for convenience according to the host organ in which they reside, e.g. lung flukes, extraintestinal tapeworms, and intestinal roundworms.

Helminths develop through egg, larval (juvenile), and adult stages. Knowledge of the different stages in relation to their growth and development is the basis for understanding the epidemiology and pathogenesis of helminth diseases, as well as for the diagnosis and treatment of patients harbouring these parasites.

Platyhelminths and nematodes that infect humans have similar anatomic features that reflect common physiologic requirements and functions. The outer covering of helminths is the cuticle or tegument. Prominent external structures of flukes and cestodes are acetabula (suckers) or bothria (false suckers). Male nematodes of several species possess accessory sex organs that are external modifications of the cuticle. Internally, the alimentary, excretory, and reproductive systems can be identified by an experienced observer. Tapeworms are unique in lacking an alimentary canal. This lack means that nutrients must be absorbed through the tegument. The blood flukes and nematodes are bisexual. All other flukes and tapeworm species that infect humans are hermaphroditic. With few exceptions, adult flukes, cestodes, and nematodes produce eggs that are passed in excretions or secretions of the host. The various stages and their unique characteristics will be reviewed in more detail as each major group of helminths is considered.

Flukes (Trematodes)

The structure of flukes is summarised in Figs 22.1 and 22.2. A dorsoventrally flattened body, bilateral symmetry, and a definite anterior end are features of platyhelminths in general and of trematodes specifically. Flukes are leaf-shaped, ranging in length from a few millimetres to 7 to 8 cm. The tegument is morphologically and physiologically complex. Flukes possess an oral sucker around the mouth and a ventral sucker or acetabulum that can be used to adhere to host tissues. A body cavity is lacking. Organs are embedded in specialised connective tissue or parenchyma. Layers of somatic muscle permeate the parenchyma and attach to the tegument.

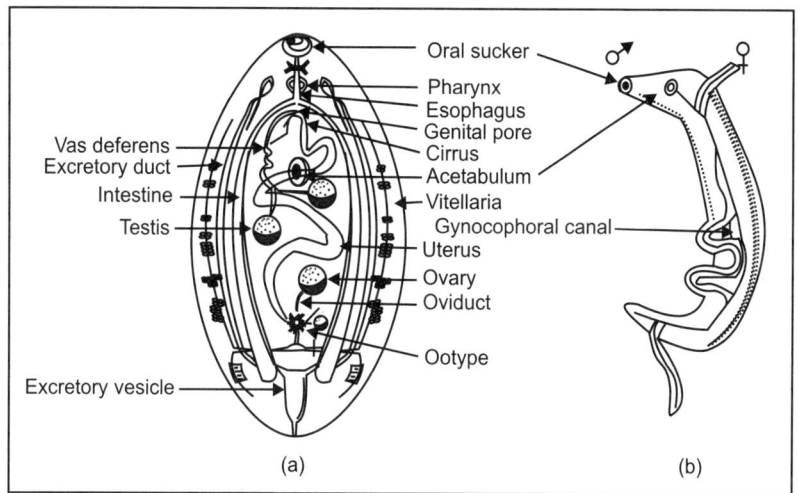

Fig. 22.1. Structure of flukes (a) hermaphroditic fluke, (b) bisexual fluke.

Flukes have a well-developed alimentary canal with a muscular pharynx and esophagus. The intestine is usually a branched tube (secondary and tertiary branches may be present) consisting of a single layer of epithelial cells. The main branches may end blindly or open into an excretory vesicle. The excretory vesicle also accepts the two main lateral collecting ducts of the excretory system, which is of a protonephridial type with flame cells. A flame cell is a hollow, terminal excretory cell that contains a beating (flamelike) group of cilia. These cells, anchored in the parenchyma, direct tissue filtrate through canals into the two main collecting ducts.

Except for the blood flukes, trematodes are hermaphroditic, having both male and female reproductive organs in the same individual. The male organ consists usually of two testes with accessory glands and ducts leading to a cirrus or penis equivalent, that extends into the common genital atrium. The female gonad consists of a single ovary with a seminal receptacle and vitellaria, or yolk glands, that connect with the oviduct as it expands into an ootype. The tubular uterus extends from the ootype and opens into the genital atrium. Both self- and cross-fertilisation occur. The components of the egg are assembled in the ootype. Eggs pass through the uterus into the genital atrium and exit ventrally through the genital pore. Fluke eggs, except for those of schistosomes, are operculated (have a lid).

The blood flukes or schistosomes are the only bisexual flukes that infect humans (Fig. 22.1). Although the sexes are separate, the general body structure is the same as that of hermaphroditic flukes. Within the definitive host, the male and female worms inhabit the lumen of blood vessels and are found in close physical association.

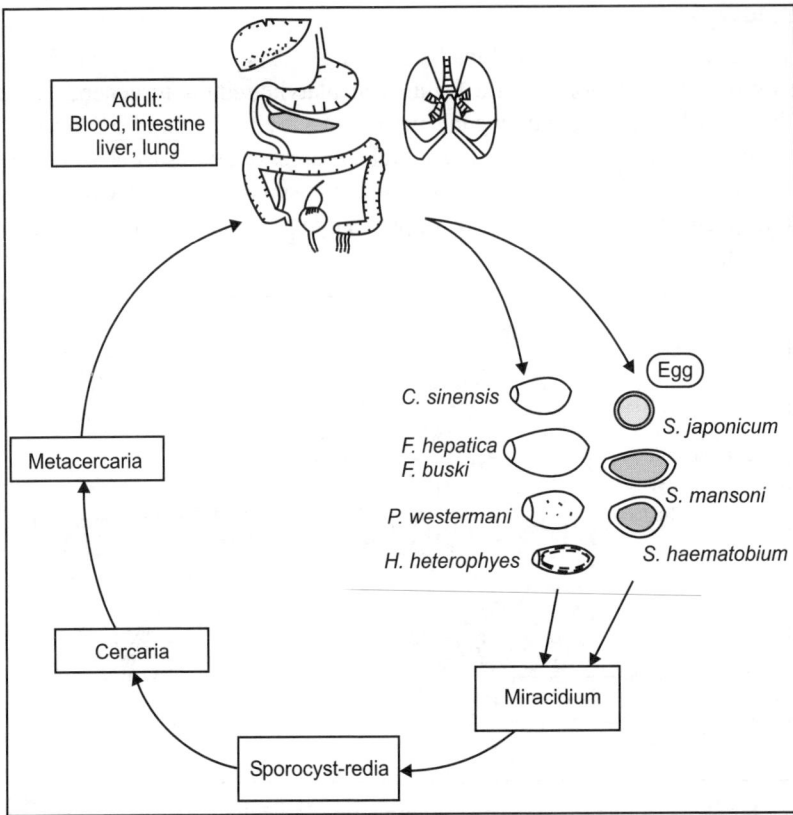

Fig. 22.2. Generalised life cycle of flukes. All cycles involve snails as intermediate hosts. Hermaphroditic flukes—*Clonorchis sinensis, Fasiolopsis buski, Paragonimys westermani,* and *Heterophytes heterophyes.* Metacercaria are infective for humans. Bisexual flukes: *Schistosoma japonicum, S. mansoni,* and *S. haematobium.* Cercariae are infective for humans.

The female lies within a tegumental fold, the gynecophoral canal, on the ventral surface of the male. The medically important flukes belong to the taxonomic category Digenea. This group of flukes has a developmental cycle requiring at least two hosts, one being a snail intermediate host. Depending on the species, other intermediate hosts may be involved to perpetuate the larval form that infects the definitive human host. Flukes go through several larval stages, each with a specific name, before reaching adulthood. Taking into account variations among species (Fig. 22.2), a generalised life cycle of digenetic flukes runs the following course. Eggs are passed in the feces, urine or sputum of humans and reach an aquatic environment. The eggs hatch, releasing ciliated larvae or miracidia, which either penetrate or are eaten by a snail intermediate host. In rare instances land snails may serve as intermediate hosts. A saclike sporocyst or redia stage develops from a miracidium within the tissues of the snail. The sporocyst gives rise either to rediae or to a daughter sporocyst stage. In turn, from the redia or daughter sporocyst, cercariae develop asexually and migrate out of the snail tissues to the external environment, which is usually aquatic.

The cercariae, which may possess a tail for swimming, develop further in one of three ways. They either penetrate the definitive host and transform directly into adults or penetrate a second intermediate host and develop as encysted metacercariae or they encyst on a substrate, such as vegetation, and develop there as metacercariae. When a metacercarial cyst is ingested, digestion of the cyst liberates an immature fluke that migrates to a specific organ site and develops into an adult worm.

Tapeworms (Cestodes)

As members of the platyhelminths, the cestodes or tapeworms, possess many basic structural characteristics of flukes, but also show striking differences. Figure 22.3 shows the general features of the structure and development of tapeworms.

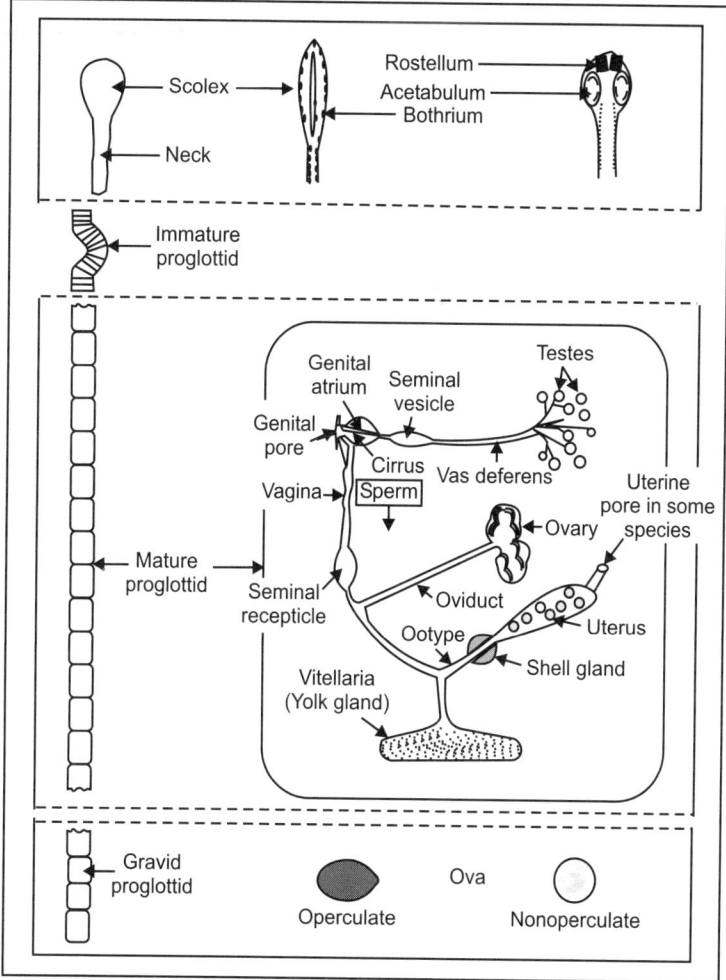

Fig. 22.3. Structure of tapeworms.

Whereas flukes are flattened and generally leaf-shaped, adult tapeworms are flattened, elongated, and consist of segments called proglottids. Tapeworms vary in length from 2 to 3 mm to 10 m, and may have three to several thousand segments.

Anatomically, cestodes are divided into a scolex or head, which bears the organs of attachment, a neck that is the region of segment proliferation, and a chain of proglottids called the strobila. The strobila elongates as new proglottids form in the neck region. The segments nearest the neck are immature (sex organs not fully developed) and those more posterior are mature. The terminal segments are gravid, with the egg-filled uterus as the most prominent feature.

The scolex contains the cephalic ganglion or 'brain', of the tapeworm nervous system. Externally, the scolex is characterised by holdfast organs. Depending on the species, these organs consist of a rostellum, bothria or acetabula. A rostellum is a retractable, conelike structure that is located on the anterior end of the scolex, and in some species is armed with hooks. Bothria are long, narrow, weakly muscular grooves that are characteristic of the pseudophyllidean tapeworms. Acetabula (suckers like those of digenetic trematodes) are characteristic of cyclophyllidean tapeworms.

A characteristic feature of adult tapeworm is the absence of an alimentary canal, which is intriguing since all of these adult worms inhabit the small intestine. The lack of an alimentary tract means that substances enter the tapeworm across the tegument. This structure is well adapted for transport functions, since it is covered with numerous microvilli resembling those lining the lumen of the mammalian intestine. The excretory system is of the flame cell type.

Cestodes are hermaphroditic, each proglottid possessing male and female reproductive systems similar to those of digenetic flukes. However, tapeworms differ from flukes in the mechanism of egg deposition. Eggs of pseudophyllidean tapeworms exit through a uterine pore in the center of the ventral surface rather than through a genital atrium, as in flukes. In cyclophyllidean tapeworms, the female system includes a uterus without a uterine pore (Fig. 22.3).

Thus, the cyclophyllidean eggs are released only when the tapeworms shed gravid proglottids into the intestine. Some proglottids disintegrate, releasing eggs that are voided in the feces, whereas other proglottids are passed intact.

The eggs of pseudophyllidean tapeworms are operculated, but those of cyclophyllidean species are not. Eggs of all tapeworms, however, contain at some stage of development an embryo or oncosphere. The oncosphere of pseudophyllidean tapeworms is ciliated externally and is called a coracidium. The coracidium develops into a procercoid stage in its micro-crustacean first immediate host and then into a plerocercoid larva in its next intermediate host which is a vertebrate. The plerocercoid larva develops into an adult worm in the definitive (final) host. The oncosphere of cyclophyllidean tapeworms, depending on the species, develops into a cysticercus larva, cysticercoid larva, coenurus larva or hydatid larva (cyst) in specific intermediate hosts. These larvae, in turn, become adults in the definitive host.

Roundworms (Nematodes)

Figure 22.4 shows the structure of nematodes. In contrast to platyhelminths, nematodes are cylindrical rather than flattened; hence the common name roundworm. The body wall is composed of an outer cuticle that has a noncellular, chemically complex structure, a thin hypodermis, and musculature. The cuticle in some species has longitudinal ridges called alae. The bursa, a flaplike extension of the cuticle on the posterior end of some species of male nematodes, is used to grasp the female during copulation.

The cellular hypodermis bulges into the body cavity or pseudocoelom to form four longitudinal cords—a dorsal, a ventral, and two lateral cords—which may be seen on the surface as lateral lines. Nuclei of the hypodermis are located in the region of the cords. The somatic musculature lying beneath the hypodermis is a single layer of smooth muscle cells. When viewed in cross-section, this layer can be seen to be separated into four zones by the hypodermal cords. The musculature is innervated by extensions of muscle cells to nerve trunks running anteriorly and posteriorly from ganglion cells that ring the midportion of the esophagus.

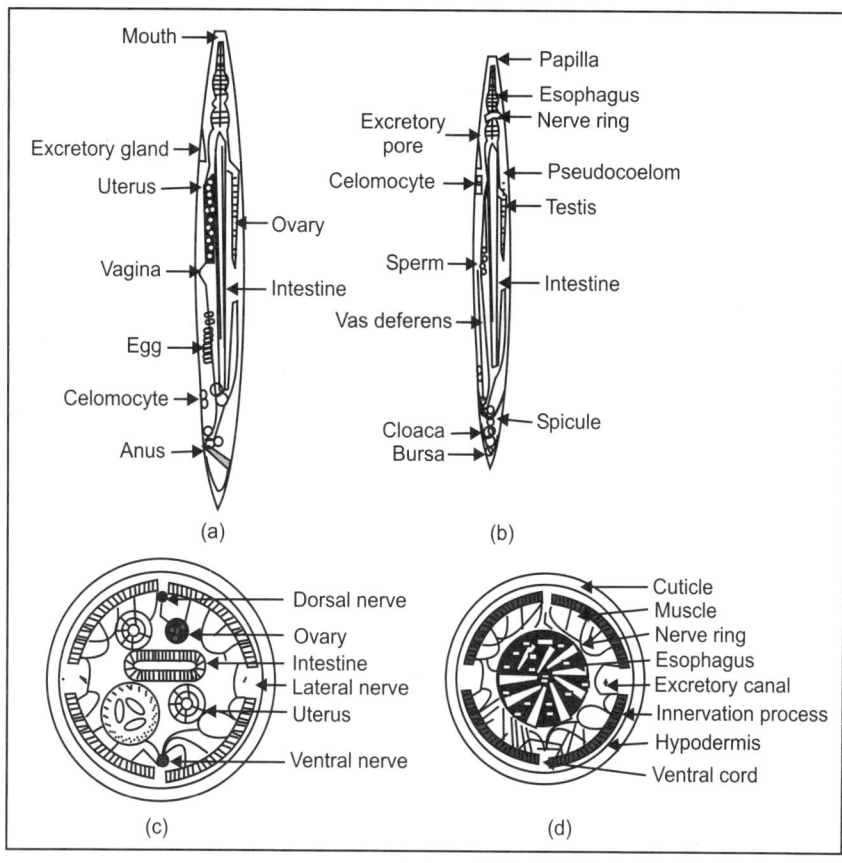

Fig. 22.4. Structure of nematodes (a) female, (b) male. Transverse sections through the midregion of the female worm (c) and through the esophageal region (d).

The space between the muscle layer and viscera is the pseudocoelom, which lacks a mesothelium lining. This cavity contains fluid and two to six fixed cells (celomocytes) which are usually associated with the longitudinal cords. The function of these cells is unknown. The alimentary canal of roundworms is complete, with both mouth and anus. The mouth is surrounded by lips bearing sensory papillae (bristles). The esophagus, a conspicuous feature of nematodes, is a muscular structure that pumps food into the intestine; it differs in shape in different species. The intestine is a tubular structure composed of a single layer of columnar cells possessing prominent microvilli on their luminal surface.

The excretory system of some nematodes consists of an excretory gland and a pore located ventrally in the mid-esophageal region. In other nematodes this structure is drawn into extensions that give rise to the more complex tubular excretory system, which is usually H-shaped, with two anterior limbs and two posterior limbs located in the lateral cords. The gland cells and tubes are thought to serve as absorptive bodies, collecting wastes from the pseudocoelom, and to function in osmoregulation.

Nematodes are usually bisexual. Males are usually smaller than females, have a curved posterior end, and possess (in some species) copulatory structures, such as spicules (usually two), a bursa or both. The males have one or (in a few cases) two testes, which lie at the free end of a convoluted or recurved tube leading into a seminal vesicle and eventually into the cloaca.

The female system is tubular also, and usually is made up of reflexed ovaries. Each ovary is continuous, with an oviduct and tubular uterus. The uteri join to form the vagina, which in turn opens to the exterior through the vulva.

Copulation between a female and a male nematode is necessary for fertilisation except in the genus *Strongyloides*, in which parthenogenetic development occurs (i.e. the development of an unfertilised egg into a new individual). Some evidence indicates that sex attractants (pheromones) play a role in heterosexual mating. During copulation, sperm is transferred into the vulva of the female. The sperm enters the ovum and a fertilisation membrane is secreted by the zygote. This membrane gradually thickens to form the chitinous shell. A second membrane, below the shell, makes the egg impervious to essentially all substances except carbon dioxide and oxygen. In some species, a third proteinaceous membrane is secreted as the egg passes down the uterus by the uterine wall and is deposited outside the shell. Most nematodes that are parasitic in humans lay eggs that, when voided, contain either an uncleaved zygote, a group of blastomeres or a completely formed larva. Some nematodes, such as the filariae and *Trichinella spiralis*, produce larvae that are deposited in host tissues.

The developmental process in nematodes involves egg, larval, and adult stages. Each of four larval stages is followed by a moult in which the cuticle is shed. The larvae are called second-stage larvae after the first moult, and so on (Fig. 22.5). The nematode formed at the fifth stage is the adult. Figure 22.6 summarises the life cycles of several intestinal nematodes.

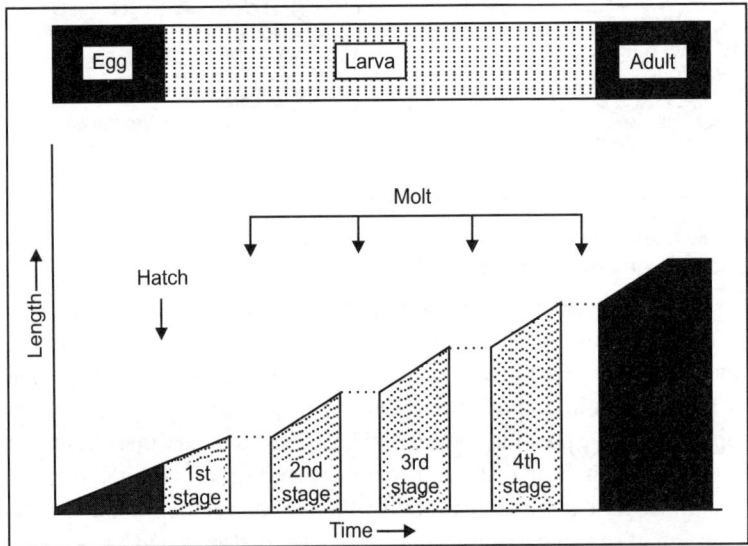

Fig. 22.5. Stages in the development of nematodes.

NEMATODE

The nematodes or roundworms (phylum Nematoda) are the most diverse phylum of pseudocoelomates, and one of the most diverse of all animals. It has been estimated that the total number of nematode species might be approximately 10,00,000. Unlike cnidarians or flatworms, roundworms have a digestive system that is like a tube with openings at both ends.

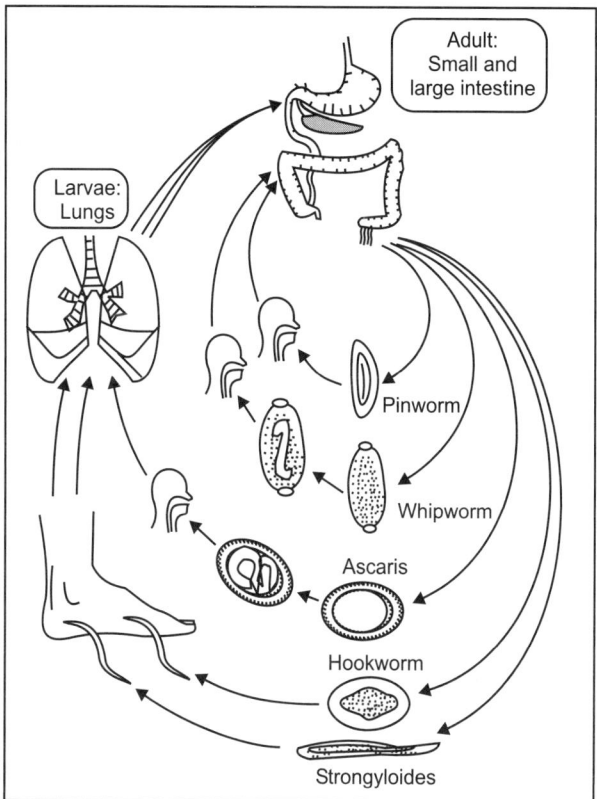

Fig. 22.6. Generalised life cycle of intestinal nematodes.

Nematodes have successfully adapted to nearly every ecosystem from marine to freshwater, from the polar regions to the tropics, as well as the highest to the lowest of elevations. They are ubiquitous in freshwater, marine, and terrestrial environments, where they often outnumber other animals in both individual and species counts, and are found in locations as diverse as mountains, deserts and oceanic trenches. They represent, for example, 90 per cent of all life on the seafloor of the earth. Their many parasitic forms include pathogens in most plants and animals (including humans). Some nematodes can undergo cryptobiosis. One group of carnivorous fungi, the nematophagous fungi, are predators of soil nematodes. They set enticements for the nematodes in the form of lassos or adhesive structures.

Taxonomy and Systematics

At the origin, the 'nematoidea' included both roundworms and horsehair worms. Along with *Acanthocephala*, *Trematoda* and *Cestoidea*, it formed the group Entozoa.

Phylogeny

The relationships of the nematodes and their close relatives among the protostomian Metazoa are unresolved. Traditionally, they were held to be a lineage of their own, but in the 1990s it was proposed that they form a clade together with moulting animals such as arthropods. This group has been named Ecdysozoa.

Conversely, the identity of the closest living relatives of the Nematoda has always been considered to be well resolved. Morphological characters and molecular phylogenies agree with placement of the roundworms as sister taxon to the parasitic horsehair worms (Nematomorpha); together they make up the Nematoida. Together with the Scalidophora (formerly Cephalorhyncha), the Nematoida form the Introverta. It is entirely unclear whether the Introverta are, in turn, the closest living relatives of the enigmatic Gastrotricha; if so, they are considered a clade Cycloneuralia, but there is much disagreement both between and among the available morphological and molecular data. The Cycloneuralia or the Introverta—depending on the validity of the former—are often ranked as a superphylum.

Nematode systematics

Due to the lack of knowledge regarding many nematodes, their systematics is contentious. Traditionally, they are divided into two classes, the Adenophorea and the Secernentea, and initial DNA sequence studies suggested the existence of five clades:

1. Dorylaimia.
2. Enoplia.
3. Spirurina.
4. Tylenchina.
5. Rhabditina.

Nematodes are slender, worm-like animals, typically less than 2.5 millimetres (0.10 in) long. The smallest nematodes are microscopic, while free-living species can reach as much as 5 centimetres (2.0 in) and some parasitic species are larger still. The body is often ornamented with ridges, rings, warts, bristles or other distinctive structures.

Digestive system

The oral cavity is lined with cuticle, which is often strengthened with ridges or other structures, and, especially in carnivorous species, may bear a number of teeth. The mouth often includes a sharp stylet which the animal can thrust into its prey. In some species, the stylet is hollow, and can be used to suck liquids from plants or animals.

The oral cavity opens into a muscular sucking pharynx, also lined with cuticle. Digestive glands are found in this region of the gut, producing enzymes that start to break down the food. In stylet-bearing species, these may even be injected into the prey.

Excretory system

Nitrogenous waste is excreted in the form of ammonia through the body wall, and is not associated with any specific organs. However, the structures for excreting salt to maintain osmoregulation are typically more complex.

In many marine nematodes, there are one or two unicellular renette glands that excrete salt through a pore on the underside of the animal, close to the pharynx. In most other nematodes, these specialised cells have been replaced by an organ consisting of two parallel ducts connected by a single transverse duct. This transverse duct opens into a common canal that runs to the excretory pore.

Nervous system

Four nerves run the length of the body on the dorsal, ventral, and lateral surfaces. Each nerve lies within a cord of connective tissue lying beneath the cuticle and between the muscle cells. The ventral nerve is the largest, and has a double structure forward of the excretory pore. The dorsal nerve is responsible for motor control, while the lateral nerves are sensory, and the ventral combines both functions.

At the anterior end of the animal, the nerves branch from a dense circular nerve ring surrounding the pharynx, and serving as the brain. Smaller nerves run forward from the ring to supply the sensory organs of the head.

Reproduction

Most nematode species are dioecious, with separate male and female individuals. Both sexes possess one or two tubular gonads. In males, the sperm are produced at the end of the gonad, and migrate along its length as they mature. The testes each open into a relatively wide sperm duct and then into a glandular and muscular ejaculatory duct associated with the cloaca. In females, the ovaries each open into an oviduct and then a glandular uterus. The uteri both open into a common vagina, usually located in the middle of the ventral surface.

Reproduction is usually sexual. Males are usually smaller than females (often much smaller) and often have a characteristically bent tail for holding the female for copulation. During copulation, one or more chitinised spicules move out of the cloaca and are inserted into genital pore of the female. Amoeboid sperm crawl along the spicule into the female worm. Nematode sperm is thought to be the only eukaryotic cell without the globular protein G-actin.

Eggs may be embryonated or unembryonated when passed by the female, meaning that their fertilised eggs may not yet be developed. A few species are known to be ovoviviparous. The eggs are protected by an outer shell, secreted by the uterus. In free-living roundworms, the eggs hatch into larvae, which appear essentially identical to the adults, except for an underdeveloped reproductive system; in parasitic roundworms, the life cycle is often much more complicated.

Nematodes as a whole possess a wide range of modes of reproduction. Some nematodes, such as *Heterorhabditis* spp., undergo a process called *endotokia matricida*: intrauterine birth causing maternal death. Some nematodes are hermaphroditic, and keep their self-fertilised eggs inside the uterus until they hatch. The juvenile nematodes will then ingest the parent nematode. This process is significantly promoted in environments with a low or reducing food supply.

The nematode model species *Caenorhabditis elegans* and *C. briggsae* exhibit androdioecy, which is very rare among animals. The single genus *Meloidogyne* (root-knot nematodes) exhibit a range of reproductive modes including sexual reproduction, facultative sexuality (in which most, but not all, generations reproduce asexually), and both meiotic and mitotic parthenogenesis.

The genus *Mesorhabditis* exhibits an unusual form of parthenogenesis, in which sperm-producing males copulate with females, but the sperm do not fuse with the ovum. Contact with the sperm is essential for the ovum to begin dividing, but because there is no fusion of the cells, the male contributes no genetic material to the offspring, which are essentially clones of the female.

Free-living species

In free-living species, development usually consists of four molts of the cuticle during growth. Different species feed on materials as varied as algae, fungi, small animals, fecal matter, dead organisms and living tissues. Free-living marine nematodes are important and abundant members of the meiobenthos. They play an important role in the decomposition process, aid in recycling of nutrients in marine environments and are sensitive to changes in the environment caused by pollution. One roundworm of note is *Caenorhabditis elegans*, which lives in the soil and has found much use as a model organism.

C. elegans has had its entire genome sequenced, as well as the developmental fate of every cell determined, and every neuron mapped.

Parasitic species

Nematodes commonly parasitic on humans include ascarids (*Ascaris*), filarias, hookworms, pinworms (*Enterobius*) and whipworms (*Trichuris trichiura*). The species *Trichinella spiralis*, commonly known as the trichina worm, occurs in rats, pigs, and humans, and is responsible for the disease trichinosis. *Baylisascaris* usually infests wild animals but can be deadly to humans as well. *Dirofilaria immitis* are Heartworms known for causing Heartworm disease by inhabiting the hearts, arteries, and lungs of dogs and some cats. *Haemonchus contortus* is one of the most abundant infectious agents in sheep around the world, causing great economic damage to sheep farms. In contrast, entomopathogenic nematodes parasitise insects and are considered by humans to be beneficial. One form of nematode is entirely dependent upon fig wasps, which are the sole source of fig fertilisation. They prey upon the wasps, riding them from the ripe fig of the wasp's birth to the fig flower of its death, where they kill the wasp, and their offspring await the birth of the next generation of wasps as the fig ripens.

A newly discovered parasitic tetradonematid nematode, *Myrmeconema neotropicum*, apparently induces fruit mimicry in the tropical ant *Cephalotes atratus*. Infected ants develop bright red gasters, tend to be more sluggish, and walk with their gasters in a conspicuous elevated position. These changes likely cause frugivorous birds to confuse the infected ants for berries and eat them. Parasite eggs passed in the bird's feces are subsequently collected by foraging *Cephalotes atratus* and are fed to their larvae, thus completing the life cycle of *Myrmeconema neotropicum*.

Plant parasitic nematodes include several groups causing severe crop losses. The most common genera are *Aphelenchoides* (foliar nematodes), *Ditylenchus*, *Globodera* (potato cyst nematodes), *Heterodera* (soyabean cyst nematodes), *Longidorus*, *Meloidogyne* (root-knot nematodes), *Nacobbus*, *Pratylenchus* (lesion nematodes), *Trichodorus* and *Xiphinema* (dagger nematodes). Several phytoparasitic nematode species cause histological damages to roots, including the formation of visible galls (e.g. by root-knot nematodes), which are useful characters for their diagnostic in the field. Some nematode species transmit plant viruses through their feeding activity on roots. One of them is *Xiphinema index*, vector of GFLV (Grapevine Fanleaf Virus), an important disease of grapes.

Agriculture and horticulture

Depending on the species, a nematode may be beneficial or detrimental to plant health. From agricultural and horticulture perspectives, there are two categories of nematode: predatory ones, which will kill garden pests like cutworms, and pest nematodes, like the root-knot nematode, which attack plants and those that act as vectors spreading plant viruses between crop plants. Predatory nematodes can be bred by soaking a specific recipe of leaves and other detritus in water, in a dark, cool place, and can even be purchased as an organic form of pest control.

Rotations of plants with nematode resistant species or varieties is one means of managing parasitic nematode infestations. For example, marigolds, grown over one or more seasons (the effect is cumulative), can be used to control nematodes. Another is treatment with natural antagonists such as the fungus *Gliocladium roseum*. Chitosan is a natural biocontrol that elicits plant defense responses to destroy parasitic cyst nematodes on roots of soyabean, corn, sugar beets, potatoes and tomatoes without harming beneficial nematodes in the soil. Furthermore soil steaming is an efficient method to kill nematodes before planting crop.

PROTOZOA

Protozoa are single-celled eukaryotes (organisms whose cells have nuclei) that commonly show characteristics usually associated with animals, most notably mobility and heterotrophy.

They are often grouped in the kingdom Protista together with the plant-like algae and fungus-like water moulds and slime moulds. In some newer schemes, however, most algae are classified in the kingdoms Plantae and Chromista, and in such cases the remaining forms may be classified as a kingdom protozoa. The name is misleading, since they are not animals (with the possible exception of the Myxozoa). Protozoa have traditionally been divided on the basis of locomotion.

Most protozoans are too small to be seen with the naked eye—most are around 0.01–0.05 mm, although forms up to 0.5 mm are still fairly common—but can easily be found under a microscope.

1. Protist: Protists are a heterogeneous group of living things, comprising those eukaryotes that are neither animals, plants, nor fungi.
2. Amoeba: Amoeba (also spelled ameba) is a genus of protozoa that moves by means of temporary projections called pseudopods.
3. Food chain: Food chains and food webs and/or food networks describe the feeding relationships between species in a biotic community.
4. Biological life cycle: A life cycle is a period involving one generation of an organism through means of reproduction.

Giardia Lamblia

Giardia lamblia (synonymous with *Lamblia intestinalis* and *Giardia duodenalis*) is a flagellated protozoan parasite that colonises and reproduces in the small intestine, causing giardiasis. The giardia parasite attaches to the epithelium by a ventral adhesive disc, and reproduces via binary fission. Giardiasis does not spread via the bloodstream, nor does it spread to other parts of the gastro-intestinal tract, but remains confined to the lumen of the small intestine. Giardia trophozoites absorb their nutrients from the lumen of the small intestine, and are anaerobes. If the organism is split and stained, it has a very characteristic pattern that resembles a familiar 'smiley face' symbol.

Chief pathways of human infection include ingestion of untreated sewage, a phenomenon particularly common in many developing countries; contamination of natural waters also occurs in watersheds where intensive grazing occurs.

Giardia infects humans, but is also one of the most common parasites infecting cats, dogs and birds. Mammalian hosts also include cows, beavers, deer, and sheep.

Transmission

Giardia infection can occur through ingestion of dormant cysts in contaminated water, food or by the faecal-oral route (through poor hygiene practices). The Giardia cyst can survive for weeks to months in cold water, and therefore can be present in contaminated wells and water systems, especially stagnant water sources such as naturally occurring ponds, storm water storage systems, and even clean-looking mountain streams. They may also occur in city reservoirs and persist after water treatment, as the Giardia cysts are resistant to conventional water treatment methods such as chlorination and ozonolysis. Zoonotic transmission is also possible, and therefore Giardia infection is a concern for people camping in the wilderness or swimming in contaminated streams or lakes, especially the artificial lakes formed by beaver dams (hence the popular name for giardiasis, 'Beaver Fever').

In addition to waterborne sources, fecal-oral transmission can also occur, for example in day care centres, where children may have poor hygiene practices. Those who work with children are also at risk of being infected, as are family members of infected individuals. Not all Giardia infections are symptomatic, and many people can unknowingly serve as carriers of the parasite.

Life cycle

The life cycle begins with a noninfective cyst being excreted with the feces of an infected individual. The cyst is hardy, providing protection from various degrees of heat and cold, desiccation, and infection from other organisms. A distinguishing characteristic of the cyst is four nuclei and a retracted cytoplasm. Once ingested by a host, the trophozoite emerges to an active state of feeding and motility.

After the feeding stage, the trophozoite undergoes asexual replication through longitudinal binary fission. The resulting trophozoites and cysts then pass through the digestive system in the faeces. While the trophozoites may be found in the faeces, only the cysts are capable of surviving outside of the host (Fig. 22.7).

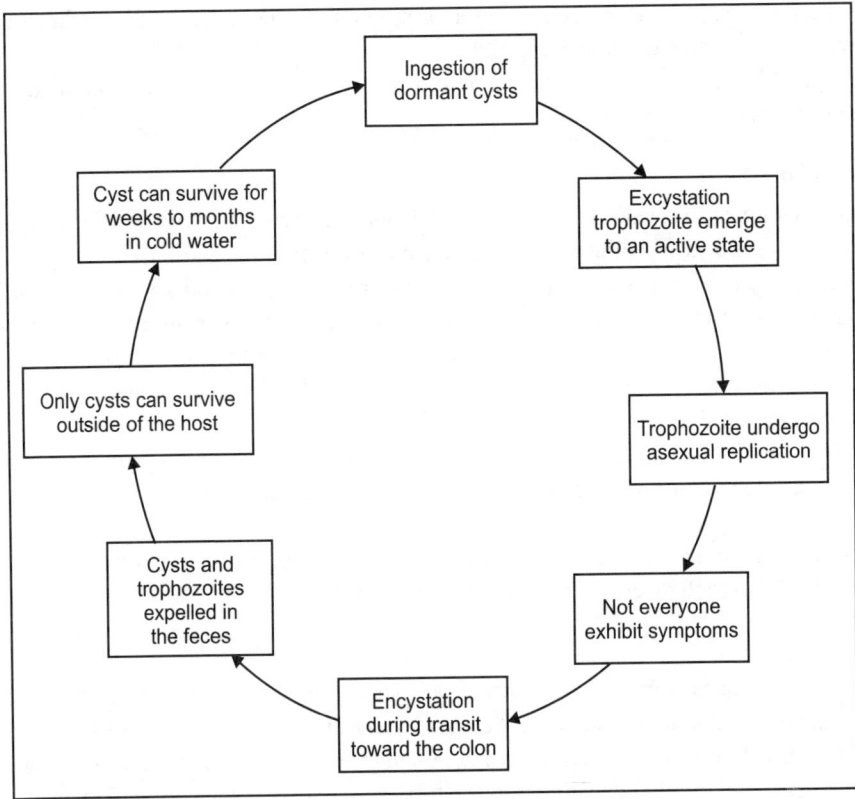

Fig. 22.7. Parasite life cycle.

Distinguishing features of the trophozoites are large karyosomes and lack of peripheral chromatin, giving the two nuclei a halo appearance. Cysts are distinguished by a retracted cytoplasm. This protozoan lacks mitochondria, although the discovery of the presence of mitochodrial remnants organelles in one recent study 'indicate that Giardia is not primitively amitochondrial and that it has retained a functional organelle derived from the original mitochondrial endosymbiont'. This organelle is now termed a mitosome. Nomenclature for Giardia species is difficult, as humans and other animals appear to have morphologically identical parasites.

Colonisation of the gut results in inflammation and villous atrophy, reducing the gut's absorptive capability. In humans, infection is symptomatic only about 50 per cent of the time, and protocol for treating asymptomatic individuals is controversial. Symptoms of infection include (in order of frequency) diarrhea, malaise, excessive gas (often flatulence or a foul or sulphuric-tasting belch, which has been known to be so nauseating in taste that it can cause the infected person to vomit), steatorrhoea (pale, foul smelling, greasy stools), epigastric pain, bloating, nausea, diminished interest in food, possible (but rare) vomiting which is often violent, and weight loss. Pus, mucus and blood are not commonly present in the stool. It usually causes 'explosive diarrhea' and while unpleasant, is not fatal. In healthy individuals, the condition is usually self-limiting, although the infection can be prolonged in patients who are immunocompromised, or who have decreased gastric acid secretion.

People with recurring Giardia infections, particularly those with a lack of IgA, may develop chronic disease. Lactase deficiency may develop in an infection with Giardia, however this usually does not persist for more than a few weeks, and a full recovery is the norm.

Some studies have shown that giardiasis should be considered as a cause of vitamin B_{12} deficiency, this a result of the problems caused within the intestinal absorption system.

Treatment and Diagnosis

Giardia lamblia infection in humans is frequently misdiagnosed. Accurate diagnosis requires an antigen test or, if that is unavailable, an ova and parasite examination of stool. Multiple stool examinations are recommended, since the cysts and trophozoites are not shed consistently. Given the difficult nature of testing to find the infection, including many false negatives, some patients should be treated on the basis of empirical evidence; treating based on symptoms. Human infection is conventionally treated with metronidazole, tinidazole or nitazoxanide. Although Metronidazole is the current first-line therapy, it is mutagenic in bacteria and carcinogenic in mice, so should be avoided during pregnancy.

It has not directly been linked to causing cancer in humans, only in other mammals, therefore appears safe. One of the most common alternative treatments is berberine sulphate (found in Oregon grape root, goldenseal, yellowroot, and various other plants). Berberine has been shown to have an antimicrobial and an antipyretic effect. Berberine compounds cause uterine stimulation, and so should be avoided in pregnancy. Continuously high dosing of berberine may lead to bradycardia and hypotension in some individuals.

Treatment in animals

Cats can be cured easily, lambs usually simply lose weight, but in calves the parasites can be fatal and often are not responsive to antibiotics or electrolytes. Carriers among calves can also be asymptomatic. Dogs have a high infection rate, as 30 per cent of the population under one year old are known to be infected in kennels. The infection is more prevalent in puppies than in adult dogs. This parasite is deadly for chinchillas, so extra care must be taken by providing them with safe water. Infected dogs can be isolated and treated, or the entire pack at a kennel can be treated together regardless.

Entamoeba Histolytica

Entamoeba histolytica is an anaerobic parasitic protozoan, part of the genus Entamoeba. Predominantly infecting humans and other primates, E. histolytica is estimated to infect about 50 million people worldwide. Previously, it was thought that 10 per cent of the world population was infected, but these figures predate the recognition that at least 90 per cent of these infections were due to a second species, *E. dispar*. Mammals such as dogs and cats can become infected transiently, but are not thought to contribute significantly to transmission.

The active (trophozoite) stage exists only in the host and in fresh loose feces; cysts survive outside the host in water, soils and on foods, especially under moist conditions on the latter. The cysts are readily killed by heat and by freezing temperatures, and survive for only a few months outside of the host. Symptoms can include fulminating dysentery, bloody diarrhea, weight loss, fatigue, abdominal pain, and amoeboma. The amoeba can actually 'bore' into the intestinal wall, causing lesions and intestinal symptoms, and it may reach the blood stream. From there, it can reach different vital organs of the human body, usually the liver, but sometimes the lungs, brain, spleen, etc. A common outcome of this invasion of tissues is a liver abscess, which can be fatal if untreated. Ingested red blood cells are sometimes seen in the amoeba cell cytoplasm. *E. histolytica* may modulate the virulence of certain human viruses and is itself a host for its own viruses.

Diagnosis

It can be diagnosed by stool samples but it is important to note that certain other species are impossible to distinguish by microscopy alone. Trophozoites may be seen in a fresh fecal smear and cysts in an ordinary stool sample. ELISA or RIA can also be used.

TOXIGENIC ALGAE

Although strictly speaking the term algae should now used as a collective term for a number of photosynthetic eukaryotic phyla, for the purposes of this section the prokaryotic cyanobacterium or blue-green algae, will also be included. A number of planktonic and benthic algae can produce very toxic compounds which may be transported to filter-feeding shellfish such as mussels and clams or small herbivorous fish which are food for larger carnivorous fish.

Dinoflagellate Toxins

Dinoflagellates are microscopic, (usually) unicellular, flagellated, often photosynthetic protists, commonly regarded as 'algae' (division dinoflagellata). They are characterised by a transverse flagellum that encircles the body (often in a groove known as the cingulum) and a longitudinal flagellum oriented perpendicular to the transverse flagellum. This imparts a distinctive spiral to their swimming motion. Both flagella are inserted at the same point in the cell wall, by convention defining the ventral surface. This point is usually slightly depressed, and is termed the sulcus. In heterotrophic dinoflagellates (ones that eat other organisms), this is the point where a conical feeding structure, the peduncle, is projected in order to consume food.

Dinoflagellates possess a unique nuclear structure at some stage of their life cycle—a dinokaryotic nucleus (as opposed to eukaryotic or prokaryotic), in which the chromosomes are perminently condensed. The cell wall of many dinoflagellates is divided into plates of cellulose (armour) within amphiesmal vesicles, known as a theca. These plates form a distinctive geometry/topology known as tabulation, which is the main means for classification.

Both heterotrophic (eat other organisms) and autotrophic (photosynthetic) dinoflagellates are known. Some are both. They form a significant part of primary planktonic production in both oceans and lakes. Most dinoflagellates go through moderately complex life cycles involving several steps, both sexual and asexual, motile and nonmotile. Some species form cysts composed of sporopollenin (an organic polymer), and preserve as fossils. Often the tabulation of the cell wall is somehow expressed in the shape and/or ornamentation of the cyst. Besides being important primary producers, and therefore an important part of the food chain, dinoflagellates are also known for producing nasty toxins, particularly when they occur in large numbers, called 'red tides' because the cells are so abundant they make the water change colour. Besides being bad for a large range of marine life, red tides can also introduce non-fatal or fatal amounts of toxins into animals (particularly shellfish) that may be eaten by humans, who are also affected by the toxins. Many of these toxins are quite potent, and if not fatal, can still cause neurological and all sorts of other nasty effects.

CYANOBACTERIAL TOXINS

The cyanotoxins are a diverse group of natural toxins, both from the chemical and the toxicological points of view. In spite of their aquatic origin, most of the cyanotoxins that have been identified to date appear to be more hazardous to terrestrial mammals than to aquatic biota. Cyanobacteria produce a variety of unusual metabolites, the natural function of which is unclear, although some, perhaps only coincidentally, elicit effects upon other biota. Research has primarily focused on compounds that impact upon humans and livestock, either as toxins or as pharmaceutically useful substances. Further ranges of nontoxic products are also being found in cyanobacteria and the biochemical and pharmacological properties of these are totally unknown.

Analytical methods suitable for quantitative toxin determination only became available in the late 1980s, but studies of specific cyanotoxins have been increasing since then. The results of both approaches indicate that neurotoxins are generally less common, except perhaps in some countries where they frequently cause lethal animal poisonings. In contrast, the cyclic peptide toxins (microcystins and nodularins) which primarily cause liver injury are more widespread and are very likely to occur if certain taxa of cyanobacteria are present. For assessing the health risk caused by cyanotoxins, an understanding of their persistence and degradation in aquatic environments is of crucial importance. Because effects on aquatic biota may be relevant issues for water managers, and because public concern could raise questions in this field for practitioners.

Mechanisms of cyanobacterial toxicity currently described and understood are very diverse and range from hepatotoxic, neurotoxic and dermatotoxic effects to general inhibition of protein synthesis. To assess the specific hazards of cyanobacterial toxins it is necessary to understand their chemical and physical properties, their occurrence in waters used by people, the regulation of their production, and their fate in the environment.

Cyanotoxins fall into three broad groups of chemical structure: cyclic peptides, alkaloids and lipopolysaccharides (LPS).

Globally the most frequently found cyanobacterial toxins in blooms from fresh and brackish waters are the cyclic peptide toxins of the microcystin and nodularin family. They pose a major challenge for the production of safe drinking water from surface waters containing cyanobacteria with these toxins. In mouse bioassays, which traditionally have been used to screen toxicity of field and laboratory samples, cyanobacterial hepatotoxins (liver toxins) cause death by liver haemorrhage within a few hours of the acute doses. Microcystins have been characterised from planktonic *Anabaena*, *Microcystis*, *Oscillatoria* (*Planktothrix*), *Nostoc*, and *Anabaenopsis* species, and from terrestrial *Hapalosiphon* genera. Nodularin has been characterised only from *Nodularia spumigena*.

MYCOTOXIN

A mycotoxin is a toxic secondary metabolite produced by organisms of the fungus kingdom, commonly known as moulds. The term 'mycotoxin' is usually reserved for the toxic chemical products produced by fungi that readily colonise crops. Most fungi are aerobic (use oxygen) and are found almost everywhere in extremely small quantities due to the minute size of their spores. They consume organic matter wherever humidity and temperature are sufficient. One mould species may produce many different mycotoxins and/or the same mycotoxin as another species.

Where conditions are right, fungi proliferate into colonies and mycotoxin levels become high. The reason for the production of mycotoxins is not yet known; they are neither necessary for growth nor the development of the fungi. Because mycotoxins weaken the receiving host, the fungus may use them as a strategy to better the environment for further fungal proliferation. The production of toxins depends on the surrounding intrinsic and extrinsic environments and the toxins vary greatly in their severity, depending on the organism infected and its susceptibility, metabolism, and defense mechanisms. Some of the health effects found in animals and humans include death, identifiable diseases or health problems, weakened immune systems without specificity to a toxin, and as allergens or irritants. Some mycotoxins are harmful to other micro-organisms such as other fungi or even bacteria; penicillin is one example. It has been suggested that mycotoxins in stored animal feed are the cause of apparent sex change in hens. Mycotoxins can appear in the food chain as a result of fungal infection of crops, either by being eaten directly by humans or by being used as livestock feed. Mycotoxins greatly resist decomposition or being broken down in digestion, so they remain in the food chain in meat and dairy products. Even temperature treatments, such as cooking and freezing, do not destroy mycotoxins.

Although various wild mushrooms contain an assortment of poisons that are definitely fungal metabolites causing noteworthy health problems for humans, they are rather arbitrarily excluded from discussions of mycotoxicology. In such cases the distinction is based on the size of the producing fungus and human intention. Mycotoxin exposure is almost always accidental whereas with mushrooms improper identification and ingestion causing mushroom poisoning is commonly the case. Ingestion of misidentified mushrooms containing mycotoxins may result in hallucinations. The cyclopeptide-produced Amanita phalloide is well known for its toxic potential and is responsible for approximately 90 per cent of all mushroom fatalities. The other primary mycotoxin groups found in mushrooms include: orellanine, monomethylhydrazine, disulphiram-like, hallucinogenic indoles, muscarinic, isoxazole, and gastrointestinal (GI)-specific irritants.

Food-based mycotoxins were studied extensively worldwide throughout the 20th century. In Europe, statutory levels of a range of mycotoxins permitted in food and animal feed are set by a range of European directives and Commission regulations. The US Food and Drug Administration has regulated and enforced limits on concentrations of mycotoxins in foods and feed industries since 1985. It is through various compliance programs that the FDA monitors these industries to guarantee that mycotoxins are kept at a practical level. These compliance programs sample food products including peanuts and peanut products, tree nuts, corn and corn products, cottonseed, and milk. There is still a lack of sufficient surveillance data on some mycotoxins that occur in the US which is largely due to the lack of reliable analytical methods.

Major Groups

Aflatoxins

Aflatoxins are a type of mycotoxin produced by *Aspergillus* species of fungi, such as *A. flavus* and *A. parasiticus*. The umbrella term aflatoxin refers to four different types of mycotoxins produced, which are B1, B2, G1, and G2. Aflatoxin B1, the most toxic, is a potent carcinogen and has been directly correlated to adverse health effects, such as liver cancer, in many animal species. Aflatoxins are largely associated with commodities produced in the tropics and subtropics, such as cotton, peanuts, spices, pistachios and maize.

Ochratoxin

Ochratoxin is a mycotoxin that comes in three secondary metabolite forms, A, B, and C. All are produced by *Penicillium* and *Aspergillus* species. The three forms differ in that Ochratoxin B (OTB) is a nonchlorinated form of Ochratoxin A (OTA) and that Ochratoxin C (OTC) is an ethyl ester form Ochratoxin A. *Aspergillus ochraceus* is found as a contaminant of a wide range of commodities including beverages such as beer and wine. *Aspergillus carbonarius* is the main species found on vine fruit, which releases its toxin during the juice making process. OTA has been labelled as a carcinogen and a nephrotoxin, and has been linked to tumours in the human urinary tract, although research in humans is limited by confounding factors.

Citrinin

Citrinin is a toxin that was first isolated from *Penicillium citrinum*, but has been identified in over a dozen species of *Penicillium* and several species of *Aspergillus*. Some of these species are used to produce human foodstuffs such as cheese (*Penicillium camemberti*), sake, miso, and soya sauce (*Aspergillus oryzae*). Citrinin is associated with yellow rice disease in Japan and acts as a nephrotoxin in all animal species tested. Although it is associated with many human foods (wheat, rice, corn, barley, oats, rye, and food coloured with Monascus pigment) its full significance for human health is unknown. Citrinin can also act synergistically with Ochratoxin A to depress RNA synthesis in murine kidneys.

Ergot alkaloids

Ergot alkaloids are compounds produced as a toxic mixture of alkaloids in the sclerotia of species of Claviceps, which are common pathogens of various grass species. The ingestion of ergot sclerotia from infected cereals, commonly in the form of bread produced from contaminated flour, cause ergotism the human disease historically known as St. Anthony's Fire. There are two forms of ergotism gangrenous affecting blood supply to extremities and convulsive which affects the central nervous system. Modern methods of grain cleaning have significantly reduced ergotism as a human disease, however it is still an important veterinarian problem. Ergot alkaloids have been used pharmaceutically.

Patulin

Patulin is a toxin produced by the *P. expansum*, *Aspergillus*, *Penicillium*, and *Paecilomyces* fungal species. *P. expansum* is especially associated with a range of mouldy fruits and vegetables, in particular rotting apples and figs. It is destroyed by the fermentation process and so is not found in apple beverages, such as cider. Although patulin has not been shown to be carcinogenic, it has been reported to damage the immune system in animals.

Fusarium

Fusarium toxins are produced by over 50 species of Fusarium and have a history of infecting the grain of developing cereals such as wheat and maize. They include a range of mycotoxins, such as: the fumonisins, which affect the nervous systems of horses and may cause cancer in rodents; the trichothecenes, which are most strongly associated with chronic and fatal toxic effects in animals and humans; and zearalenone, which is not correlated to any fatal toxic effects in animals or humans. Some of the other major types of Fusarium toxins include: beauvercin and enniatins, butenolide, equisetin, and fusarins.

Binding Agents and Deactivators

In the feed and food industry it has become common practice to add mycotoxin binding agents such as Montmorillonite or bentonite clay in order to affectively adsorb the mycotoxins. To reverse the adverse effects of mycotoxins, the following criteria are used to evaluate the functionality of any binding additive:

1. Efficacy of active component verified by scientific data.
2. A low effective inclusion rate.
3. Stability over a wide pH range.
4. High capacity to adsorb high concentrations of mycotoxins.
5. High affinity to adsorb low concentrations of mycotoxins.
6. Affirmation of chemical interaction between mycotoxin and adsorbent.
7. Proven *in vivo* data with all major mycotoxins.
8. Nontoxic, environmentally friendly component.

Since not all mycotoxins can be bound to such agents, the latest approach to mycotoxin control is mycotoxin deactivation. By means of enzymes (esterase, epoxidase), yeast (*Trichosporon mycotoxinvorans*) or bacterial strains (Eubacterium BBSH 797), mycotoxins can be reduced during pre-harvesting contamination. Other removal methods include physical separation, washing, milling, heat-treatment, radiation, extraction with solvents, and the use of chemical or biological agents. Irradiation methods have proven to be effective treatment against mould growth and toxin production.

Other Aspergillus Toxins

Sterigmatocystin is a poison of the type dermatoxin, from the fungi genus *Aspergillus*. It appears on crusts of cheese with mould.

Sterigmatocystin is a toxic metabolite structurally closely related to the aflatoxins (compare general fact sheet number 2), and consists of a xanthone nucleus attached to a bifuran structure. Sterigmatocystin is mainly produced by the fungi *Aspergillus nidulans* and *A. versicolour*. It has been reported in mouldy grain, green coffee beans and cheese although information on its occurrence in foods is limited. It appears to occur much less frequently than the aflatoxins, although analytical methods for its determination have not been as sensitive until recently, and so it is possible that small concentrations in food commodities may not always have been detected. Although it is a potent liver carcinogen similar to aflatoxin B1, current knowledge suggests that it is nowhere near as widespread in its occurrence. If this is the true situation it would be justified to consider sterigmatocystin as no more than a risk to consumers in special or unusual circumstances. A number of closely related compounds such o-methyl sterigmatocystin are known and some may also occur naturally.

Mycotoxins of *Penicillium*

Penicillium is much more common as a spoilage mould in Europe than *Aspergillus* with species such as *P. italicum* and *P. digitatum* causing blue and green mould respectively of oranges, lemons and grapefruits, *P. expansum* causing a soft rot of apples, and several other species associated with the moulding of jams, bread and cakes.

Penicillium Roqueforti

Penicillium roqueforti is a common saprotrophic fungus from the family Trichocomaceae. Widespread in nature, it can be isolated from soil, decaying organic matter, and plants. The major industrial use of this fungus is the production of blue cheeses, flavouring agents, antifungals, polysaccharides, proteases and other enzymes. The fungus has been a constituent of Roquefort, Stilton, Danish blue and other blue cheeses eaten by humans since about 50 AD; blue cheese is mentioned in literature as far back as AD 79, when Pliny the Elder remarked upon its rich flavour.

Classification

They were grouped into different species based on phenotypic differences, but later combined into one species by Raper and Thom. The *P. roqueforti* group got a reclassification in 1996 thanks to molecular analysis of ribosomal DNA sequences. Formerly divided into two varieties—cheese-making (*P. roqueforti* var. *roqueforti*) and patulin-making (*P. roqueforti* var. *carneum*), *P. roqueforti* was reclassified into three species named *P. roqueforti*, *P. carneum* and *P. paneum*.

   As this fungus does not form visible fruiting bodies, descriptions are based on macromorphological characteristics of fungal colonies growing on various standard agar media, and on microscopic characteristics. When grown on Czapek yeast autolysate (CYA) agar or yeast-extract sucrose (YES) agar, *P. roqueforti* colonies are typically 40 mm in diameter, olive brown to dull green (dark green to black on the reverse side of the agar plate), with a velutinous texture. Grown on malt extract (MEA) agar, colonies are 50 mm in diameter, dull green in colour (beige to greyish green on the reverse side), with arachnoid (with many spider-web-like fibres) colony margins. Another characteristic morphological feature of this species includes the production of asexual spores in phialides with a distinctive brush-shaped configuration. *P. roqueforti* is known to be one of the most common spoilage moulds of silage. It is also one of several different moulds that can spoil bread.

FUSARIUM

Fusarium is a large genus of filamentous fungi widely distributed in soil and in association with plants. Most species are harmless saprobes, and are relatively abundant members of the soil microbial community. Some species produce mycotoxins in cereal crops that can affect human and animal health if they enter the food chain. The main toxins produced by these *Fusarium* species are fumonisins and trichothecenes.

Pathogen

The genus includes a number of economically important plant pathogenic species. *Fusarium graminearum* commonly infects barley if there is rain late in the season. It is of economic impact to the malting and brewing industries, as well as feed barley. Fusarium contamination in barley can result in head blight, and in extreme contaminations, the barley can appear pink. The genome of this wheat and maize pathogen has been sequenced. *F. graminearum* can also cause root rot and seedling blight.

   Fusarium oxysporum f.sp. *cubense* is a fungal plant pathogen that causes Panama disease of banana (*Musa* spp.), also known as fusarium wilt of banana. Panama disease affects a wide range of banana cultivars, which are propagated asexually from offshoots and therefore have very little genetic diversity. Panama disease is one of the most destructive plant diseases of modern times, and caused the commercial disappearance of the once dominant Gros Michel cultivar. A more recent strain also affects the Cavendish cultivars used as a substitute for Gros Michel. It is considered inevitable that this susceptibility will spread globally and commercially wipe out the Cavendish cultivar, for which there are currently no acceptable replacements.

In humans

Some species may cause a range of opportunistic infections in humans. In humans with normal immune systems, fusarial infections may occur in the nails (onychomycosis) and in the cornea (keratomycosis or mycotic keratitis). In humans whose immune systems are weakened in a particular way, (neutropenia, i.e. very low neutrophils count), aggressive fusarial infections penetrating the entire body and bloodstream (disseminated infections) may be caused by members of the *Fusarium solani* complex, *Fusarium oxysporum*, *Fusarium verticillioides*, *Fusarium proliferatum* and, rarely, other fusarial species.

Biological Warfare

Mass casualties occurred in the Soviet Union in the 1930s and 1940s when *Fusarium*-contaminated wheat flour was baked into bread, causing alimentary toxic aleukia with a 60 per cent mortality rate. Symptoms began with abdominal pain, diarrhea, vomiting, and prostration, and within days, fever, chills, myalgias and bone marrow depression with granulocytopenia and secondary sepsis occurred. Further symptoms included pharyngeal or laryngeal ulceration and diffuse bleeding into the skin (petechiae and ecchymoses), melena, bloody diarrhea, hematuria, hematemesis, epistaxis, vaginal bleeding, pancytopenia and gastrointestinal ulceration.

Fusarium sporotrichoides contamination was found in affected grain in 1932, spurring research for medical purposes and for use in biological warfare. The active ingredient was found to be trichothecene T-2 mycotoxin, and it was produced in quantity and weaponised prior to the passage of the Biological Weapons Convention in 1972. The Soviets were accused of using the agent, dubbed 'yellow rain', to cause 6300 deaths in Laos, Kampuchea, and Afghanistan between 1975 and 1981. The supposed biological warfare agent was later shown to be bee feces.

Esophageal Cancer

Esophageal cancer (or oesophageal cancer) is malignancy of the esophagus. There are various subtypes, primarily squamous cell cancer (approx. 90–95 per cent of all esophageal cancer worldwide) and adenocarcinoma (approx. 50–80 per cent of all esophageal cancer in the United States). Squamous cell cancer arises from the cells that line the upper part of the esophagus. Adenocarcinoma arises from glandular cells that are present at the junction of the esophagus and stomach.

Esophageal tumours usually lead to dysphagia (difficulty swallowing), pain and other symptoms, and are diagnosed with biopsy. Small and localised tumours are treated surgically with curative intent. Larger tumours tend not to be operable and hence are treated with palliative care; their growth can still be delayed with chemotherapy, radiotherapy or a combination of the two. In some cases chemo- and radiotherapy can render these larger tumours operable. Prognosis depends on the extent of the disease and other medical problems, but is fairly poor.

Signs and symptoms

Dysphagia (difficulty swallowing) and odynophagia (painful swallowing) are the most common symptoms of esophageal cancer. Dysphagia is the first symptom in most patients. Odynophagia may also be present. Fluids and soft foods are usually tolerated, while hard or bulky substances (such as bread or meat) cause much more difficulty. Substantial weight loss is characteristic as a result of reduced appetite and poor nutrition and the active cancer. Pain behind the sternum or in the epigastrium, often of a burning, heartburn-like nature, may be severe, present itself almost daily, and is worsened by swallowing any form of food. Another sign may be an unusually husky, raspy, or hoarse sounding cough, a result of the tumour affecting the recurrent laryngeal nerve.

The presence of the tumour may disrupt normal peristalsis (the organised swallowing reflex), leading to nausea and vomiting, regurgitation of food, coughing and an increased risk of aspiration pneumonia. The tumour surface may be fragile and bleed, causing haematemesis (vomiting up blood). Compression of local structures occurs in advanced disease, leading to such problems as upper airway obstruction and superior vena cava syndrome. Fistulas may develop between the esophagus and the trachea, increasing the pneumonia risk; this condition is usually heralded by cough, fever or aspiration.

Most of the people diagnosed with esophageal cancer have late-stage disease. This is because people usually do not have significant symptoms until half of the inside of the esophagus, called the lumen, is obstructed, by which point the tumour is fairly large.

If the disease has spread elsewhere, this may lead to symptoms related to this: liver metastasis could cause jaundice and ascites, lung metastasis could cause shortness of breath, pleural effusions, etc.

Mycotoxins of Other Fungi

Claviceps purpurea

Claviceps purpurea is a fungus that grows on the ears of rye and related cereal and forage plants. Consumption of grains or seeds contaminated with the fruiting structure of this fungus, the ergot sclerotium, can cause ergotism in humans and other mammals. *C. purpurea* most commonly affects outcrossing species such as rye (its most common host), as well as triticale, wheat and barley. It affects oats only rarely.

An ergot kernel called Sclerotium clavus develops when a floret of flowering grass or cereal is infected by a spore of *C. purpurea*. The infection process mimics a pollen grain growing into an ovary during fertilisation. Because infection requires access of the fungal spore to the stigma, plants infected by *C. purpurea* are mainly outcrossing species with open flowers, such as rye (*Secale cereale*) and Alopecurus. The proliferating fungal mycelium then destroys the plant ovary and connects with the vascular bundle originally intended for feeding the developing seed. The first stage of ergot infection manifests itself as a white soft tissue (known as *Sphacelia segetum*) producing sugary honeydew, which often drops out of the infected grass florets. This honeydew contains millions of asexual spores (conidia) which are dispersed to other florets by insects or rain. Later, the *Sphacelia segetum* convert into a hard dry *Sclerotium clavus* inside the husk of the floret. At this stage, alkaloids and lipids (e.g. ricinoleic acid) accumulate in the Sclerotium.

Acremonium

Acremonium is a genus of Fungi in the Hypocreaceae family; it was previously known as 'Cephalosporium'. Acremonium species are usually slow growing and are initially compact and moist. Acremonium hyphae are fine and hyaline and produce mostly simple phialides. Their conidia are usually one-celled (i.e. ameroconidia), hyaline or pigmented, globose to cylindrical, and mostly aggregated in slimy heads at the apex of each phialide.

The genus Acremonium currently contains approximately 100 species, of which most are saprophytic, being isolated from dead plant material and soil. Many species of Acremonium are recognised as opportunistic pathogens of man and animals, causing mycetoma, onychomycosis, and hyalohyphomycosis. Clinical manifestations of hyalohyphomycosis caused by Acremonium include arthritis, osteomyelitis, peritonitis, endocarditis, pneumonia, cerebritis and subcutaneous infection.

The cephalosporins, a class of β-lactam antibiotics, were originally derived from Acremonium (which was previously known as 'Cephalosporium').

Enterovirus

Enteroviruses are a genus of (+)ssRNA viruses associated with several human and mammalian diseases. Serologic studies have distinguished 66 human enterovirus serotypes on the basis of antibody neutralisation tests. Additional antigenic variants have been defined within several of the serotypes on the basis of reduced or nonreciprocal cross-neutralisation between variant strains. On the basis of their pathogenesis in humans and animals, the enteroviruses were originally classified into four groups, polioviruses, Coxsackie A viruses (CA), Coxsackie B viruses (CB), and echoviruses, but it was quickly realised that there were significant overlaps in the biological properties of viruses in the different groups. Enteroviruses isolated more recently are named with a system of consecutive numbers: EV68, EV69, EV70, and EV71, etc.

Enteroviruses affect millions of people worldwide each year, and are often found in the respiratory secretions (e.g. saliva, sputum or nasal mucus) and stool of an infected person. Historically, poliomyelitis was the most significant disease caused by an enterovirus, Poliovirus. There are 62 non-polio enteroviruses that can cause disease in humans: 23 Coxsackie A viruses, 6 Coxsackie B viruses, 28 echoviruses, and 5 other enteroviruses. Poliovirus, as well as coxsackie and echovirus are spread through the fecal-oral route. Infection can result in a wide variety of symptoms ranging from mild respiratory illness (common cold), hand, foot and mouth disease, acute haemorrhagic conjunctivitis, aseptic meningitis, myocarditis, severe neonatal sepsis-like disease, and acute flaccid paralysis.

Enteroviruses are members of the picornavirus family, a large and diverse group of small RNA viruses characterised by a single positive-strand genomic RNA. All enteroviruses contain a genome of approximately 7500 bases and are known to have a high mutation rate due to low-fidelity replication and frequent recombination. After infection of the host cell, the genome is translated in a cap-independent manner into a single polyprotein, which is subsequently processed by virus-encoded proteases into the structural capsid proteins and the nonstructural proteins, which are mainly involved in the replication of the virus.

BOVINE SPONGIFORM ENCEPHALOPATHY

Bovine spongiform encephalopathy (BSE) is a transmissible, neurodegenerative, fatal brain disease of cattle. The disease has a long incubation period of four to five years, but ultimately is fatal for cattle within weeks to months of its onset. BSE first came to the attention of the scientific community in November 1986 with the appearance in cattle of a newly-recognised form of neurological disease in the United Kingdom (UK).

Source of the Epidemic

1. Epidemiological studies conducted in the UK suggest that the source of BSE was cattle feed prepared from bovine tissues, such as brain and spinal cord, that was contaminated by the BSE agent.
2. Speculation as to the cause of the appearance of the agent causing the disease has ranged from spontaneous occurrence in cattle, the carcasses of which then entered the cattle food chain, to entry into the cattle food chain from the carcasses of sheep with a similar disease, scrapie.

Cause

1. BSE in the brain affects the brain and spinal cord of cattle. Lesions are characterised by sponge-like changes visible with an ordinary microscope.
2. The agent is highly stable, resisting freezing, drying and heating at normal cooking temperatures, even those used for pasteurisation and sterilisation.
3. The nature of the BSE agent is still a matter of debate. According to the prion theory, the agent is composed largely, if not entirely, of a self-replicating protein, referred to as a prion. Another theory argues that the agent is virus-like and possesses nucleic acids which carry genetic information. Strong evidence collected over the past decade supports the prion theory, but the ability of the BSE agent to form multiple strains is more easily explained by a virus-like agent.

Cases of BSE

1. Between November 1986 and November 2002, 1,81,376 cases of BSE were confirmed in the UK.
2. Since 1989, when the first BSE case was reported outside the UK, relatively small numbers of BSE cases (in total 3286) have also been reported in native cattle in Austria, Belgium, Czech Republic, Denmark, Finland, France, Germany, Greece, Ireland, Israel, Italy, Japan, Liechtenstein, Luxembourg, Netherlands, Poland, Portugal, Slovakia, Spain and Switzerland. However, all but 206 cases have been reported in six countries—France, Germany, Ireland, Portugal, Spain and Switzerland.
3. Since the introduction of monitoring programs to detect BSE in dead and slaughtered cattle, 12 countries have found their first native case (Austria, Czech Republic, Finland, Germany, Greece, Israel, Italy, Japan, Poland, Slovakia, Slovenia, Spain). Small numbers of cases have also been reported in Canada, the Falkland Islands (Islas Malvinas) and Oman, but solely in animals imported from the UK. The International Office for Epizootic Diseases (OIE) reports these cases on their web site: www.oie.int.

Measures Taken to Prevent the Spread of BSE

1. In July 1988, the UK banned the use of ruminant proteins in the preparation of animal feed. The use in the food chain of bovine offals considered to pose a potential risk to humans was also banned in the UK in 1989. The list of banned bovine offals was revised and expanded on several occasions as new information became available. In 1994, the EU banned mammalian MBM to ruminants, however, the measures taken, the date of implementation and the extent of enforcement vary from country to country. In 2001, because of the continued risk from cross contamination, the EU introduced a total feed ban (e.g. ban on feeding MBM to all farm animals).
2. Starting in 1996, bans prevented the sale of food and food products containing beef from the UK to other countries. Other products (e.g. tallow, gelatin) derived from bovine tissues were also prohibited from sale from the UK to other countries. However, in 1999 the European Union (EU) lifted the ban for meat fulfilling specific requirements; for example, de-boned beef from animals from farms where there have been no cases of BSE and where the animals are less than 30 months of age at slaughter.
3. Cattle are continuously monitored for BSE and BSE is decreasing in the UK. The number of reports of BSE in the UK began to decline in 1992 and has continuously declined year by year since then. New monitoring programs using newly developed tests for the diagnosis of BSE in dead and slaughtered cattle have been introduced throughout the EU. Use of these tests led to the first cases of BSE being detected in 12 countries.

Transmissible Spongiform Encephalopathies in Animals

Transmissible spongiform encephalopathies (TSEs) are diseases characterised by spongy degeneration of the brain with severe and fatal neurological signs and symptoms. BSE is one of several different forms of transmissible brain disease affecting a number of animal species. Scrapie is a common disease in sheep and goats. Mink and North American mule deer and elk can contract TSEs. A neurological disease in household cats and in ruminant and feline species in zoos has been linked to BSE; most cases in such animals appear to have occurred in the UK.

Creutzfeldt-Jakob Disease

1. While several human TSEs exist, Creutzfeldt-Jakob disease (CJD) is the prototype human TSE. CJD occurs in a form associated with a hereditary predisposition (approximately 5–10 per cent of all cases) and in a more common, sporadic form that accounts for 85–90 per cent of cases.
2. A small percentage of cases (less than 5 per cent) are iatrogenic (resulting from the accidental transmission of the causative agent via contaminated surgical equipment or as a result of cornea or dura mater transplants). It has also been shown that CJD can be transmitted to humans as a result of treatment with natural human growth hormone. Replacement of natural human growth hormone by recombinant growth hormone has alleviated this risk.

Variant Creutzfeldt-Jakob Disease

1. A newly recognised form of CJD, variant Creutzfeldt-Jakob disease (vCJD), was first reported in March 1996 in the UK (cf. WHO Fact Sheet N° 180 on variant Creutzfeldt-Jakob disease). In contrast to the classical forms of CJD, vCJD has affected younger patients (average age 29 years, as opposed to 65 years), has a relatively longer duration of illness (median of 14 months as opposed to 4.5 months) and is strongly linked to exposure, probably through food, to BSE. Recent studies have confirmed that vCJD is distinct from sporadic and acquired CJD.
2. From October 1996 to November 2002, 129 cases of vCJD have been reported in the UK, six in France and one each in Canada, Ireland, Italy and the United States of America. Insufficient information is available at present to make any precise prediction about the future number of vCJD cases.
3. Since few countries have surveillance systems, the geographical distribution of the incidence of vCJD needs to be better defined.
4. Similarities observed between the strain of the agent responsible for vCJD and those of BSE and closely related agents transmitted naturally and experimentally to different animal species, are consistent with the hypothesis discussed during two 1996 WHO consultations: that the cluster of vCJD cases is due to the same agent that caused BSE in cattle.

WHO and Recommendations to Reduce Exposure to the BSE Agent

1. All countries must prohibit the use of ruminant tissues in ruminant feed and must exclude tissues that are likely to contain the BSE agent from any animal or human food chain. BSE eradication was recommended during a WHO consultation held in December 1999.
2. All countries are encouraged to conduct risk assessments to determine if they are at risk for BSE in sheep and goats. It is advised that any tissue which may come from deer or elk with Chronic Wasting Disease (CWD, a transmissible spongiform disease of North American mule deer and elk) is not used in animal or human food; however, at this time there is no evidence to suggest that CWD in deer and elk can be transmitted to humans.

3. No infectivity has yet been detected in skeletal muscle tissue. Reassurance can be provided by removal of visible nervous and lymphatic tissue from meat (skeletal muscle).

4. Milk and milk products are considered safe. Tallow and gelatine are considered safe if prepared by a manufacturing process which has been shown experimentally to inactivate the transmissible agent and, if prepared from specifically identified tissues or from cattle without risk of exposure to BSE.

5. Human and veterinary vaccines prepared from bovine materials may carry the risk of transmission of animal TSE agents. The pharmaceutical industry should ideally avoid the use of bovine materials and materials from other animal species in which TSEs naturally occur. If absolutely necessary, bovine materials should be obtained from countries which have a surveillance system for BSE in place and which report either zero or only sporadic cases of BSE. These precautions apply to the manufacture of cosmetics as well.

CONTROL OF FOODBORNE VIRUSES

There are two main foodborne virus infections. These are viral gastroenteritis caused by small round structured viruses (SRSV) of the Norwalk group and hepatitis A. Both infections are normally transmitted directly from person-to-person, but on occasions they may also be foodborne or waterborne viruses do not multiply or produce toxins in foods, and foods merely act as vehicles for their passive transfer. Foods may be contaminated by infected food-handlers, and outbreaks frequently involve cold foods that require much handling during preparation. Foods may also be contaminated in their growing and harvesting areas by sewage polluted water, and molluscan shellfish have been particularly implicated. PCR and ELISA based methods are being developed for detection and typing of viruses in patients and also in food samples. Sensitive detection methods should facilitate the design of improved food processing methods to ensure virus-free food.

There are two main foodborne viral infections, namely viral gastroenteritis and hepatitis A. Foodborne incidents of viral gastroenteritis are nearly all caused by just one of the viruses, commonly known as small round structured viruses (SRSV) or Norwalk-like viruses. The other well-known gastroenteritis viruses, such as rotavirus and astrovirus, are only rarely implicated in foodborne outbreaks. Food and waterborne outbreaks of hepatitis A are infrequently reported. Both viral gastroenteritis and hepatitis A are most usually transmitted directly from person-to-person, and food or waterborne transmission appears to be responsible for only a small proportion of incidents.

Unlike bacteria, viruses do not multiply or produce toxins in foods. Food or water merely act as vehicles for their passive transfer. The true incidence of foodborne viral transmission is undetermined, but probably grossly under-reported. As a result of the rising numbers of food poisoning reports in recent years, the Advisory Committee on the Microbiological Safety of Food (ACMSF) was set-up. A report from this committee was published in 1998, identifying the problems associated with foodborne viral infections and areas of research required.

Routes of Contamination

Foods may be contaminated with viruses in two main ways. Firstly, they may be contaminated at source in their growing and harvesting areas, usually by coming into contact with polluted water. Shellfish have been a particular problem and have been implicated in many outbreaks worldwide. Secondly, foods may be contaminated during handling and preparation, often from infected food-handlers.

Shellfish

It is the bivalve molluscs—including oysters, mussels, clams and cockles—that are mainly involved in transmitting viral illness, and in fact most illness associated with these shellfish is viral. In the period 1992–1997, 42 outbreaks associated with consumption of oysters in England and Wales were reported to the PHLS Communicable Disease Surveillance Centre (CDSC). Of these, 17 outbreaks were caused by SRSV and one outbreak by an astrovirus.

The remaining 24 outbreaks were of unknown aetiology, but mostly had the characteristic features of viral gastroenteritis. Of 119 oyster-associated outbreaks reported since 1982, only two are known to have been caused by a bacterial pathogen.

The bivalve molluscs live in shallow, coastal and estuarine waters which are frequently polluted with sewage. They feed by filtering particulate matter from the large volumes of water passing over their gills, and this can include potentially pathogenic micro-organisms. Although human viruses do not replicate in shellfish, they can be concentrated within the molluscs to higher concentrations than occur within the surrounding water up to 100-fold. Cockles, mussels and clams are only lightly cooked and frequently oysters are consumed raw.

Fruit and vegetables

There is the potential for fruits, vegetables and salad items to be contaminated with polluted water and sewage sludge during irrigation and fertilisation. Although several outbreaks of viral gastroenteritis have been attributed to salad items, contamination on these occasions is usually thought to have occurred at the time of preparation.

Soft fruits believed to have been contaminated at their source, have been implicated in outbreaks of hepatitis A, and there has been one report of viral gastroenteritis due to SRSV and associated with raspberries affecting 300 people in Canada in 1997.

Food-handlers

Viruses causing gastroenteritis and hepatitis A are infectious in very low doses, and thus are spread very easily from infected persons. It is now recognised that outbreaks arising from food contamination by infected food handlers are common occurrences. Cold items, such as sandwiches and salads that require much handling during preparation, are implicated most frequently. Without meticulous attention to personal hygiene and thorough and frequent hand-washing, faecally-contaminated fingers can contaminate food and work surfaces.

Viral Gastroenteritis

Viral gastroenteritis is usually regarded as a mild, self-limiting illness lasting 24–48 hr. Symptoms commonly include malaise, abdominal pain, pyrexia, diarrhoea and/or vomiting. Onset may be sudden and commence with projectile vomiting. This is a particular hazard where food is being prepared and laid out, as virus can be disseminated over a wide area in aerosol droplets. The viruses are usually transmitted from person-to-person via the faecal-oral route, but may also be spread by contaminated food and water causing common source outbreaks. Viruses account for 6 per cent of foodborne outbreaks and 5 per cent of waterborne outbreaks occurring in England and Wales and reported to CDSC. Secondary person-to-person transmission to close contacts is a characteristic feature of foodborne and waterborne virus outbreaks. Several different types of viruses cause gastroenteritis: the most important include rota virus, SRSV or Norwalk group viruses, astrovirus and adenovirus types 40 and 41. However, in almost all foodborne outbreaks, where a virus is identified it is an SRSV. Rotavirus and astrovirus are only rarely implicated. Adenovirus has not been associated with food or waterborne transmission.

Small round structured viruses

This group of viruses infects all age groups. There is a variable incubation period from about 12–60 hr. It occurs all year round, although in temperate climates, most infections occur over the winter months. These viruses are responsible for both sporadic cases of gastroenteritis in the community and for outbreaks in schools, hospitals, old peoples' homes, hotels and cruise ships.

SRSVs cannot be cultured and until recently detection relied on electron microscopy. This is a time-consuming technique and is not conducive to examining large numbers of specimens. It is also insensitive: it cannot be used for examining food samples and usually virus can only be detected in clinical samples if collected within 48 hr of onset of symptoms. More recently, methods of detection have been developed based on PCR assays. Virus can be detected for up to a week after onset in patients, although it is not clear whether this is infectious virus. PCR assays are sensitive enough to detect virus in shellfish, environmental samples and other foods. Such tests are only available in specialised laboratories at present and cannot be used for routine testing of food samples. There is great diversity within the SRSV group and current PCR tests do not detect all strains. Hence, electron microscopy is still necessary for the investigation of some outbreaks.

The SRSVs form a complex group of viruses. They have formally been classified with the *Caliciviridae* and now are often referred to as human caliciviruses. They are split into three broad genogroups. Two groups have the morphology of SRSVs and the third group has the classical morphology of a calicivirus and a genomic arrangement distinct from the other two groups. There are several serotypes which broadly correspond with the genotypic groups. Immunity is complex and short-lived. Persons can be infected repeatedly with the same strain. The incidence is grossly under-reported, partly due to the mild nature of the infection and partly from the difficulty in detecting and identifying the virus (Table 22.1).

Table 22.1. Under-reporting of foodborne virus outbreaks.

SRSV	Short incubation period of 12–60 hr. But mild illness—hence not reported virus only readily detected for 48 hr from onset.
Hepatitis A	Incubation period 3–6 weeks hence difficult to identify food source.

Viral antigen has been produced by expression of virus capsids in insect cells or yeast cells, and is providing material for development of ELISA-based detection tests. However, these only select for a very few strains and are not available for routine use at present.

Rotavirus

Rotaviruses mainly infect young children. It is estimated that they may cause 1 million deaths a year in children under 5 years of age, mostly in nonindustrialised countries. In industrialised countries deaths are relatively rare, but rotavirus gastroenteritis is the most frequent reason for admission of young children to hospital. Foodborne and particularly waterborne spread are probably a significant mode of transmission in nonindustrialised countries, but in industrialised countries reports are rare. Although rotavirus has been detected in shellfish, so far there have been no reports of illness from this source.

Astrovirus

The astroviruses form a morphologically distinct group of viruses, and are named from the five or six point star seen by electron microscopy on the surface of some particles. Astroviruses are normally associated with gastroenteritis in young children, often under 1 year of age. Adults are infected infrequently, although outbreaks have been reported in the elderly. Astroviruses have been seen in some adults following the consumption of shellfish or contaminated water, but these incidents appear comparatively rare.

Parvovirus

Small round viruses measuring 20–26 nm in diameter and with the characteristics of parvoviruses have been observed in outbreaks of gastroenteritis, but their role as causative agents in humans remains uncertain. Parvoviruses do cause other illnesses in humans and are an important causes of gastroenteritis in some animal species. Parvoviruses have been observed in school outbreaks of winter vomiting disease and in a number of outbreaks associated with the consumption of shellfish. Parvovirus-like particles have been detected occasionally in shellfish that have been implicated in illness and where similar virus has been found in patients. Reports of parvovirus in association with gastroenteritis are infrequent and there have been few studies on the nature and role of these viruses.

Hepatitis

There are two types of enterically transmitted hepatitis—hepatitis A and hepatitis E.

Hepatitis A

Food and waterborne outbreaks of hepatitis A have been recognised for over 40 years, but are infrequently reported. Between 1992 and 1997, 228 outbreaks occurring in England and Wales were reported to CDSC, but only one of these was known to be foodborne. That outbreak was associated with shellfish. The incubation period is 2–6 weeks making it difficult to associate the source of infection with a particular food item or even recognise an outbreak (Table 22.1). Like viral gastroenteritis, transmission is via the faecal-oral route, although with hepatitis the main site of viral replication is the liver.

The epidemiology of food-borne hepatitis A is similar to that of viral gastroenteritis. Contaminated shellfish have been the cause of many outbreaks worldwide. In one notable outbreak in Shanghai in 1988, over 3,00,000 people were infected after eating inadequately cooked clams. Cases of viral gastroenteritis were also reported in the proceeding month indicating the gross sewage pollution of the shellfish waters. Outbreaks are not just confined to nonindustrialised countries, but also continue to be reported from Europe, North America and Australia. Soft fruits, particularly strawberries and raspberries, and lettuce contaminated at source have been implicated in outbreaks. Some outbreaks have originated from infected food-handlers. Virus excretion may commence up to a week before symptoms are apparent, making control difficult.

There is only one serotype of hepatitis A. Once infected immunity is life-long. An effective vaccine is available, but is not used widely. Incidence in industrialised countries has fallen in recent years and hence a susceptible population has built up. As endemic infection declines, it is possible that an increase in foodborne outbreaks will be seen.

Hepatitis E

Hepatitis E, has been associated with large waterborne outbreaks in some nonindustrialised countries, notably in Asia, Africa and Central America. Foodborne transmission has been suggested, but not proved conclusively. Illness appears more severe than hepatitis A, particularly in pregnant women where a death rate of 17–33 per cent has been observed. Secondary person-to-person transmission is estimated at only 0.7–8 per cent. The primary source of infection appears to be contaminated water rather than person-to-person spread. Hence, control should be directed at improving the quality of water supplies. Cases in the UK are reported infrequently and are mainly imported from endemic areas.

Tickborne Encephalitis

Tickborne encephalitis is possibly the only known viral zoonosis that is transmitted via food. It occurs in Eastern Europe. Goats, sheep and cattle bitten by infected ticks become infected with the virus which is then shed in their milk. Outbreaks have occurred from the consumption of raw milk or products made from unpasteurised milk. These incidents are fortunately rare, because of the limited distribution of the appropriate ticks.

Virus Survival

Gastroenteritis viruses and hepatitis viruses survive extremely well in the environment. There is little precise information on the stability of SRSVs since they cannot be cultured. Most information comes from epidemiological observations and limited studies of infectivity in volunteers. Some strains of hepatitis A and rotavirus have been cultured in the laboratory and there have been a small number of experimental studies on their stability. Of all the enteric viruses, however, SRSVs and hepatitis A virus seem to be the most resistant to inactivation. Observations and studies on readily culturable enteroviruses, such as poliovirus and Coxsackie viruses cannot be used to predict the survival of SRSV or hepatitis A virus.

Viruses that infect via the gastrointestinal tract are acid stable. Hence they survive food processing and preservation conditions designed to produce the low pH that inhibits bacterial and fungal spoilage organisms (e.g. pickling in vinegar and fermentation processes that produce foods such as yoghurt). Outbreaks of viral gastroenteritis have been associated with cockles pickled in brine and vinegar. Both SRSVs and hepatitis A virus retain infectivity after exposure to acidity levels below pH 3.

Most viruses remain infectious after refrigeration and freezing. Frozen foods that have not received further cooking have been implicated in a number of incidents of both viral gastroenteritis and hepatitis A. Gastroenteritis viruses and hepatitis viruses are inactivated by normal cooking processes, but are not always inactivated in shellfish given only minimal heat treatment. Both SRSVs and hepatitis A virus retain infectivity after heating to 60°C for 30 min. It is uncertain that they would be inactivated completely in many pasteurisation processes. These viruses survive on inanimate surfaces, on hands and in dried faecal suspensions. Lingering outbreaks have occurred in hospitals, in residential homes and on cruise ships, probably as a result of environmental contamination. SRSVs have been detected by PCR in environmental swabs from hospital lockers and hotel carpets supposedly cleaned after incidents of vomiting.

There are conflicting reports on the effectiveness of disinfectants. Chlorine-based disinfectants are usually considered the most effective against enteric viruses. However, SRSVs and hepatitis A appear resistant to levels of chlorine present in drinking water, equivalent to free residual chlorine of 0.5–1 mg/l. SRSVs are inactivated by 10 mg chlorine/l, which is the concentration used to treat a water supply after a contamination incident. In the US, a level of 5 mg chlorine/l with a contact time of 1 min. is recommended for inactivation of hepatitis A. Sodium hypochlorite, 2 per cent glutaraldehyde and quarternary ammonium compounds with hydrochloric acid have been shown to reduce the infectivity of hepatitis A virus, but there are no comparative data for SRSVs. Clearly, there is a need for further studies on disinfection of these persistent organisms.

Control

A major factor in the contamination of food and water is sewage pollution. Ideally, there would be no sewage discharge into the coastal waters and rivers, thus preventing contamination of shellfish growing areas. Sewage sludge is applied to agricultural land, with the benefit that useful plant nutrients and organic matter are recycled to the soil. The UK government is proposing more stringent controls for harvesting vegetables from land where conventionally processed sewage sludge is applied and that spread of untreated sewage sludge on agricultural land should cease at the earliest. Viruses from sewage deposited on land do not bind with soil particles and can enter groundwaters, leading to contamination of water sources. Hepatitis A virus has been recovered from a groundwater source associated with an outbreak.

Shellfish

Pollution of coastal waters is unfortunately a reality, and shellfish harvested from all but the cleanest waters are required to undergo treatment as laid down in the European Union Directive on Shellfish Hygiene.

Some molluscs, such as cockles, are subject to a brief heat treatment by boiling or steaming. Thorough cooking will destroy contaminating viruses, but also cause shrinkage of the shellfish meat rendering it tough and unpalatable. Many outbreaks have resulted from consumption of inadequately cooked shellfish. Heat treatment studies in the UK led to recommendations, in 1988, that the internal temperature of shellfish meat should be raised to 90°C and be maintained for 1.5 min. These conditions are known to inactivate hepatitis A virus, but still achieve a commercially acceptable product. Continued surveillance has shown that there have been no recorded incidents of viral illness—either hepatitis A or viral gastroenteritis—from shellfish treated according to these recommendations. More recent laboratory studies have indicated that these conditions will also readily inactivate SRSVs.

Some shellfish taken from polluted water are treated by relaying and depuration. This particularly applies to oysters that may be eaten raw. Relaying involves moving shellfish from their original growing site to an area of cleaner water, where they are left for several weeks or months. The level of microbial contamination in the shellfish falls as micro-organisms are washed out during the normal feeding process. Depuration depends on the same principle, but the shellfish are placed in land-based tanks, usually for about 48 hr. *Escherichia coli,* the usual indicator of contamination, is virtually eliminated during this period, but viruses can remain for several weeks. There is no guarantee that shellfish that appear safe in bacteriological tests are necessarily free of viruses and, at present, there is no satisfactorily indicator system for viruses.

Detection of viruses in shellfish is technically difficult. Extraction of infectious virus or viral RNA is a complex and unreliable procedure. SRSVs and hepatitis A virus have been detected in shellfish implicated in outbreaks or harvested from polluted beds, but routine testing for viruses in shellfish is not feasible.

Food-handlers

The other major source of contamination is from infected persons handling and preparing food. Persons with symptoms should be excluded from food handling. However, food-handlers with only very minimal symptoms have been implicated in transmission of SRSVs. Recommendations that food-handlers should be allowed to return to work 48 hr after symptoms have ceased appear to work satisfactorily. These recommendations were based on the rapid decrease in virus excretion observed by electron microscopy. Using more sensitive PCR assays, SRSVs can be detected for longer periods than by electron microscopy and, in some instances, for up to a week after onset of symptoms. It is not clear if persons shedding virus detectable by PCR are infectious, but recommendations on how long to exclude people from work needs to be kept under review.

If vomiting occurs, virus can be spread over a wide area in aerosol droplets. Uncovered food, that is not to receive further cooking, should be discarded. The environment should be thoroughly cleaned, including work surfaces, sinks and door handles.

Control of food-borne viral illness largely depends on strict attention to normal good hygienic practice in the kitchen and serving areas. Salad items, fruits and raw vegetables should be washed thoroughly. Cross contamination from uncooked shellfish should be regarded as a potential hazard.

The Future

The key element in reducing foodborne spread of viruses is continued surveillance and awareness. Meticulous attention to good food-handling practices and education, to prevent people with even the mildest symptoms handling food, is essential. Development of sensitive and easily used detection tests are required for estimating the extent of foodborne viral infections and their control.

Sensitive detection tests will give more accurate estimates on the length of time a person excretes virus and hence better informed advice can be formulated on factors such as how long food-handlers should be excluded from work.

Expression of recombinant virus capsids in yeast and insect cells has the potential to provide large quantities of noninfectious viral antigen. These antigens are already being used in a few laboratories for the development of ELISA-based diagnostic assays and commercial kits for detecting a wide range of SRSVs are already being evaluated. It is likely that user-friendly diagnostic tests for specimens from patients soon will be widely available. Routine detection of virus contaminants in foods is more difficult. Current methods for extraction of viruses from shellfish are inefficient and unsatisfactory. Extraction of viruses from other types of food, where there is just surface contamination, does not present such a challenge, but the number of virus particles present in food, as compared to specimens from patients, is very low and available detection tests may not always be sufficiently sensitive.

Recombinant capsid proteins provide a relatively safe, noninfectious source of viral antigens. These antigens could be used for assessing and improving food-processing methods including depuration conditions for shellfish. They could also be used, for instance, in assessing the efficacy of washing salads, vegetables and fruit for the ready-to-eat market. Vaccine for hepatitis A is already available and consideration is being given to licensing of rotavirus vaccines. No vaccines have been developed for SRSVs. Recombinant capsid antigens of SRSVs expressed by baculovirus or yeast cells can be purified in large quantities. They are highly immunogenic and stable at low pH, which offers the potential for development of vaccines. Studies to express SRSV capsid antigens in transgenic plants, such as tobacco leaves and potato tubers, are underway. It has been shown that these antigens are immunogenic in mice, thus offering further potential for the development of oral vaccines.

Chapter 23

Investigation of Foodborne Disease Outbreaks

INTRODUCTION

The investigation and control of foodborne disease outbreaks are multi-disciplinary tasks requiring skills in the areas of clinical medicine, epidemiology, laboratory medicine, food microbiology and chemistry, food safety and food control, and risk communication and management. Many outbreaks of foodborne disease are poorly investigated, if at all, because these skills are unavailable or because a field investigator is expected to master them all single-handedly without having been trained.

These guidelines have been written for public health practitioners, food and health inspectors, district and national medical officers, laboratory personnel and others who may undertake or participate in the investigation and control of foodborne disease outbreaks.

While the chapter focuses on practical aspects of outbreak investigation and control, it also provides generic guidance that can be adapted to individual countries and local requirements. At the field level it will be valuable in initial epidemiological, environmental and laboratory investigations, in implementation of appropriate control measures, and in alerting investigators to the need to seek assistance for more complex situations. At national and regional levels, the guidelines will assist decision-makers in identifying and coordinating resources and in creating an environment appropriate for the successful management of foodborne disease outbreaks.

Despite a clear focus on foodborne diseases, much of the material in these guidelines is also applicable to the investigation of outbreaks of other communicable and noncommunicable diseases.

PRACTICAL GUIDE

This practical guide summarises the steps that may be required during an outbreak investigation and which are dealt with in more detail in the subsequent sections. The purpose of this summary is to give a brief overview of the investigatory steps required and may serve as checklist. It is recognised that not all settings where outbreaks occur will have the necessary infrastructure to complete all steps described but efforts should be made to do so. The steps are presented in approximately chronological order but different situations will demand changes from this order. In practice, some steps will be carried out simultaneously, others will be required throughout the whole process while some may not be required at all.

Preliminary Assessment of the Situation

1. Consider whether or not the cases have the same illness (or different manifestations of the same disease).

2. Determine whether there is a real outbreak by assessing the normal background activity of disease.
3. Conduct in-depth interviews with initial cases.
4. Collect clinical specimens from cases.
5. Identify factors common to all or most cases.
6. Conduct site investigation at implicated premises.
7. Collect food specimens when appropriate.
8. Formulate preliminary hypotheses.
9. Initiate control measures as appropriate.
10. Decide whether to convene a formal outbreak control team.
11. Make a decision about the need for further investigation.

Communication

1. Consider the best routes of communication with colleagues, patients and the public.
2. Ensure accuracy and timeliness. Include all those who need to know.
3. Use mass media constructively.

Descriptive Epidemiology

1. Establish case definitions for confirmed and probable cases.
2. Identify as many cases as possible.
3. Collect data from affected persons on a standardised questionnaire.
4. Categorise cases by time, place and person.
5. Determine who is at risk of becoming ill.
6. Calculate attack rates.

GUIDELINES FOR REPORTING SUSPECTED OUTBREAK-RELATED ILLNESSES

If an individual is suspected of having a foodborne illness, the health care provider should:

1. Collect clinical samples for laboratory analysis: (stool specimens from up to 10 persons in a suspected outbreak can be tested). If suspected food item(s) are available, instruct the individual not to ingest or discard food, but to keep it refrigerated. Arrangements will be made to collect and analyse the food samples pending further investigation. Arrangements must be made for the Local Health Department (LHD) to collect and hold the food items under refrigeration. Questions regarding sample collecting/testing of food samples should be directed to the approved laboratory.
2. Inquire whether there are other ill persons.
3. Immediately contact the communicable disease epidemiology section.

Please provide the following information:

1. Brief description of situation.
2. Names of ill persons.
3. Address, telephone number.
4. Age, sex.
5. Onset of symptoms (date, time).
6. Description of symptoms.
7. Hospitalisation status.

8. Other available information (other ill persons, possible food sources, etc.).
9. Name of physician (if different than reporter), address, telephone number.

Roles and Responsibilities

Food worker

1. Maintain good personal hygiene, including frequent and thorough hand washing practices.
2. Practice good food handling procedures.
3. Notify employers of illness, and exclude self from work when ill with gastrointestinal symptoms (e.g. abdominal cramping, vomiting, diarrhea, jaundice), optimally for 48–72 hours following resolution of symptoms. This may also apply when the food worker has exposed skin lesions.
4. Fully cooperate with LHD during investigations of foodborne illness.

Food establishment licensee

1. Train employees and management as to proper food handling practices and hand washing.
2. Exclude employees with apparent gastrointestinal illness or exposed skin lesions from work.
3. Avoid practices that punish or discourage employees from reporting illness.
4. Cooperate with LHDs during investigations of foodborne illness.
5. Provide adequate toilet and hand washing facilities for employees and ensure proper use.

Physicians, health care providers

1. Report to LHD by telephone immediately upon recognition of a suspected outbreaks. Although not required by law, the physician should consider contacting the LHD regarding any person with a communicable enteric disease that they know works as a food worker.
2. Cooperate with LHD in the investigation and control of an outbreak, including collecting specimens if requested.
3. Encourage patients to adhere to the prevention and control recommendations of the LHD.

Local health department

1. Conduct the initial investigation of a suspected outbreak. The investigation should be directed by the LHD in whose jurisdiction the outbreak originated.
2. Provide direction to food establishment operators regarding the application and removal of food employee exclusions and restrictions.
3. Immediately notify the CDES and/or LHS&EMS Regional Office of any outbreak as early in the investigation as possible.
4. Request assistance of the CDES and/or LHS&EMS Regional Office, if needed, to control the spread of the outbreak.
5. Obtain clinical and environmental specimens, conduct interviews, compile line lists, record onset times and other important epidemiologic data.
6. Provide education to food workers regarding proper food handling and personal hygiene.
7. Complete a foodborne or waterborne outbreak report and mail a copy to CDES (This may be done in conjunction with the CDES).
8. Maintain an ongoing foodborne disease complaint file or log.
9. Assume costs of the investigation. BCDP will cover expenses incurred by CDES staff when on-site.

Bureau of local health support and emergency medical services — regional office director and staff

1. Provide assistance in coordinating outbreak investigations (especially those involving multiple jurisdictions) and ensure the involvement of all appropriate local agencies.
2. Provide consultation and obtain appropriate technical assistance for the LHD in epidemiologic investigation of disease outbreaks.
3. Assign appropriate regional staff (e.g. public health nurses, sanitarians, nutritionists, educators, regional staff) to participate in investigations, as needed.
4. Notify CDES of all investigations, and other agencies as necessary.
5. Assist the LHDs in completing outbreak investigations, initiating control measures, and submitting the DPH and/or CDC report forms to CDES.

Regional public health sanitarian or agency sanitarian

1. Coordinate environmental investigation with epidemiologic investigations being conducted by LHDs.
2. Inspect establishment and enforce rules pertaining to the regulation of hotels, tourist rooming houses, bed and breakfast establishments, restaurants, food and beverage machines, vending commissaries, campgrounds, public swimming pools, recreational and educational camps.
3. Conduct or direct a complete sanitation investigation of the facility or site of a suspected outbreak. Do a Hazard Analysis and Critical Control Points (HACCP) investigation for implicated food(s).
4. Collect food, water, and other specimens as needed.
5. Consult and participate (as needed) in investigations of outbreaks not specifically involving licensed facilities or sites.
6. Send copy of the sanitarian's inspection report and narrative of inspection to LHD and CDES.

Bureau of communicable diseases and preparedness/communicable disease epidemiology section

1. Provide consultation and technical assistance to regional office staff and LHD staff in the epidemiologic investigation of disease outbreaks.
2. Provide guidelines for the epidemiologic investigation and control of a specific outbreak consistent with state and national objectives, current policy, and current medical and scientific literature.
3. Determine whether a particular outbreak warrants further epidemiologic investigation and the nature and extent of additional epidemiologic or laboratory data required.
4. Keep BEOH and regional offices informed of the progress of any outbreak investigation.
5. Identify and arrange for additional staff and material resources from the BCDP if an outbreak exceeds the resource capacity of the LHD and the regional office.
6. Provide advice on collection of food, water or other specimens in coordination with WSLH and/or DATCP/BLS.
7. Recommend and request implementation of control measures.
8. Maintain and distribute surveillance information and summary reports relating to outbreaks to LHDs, regional offices, physicians and other agencies.
9. Provide training materials instructive in the methods of outbreak investigations.

Bureau of environmental and occupational health

1. Provide technical assistance, training and support to regional offices and agent health departments, when requested, regarding the investigation and follow-up of outbreaks related to the above-mentioned licensed establishments.
2. Contract with LHD agents to provide investigation services for the above-mentioned establishments and facilities within their jurisdiction.

Bureau of quality assurance

1. Conduct surveys and complaint-related investigations of nursing homes, general and special hospitals, home health agencies and other health care providers to determine compliance with state licensure rules.
2. Conduct epidemiologic investigations, in cooperation with the LHD, at a health care facility when an outbreak is suspected to determine the cause and prevent further infections.
3. Evaluate the facility's infection control techniques, food handling techniques, communicable disease-related procedures and communicable diseases reporting to assure that the measures comply with appropriate state and federal regulations and are properly implemented.
4. Take enforcement actions in the event the facility fails to comply with appropriate rules, regulations and procedures.

Steps in Investigating an Outbreak

Prompt response to food or water-related complaints is the foundation of a successful investigation. Important steps and information necessary to determine the initiation and extent of an investigation include examination of test results and preliminary evidence such as onset times, symptoms and duration of illness, development of hypotheses, assessment of the magnitude of the problem, and evaluation of available resources.

Once an outbreak has been identified, immediately notify the CDES and/or the BLHS&EMS Regional Office, especially if there are cases from outside the jurisdiction of the LHD. These offices may assist in coordinating the investigation, assist in the investigation if requested by the LHD, and can be consulted on collection of food, clinical, or environmental specimens. The procedure for the investigation and determination of the existence of an outbreak is reasonably standard regardless of the disease being investigated. The steps listed below are not sequential and some contingency planning can be done before an outbreak. The steps in this procedure include:

1. Preparation for a detailed epidemiologic investigation.
2. Establish the existence of an outbreak or epidemic.
3. Verify diagnosis.
4. Formulate a tentative hypothesis.
5. Put control measures into operation.
6. Conduct the investigation.
7. Relate the outbreak to time, place and person.
8. Analyse and interpret data.
9. Test hypothesis and formulate conclusions.
10. Prepare a final report of the investigation.

Preparation for a detailed epidemiologic investigation

Although the steps in investigating an outbreak are not always implemented sequentially, planning an epidemiologic investigation may be considered as the initial step in the process because part of the planning can be done before an outbreak occurs. The LHD can begin by training personnel in how to compile line lists, develop questionnaires, conduct interviews, and use EPI-INFO. The LHD should have 6–8 stool culture kits on hand or readily available should an outbreak occur because in most cases stool specimens must be collected within 72 hours of onset of illness to isolate and identify certain pathogens (e.g. *Clostridium perfringens, Bacillus cereus, Staphylococcus aureus*). Lists of contacts such as administrative contacts, additional personnel, sanitarians, regional contacts, physicians, clinical laboratories or other persons who may become involved in outbreak investigations should be assembled. Resource materials describing signs and symptoms, incubation times and specifics regarding specimen collection and appropriate kits to be used should be maintained and readily available to those processing the initial calls. This may help in formulating an initial hypothesis. It is also very important for the LHD to realise in advance the limits of the LHD's resources. It is critical to determine at the beginning of an outbreak investigation whether the LHD has the resources to properly conduct the investigation. If an outbreak investigation requires additional resources, they should immediately notify the CDES and/or the regional office.

Once the investigation is underway, the proper clinical specimens should be collected as soon as possible before patients recover and become less likely to submit specimens, and before the general interest in the investigation wanes. All suspected outbreaks should be examined and a determination made regarding the feasibility of conducting an investigation even if the time to collect proper clinical specimens has passed. This is done in order to determine the source of the outbreak and to prevent similar outbreaks from recurring.

Establish the existence of an outbreak or epidemic

Establish the existence of an outbreak by comparing the incidence of the disease in a specified population during a comparable previous time period or when point source outbreaks occur. Be familiar with disease trends in the community and determine whether there actually is a higher than expected number of cases in a community. This can be done through diligent public health surveillance that provides an accurate assessment of the status of the health of the community and helps to determine any increases or decreases in communicable diseases in the local population. Surveillance data should be reviewed by the LHD on a regular basis to become familiar with the status of all communicable diseases in the area of jurisdiction. Be aware of artificial causes of increases such as: (i) changes in local reporting, (ii) changes in case definitions of reportable diseases, (iii) increased local or national interest in particular diseases, (iv) new physicians in the area, (v) new diagnostic procedures which might identify new or existing infectious agents, and (vi) increased populations or new arrivals into the area.

Verify diagnosis

Analyse clinical histories of cases and have laboratory tests performed in order to confirm the etiologic agent associated with the illness. Clinical, laboratory and epidemiologic evidence should be considered. Verify that laboratory results are consistent with the clinical evidence as laboratory errors sometimes occur. In verifying the diagnosis, it is crucial to collect clinical and environmental samples as soon as possible because many etiologic agents become more difficult to isolate with time (e.g., *Bacillus cereus, Clostridium perfringens, Staphylococcus aureus*). As case-patients begin to recover they may become more reluctant to submit clinical samples. Also, when delay occurs, environmental samples are more likely to be discarded or disinfected.

Formulate a tentative hypothesis

Formulate a tentative hypothesis to explain the most likely cause of illness, etiologic agent, vehicle, and distribution of cases. Hypothesis generating is an ongoing process. It may begin with the first phone call. This hypothesis may be based on known incubation periods, symptoms, duration of illness or foods eaten, as well as knowledge about the various agents responsible for outbreaks. The tentative hypothesis directs the course of an investigation and control measures, and is tested by data gathered during the investigation. Develop several hypotheses if necessary. A series of hypotheses may evolve during an investigation. First, facts are examined and broad hypotheses are formulated. As more facts are gathered, a more specific hypothesis may be formulated. Confirm the diagnosis if laboratory testing has been completed. Examine case histories to determine if there are common exposures, or if signs and symptoms and onset of illness are consistent with etiologic agents. Next, additional facts to test the new hypothesis are gathered. The cycle is continued as necessary. Consult the CDES if your LHD needs assistance generating hypotheses.

Put control measures into operation

The priority during each investigation should be to implement effective control measures. This should be done early in the course of the investigation based on the initial hypotheses. Factors to consider when determining the most effective control measures include the extent of the illness, who was affected, when and where did the critical exposure take place, what was the vehicle, how was the disease transmitted, what is the etiologic agent and whether or not there is a potential for ongoing or future transmission. Control measures should focus on specific agents, sources or reservoirs of infection and should be targeted to interrupt the transmission of disease or reduce exposure to disease. These measures should be instituted as soon as possible to control the current problem and demonstrate to the community that efforts are being made to control the problem. Use the information collected during the investigation to control the current situation and to prevent future problems in the community.

Conduct the investigation

1. Prepare a line list of ill persons listing signs, symptoms, onset times, duration of illness.
2. Gather appropriate community and environmental information; investigate potential sources of the responsible agent and factors that may have contributed to the outbreak.
3. Obtain clinical specimens (usually stool specimens) from up to 10 ill case patients for laboratory analysis of enteric pathogens.
4. When possible, obtain samples of implicated food or environmental samples for laboratory analysis. Hold these samples under refrigeration until a known etiologic agent has been identified.

Relate the outbreak to time, place and person

If an outbreak occurs following a common meal or exposure (e.g. wedding, parties), conduct a survey of known cases to investigate commonalties, such as onset of illness (time), population characteristics (e.g. age, gender) (person) and where they could have been infected or exposed (place). If an outbreak does not have an established common meal or exposure (e.g. an increase of cases of illness in a community within a close time frame), it may be necessary to start with an informational or a more general survey in order to select case patients. Develop a questionnaire and perform a case-control study or cohort study. It is imperative to interview non-ill (control) persons who are similar or had similar experiences regarding time and place to those ill. Obtain identifying information (name, address, telephone number, etc.); demographic information (age, sex, race, occupation or group characteristics); and clinical information (symptoms, onset times, and duration of illness).

Analyse and interpret data

Summarise field investigations. Compare and interpret all information collected and results of tests conducted. Construct epidemic curves to detect the course of the outbreak and to determine if the illness originated from a single source or is on going, calculate attack rates, develop appropriate tables and charts, apply statistical tests (EPI-INFO software) and interpret the cumulative data. Define the geographic extent of the outbreak and the population at risk.

Test hypothesis and formulate conclusions

Accept or reject the hypothesis on the basis of the available data and appropriate statistical analysis. For a hypothesis to be accepted, the patterns of disease must fit the nature of the agent, its source, its mode of transmission, and the contributory factors that allowed the outbreak to occur. If the hypothesis is rejected, another hypothesis should be developed and additional data gathered in order to test this new hypothesis. A more systematic study can be conducted as needed to improve the sensitivity and specificity of the findings, establish the true number of cases, and assist in arriving at more definitive conclusions.

Prepare a final report of the investigation

Investigations should be summarised as soon as completed and a final report sent to the CDES. These can also be done with the assistance of the CDES. These final reports serve as a record of the rationale and provide documentation for the activities conducted during the investigation. The final report can also be used to improve future investigations and prevention measures. The report should follow the usual scientific format of introduction, background, methods, results, discussion, references and recommendations. Do not use the names of case-patients. The names of LHD personnel or authorised personnel involved in the investigation may be included. The names of facilities or locations where the outbreak occurred may be included at the discretion of the LHD.

The background is a short paragraph describing why the outbreak investigation was initiated and may include who was affected, how many people were ill and how many exposed, where the outbreak occurred, the severity and clinical presentation of the cases. Note whether or not the outbreak involved a particular setting or social event (e.g. school, restaurant, wedding, festival) or to particular population (e.g. nursing home, day care center).

The methods section should list how cases were identified, how questionnaires were developed, methods used to collect data, as well as clinical and environmental samples, laboratory tests performed, statistical methods (e.g. EPI-INFO software), control methods instituted, and other features of the investigations used during the outbreak investigation.

The results section should list what was discovered in the investigation, results of laboratory testing of clinical or environmental samples, results of the epidemiologic investigation, the sanitarian's report, statistical results, epi-curves, tables, charts and other studies used during the investigation.

The discussion should briefly summarise the findings of the investigation. Evaluate the control and methods used in the investigation. Were they successful? Could they be instituted in similar outbreaks in the future or how should they be changed? What problems were encountered by the LHD? Is the current surveillance program sufficient to identify and control future outbreaks? List any important or unique aspects of the outbreak or a specific disease agent uncovered during the investigation.

Collection of clinical samples

One of the most important factors in the identification of etiologic agents responsible for foodborne or waterborne disease outbreaks is the collection of clinical samples as early in the course of the investigation as possible. This is especially true for those agents that may only be shed for several days such as *Clostridium perfringens*, *Bacillus cereus* or *Staphylococcus aureus*. The LHD should provide the CDES with a name for the outbreak (preceded by the county name) so that all associated clinical and environmental samples can be identified and located under the same identifying name. It is also important for the laboratory to be notified about these specimens as early as possible because several of these agents require special plating media that may need to be ordered before the samples reach the laboratory.

Clinical samples

Collect clinical specimens (usually stools) from up to 10 ill cases for laboratory analysis of enteric bacteria and viral pathogens. The amount of sample required for bacterial and viral testing is less than for parasites. For parasite testing a walnut-sized portion of stool is submitted in formalin. For bacterial and norovirus testing, about 15 ml of stool in a Kit #10 will suffice. Do not overfill and follow the directions on the specimen container. Rectal swabs are not preferred.

COLLECTION AND HANDLING OF FOOD SAMPLES

Food Sampling

1. Food specimens are tested only after a foodborne pathogen has been isolated or its toxin identified from clinical patient specimens. However, suspected foods should be collected by the LHD as early in the investigation as possible. Foods should be refrigerated, not frozen. If the food item was already frozen, hold it in the freezer until a determination can be made about testing. Freezing causes significant loss of viability for certain organisms.

2. If available, the sanitarian or LHD staff should obtain a sample of the implicated food(s). If none is available, obtain an associated sample (same lot or batch).

3. If the volume of the implicated food sample is less than 200 grams (1/2 lb.), the whole sample should be collected and submitted in its original container. (Be sure that the container is leakproof!). If the volume of sample is greater than 200 grams, obtain a 200 gram sample. Sampling should be representative (i.e. taken from food throughout the sample, not just one portion of the sample).

4. Samples should be labelled with the name of the outbreak or establishment where the sample was collected, type of specimen, time and date of collection, a unique sample number and the investigating official's initials. All food samples should be held under refrigeration until clinical specimens have been tested. If clinical samples on case patients are negative or not tested, food samples are not tested unless there is compelling epidemiologic evidence incriminating a particular food item. Laboratory procedures for the isolation of microbial foodborne disease agents are complicated and time consuming. It is important the laboratory has good epidemiologic information before analysing food samples to insure a proper analysis.

5. If the sample being submitted is a commercial food, the name of the manufacturer or processor, code or lot number, and other identifying characteristics are important. If still available, it is important to submit the original food container.
6. If a clinical specimen from at least one ill individual is positive for a foodborne pathogen, food samples should then be transported to the laboratory on ice or under refrigeration as rapidly as possible in order to maintain the population of organisms present.
7. If food kit #32 is not available, an insulated container with frozen kool-pacs or ice cans should be used when shipping samples to the laboratory.

Laboratory Testing and Interpretation

1. With some microbial agents of foodborne disease, it is necessary that large numbers of the organisms be present in a food for it to be hazardous. Examples of these agents would be: *Bacillus cereus*, *Clostridium perfringens* and *Staphylococcus aureus*. Usually 10^6 organisms per gram of food are necessary before there is a danger of food poisoning from these agents. For these kinds of agents the laboratory reports the number of organisms present per gram of food, and whether or not this would be considered a significant level. If *S. aureus* is identified, the laboratory will also examine the isolates for enterotoxin production.
2. With other bacteria, any number of organisms present in a ready-to-eat food may be significant. Examples of such agents are *Salmonella*, *Shigella*, *Campylobacter*, and *Yersinia*. For these kinds of agents, the laboratory reports their presence or absence. Their presence in a ready-to-eat food should be considered significant.

Food Sample Kit

1. Mailing container and contents.
2. Other materials.
3. Cost.
4. Replacement.

Preparing a Final Report

Purpose

1. To document the progression and rationale behind activities in the investigation.
2. To document information in case of potential legal issues.
3. To provide a reference for education and improve investigations and prevention methods for future outbreaks.

Background

1. What was the setting in which the problem occurred or what were the circumstances initiating the investigation? Were any special events surrounding the outbreak?
2. Who was involved in the outbreak? (Do not use names of case-patients or contacts. The names of LHD personnel or authorised personnel involved in the investigation may be included. The names of facilities or locations where FBO/WBOs occurred may be included at the discretion of the LHD.)
3. Demographic setting (age, gender, occupation, etc.).
4. How many exposed? How many people were ill? (Those meeting the case definition).

5. What was the severity and clinical picture of cases? (e.g. # ill, # hospitalised, # fatalities, list of symptoms, unusual clinical cases or onset times).
6. Where did it occur? Relevant geography (e.g. home environment, work environment, school environment).
7. Is it an ongoing problem?

Methods

1. What control methods were employed? Was an inspection of the facility conducted?
2. What lab tests were done? What was the rationale for these tests (clinical? epidemiological?).
3. How was the data analysed? (e.g. line lists, epi-curves, EPI-Info software).
4. Include a copy of the questionnaire used. Who developed and administered questionnaire?

Results

1. What did the investigation reveal? (What was the etiologic agent? What was the vehicle? What was the primary problem? Has it been resolved?).
2. What did the sanitarian's report reveal? (Did environmental factors contribute to the outbreak?).
3. Laboratory results. (Clinical or environmental samples. Do they support the hypotheses?).
4. Epidemic curve, charts, etc. (Indication of source? Time of exposure?).
5. Statistical analysis. (What sources were statistically associated with illness?).

Discussion

1. Were the control measures effective and would they be effective in future outbreaks?
2. Were there any important or unusual outcomes or findings?.
3. Assess current surveillance procedures (Are current surveillance strategies effective enough to detect a similar outbreak in the future? What methods need to be enhanced or curtailed?).
4. Summarise important aspects of the investigation (What important elements were learned from this investigation that could be used by the LHD or other LHDs).

The following sections within this section will discuss and provide examples of the components of a final report for an outbreak investigation. The information is then compiled into a narrative report. The narrative report provides valuable information following an outbreak investigation. The narrative report may be beneficial to the LHD by documenting the rationale for activities undertaken during the investigation, providing documentation for potential legal issues, and information that may be used to improve future investigations, recognise future outbreaks and plan prevention strategies. In addition, the narrative report may increase information already known about enteric diseases, their etiologic agents, vehicles of infection, and changes in the nature of the diseases.

Components of a final report: Example of a line listing for a FBO investigation

Line list

A table listing case identifiers, age, gender, onset time, incubation period, duration of illness, symptoms, or any other information which facilitates comparisons of many characteristics for possible similarities or associations. The line list is started early in the investigation and consists of a detailed listing of cases, line by line, and may include demographic features, occupation, special activities or any other variables which might be associated with the outbreak. Each column represents an important variable and each row represents a different case.

A line list provides the data needed to construct an epi curve (Table 23.1).

Table 23.1. A line list provides the data needed to construct an epi curve.

No.	Age	M/F	Oset	Time	N	V	D	BD	AC	Fe	HA	Ch	Fa
1	25	M	20-Dec	16:00	+	+	+	+	+	+	+	−	+
2	35	M	21-Dec	19:00	+	−	+	+	+	+	−	−	−
3	48	F	21-Dec	6:00	+	−	+	−	+	+	+	−	+
4	33	M	20-Dec	23:00	−	−	+	−	+	−	−	−	−
5	56	M	21-Dec	7:00	+	+	+	−	+	+	+	+	+

M/F = Gender; Onset = Onset day of illness; Time = Time of day; N = Nausea; V = Vomiting; D = Diarrhea; BD = Bloody diarrhea; AC = Abdominal cramps; Fe = Fever; HA = Headache; Ch = Chills; Fa = Fatigue.

Considerations when Reporting on an Outbreak Related to Restaurants, Weddings or Banquets

Eating establishments

1. Did the eating establishment have a history of violations or food complaints?
2. Did the facility maintain an accurate record of food workers missing work due to illness? Were any workers ill at the time of the outbreak? Were there any illnesses in the families of food workers?
3. Did the facility have a policy regarding ill food workers? Any exclusions?
4. Was the schedule of staff working at the time of, or shortly before the outbreak available?
5. Did food workers wear disposable gloves?
6. Were there adequate hand washing facilities available?
7. Before the outbreak, did the facility change the menu or serve unusual food items? Offer any specials?
8. Were invoices of suspect foods available and obtained if tracebacks were warranted?
9. Were foods prepared ahead in batches or precooked (e.g. roasts)?
10. Were foods held at room temperature before food preparation (e.g. pooled eggs for omelets)?
11. Did facility use municipal or well water (If well, record of last well test available)?
12. Were there opportunities for cross contamination of foods during food handling?
13. Were there opportunities for cross contamination of foods in coolers (e.g. poultry dripping on lettuce)?
14. Were there opportunities for cross contamination or back flow from the plumbing system?

Additional comments for weddings or banquets

1. Is a table arrangement available? Location of buffet lines?
2. How was food prepared? (In batches? Precooked portions? Uniform cooking facilities? How long were foods held before serving?, etc.).
3. Was food left out on the buffet tables? How long?
4. Were meals cooked in-house or catered? (If catered, see restaurant recommendations.)
5. Are there leftover food items available?
6. Can illnesses be linked to rehearsal dinner? (Location? Time? Foods? etc.)
7. Were there any other social events in conjunction with the wedding or banquet? (e.g. happy hour, hotel parties, brunches.)

8. Hotel arrangements? (foods, parties, swimming pool or whirlpools, room numbers, ice machines, etc.)

Private Water Systems

Wells

For those individuals with a private water system, usually a well, the responsibility for testing resides with the individuals who own the well site. Annual testing of wells is recommended, especially if the well is located near sources of potential contamination. Even if the water is currently safe, routine testing provides a water quality record if problems arise. Routine testing should include screening for coliform bacteria and *E. coli*, nitrates, lead, copper, and triazines.

Circumstances for which more frequent testing (both bacteriological and chemical) would be recommended include: a well located near septic fields, a dump, landfill, factory, underground storage tank or a mining operation, intensive agriculture or livestock operations, or when a consumer of the water is pregnant. Natural disasters such as flooding may also necessitate water testing. If flooding occurs, bottled water or water brought to a 'rolling boil' for one minute should be used until the well can be tested and, if necessary, disinfected. Consideration should be given to the fact that boiling water will concentrate nitrate levels if the water is consumed by pregnant women or infants.

Collection of potable water from wells

1. Locate a sample tap near the well, preferably not a swing, leaky or outside faucet. Remove any screens or aerators from the tap.
2. Sterilise metal taps by heating with a flame (e.g. butane lighter, propane torch, alcohol lamp). Eliminate this step for plastic or partially plastic taps.
3. Allow the water to run for several minutes. Do not change the flow rate, do not shut the faucet off, and do not wipe or wash the faucet prior to sample collection.
4. Do not open the bottle until ready to collect the sample. Take care not to touch the top of the collection bottle or inside of the cap. Fill the bottle to within ½ inch of top.

Possible sources of bacterial contamination of wells

1. Not following sampling instructions properly.
2. Insects getting into the well through non-vermin-proof cap or seal or a loose well cap.
3. The well casing is not properly sealed into the rock formation.
4. The well casing does not terminate at least 12 inches above the ground.
5. The well terminates in a nonconforming pit, which may be subject to flooding or seepage from groundwater.
6. Contamination of new wells because the drill hole becomes contaminated through dirty tools, pipe and drilling water.
7. Recent repairs or construction to the plumbing system may contaminate the system.
8. Flooding or other natural disasters.

Disinfection of the well and water system

Wells may be disinfected once an inspection has determined that the water system is free from any continual contamination (Fig. 23.1).

1. Mix one gallon of household laundry bleach with 100 gallons of water. If the well is more than 150 feet deep, mix two gallons of bleach with 200 gallons of water. If there is no container large

enough to mix the solution, it can be made up 25 gallons at a time in four clean plastic garbage cans.

2. Remove the cap from the well and pour the entire bleach and water solution into the well in rapid succession.

3. Rinse down the sides of the well casing with a garden hose for five to 10 minutes. The rinse water should be from a hose on the water system being disinfected. This procedure circulates the bleach through the water system to insure better disinfection.

4. If the plumbing system is to be disinfected, turn on all the cold water taps until you smell the bleach, then turn the taps off.

5. Let the bleach remain in the system for at least eight hours (preferably 24 hours).

6. Pump all the bleach out of the water system by running the water through a garden hose to an area where the bleach will not damage lawns, shrubs or septic systems. Pump until the bleach odour is no longer apparent.

7. Two or three days after the disinfection, a water sample from the well should be submitted for bacteriological analysis. One month after the disinfection, a sample from the well should be submitted for bacteriological analysis to assure the well is maintaining safe, quality water.

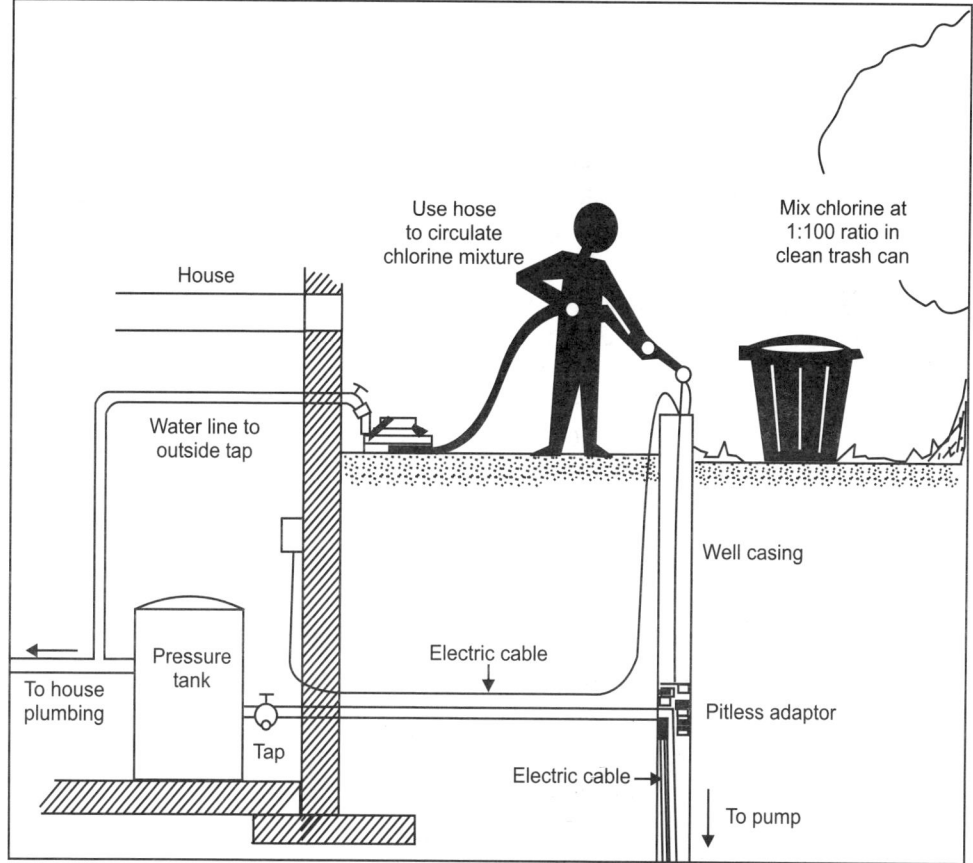

Fig. 23.1. Disinfection of well and water system.

Collection of Water from Swimming Pools and Whirlpools for Bacterial Enteric Pathogens

Testing for specific pathogenic bacteria or parasites is not routinely available or practical in recreational waters such as swimming pools or whirlpools. Therefore, when investigating a WBO, water quality may be determined by testing for the presence or absence of coliform bacteria. In addition to testing following a suspected WBO, proprietors of licensed public pools are encouraged to routinely sample for bacteriologic contamination. Sample the pool during a period of average use, dependent on individual pool usage. Using a sweeping motion, collect a sample from a depth of 18 inches. Please ensure that the chlorine neutralising substance is not rinsed from the bottle.

In addition to these procedures, swabs from skimmers, filters, and drains may also be used for investigations of outbreaks of *Pseudomonas folliculitis* outbreaks involving swimming pools or whirlpools.

Collection of Water from Swimming Pools and Whirlpools for *Legionella*

1. Sand filters:
   (a) Collect approximately 5 teaspoons of sand from the filter and place in a sterile 200 ml bottle (or two 100 ml bottles) containing sodium thiosulphate.
   (b) Fill the bottle(s) with water from filter casing to within 1″ of the top of the bottle.
   (c) Indicate on a laboratory requisition 'sand filter' for *Legionella* testing.
2. Diatomaceous earth and cartridge filters.
   (a) Consult with the BCDP or BEOH staff before collecting these specimens.

Swimming Pools and Whirlpools Contaminated with *Cryptosporidium*

Because of the large number of oocysts shed by symptomatic persons and high infectivity of *Cryptosporidium*, even limited fecal contamination could result in sufficient oocyst concentrations in localised areas of a pool to cause additional human infections. Since *Cryptosporidium* oocysts are very small (4–6 microns) and resistant to chlorine (The chlorine CT* of 9600 needed to kill *Cryptosporidium* oocysts is approximately 640 times greater than required for *Giardia* cysts), rapid sand filters and recommended chlorine levels commonly used in swimming pools may not be effective in removing *Cryptosporidium* oocysts. However, a well-maintained fine-grade diatomaceous earth (DE) filtration system may remove *Cryptosporidium*. If the swimming pool is believed to be fecally contaminated, the pool should be closed until the chlorine level and contact time is sufficient to kill *Giardia* cysts. Draining the pool and replacing contaminated filter media in filters are not considered effective against *Cryptosporidium*. Maintaining the high level chlorine necessary to kill *Cryptosporidium* in swimming pools is not feasible; therefore, such recreational water used should be recognised as a potential increased risk for cryptosporidiosis in immunocompromised persons. In systems that use DE filters, one option may be to close contaminated pools until relatively complete filtration has occurred (typically three turnovers or approximately one day).

SECTION VI

Food Sanitation and Public Health

Chapter 24

Microbiology in Food Sanitation

INTRODUCTION

Sanitation is the hygienic means of promoting health through prevention of human contact with the hazards of wastes. Hazards can be either physical, microbiological, biological or chemical agents of disease. Wastes that can cause health problems are human and animal feces, solid wastes, domestic waste-water (sewage, sullage, greywater), industrial wastes, and agricultural wastes. Hygienic means of prevention can be by using engineering solutions (e.g. sewerage and waste-water treatment), simple technologies (e.g. latrines, septic tanks) or even by personal hygiene practices (e.g. simple handwashing with soap).

The World Health Organisation states that:

'Sanitation generally refers to the provision of facilities and services for the safe disposal of human urine and faeces. Inadequate sanitation is a major cause of disease worldwide and improving sanitation is known to have a significant beneficial impact on health both in households and across communities. The word 'sanitation' also refers to the maintenance of hygienic conditions, through services such as garbage collection and waste-water disposal.

Food sanitation refers to the hygienic measures for ensuring food safety.

WASTE-WATER SANITATION

Waste-water Collection

The standard sanitation technology in urban areas is the collection of waste-water in sewers, its treatment in waste-water treatment plants for reuse or disposal in rivers, lakes or the sea. Sewers are either combined with storm drains or separated from them as sanitary sewers. Combined sewers are usually found in the central, older parts or urban areas. Heavy rainfall and inadequate maintenance can lead to combined sewer overflows or sanitary sewer overflows, i.e. more or less diluted raw sewage being discharged into the environment. Industries often discharge waste-water into municipal sewers, which can complicate waste-water treatment unless industries pre-treat their discharges.

The high investment cost of conventional waste-water collection systems are difficult to afford for many developing countries. Some countries have therefore promoted alternative waste-water collection systems such as condominial sewerage, which uses smaller diameter pipes at lower depth with different network layouts from conventional sewerage.

Waste-water treatment

In developed countries treatment of municipal waste-water is now widespread, but not yet universal. In developing countries most waste-water is still discharged untreated into the environment.

Reuse of waste-water

The reuse of untreated waste-water in irrigated agriculture is common in developing countries. The reuse of treated waste-water in landscaping (especially on golf courses), irrigated agriculture and for industrial use is becoming increasingly widespread. In many peri-urban and rural areas households are not connected to sewers. They discharge their waste-water into septic tanks or other types of on-site sanitation.

Ecological sanitation

Ecological sanitation is sometimes presented as a radical alternative to conventional sanitation systems. Ecological sanitation is based on composting or vermicomposting toilets where an extra separation of urine and feces at the source for sanitisation and recycling has been done. It thus eliminates the creation of blackwater and eliminates fecal pathogens from any still present waste-water (urine). If ecological sanitation is practiced municipal waste-water consists only of greywater, which can be recycled for gardening. However, in most cases greywater continues to be discharged to sewers.

Sanitation and public health

The importance of waste isolation lies in an effort to prevent water and sanitation related diseases, which afflicts both developed countries as well as developing countries to differing degrees. It is estimated that up to 5 million people die each year from preventable waterborne disease, as a result of inadequate sanitation and hygiene practices. The affects of sanitation have also had a large impact on society. Published in *Griffins Public Sanitation* proven studies show that higher sanitation produces more attractiveness.

Solid Waste Disposal

Disposal of solid waste is most commonly conducted in landfills, but incineration, recycling, composting and conversion to biofuels are also avenues. In the case of landfills, advanced countries typically have rigid protocols for daily cover with topsoil, where underdeveloped countries customarily rely upon less stringent protocols. The importance of daily cover lies in the reduction of vector contact and spreading of pathogens. Daily cover also minimises odour emissions and reduces windblown litter. Likewise, developed countries typically have requirements for perimeter sealing of the landfill with clay-type soils to minimise migration of leachate that could contaminate groundwater (and hence jeopardise some drinking water supplies).

For incineration options, the release of air pollutants, including certain toxic components is an attendant adverse outcome. Recycling and biofuel conversion are the sustainable options that generally have superior life cycle costs, particularly when total ecological consequences are considered. Composting value will ultimately be limited by the market demand for compost product.

SANITATION IN THE FOOD INDUSTRY

Sanitation within the food industry means to the adequate treatment of food-contact surfaces by a process that is effective in destroying vegetative cells of micro-organisms of public health significance, and in substantially reducing numbers of other undesirable micro-organisms, but without adversely affecting the product or its safety for the consumer (US Food and Drug Administration, Code of Federal Regulations, 21CFR110, USA). Sanitation Standard Operating Procedures are indispensable for food industries in US, which are regulated by 9 CFR part 416 in conjunction with 21 CFR part 178.1010. Similarly in Japan, food hygiene has to be reached through the compliance of Food Sanitation Law.

Additionally, in the food and biopharmaceutical industries, the term sanitary equipment means equipment that is fully cleanable using clean-in-place (CIP), and sterilisation in place (SIP) procedures: that is fully drainable from cleaning solutions and other liquids. The design should have a minimum amount of deadleg or areas where the turbulence during cleaning is not enough to remove product deposits. In general, to improve cleanability, this equipment is made from Stainless Steel 316L, (an alloy containing small amounts of molybdenum). The surface is usually electropolished to an effective surface roughness of less than 0.5 micrometre, to reduce the possibility of bacterial adhesion to the surface.

Bacteriological Water Analysis

Bacteriological water analysis is a method of analysing water to estimate the numbers of bacteria present and, if needed, to find out what sort of bacteria they are. It is a microbiological analytical procedure which uses samples of water and from these samples determines the concentration of bacteria. It is then possible to draw inferences about the suitability of the water for use from these concentrations. This process is used, for example, to routinely confirm that water is safe for human consumption or that bathing and recreational waters are safe to use. The interpretation and the action trigger levels for different waters vary depending on the use made of the water. Very stringent levels applying to drinking water whilst more relaxed levels apply to marine bathing waters where much lower volumes of water are expected to be ingested by users. The common feature of all these routine screening procedures is that the primary analysis is for indicator organisms rather than the pathogens that might cause concern. Indicator organisms are bacteria such as nonspecific coliforms, *Escherichia coli* and *Pseudomonas aeruginosa* that are very commonly found in the human or animal gut and which, if detected, may suggest the presence of sewage. Indicator organisms are used because even when a person is infected with a more pathogenic bacteria, they will still be excreting many millions times more indicator organisms than pathogens. It is, therefore, reasonable to surmise that if indicator organism levels are low, then pathogen levels will be very much lower or absent. Judgements as to suitability of water for use are based on very extensive precedents and relate to the probability of any sample population of bacteria being able to be infective at a reasonable statistical level of confidence.

Analysis is usually performed using culture, biochemical and sometimes optical methods. When indicator organisms levels exceed preset triggers, specific analysis for pathogens may then be undertaken and these can be quickly detected (where suspected) using specific culture methods or molecular biology.

Methodologies

Because the analysis is always based on a very small sample taken from a very large volume of water, all methods rely on statistical principles.

Multiple tube method

One of the oldest methods is called the multiple tube method. In this method a measured sub-sample (perhaps 10 ml) is diluted with 100 ml of sterile growth medium and an aliquot of 10 ml is then decanted into each of ten tubes. The remaining 10 ml is then diluted again and the process repeated. At the end of 5 dilutions this produces 50 tubes covering the dilution range of 1:10 through to 1:10000. The tubes are then incubated at a preset temperature for a specified time and at the end of the process the number of tubes with growth in is counted for each dilution. Statistical tables are then used to derive the concentration of organisms in the original sample. This method can be enhanced by using indicator medium which changes colour when acid forming species are present and by including a tiny inverted tube in each sample tube. This inverted tube catches any gas produced. The production of gas at 37°C is a strong indication of the presence of *Escherichia coli*.

ATP testing

An ATP test is the process of rapidly measuring active micro-organisms in water through detection of a molecule called Adenosine Triphosphate or ATP.

ATP is a molecule found only in and around living cells, and as such it gives a direct measure of biological concentration and health. ATP is quantified by measuring the light produced through its reaction with the naturally-occurring firefly enzyme Luciferase using a Luminometer. The amount of light produced is directly proportional to the amount of biological energy present in the sample.

Second generation ATP tests are specifically designed for water, waste-water and industrial applications where, for the most part, samples contain a variety of components that can interfere with the ATP assay.

Plate count

The plate count method relies on bacteria growing a colony on a nutrient medium so that the colony becomes visible to the naked eye and the number of colonies on a plate can be counted. To be effective, the dilution of the original sample must be arranged so that on average between 30 and 300 colonies of the target bacterium are grown. Fewer than 30 colonies makes the interpretation statistically unsound whilst greater than 300 colonies often results in overlapping colonies and imprecision in the count. To ensure that an appropriate number of colonies will be generated several dilutions are normally cultured.

The laboratory procedure involves making serial dilutions of the sample (1:10, 1:100, 1:1000, etc.) in sterile water and cultivating these on nutrient agar in a dish that is sealed and incubated. Typical media include plate count agar for a general count or MacConkey agar to count gram-negative bacteria such as *E. coli*. Typically one set of plates is incubated at 22°C and for 24 hours and a second set at 37°C for 24 hours. The composition of the nutrient usually includes reagents that resist the growth of nontarget organisms and make the target organism easily identified, often by a colour change in the medium. Some recent methods include a fluorescent agent so that counting of the colonies can be automated. At the end of the incubation period the colonies are counted by eye, a procedure that takes a few moments and does not require a microscope as the colonies are typically a few millimetres across.

Membrane filtration

Most modern laboratories use a refinement of total plate count in which serial dilutions of the sample are vacuum filtered through purpose made membrane filters and these filters are themselves laid on nutrient medium within sealed plates. The methodology is otherwise similar to conventional total plate counts. Membranes have a printed millimetre grid printed on and can be reliably count a much greater number of colonies under a binocular microscope.

Pour plates

When the analysis is looking for bacterial species that grow poorly in air, the initial analysis is done by mixing serial dilutions of the sample in liquid nutrient agar which is then poured into bottles which are then sealed and laid on their sides to produce a sloping agar surface. Colonies that develop in the body of the medium can be counted by eye after incubation.

The total number of colonies is referred to as the total viable count (TVC). The unit of measurement is cfu/ml (or colony forming units per millilitre) and relates to the original sample. Calculation of this is a multiple of the counted number of colonies multiplied by the dilution used.

Pathogen analysis

When samples show elevated levels of indicator bacteria, further analysis is often undertaken to look for specific pathogenic bacteria. Species commonly investigated in the temperate zone include *Salmonella typhi* and *Salmonella typhimurium* depending on the likely source of contamination investigation may also extend to organisms such as *Cryptosporidium* spp. In tropical areas analysis of *Vibrio cholerae* is also routinely undertaken.

WATER MICROBIOLOGY

Water microbiology is concerned with the micro-organisms that live in water or can be transported from one habitat to another by water. Water can support the growth of many types of micro-organisms. This can be advantageous. For example, the chemical activities of certain strains of yeasts provide us with beer and bread. As well, the growth of some bacteria in contaminated water can help digest the poisons from the water.

However, the presence of other disease causing microbes in water is unhealthy and even life threatening. For example, bacteria that live in the intestinal tracts of humans and other warm blooded animals, such as *Escherichia coli*, *Salmonella*, *Shigella*, and *Vibrio*, can contaminate water if feces enters the water. Contamination of drinking water with a type of *Escherichia coli* known as O157:H7 can be fatal. The contamination of the municipal water supply of Walkerton, Ontario, Canada in the summer of 2000 by strain O157:H7 sickened 2000 people and killed seven people.

The intestinal tract of warm-blooded animals also contains viruses that can contaminate water and cause disease. Examples include rotavirus, enteroviruses, and coxsackievirus. Another group of microbes of concern in water microbiology are protozoa. The two protozoa of the most concern are *Giardia* and *Cryptosporidium*. They live normally in the intestinal tract of animals such as beaver and deer. *Giardia* and *Cryptosporidium* form dormant and hardy forms called cysts during their life cycles. The cyst forms are resistant to chlorine, which is the most popular form of drinking water disinfection, and can pass through the filters used in many water treatment plants. If ingested in drinking water they can cause debilitating and prolonged diarrhea in humans, and can be life threatening to those people with impaired immune systems. *Cryptosporidium* contamination of the drinking water of Milwaukee, Wisconsin with in 1993 sickened more than 4,00,000 people and killed 47 people.

Many micro-organisms are found naturally in fresh and saltwater. These include bacteria, cyanobacteria, protozoa, algae, and tiny animals such as rotifers. These can be important in the food chain that forms the basis of life in the water. For example, the microbes called cyanobacteria can convert the energy of the sun into the energy it needs to live. The plentiful numbers of these organisms in turn are used as food for other life. The algae that thrive in water is also an important food source for other forms of life.

A variety of micro-organisms live in freshwater. The region of a water body near the shoreline (the littoral zone) is well lighted, shallow, and warmer than other regions of the water. Photosynthetic algae and bacteria that use light as energy thrive in this zone. Further away from the shore is the limnitic zone.

Photosynthetic microbes also live here. As the water deepens, temperatures become colder and the oxygen concentration and light in the water decrease. Now, microbes that require oxygen do not thrive. Instead, purple and green sulphur bacteria, which can grow without oxygen, dominate. Finally, at the bottom of freshwaters (the benthic zone), few microbes survive. Bacteria that can survive in the absence of oxygen and sunlight, such as methane producing bacteria, thrive.

Saltwater presents a different environment to micro-organisms. The higher salt concentration, higher pH, and lower nutrients, relative to freshwater, are lethal to many micro-organisms. But, salt loving (halophilic) bacteria abound near the surface, and some bacteria that also live in freshwater are plentiful (i.e. *Pseudomonas* and *Vibrio*). Also, in 2001, researchers demonstrated that the ancient form of microbial life known as archaebacteria is one of the dominant forms of life in the ocean. The role of archaebacteria in the ocean food chain is not yet known, but must be of vital importance.

Another micro-organism found in saltwater are a type of algae known as dinoflagellelates. The rapid growth and multiplication of dinoflagellates can turn the water red. This 'red tide' depletes the water of nutrients and oxygen, which can cause many fish to die. As well, humans can become ill by eating contaminated fish. Water can also be an ideal means of transporting micro-organisms from one place to another. For example, the water that is carried in the hulls of ships to stabilise the vessels during their ocean voyages is now known to be a means of transporting micro-organisms around the globe. One of these organisms, a bacterium called Vibrio cholerae, causes life threatening diarrhea in humans.

Drinking water is usually treated to minimise the risk of microbial contamination. The importance of drinking water treatment has been known for centuries. For example, in pre-Christian times the storage of drinking water in jugs made of metal was practiced. Now, the antibacterial effect of some metals is known. Similarly, the boiling of drinking water, as a means of protection of water has long been known.

Chemicals such as chlorine or chlorine derivatives has been a popular means of killing bacteria such as *Escherichia coli* in water since the early decades of the twentieth century. Other bacteria-killing treatments that are increasingly becoming popular include the use of a gas called ozone and the disabling of the microbe's genetic material by the use of ultraviolet light. Microbes can also be physically excluded form the water by passing the water through a filter. Modern filters have holes in them that are so tiny that even particles as miniscule as viruses can be trapped.

An important aspect of water microbiology, particularly for drinking water, is the testing of the water to ensure that it is safe to drink. Water quality testing can be done in several ways. One popular test measures the turbidity of the water. Turbidity gives an indication of the amount of suspended material in the water. Typically, if material such as soil is present in the water then micro-organisms will also be present. The presence of particles even as small as bacteria and viruses can decrease the clarity of the water. Turbidity is a quick way of indicating if water quality is deteriorating, and so if action should be taken to correct the water problem.

In many countries, water microbiology is also the subject of legislation. Regulations specify how often water sources are sampled, how the sampling is done, how the analysis will be performed, what microbes are detected, and the acceptable limits for the target micro-organisms in the water sample. Testing for microbes that cause disease (i.e. *Salmonella typhymurium* and *Vibrio cholerae*) can be expensive and, if the bacteria are present in low numbers, they may escape detection. Instead, other more numerous bacteria provide an indication of fecal pollution of the water. *Escherichia coli* has been used as an indicator of fecal pollution for decades. The bacterium is present in the intestinal tract in huge numbers, and is more numerous than the disease-causing bacteria and viruses. The chances of detecting *Escherichia coli* is better than detecting the actual disease causing micro-organisms. *Escherichia coli* also had the advantage of not being capable of growing and reproducing in the water (except in the warm and food-laden waters of tropical countries). Thus, the presence of the bacterium in water is indicative of recent fecal pollution. Finally, *Escherichia coli* can be detected easily and inexpensively.

Drinking Water Microbiology

Water is indispensable for life. The basic human physiological requirement for water is about 2.5 litres per day. This drinking water should be free from chemical as well as microbial contaminants, since the potential of contaminated water to transmit diseases is very high. For instance, a person with cholera excretes about 1013 bacteria each day. The infectious dose for cholera pathogen is 106 cells. Thus, on average, an infected person can transmit the disease to about ten million people. Drinking water is obtained from different sources like well, river and surface waters. Various impurities, from branches of trees to invisible micro-organisms, may occur in these waters and have to be removed before the water is supplied to the public. To render the water safe for drinking it has to be treated properly. Although there occur some similarities between sewage treatment and drinking water treatment, they are entirely different from each other. Bacteriological quality of drinking-water is given in Table 24.1.

Table 24.1. Bacteriological quality of drinking-water[a].

Organisms	Guideline value
All water intended for drinking	
E. coli or thermotolerant coliform bacteria[b,c]	Must not be detectable in any 100 ml sample
Treated water entering the distribution system	
E. coli or thermotolerant coliform bacteria[b]	Must not be detectable in any 100 ml sample
Total coliform bacteria	Must not be detectable in any 100 ml sample
Treated water in the distribution system	
E. coli or thermotolerant coliform bacteria[b]	Must not be detectable in any 100 ml sample
Total coliform bacteria	Must not be detectable in any 100 ml sample. In the case of large supplies, where sufficient samples are examined, must not be present in 95 per cent of samples taken throughout any 12 month period

[a]Immediate investigative action must be taken if either *E. coli* or total coliform bacteria are detected. The minimal action in the case of total coliform bacteria is repeat sampling; if these bacteria are detected in the repeat sample, the cause must be determined by immediate further investigation.

[b]Although *E. coli* is the more precise indicator of faecal pollution, the count of thermotolerant coliform bacteria is an acceptable alternative. If necessary, proper confirmatory tests must be carried out. Total coliform bacteria are not acceptable indicators of the sanitary quality of rural water supplies, particularly in tropical areas where many bacteria of no sanitary significance occur in almost all untreated supplies.

[c]It is recognised that, in the great majority of rural water supplies in developing countries, faecal contamination is widespread. Under these conditions, the national surveillance agency should set medium-term targets for the progressive improvement of water supplies.

Plant Water

All water that comes into contact with foods should meet the bacteriological standards for drinking water, and preferably all freshwater at the plant should be that good. But this water also should be satisfactory from a bacteriological standpoint for use with the particular food being processed. A water supply may be adjudged potable yet be unsatisfactory for use with a food. Thus, for example, water containing appreciable numbers of psychrotrophs of the genera *Pseudomonas* or *Alcaligenes* might be unsatisfactory without treatment in a dairy plant making butter or cottage cheese. The slimy growth of iron bacteria in water supplies often leads to trouble in the food plant.

More likely to be important is the chemical composition of the water, which must be suited to the use to be made of it. Thus hard water is undesirable in pea canning and in brewing; iron and manganese are bad in beet canning and in brewing; excessive organic matter may lead to off-flavours, etc.

Of special interest in canning factories is the bacteriology of the water in which the cans of processed foods are cooled after their heat treatment. If this water contains micro-organisms able to spoil the food, it can enter defective cans through minute leaks and increase the percentage of cans of food spoiling during storage. Many canneries routinely chlorinate the cooling water to reduce or eliminate this problem.

The shortage of water in many food plants has necessitated reuse of part of the water, and micro-organisms may build up in such reused water. Water employed for the final rinse of a food must be fresh and potable, but after use it may be returned for soaking, first wash or fluming, preferably after treatment with chlorine, chlorine dioxide or a similar germicide.

In-plant or continuous chlorination beyond the break point (the point where the chlorine demand has been satisfied) to a residual of 5 to 7 ppm of chlorine is employed for continuous application to areas and equipment where slime bacteria may be a problem, e.g. conveyors or belts, can coolers, product washers, and flumes. The chlorinated water may be applied as a spray or parts of equipment may be immersed. When operations cease, chlorinated water may be applied to fillers, peelers, dicers, and similar equipment. Contaminated or polluted water lines are held filled with chlorinated water containing 50 to 100 ppm of chlorine for 12 to 48 hr, the strength of chlorine and length of time depending on the extent of pollution. Ice used in contact with foods should meet the bacteriological requirements for potable water. Much work has been done on the incorporation of bacteriostatic or bactericidal chemicals in water and in ice to aid in food preservation. It has been noted previously that a chlortetracycline or oxytetracycline dip for dressed poultry had been approved, but approval was later revoked; however, these antibiotics may be incorporated in ice to be applied to fish and other seafood.

SEWAGE AND WASTE-WATER TREATMENT

Human activities generate a tremendous volume of sewage and waste-water that require treatment before discharge into waterways. Often this waste-water contains excessive amounts of nitrogen, phosphorus, and metal compounds, as well as organic pollutants that would overwhelm waterways with an unreasonable burden. Waste-water also contains chemical wastes that are not biodegradable, as well as pathogenic micro-organisms that can cause infectious disease.

The chemical and biological waste in sewage and water must be broken down before it is deposited to the soil and environment. This breakdown can effectively be controlled by managing the microbial population in waters and encouraging micro-organisms to digest the organic matter. The water must then be purified before it is considered fit to drink. Water taken from ground sources must also be treated before consumption.

Water Purification

To purify water for drinking, a number of processes are conducted to reduce the microbial population and maintain that population at a safe level. First, the solid matter is allowed to settle out in a sedimentation tank. Flocculating materials such as alum are used to drag micro-organisms to the bottom of the tank. Then the filtration process is begun. Water is filtered through either a slow sand filter or a rapid sand filter. These processes remove 99 per cent of the micro-organisms. The slow sand filter is composed of finer grains of sand, and the filtration process takes longer than in the rapid sand filter, where larger grains are used. Many communities then purify the water by chlorination. When added to water, chlorine maintains the low microbial count and ensures that the water remains safe for drinking purposes. Chlorine gas or hypochlorite (NaOCl) is used for chlorination purposes. The water is chlorinated until a slight residue of chlorine remains.

Sewage Treatment

Sewage treatment involves a more complex set of procedures than are needed for water purification because the volume of organic matter and the variety of micro-organisms are much greater. The first treatment or primary treatment, of sewage and waste-water involves the removal in settling tanks of particulate matter such as plant waste. The solids that sediment are strained off, and the sludge is collected to be burned or buried in landfills. Alternatively, it can be treated in an anaerobic sludge-digesting tank.

During the secondary treatment of waste-water and sewage, the microbial population of liquid and sludge waste is reduced. In the anaerobic sludge digester, micro-organisms break down the organic matter of proteins, lipids, and cellulose into smaller substances for metabolism by other organisms. Results of these breakdowns include organic acids, alcohols, and simple compounds. Methane gas is produced in the sludge tank, and it can be burned as a fuel to operate the waste treatment facility. The remaining sludge is incinerated or buried in a landfill, and its fluid is recycled and purified (Fig. 24.1).

In aerobic secondary sewage treatment, the fluid waste is aerated and then passed through a trickling filter. In this process, the liquid waste is sprayed over a bed of crushed rocks, tree bark or other filtering material. Colonies of bacteria, fungi, and protozoa grow in the bed and act as secondary filters to remove organic materials. The micro-organisms metabolise organic compounds and convert them to carbon dioxide, sulphate, phosphates, nitrates, and other ions.

The material that comes through the filter has been 99 per cent cleansed of micro-organisms. Liquid waste can also be treated in an activated digester after it has been vigorously aerated. Slime-forming bacteria form masses that trap other micro-organisms to remove them from the water. Treatment for several hours reduces the microbial population significantly, and the clear fluid is removed for purification. The sludge is placed in a landfill or at sea.

In the tertiary treatment of sewage, the fluid from the secondary treatment process is cleansed of phosphate and nitrate ions that might cause pollution. The ions are precipitated as solids, often by combining them with calcium or iron, and the ammonia is released by oxidising it to nitrate in the nitrification process. Adsorption to activated charcoal removes many organic compounds such as polychlorinated biphenyls (PCBs), a chemical pollutant.

The home septic system is a waste treatment facility on a small scale. In a septic tank, household sewage is digested by anaerobic bacteria, and solids settle to the bottom of the tank. Solid waste is carried out of the outflow apparatus into the septic field beneath the ground. The water seeps out through holes in tiles and enters the soil, where bacteria complete the breakdown processes. A similar process occurs in cesspools, except that sludge enters the ground at the bottom of the pool and liquids flow out through the sides of the pool.

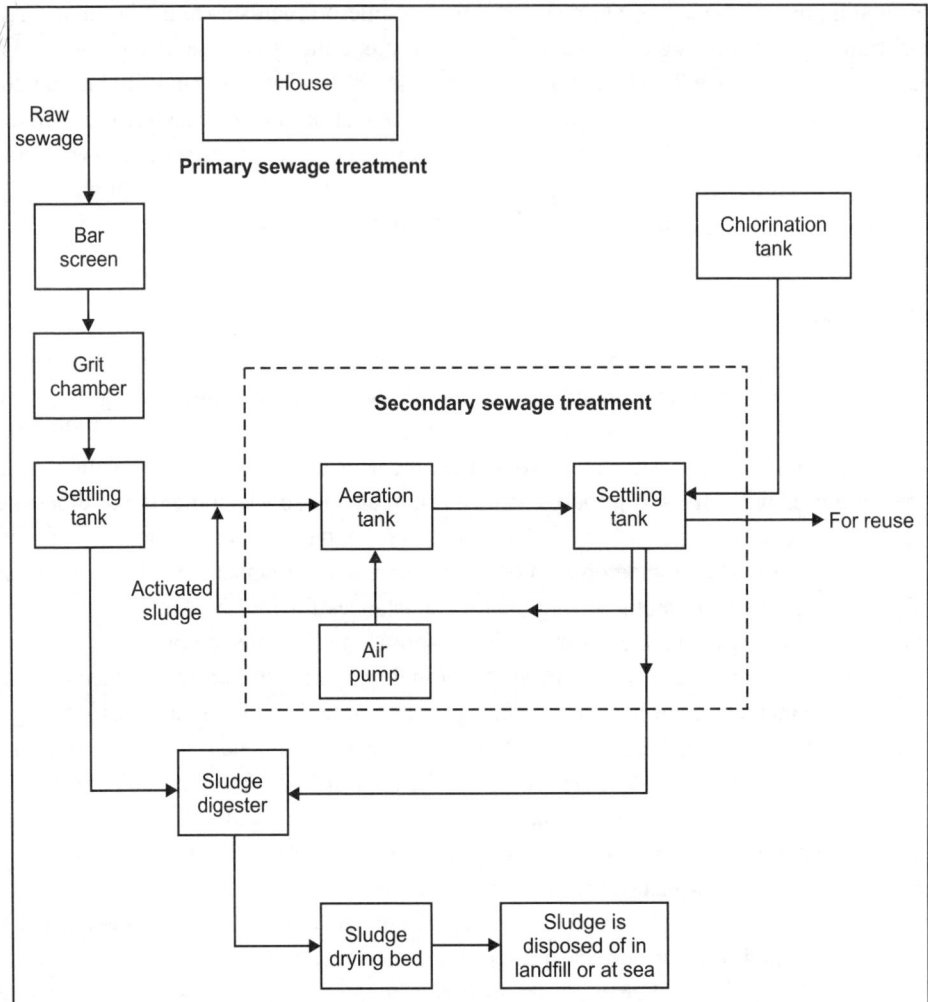

Fig. 24.1. A view of the methods used in sewage treatment in a large municipality. Primary treatment is represented by the steps preceding secondary treatment, and tertiary treatment is performed in the chlorination tank at the conclusion of the process.

Fundamental Microbiology of Sewage

The purpose of this section is to provide a fundamental background on the relationship between microbes, waste-water, and waste-water treatment, i.e. why are we concerned about microbes in waste-water, what role do they play in waste-water treatment, and what happens when 'clean' water is released into the environment.

Pathogenic waste-water microbiology

Waste-water, by its nature, is teaming with microbes. Many of these microbes are necessary for the degradation and stabilisation of organic matter and thus are beneficial. On the other hand, waste-water may also contain pathogenic or potentially pathogenic micro-organisms, which pose a threat to public health. By definition, a pathogen is an organism capable of inflicting damage on its host. Waterborne and water-related diseases caused by pathogenic microbes are among the most serious threats to public health today. Up to 35 per cent of the potential productivity of developing nations is lost because of waterborne disease. Waterborne diseases whose pathogens are spread by the fecal-oral route (with water as the intermediate medium) can be caused by bacteria, viruses, and parasites (including protozoa, worms, and rotifers). Many of the most common pathogenic micro-organisms are described in the Bad Bug Book website maintained by the Food and Drug Administration. Dr. Charles Hagedorn at Virginia Polytechnic Institute has several informative websites including waste-water testing and waste-water Microbes where many of the pathogenic micro-organisms discussed are more fully described.

Bacteria are defined as any of the one-celled prokaryotic organisms, which vary in morphology and nutritional requirements and may be free-living, saprophytic, or pathogenic. The major bacterial pathogens and their associated diseases are given in Table 24.2.

Table 24.2. The major bacterial pathogens and their associated diseases.

Bacterial pathogens	Related disease
Salmonella	Salmonellosis
S. typhimurium	Typhoid fever
Shigella	Shigellosis
Enterococcus (Fecal streptococci)	Diarrhea
E. coli (Fecal Coliform)	Diarrhea
Vibro cholerae	Cholera
Camplyobacter jejuni	Gastroenteritis

Viruses are defined as genetic elements, containing either DNA or RNA and a protein capsid membrane, which are able to alternate between intracellular and extracellular states, the latter being the infectious state. Over 100,000 different viral types have been identified in human feces, and therefore, there is a direct correlation between contact with improperly disposed of treated waste and diarrheal disease. Among the viral pathogens listed below are over 120 enteric viruses, all pathogenic to humans requiring low infectious doses. The major viral pathogens and their associated diseases are given in Table 24.3.

Table 24.3. The major viral pathogens and their associated diseases.

Viral pathogens	Related disease
Hepatitis A	Hepatitis
Norwalk-like agents	Gastroenteritis
Virus-like 27 nanometre particles	Gastroenteritis
Rotavirus	Gastroenteritis and polio

Diarrhea is one of the most common features of waterborne disease. Fecal pollution is one of the primary contributors to diarrhea. In this country, we tend to think of diarrhea as primarily a nuisance. Diarrhea, however, causes dehydration that if not properly treated, can ultimately lead to death. In fact globally, 42,00,000 deaths per year are attributed to diarrhea caused mainly by bacteria and viruses. A person infected with a disease-causing virus may excrete up to 106 (10,00,000) infectious particles per gram of feces. When you stop to consider that potentially, it only takes 1 virus particle to cause disease, the capacity for disaster with untreated or improperly treated waste is enormous. Examples of bacteria commonly associated with diarrheal disease are *Shigella dysenteriae* and *Salmonella typhi*. Two protozoans commonly associated with diarrheal disease are *Giardia lamblia* (responsible for the most widespread protozoan caused disease in the world) and members of the genus *Cryptosporidium*.

Parasites are defined as organisms that grow, feed, and live on or in another organism to whose survival it contributes nothing. The three most important protozoal pathogens in temperate zone countries are give below.

Indicators and detection

Water quality, and its threat to public health, has inspired development of tests designed to measure its suitability for drinking, bathing, and release back to the environment. Water that looks clear and pure may be contaminated with pathogenic micro-organisms. For example, 10^5 (1,00,000) bacteria per millilitre of water is invisible to the naked eye. Therefore, even water that appears 'pure' must be tested to ensure that it contains no micro-organisms that might cause disease. On the other hand there are so many potential pathogens that it is impractical to test for them all. Because of this, tests have been developed for indicator organisms. These are organisms that are present in feces (or sewage), survive as long as pathogenic organisms, and are easy to test for at relatively low cost.

Indicator organisms indicate that fecal pollution has occurred and microbial pathogens might be present. Total and fecal coliforms, and the enterocci—fecal streptocci are the indicator organisms currently used in the public health arena. Coliform bacteria include all aerobic and facultative anaerobic, gram-negative, nonspore-forming, rod-shaped bacteria that ferment lactose with gas formation. There are three groupings of coliform bacteria used as standards: total coliforms (TC), fecal coliforms (FC) and *Escherichia coli*. Total coliforms are the broadest grouping including *Escherichia*, *Enterobacter*, *Klebsiella*, and *Citrobacter*.

These are found naturally in the soil, as well as in feces. Fecal coliforms are the next widest grouping, which includes many species of bacteria commonly found in the human intestinal tract. Usually between 60 and 90 per cent of total coliforms are fecal coliforms. *E. coli* are a particular species of bacteria that may or may not be pathogenic but are ubiquitous in the human intestinal tract. Generally more than 90 per cent of the fecal coliform are *Escherichia* (usually written as *E. coli*). The major protozoal pathogens and their associated diseases are given in Table 24.4.

Table 24.4. The major protozoal pathogens and their associated diseases.

Protozoal pathogens	Related disease
Cryptosporidium parvum	Cryptosporidiosis
Giardia lamblia	Giardiasis
Entamoeba histolytica	Amoebic dysentery

Biological waste-water treatment

Principal goals of biological treatment

It was mentioned earlier that many of the microbes present in waste-water are beneficial. In fact, many waste-water treatment technologies are dependent on these beneficial micro-organisms for remediation of waste-water so that it won't detrimentally impact the environment. One of the primary goals of biological treatment is the removal of organic material from waste-water so that excessive oxygen consumption won't become a problem when it is released to the environment.

Another goal of biological treatment is nitrification/denitrification. Nitrification is an aerobic process in which bacteria oxidise reduced forms of nitrogen ($NH_4^+ \rightarrow NO_2^- \rightarrow NO_3^-$). Denitrification is an anaerobic process by which oxidised forms of nitrogen are reduced to gaseous forms ($NO_3^- \rightarrow NO_2^- \rightarrow N_2O$ or N_2), which can then escape into the atmosphere. This is important because the release of nitrogen to the aquatic environment can also cause eutrophication.

Immobilisation of phosphate (PO_4^{3-}) through bacterial assimilation or precipitation is important for the same reason. Another goal of biological treatment is elimination of pathogenic micro-organisms either through predation or out-competition. The oxidation/stabilisation of organic sludge is also of importance in biological treatment of waste-water.

Biochemical oxygen demand (BOD) and eutrophication

Organic material in waste-water originates from micro-organisms, plants, animals, and synthetic organic compounds. Organic materials enter waste-water in human wastes, paper products, detergents, cosmetics, and foods. They are typically a combination of carbon, hydrogen, oxygen, and nitrogen and may contain other elements. Typical waste-water contains organic matter in the forms of proteins (40 to 60 per cent), carbohydrates (25 to 50 per cent), and oils and fats (8 to 12 per cent). Waste-water may also contain small amounts of synthetic organic molecules (i.e. pesticides and solvents) which may range from simple to complex in structure.

The oxidation of organic materials in the environment can have profound effects on the maintenance of aquatic life and the aesthetic quality of waters. Biochemical oxidation reactions involve the conversion of organic material using oxygen and nutrients into carbon dioxide, water, and new cells. The equation that expresses this is:

$$\text{Organic material} + O_2 + \text{nutrients} \rightarrow CO_2 + H_2O + \text{new cells} + \text{nutrients} + \text{energy}$$

It can be seen from this equation that organisms use oxygen to breakdown carbon-based materials for assimilation into new cell mass and energy. A common measure of this oxygen use is biochemical oxygen demand (BOD). BOD is the amount of oxygen used in the metabolism of biodegradable organics. If water with a large amount of BOD is discharged into the environment, it can deplete the natural oxygen resources. Heterotrophic bacteria utilise deposited organics and O_2 at rates that exceed the oxygen-transfer rates across the water surface. This can cause anaerobic conditions, which leads to noxious odours. It can also be detrimental to aquatic life by reducing dissolved oxygen concentrations to levels that cause fish to suffocate. The end result is an overall degradation of water quality. Typical waste-water contains 110–400 mg/l BOD.

Waste-water often contains large amounts of the nutrients, particularly nitrogen and phosphorous (as phosphate- PO_4^{3-}). Typical waste-water values range from 20–85 mg/l total nitrogen and 4–15 mg/l total phosphorous. Nitrogen and phosphorous are essential for growth of all organisms and are typically limiting in the environment. Nitrogen is a complex element existing both in organic and inorganic forms. The forms of most interest from a water quality perspective are organic nitrogen (often as proteins or urea), ammonia, nitrite, nitrate, and dinitrogen. Phosphorous is found in synthetic detergents and is used for corrosion control in water supplies. Because of its increased usage, its concentration has risen from 3–4 mg/l to 10–20 mg/l since the introduction of synthetic detergents.

The introduction of large concentrations of these nutrients from untreated or improperly treated waste-water can lead to eutrophication. Eutrophication is the process by which bodies of water become rich in mineral and organic nutrients causing plant life, especially algae, to proliferate, then die and decompose thereby reducing the dissolved oxygen content and often killing off other organisms. A specific health problem associated with increased levels of nitrogen is methemoglobinemia or blue-baby syndrome. This disease is a direct result of elevated concentrations of nitrite.

Fundamentals of biological treatment

The basic mechanisms of biological treatment are the same for all treatment processes. Micro-organisms, principally bacteria, metabolise organic material and inorganic ions present in waste-water during growth. Which brings us to the fundamental differences between catabolic and anabolic processes. Catabolic processes are those biochemical processes involved in the breakdown of organic products for the production of energy or for use in anabolism. Catabolic processes are dissimilar because the reactants and products in the reaction are not incorporated into new cell mass. These reactions can be thought of as redox reactions because they involve the transfer of electrons resulting in the generation of energy to be used in cell metabolism. In contrast, anabolic processes are the biochemical processes involved in the synthesis of cell constituents from simpler molecules. These processes usually require energy and are assimilatory. That is the processes result in the incorporation of the reacting molecules or compounds into new cell mass.

A bacterial perspective of contaminant removal involves several steps. First, there must be a liquid-phase transport of the contaminant to the cell surface. Next, there must be a sorption of the contaminant to the cell surface. Third, if necessary, extracellular enzymes will hydrolyse the contaminant into subunits, which can then be transported by diffusion to and through the cytoplasmic membrane. This is the point at which dissimilatory or assimilatory processes take place resulting in a gain in energy and/or an increase in biomass. It is important to realise that biological waste-water treatment alone does not result in the regeneration of potable water.

Biofilms

The growth of bacteria in pure culture has been the mainstay of microbiology, specifically the mainstay of microbiological technique. Solid media techniques (and selective/differential media) have allowed the isolation of individual species from complex natural populations. The study of individual strains of bacteria in nutrient rich batch cultures is still the basis of microbiology today. In natural environments and in pathogenic relationships, bacteria are different than the same organisms grown *in vitro*. In natural systems, bacterial consortia (mixed populations) grow as biofilms.

Physiology of biofilm bacteria

Bacteria in the environment are described as planktonic or sessile. Planktonic bacteria are free in the environment and are committed to motility and colonisation of new surfaces. Sessile bacteria are bound within or to a surface structure. These bacteria have more active reproduction and general metabolism. Because of this, they have an increased heterotrophic potential. In other words, sessile bacteria have greater activity than the same micro-organisms dispersed in the biofilm (planktonic). This has been proven by studies describing the release of increased concentrations of $^{14}CO_2$ from a radiolabelled organic substrate by sessile micro-organisms.

Another important concept relative to micro-organisms and biofilm formation is phenotypic plasticity. This concept describes the ability of bacterial species to change their morphologies in response to the situation. To illustrate this concept, we will describe the genus *Caulobacter*, which is commonly found in oligotrophic aquatic environments. *Caulobacter* binds to surfaces via a stalk possessing a holdfast.

Spread of the biofilm occurs via motile swarmer cells which bind to surfaces, lose their flagella, and form a stalk to complete the cell cycle.

Mineral surfaces

The surfaces that bacteria bind to are not homogenous. Even on a single particle of clay, on a micrometre scale, there will be differences in charge density. In fact, the range of ionic interactions and hydrophobicity seems to be important in terms of both the bacteria forming the biofilm and for the surface upon which the biofilm is formed.

Formation of biofilms

There are three steps necessary for the formation of biofilms. First, there must be a macromolecular conditioning of the surface to be colonised. This is a purely chemical process that occurs on the order of microseconds. If you put any clean surface into the environment, low molecular weight compounds possessing their own unique hydrophilic and hydrophobic character will bind to that surface. Step two, microbial binding, is a two-step process. First, there is reversible binding (colonisation) by bacteria. Next, if the cell senses the proper conditions, irreversible binding takes place, often triggering capsule formation. Finally, there is further permanent attachment of cells and cell division leading to microcolony formation and biofilm generation.

General properties of biofilms

A biofilm consists of cells immobilised at a substratum and frequently embedded in an organic polymer matrix of microbial origin (capsule). The coverage is either uniform or non-uniform (because of microcolony formation). In the natural environment (e.g. pristine alpine streams), sessile bacterial populations are 10^3 to 10^4 times higher than planktonic bacteria. The biofilm may consist of a single monolayer up to multiple layers of bacterial cells. An example of this is algal mats which can be 300 to 400 millimetres thick. Because bacteria grow as microcolonies in biofilms (i.e. as clumps of cells) they are protected from bacteriophage, phagocytic eukaryotic micro-organisms, antibiotics, toxic heavy metals, and xenobiotics. The diffusion gradients through these microcolonies protect the inner cells from pollutants in the water, and the outer cells of the microcolony are sacrificed for the good of the population.

One important distinction of biofilms is that they can provide a variety of microenvironments, i.e. they are chemically heterogeneous throughout. They establish their own gradients of nutrients, oxygen saturation, and pH relative to the bulk environment. Because the capsule is hydrated, biofilms are greater than 95 per cent water and thus they will trap inorganic and organic material that is soluble or particulate in nature. The solid/liquid interface between the biofilm and the environment is important as well to current/flow rates.

There is a critical role of transport and transfer processes which are generally rate controlling in biofilm systems. For example, high flow rates in oligotrophic environments will be well nourished due to high transfer rates across the interface.

In natural systems, biofilms are responsible for the removal of dissolved and particulate contaminants and are important in the cycling of chemical elements. These concepts are equally important in waste-water treatment systems. Also, in the natural environment, enhanced growth may result from nutrient trapping. Another important property of biofilms is that the capsule, the bulk matrix of biofilms, acts as an ion exchange resin because it consists of anionic polymers which will bind Mg^{2+}, Ca^{2+}, and $Fe^{2+/3+}$ cations. Examples of naturally occurring biofilms include mineral, metal, and wood degrading consortia of bacteria.

Pathogen transport and survival through the subsurface

We have discussed the presence of beneficial and disease-causing micro-organisms associated with waste-water. Another topic of importance when discussing the fundamental microbiology of waste-water is the ability (or lack thereof) of pathogens to move through and survive in the subsurface. There are many reasons that this is important. In the United States, approximately 25 per cent of all water used is groundwater and approximately 50 per cent of the population relies on groundwater for drinking. The good news is that bacteria don't usually move large distances in fine textured soils (generally less than a few meters). The bad news is that they can move larger distances in coarse-textured or fractured materials. Fortunately, pathogenic micro-organisms not native to the subsurface generally don't multiply underground and will eventually die. Despite these facts, they can move far enough distances and live long enough to be of concern around waste-water disposal areas. Of special concern, saturated flow conditions lead to horizontal movement of microbes. Unsaturated conditions are optimal and lead to greater attenuation.

Microbial transport through the subsurface

There are two factors that significantly affect mobility of bacteria and viruses through the subsurface. First, the size of existing water filled pores (including cracks, fissures, and solution channels) will affect mobility. Second, the velocity of water through these pores plays an important role in micro-organism mobility. There are also two mechanisms of retention of bacteria in the subsurface.

The first mechanism is filtration. This is the trapping of particles and bacteria in pore spaces. Larger suspended particles are trapped first. These then act as a filter for progressively smaller particles and bacteria. Eventually this system will become clogged and block further transport.

The second mechanism of retention of bacteria is adsorption. This is the adhesion of bacteria (or viruses), in an extremely thin layer, to the surfaces of solid bodies. Clays are ideal for this type of bacterial retention because of their small size, layered structure, and large surface-to-volume ratio. Thus, adsorption plays a more important role in soils that contain clays.

Bacterial size also plays a role in determining whether they are more likely to be retained by adsorption or filtration. Larger bacteria are more likely to be removed by filtration, whereas smaller bacteria are more likely to be removed by adsorption.

Because of the smaller size of viruses (they are approximately 100 nanometres as opposed to the approximate 1 micrometre length of the 'typical' bacterial cell), their retention is mainly by adsorption. The isoelectric point of viruses usually ranges from pH 3 to pH 7. Below pH 3, they are generally positively charged and will be immobilised by negatively charged surfaces, and above pH 7 they are generally negatively charged and will be immobilised by positively charged surfaces. Increased salt concentrations and the presence of divalent and trivalent cations will also increase adsorption. Having said all this, rainfall can mobilise previously retained bacteria and viruses.

Microbiology of Onsite Systems

The septic tank works by a combination of sedimentation and anaerobic (without molecular oxygen) digestion. Anaerobic bacteria are responsible for the digestion. Anaerobic bacteria are non-pathogenic and are present in large numbers in the human intestine. A new supply of these bacteria are regularly added to the septic tank with each flush of human fecal material. Anaerobic digestion represents an incomplete digestion. Methane, hydrogen sulphide, and sulphur dioxide gases are produced, as well as a sludge of high molecular weight hydrocarbons. This sludge will readily decompose further when exposed to oxygen and aerobic bacteria. This further decomposition will take place in the municipal sewage treatment plant or landfill if either of these places is used to dispose of sludge pumped periodically from septic tanks. Anaerobic digestion which achieves the reduction of the contaminant load is given in Table 24.5.

Table 24.5. Anaerobic digestion achieves the reduction of the contaminant load.

Water quality parameter	% Removal in a septic tank
Biochemical oxygen demand (BOD)	15% to 50%
Total suspended solids (TSS)	25% to 45%
Settleable solids	> 90%
Enteric bacteria	10% to 40%
Enteroviruses	No significant reductions
Protozoa	No significant reductions

Aerobic digestion in the drainfield and aerobic treatment unit (ATU)

Aerobic digestion (with molecular oxygen) is far more complete. Aerobic digestion takes place in a properly constructed and maintained drainfield, as well as in an aerobic treatment device (ATU). In an ATU, the aerobic bacteria are selected out from any remaining aerobic bacteria which survive the trip through the septic tank or are facultative bacteria which can exist both with and without molecular oxygen or are random seed bacteria which are everywhere in our environment. In the soil, there are hundreds of different types of organisms that proliferate in the trenches where there is a regular supply of nutrients (septic tank effluent). Biological mats develop on the sides and bottoms of the trenches and add to a biological filtration of the effluent passing through it into the soil environment. The structure of these mats are due in part to the long filaments often growing out of several common strains of soil bacteria. If biomats are improperly managed, the growth can become so thick that the pores in the soil structure surrounding the disposal trench can become clogged. With the right balance of molecular oxygen to influent, the biological mat can be maintained as a benefit to the water treatment, and the wastes can be degraded completely to carbon dioxide and water allowing the aerobic treatment to go to completion.

Aerobic treatment in a trench or in an ATU is complete digestion and can achieve the reductions of influent contaminant levels (Table 24.6).

Table 24.6. Aerobic treatment in a trench.

Water quality parameter	% Removal in a septic tank
Biochemical oxygen demand (BOD)	75% to 90%
Chemical oxygen demand (COD)	75% to 90%
Total suspended solids (TSS)	75% to 90%
Ammonia (changed to nitrate – N)	80% to 90%
Enteric bacteria	Generally high but variable
Enteroviruses	Generally high but variable
Protozoa	Generally high but variable

Food Waste

Food waste is 'any food substance, raw or cooked, which is discarded or intended or required to be discarded', according to the legal definition of waste by the EU Commission. Since there are several definitions of waste, equally many definitions of food waste exist; professional bodies, including international organisations, state governments and secretariats may formally have their own definitions.

Sources of waste

Food production

In developing and developed countries who operate either commercial or industrial agriculture, food waste can occur at most stages of the food industry and in significant amounts. In subsistence agriculture, the amounts of food waste are unknown but are likely to be insignificant by comparison, due to the limited stages at which waste can occur, and given that food is grown for projected need as opposed to a global marketplace demand. Nevertheless, on-farm losses in storage in developing countries, particularly in Africa, can be high although the exact nature of such losses is much debated.

Research into the food industry of the United States, whose food supply is the most diverse and abundant of any country in the world, found food waste occurring at the beginning of food production. From planting, crops can be subjected to pest infestations and severe weather, which cause losses before harvest. Since natural forces (e.g. temperature and precipitation) remain the primary drivers of crop growth, losses from these can be experienced by all forms of outdoor agriculture. The use of machinery in harvesting can cause waste, as harvesters may be unable to discern between ripe and immature crops or collect only part of a crop. Economic factors, such as regulations and standards for quality and appearance, also cause food waste; farmers often harvest selectively, preferring to leave crops not to standard in the field (where they can be used as fertiliser or animal feed), since they would otherwise be discarded later.

Food processing

Food waste continues in the postharvest stage, but the amounts of postharvest loss involved are relatively unknown and difficult to estimate. Regardless, the variety of factors that contribute to food waste, both biological/environmental and socio-economical, would limit the usefulness and reliability of general figures. In storage, considerable quantitative losses can be attributed to pests and micro-organisms. This is a particular problem for countries that experience a combination of heat (around 30°C) and ambient humidity (between 70 and 90 per cent), as such conditions encourage the reproduction of insect pests and micro-organisms.

Losses in the nutritional value, caloric value and edibility of crops, by extremes of temperature, humidity or the action of micro-organisms, also account for food waste; these 'qualitative losses' are more difficult to assess than quantitative ones. Further losses are generated in the handling of food and by shrinkage in weight or volume.

Some of the food waste produced by processing can be difficult to reduce without affecting the quality of the finished product. Food safety regulations are able to claim foods which contradict standards before they reach markets. Although this can conflict with efforts to reuse food waste (such as in animal feed), safety regulations are in place to ensure the health of the consumer; they are vitally important, especially in the processing of foodstuffs of animal origin (e.g. meat and dairy products), as contaminated products from these sources can lead to and are associated with microbiological and chemical hazards.

Retail

Packaging protects food from damage during its transportation from farms and factories via warehouses to retailing, as well as preserving its freshness upon arrival. Although it avoids considerable food waste, packaging can compromise efforts to reduce food waste in other ways, such as by contaminating waste that could be used for animal feedstocks.

Retail stores can throw away large quantities of food. Usually this consists of items that have reached their sell-by date or use-by date. Most, if not all, of this food is edible at the time of disposal but stores often go to great lengths to ensure that poor or homeless people are unable to access it. On the other hand some stores work with charitable organisations to distribute food they can no longer display on their shelves. Retailers also contribute to waste as a result of their contractual arrangements with suppliers. Failure to supply agreed quantities renders farmers or processors liable to have their contracts cancelled. As a consequence they plan to produce more than actually required in order to meet the contract, in order to have a margin of error. Most of the surplus production is thrown away.

Response

Response to the problem of food waste at all social levels has varied hugely.

Prevention

One way of dealing with food waste is to reduce its creation. This attitude has been promoted by campaigns from advisory and environmental groups, and by concentrated media attention on the subject.

Psychology can be useful in helping reduce food waste. There are two ways we can reduce food waste. We can either prevent the consumer from throwing away huge amounts of waste or stop them in some way from producing so much waste. Once someone begins a certain behaviour in their lives, it is difficult to discourage this behaviour. So rather, than discouraging someone from wasting food, it is easier for someone to act as a good influence in order for them not to even begin wasting food in the first place. As a child, it is easier to establish a social norm for them so it is harder for them to change it later in their lives. We can establish a form of positive punishment to the child. For example, if a child decides to not finish their food on their plate, then the parent can scold them in order for the child to realise that the parent is disappointed or angry with them. The child may be scared so they will be less likely to throw food away. This way may work or instead negative punishment can also be useful. For example, not giving dessert to a child if they don't finish all their food. Positive punishment has been more effective according to many studies.

If an adult has established a negative behaviour it is extremely difficult for them to suddenly stop wasting too much food. Our parents are our main influence growing up so getting rid of these prints can be difficult. It is possible. We can begin with the idea of small steps at a time. Asking people to think about what they want to eat gets them thinking about how to proportion themselves. This is a smaller step compared to asking them not to take as much food. We can also start talking to them about what barriers exist in their lives.

Barriers are one of the main causes that stop people from changing their behaviours. Barriers associated with wasting food include: not wanting to get up and refill one's plate, inconvenience, and not thinking holistically. Holism involves seeing the idea of wasting less food as a whole positive effect across the world and not only themselves. People tend to see the present but forget about the effects in the future. Combining these ideas together can work to help people throw away less food which will certainly lead to a decrease in food waste piles.

Consumers can reduce their food waste output at point-of-purchase and in their home by adopting some simple measures; planning when shopping for food is important, spontaneous purchases are shown as often the most wasteful; proper knowledge of food storage reduces foods becoming inedible and thrown away.

Collection

In areas where waste collection is a public function, food waste is usually managed by the same governmental organisation as other waste collection. Most food waste is combined with general waste at the source. Separate collections, also known as Source Separated Organics, have the advantage that food wastes can be disposed of in ways not applicable to other wastes.

From the end of the 19th century through the middle of the twentieth century, many municipalities collected food waste (called 'garbage' as opposed to 'trash') separately. This was typically disinfected by steaming and fed to pigs, either on private farms or in municipal piggeries.

Separate kerbside collection of food waste is now being revived in some areas. To keep collection costs down and raise the rate of food waste segregation, some local authorities, especially in Europe, have introduced 'alternate weekly collections' of biodegradable waste (including, e.g. garden waste), which enable a wider range of recyclable materials to be collected at reasonable cost, and improve their collection rates. However, they result in a two week wait before the waste will be collected. So there is criticism that, particularly during hot weather, food waste rots and stinks, and attracts vermin. Much kitchen waste also leaves the home through garbage disposal units.

Disposal

Like other waste, food waste can be dumped, but food waste can also be fed to animals (typically swine) or it can be biodegraded by composting or anaerobic digestion, and reused to enrich soil.

Dumping food waste in a landfill causes odour as it decomposes, attracts flies and vermin, and has the potential to add biological oxygen demand (BOD) to the leachate. The EU landfill directive and waste regulations, like regulations in other countries, enjoin diverting organic wastes away from landfill disposal for these reasons. Food waste can be composted at home, avoiding central collection entirely, and many local authorities have schemes to provide subsidised composting bin systems. However, the proportion of the population willing to dispose of their food waste in that way may be limited.

Anaerobic digestion produces both useful gaseous products and a solid fibrous 'compostable' material. Anaerobic digestion plants can provide energy from waste by burning the methane created from food and other organic wastes to generate electricity, defraying the plant's costs and reducing greenhouse gas emissions. Food waste coming through the sanitary sewers from garbage disposal units is treated along with other sewage and contributes to sludge.

Commercially, food waste in the form of waste-water coming from commercial kitchens' sinks, dishwashers and floor drains is collected in holding tanks called grease interceptors to minimise flow to the sewer system. This often foul smelling waste contains both organic and inorganic waste (chemical cleaners, etc.) and may also contain hazardous hydrogen sulphide gases. It is referred to as FOG (fats, oils, and grease) waste or more commonly 'brown grease' (versus 'yellow grease' which is fryer oil that is easily collected and processed into biodiesel) and is an overwhelming problem especially in the USA, for the ageing sewer systems. Per the US EPA, Sanitary Sewer Overflows also occur due to the improper discharge of fats, oils and grease to the collection system. Overflows discharge 3–10 billion gallons of untreated waste-water annually into local waterways and up to 3700 illnesses annually are due to exposure to contamination from sanitary sewer overflows into recreational waters.

In US metropolitan areas the brown grease is taken by pumpers or grease hauling trucks to a wastewater treatment plant where they are charged to dump it. In other areas it may be taken to a landfill or it may be illegally dumped somewhere unknown, to avoid charges. This unmonitored disposal process is not only harmful for our environment and our health, it also hurts businesses who have no idea where their business waste ends up or indeed how much liquid waste is in their grease interceptor at any point in time, leaving them vulnerable to illegal dumping into their own grease trap or grease interceptor. Some companies such as Hydrologix Grease Reduction Systems Inc. now market computerised monitoring services along with *in situ* bioremediation which produces by-products of CO_2 and gray water that can safely flow into the sewer system.

Other new technologies offer *ex situ* treatment to process brown grease into some form of transportation fuel. This may not be as environmentally friendly as *in situ* treatment since it still requires vehicles to pump and transport the brown grease waste to the plants.

It is hard to estimate how much brown grease food waste is produced annually but in the US alone some think the number is in the billions of gallons. In 2009 the city of San Francisco stated it produces about 10 million gallons of brown grease a year. It is starting the first city-wide project in the US to recycle brown grease into biodiesel and other fuels.

MICROBIOLOGY OF THE FOOD PRODUCTS

To reduce contamination with micro-organisms to a minimum and obtain good keeping quality of the product, the raw materials are examined; the equipment contacting the food is adequately cleaned, sanitised, and tested; the preserving process is checked; and packaging and storage are supervised.

Ingredients

The raw product is inspected and tested for quality, but this does not necessarily involve bacteriological laboratory testing in all instances. Some of the ingredients of some products may contain numbers and kinds of micro-organisms that can affect the keeping quality of the product or even its acceptability. Some ingredients, such as sweetening agents, starch, and spices, can be purchased on specification as to maximal allowable content of micro-organisms or of numbers of certain kinds. The numbers of bacteria in ingredients are important in foods for which there are bacterial standards. Large numbers of spores of aerobes are undesirable in dry milk to be used in bread-making because of the increased risk of ropiness developing; heat-resistant spores in sugar and starch may add to the difficulty in adequately heat-processing canned vegetables to which sugar or starch is added; and large numbers of bacteria in spices may favour the spoilage of summer sausage.

The microbiology of the main raw product often is important. Excessive mould mycelium in the raw fruit, which is indicative of the presence of rotten parts, may lead to condemnation of the canned or frozen product. Large numbers of thermoduric bacteria in raw milk may yield a pasteurised milk that will not meet the bacterial standards for numbers as estimated by the standard platecount method. Large numbers of bacteria on vegetables or in fruits may indicate inferiority that will carryover into the frozen product. Laboratory examination may be employed to detect these undesirable organisms and estimate their numbers. Often there is opportunity for micro-organisms to grow in a food product during handling and processing in the plant. Examples are the buildup of thermophiles where foods are kept hot, as in forewarmers and blanchers, and increases in total numbers of bacteria in vegetables between blanching and freezing. Line samples may be tested in the laboratory to ascertain where appreciable growth of micro-organisms is taking place.

Packaging Materials

Packaging materials are a possible source of contamination of foods with micro-organisms, but ordinarily, the penetrability of nonmetallic materials to moisture and to gases is of more significance in the preservation of foods than the microbiology of these materials, for they harbour mostly low numbers of innocuous micro-organisms or no organisms. Also, as indicated previously, wrappers may be treated or impregnated with bacteriostatic or fungistatic compounds, e.g. cheese wraps with sorbic or caprylic acid. Paper and paperboard used for milk cartons contain mostly bacilli and micrococci, and occasionally other rods, actinomycetes, and mould spores, but no organisms of public health significance. Wax paper is practically sterile as produced, as are most plastic packaging materials. All packaging materials should be protected from contamination with dust or other sources of micro-organisms in handling.

According to federal regulations a food is deemed to be adulterated 'if its container is composed, in whole or in part, of any poisonous or deleterious substance which render its contents injurious to health'.

Food Safety and Environmental Services

Cleaning and sanitising program

Since cleaning and sanitising may be the most important aspect of a sanitation program, sufficient time should be given to outline proper procedures, and parameters. Detailed procedures must be developed for all food-product contact surfaces (equipment, utensils, etc.) as well as for non-product surfaces such as: non-product portions of equipment, overhead structures, shield, walls, ceilings, lighting devices, refrigeration units, heating, ventilation and air conditioning (HVAC) systems, and anything else which could impact food safety. Cleaning frequency must be clearly defined for each process line (i.e. daily, after production runs, or more often, if necessary). The type of cleaning required must also be identified. The objective of cleaning and sanitising food contact surfaces is to remove food (nutrients) which bacteria need to grow, and to kill those bacteria which are present. It is important that the clean, sanitised equipment and surfaces drain dry and are stored dry so as to prevent bacteria growth. Necessary equipment (brushes, etc.) must also be clean and stored in a clean, sanitary manner.

Cleaning/sanitising procedures must be evaluated for adequacy through evaluation and inspection procedures. Adherence to prescribed written procedures (inspection, swab testing, direct observation of personnel) should be continuously monitored, and records maintained to evaluate long-term compliance.

The correct order of events for cleaning/sanitising of food product contact surfaces is:
1. Rinse.
2. Clean.
3. Rinse.
4. Sanitise.

Definitions

Cleaning

Cleaning is the complete removal of food soil using appropriate detergent chemicals under recommended conditions. It is important that personnel involved have a working understanding of the nature of the different types of food soil and the chemistry of its removal.

Cleaning methods

Equipment can be categorised with regard to cleaning method as follows:
1. Mechanical cleaning: Often referred to as clean-in-place (CIP). Require no disassembly or partial disassembly.

2. Clean-out-of-Place (COP): Can be partially disassembled and cleaned in specialised COP pressure tanks.
3. Manual cleaning: Requires total disassembly for cleaning and inspection.

Sanitisation

It is important to differentiate and define certain terminology:

1. Sterilise refers to the statistical destruction and removal of all living organisms.
2. Disinfect refers to inanimate objects and the destruction of all vegetative cells (not spores).
3. Sanitise refers to the reduction of micro-organisms to levels considered safe from a public health viewpoint.

Appropriate and approved sanitisation procedures are processes and, thus, the duration or time as well as the chemical conditions must be described. The official definition (Association of Official Analytical Chemists) of sanitising for food product contact surfaces is a process which reduces the contamination level by 99.999 per cent (5 logs) in 30 sec.

The official definition for non-product contact surfaces requires a contamination reduction of 99.9 per cent (3 logs). The standard test organisms used are: *Staphylococcus aureus* and *Escherichia coli*.

General types of sanitisation include:

1. Thermal sanitisation involves the use of hot water or steam for a specified temperature and contact time.
2. Chemical sanitisation involves the use of an approved chemical sanitiser at a specified concentration and contact time.

Good Manufacturing Practice

Good manufacturing practice (GMP) is part of a quality system covering the manufacture and testing of pharmaceutical dosage forms or drugs and active pharmaceutical ingredients, diagnostics, foods, pharmaceutical products, and medical devices. GMPs are guidelines that outline the aspects of production and testing that can impact the quality of a product.

Although there are a number of them, all guidelines follow a few basic principles.

1. Manufacturing processes are clearly defined and controlled. All critical processes are validated to ensure consistency and compliance with specifications.
2. Manufacturing processes are controlled, and any changes to the process are evaluated. Changes that have an impact on the quality of the drug are validated as necessary.
3. Instructions and procedures are written in clear and unambiguous language.
4. Operators are trained to carry out and document procedures.
5. Records are made, manually or by instruments, during manufacture that demonstrate that all the steps required by the defined procedures and instructions were in fact taken and that the quantity and quality of the drug was as expected. Deviations are investigated and documented.
6. Records of manufacture (including distribution) that enable the complete history of a batch to be traced are retained in a comprehensible and accessible form.
7. The distribution of the drugs minimises any risk to their quality.
8. A system is available for recalling any batch of drug from sale or supply.
9. Complaints about marketed drugs are examined, the causes of quality defects are investigated, and appropriate measures are taken with respect to the defective drugs and to prevent recurrence.

GMP guidelines are not prescriptive instructions on how to manufacture products. They are a series of general principles that must be observed during manufacturing. When a company is setting up its quality program and manufacturing process, there may be many ways it can fulfil GMP requirements. It is the company's responsibility to determine the most effective and efficient quality process.

GMPs are enforced in the United States by the US FDA, under Section 501(B) of the 1938 Food, Drug, and Cosmetic Act (21USC351). The regulations use the phrase 'current good manufacturing practices' (cGMP) to describe these guidelines. Courts may theoretically hold that a drug product is adulterated even if there is no specific regulatory requirement that was violated as long as the process was not performed according to industry standards. As of June 2010, the same CGMP requirements apply to all manufacturers of dietary supplements.

Regulatory agencies (including the FDA in the US and regulatory agencies in many European nations) are authorised to conduct unannounced inspections, though some are scheduled. FDA routine domestic inspections are usually unannounced, but must be conducted according to 704(A) of the FD&C Act (21USC374), which requires that they are performed at a 'reasonable time'. Courts have held that any time the firm is open for business is a reasonable time for an inspection.

Other good practices

Other good-practice systems, along the same lines as GMP, exist:
1. Good laboratory practice (GLP), for laboratories conducting non-clinical studies (toxicology and pharmacology studies in animals).
2. Good clinical practice (GCP), for hospitals and clinicians conducting clinical studies on new drugs in humans.
3. Good regulatory practice (GRP), for the management of regulatory commitments, procedures and documentation.

Collectively, these and other good-practice requirements are referred to as 'GxP' requirements, all of which follow similar philosophies. (Other examples include good agriculture practices, good guidance practices, and good tissue practices.) In the US, medical device manufacturers must follow what are called 'quality system regulations' which are deliberately harmonised with ISO requirements, not cGMPs.

Chapter 25

Food Control

INTRODUCTION

Producing a food supply that is safe and of good quality is a prerequisite to successful domestic and international food trade and a key to sustainable development of national agricultural resources. All consumers have the right to expect and demand good-quality and safe food at affordable prices. This right was recognised by the participants at the United Nations Conference on Food and Agriculture, held in Hot Springs, Virginia, United States in 1943, which laid the foundation for the creation of FAO. The conference called on FAO 'to assist governments to extend and improve standards of nutrient content and purity of all important foods'.

The United Nations General Assembly, through its Resolution 39/248 of 9 April 1985, adopted guidelines for consumer protection which provide a framework for governments, particularly those of developing countries, to use in elaborating and strengthening consumer protection policies and legislation. The guidelines state that 'When formulating national policies and plans with regard to food, governments should take into account the need of all consumers for food security and should support and, as far as possible, adopt standards from the Food and Agriculture Organisation of the United Nations and the World Health Organisation Codex Alimentarius or, in their absence, other generally accepted international food standards. Governments should maintain, develop or improve food safety measures, including, *inter alia*, safety criteria, food standards and dietary requirements and effective monitoring, inspection and evaluation mechanisms.'

Following the 1962 creation of the Codex Alimentarius Commission and the establishment of its subsidiary bodies, it became clear that without substantial participation of developing countries in the commission's work, the international character of the Joint FAO/World Health Organisation (WHO) Food Standards Program might be jeopardised.

Therefore, FAO created the Food Control and Consumer Protection Group, with the main objective of assisting developing member countries in establishing and/or strengthening their national food control systems, thus to enable them to participate more actively in international standardisation activities. The new group would provide expert advice to the Codex Alimentarius Commission on various issues related to the quality and safety of foods.

The Food Control and Consumer Protection Group together with the Codex Secretariat formed the Food Standards and Food Science Service, renamed in 1985 as the Food Quality and Standards Service. In 1994, after the Uruguay Round of the General Agreement on Tariffs and Trade (GATT) negotiations ended, the new Food Quality Liaison Group was added to this service.

NEED FOR FOOD CONTROL

The world has witnessed unprecedented progress in agricultural production and in food science and technology over the past 50 years, which has had a profound impact on the way in which food is produced, processed, stored, distributed and consumed. The changes have contributed to a sizeable increase in the amount of food that is available globally and to a general improvement of the nutritional status of people worldwide, although malnutrition still persists among poor population groups. At the same time, as new production, processing and preservation techniques are used at farm level and in food processing plants to increase productivity, prolong shelf-life or improve the organoleptic and nutritional properties of food products, concern has grown among consumers about the quality and safety of the food supply.

The contamination of the environment with industrial pollutants which find their way into the food chain has escalated consumer anxiety over the safety of food. Furthermore, the rapid development of international food trade and the expansion of food distribution systems has increased the potential for the spread of foodborne diseases and zoonoses.

For these reasons, it has become essential that every nation establish an effective food control infrastructure capable of ensuring maximum consumer protection and promoting fair practices in food trade. Such an infrastructure, when accompanied by a reliable program of export inspection and certification, can add value to exported food products and help in national development efforts. An effective national strategy on food control should take into account the development needs of the country and assist in programs for increased food production, improved processing and reduction of food losses.

WORK OF FAO

Ten years after FAO's food control work had its origins at the Hot Springs Conference of 1945. FAO, with WHO, established the Joint FAO/WHO Expert Committee on Food Additives (JECFA) to evaluate the safety and efficacy of additives used in food production. This was followed by joint efforts of FAO and WHO to establish worldwide standards for milk and milk products in 1958 and the creation of the Codex Alimentarius Commission under the Joint FAO/WHO Food Standards Program in 1962. Direct assistance to developing countries in food control began in the 1960s.

What is Food Control?

An effective food control system has the following fundamental components:
1. Laws and regulations: There must be a basic food quality and safety law supplemented by detailed regulations requiring, among other things, sound hygienic practices along the food chain, the establishment of food standards, safe use of food additives and pesticides and informative labelling that will not mislead or deceive consumers.
2. Inspection and analysis: For effective administration of the laws and regulations, an organisation of technical administrative officers, food inspectors and analysts is needed, with adequate food laboratories and other facilities.
3. Certification and reporting: A credible reporting or certification system is needed to give the producer and the purchaser confidence in the food control system.
4. Information: The consumer must be made aware of food problems through information and education, especially on proper food handling and storage. The consumer is an effective partner in food control activities.

5. Quality control: Food producers, processors and marketers must be aware of and implement strict quality control procedures at all levels of the food chain to ensure that consumers receive good-quality and safe foods at all times.
6. Cooperation: Food producers, processors and handlers must cooperate with enforcement agencies to ensure food safety and quality.

Specialist advice

FAO provides specialist advice on the quality and safety of foods, especially in regard to food additives, contaminants and residues of chemicals used during agricultural and livestock production.

Additives

The use of food additives is stimulated by the need to maintain the physical and nutritional quality of food during shipment, storage and distribution and the need to meet the requirements of consumers in terms of the attractiveness of the food and its other characteristics. However, the potential use of additives to mask deficiencies in food quality, coupled with a better understanding of the possible negative effects of long-term exposure to small amounts of chemicals, has led countries to control the use of chemicals in food and to limit this use to chemicals that can be shown to be safe and effective in their intended use. The control of the use of food additives is therefore an important element of national food control systems.

JECFA provides essential advice to member countries of FAO and WHO on the safety of additives and on the specifications of purity to which such additives must conform. This independent scientific committee of experts has been active since 1956, and its work remains a world reference point for determining the acceptance of food additives. To date, some 800 food additives have been evaluated by JECFA, and the results of these evaluations have been published and distributed to professionals worldwide.

Contaminants

JECFA evaluates environmental and industrial contaminants such as lead, mercury and aflatoxins to determine how the contamination enters the food supply, what levels of intake are safe and how the intake of the contaminants can be minimised and controlled. The committee has evaluated several contaminants and established the acceptable daily intake (ADI) for them.

Residues

Biologically active chemicals are used in agricultural and livestock production to protect against disease, infestation and resulting production losses, as well as to improve production rates. Residues of these chemicals may remain in food. Maximum residue levels (MRLs) which are determined to be safe are established by JECFA for veterinary drugs and related compounds and by the Joint FAO/WHO Meeting on Pesticide Residues (JMPR) for pesticides. At present, some 50 veterinary drugs have been evaluated and more than 1200 MRLs have been established for pesticide residues.

Food contamination and residues monitoring

Food contamination continues to be a serious problem around the world. Surveillance of chemical and biological contaminants in foods is important not only for public health but also because of the negative economic impact of contamination. Excessive levels of aflatoxin or pesticide residues are often a cause of food export/import rejections in international food trade. Since 1975, FAO, WHO and the United Nations Environment Program (UNEP) have been operating the Food Contamination Monitoring Program, which provides information to member countries on the extent of environmental contamination of food including that due to persistent pesticides. The program also follows the global trends of food contamination problems to devise and implement corrective measures. FAO advises collaborating centres on quality assurance programs designed to ensure accuracy and reproducibility in laboratory analysis; as of 1995 there are 42 such centres.

Other matters

FAO provides expert advice to member countries and to the Codex Alimentarius Commission on different issues related to food quality and safety. Advice is provided through the convening of expert consultations and meetings on specific technical questions. At these meetings, top scientists from various parts of the world debate the subject and reach agreement on a recommended course of action. A number of such consultations and meetings have been convened by FAO, some in collaboration with other agencies such as WHO, UNEP and the International Atomic Energy Agency (IAEA). The most recent subjects considered by expert groups include: assessment of protein quality; determination of radionuclide contamination; establishment of a sampling plan for aflatoxin analysis in peanuts and corn; consumer participation in food control; application of Hazard Analysis Critical Control Points (HACCP) in food control; risk assessment in setting of food standards; and technology and quality control of food fortification.

Publications

An important aspect of FAO's work is the production and dissemination among professionals and policy-makers of technical and policy advisory publications. In the field of food quality control, a wide range of such publications has been developed and published by FAO, at times in collaboration with other agencies. The publications include guidelines and manuals covering different aspects of food control and food safety such as management of food control programs, food inspection, food analysis, prevention of mycotoxin contamination, food laboratory design and management and analytical quality assurance. Of particular interest to developing countries is the Guidelines for developing an effective national food control system prepared by FAO and WHO as part of a UNEP project; this publication is a valuable reference for member countries working to develop and modernise their national food control infrastructures.

Food control in developing countries

The development and strengthening of an integrated national food control system and the establishment of food contaminant control and monitoring programs at the national, regional and international levels have received particular attention in FAO programs during the past 20 years. Technical assistance in food control, in the form of project implementation, consultation, training and/or other advisory services, has been provided to more than 60 countries in Europe, Latin America and the Caribbean, the Near East, Africa and Asia and the Pacific. A few of FAO's recent activities are highlighted below to provide a general idea of the work being carried out to meet the technical assistance needs of developing countries in the field of food quality control.

Development of national strategies

To provide a certain measure of coherence in national food quality control systems and programs, FAO has assisted countries in reviewing their food control systems and activities and in formulating strategies to improve food quality and consumer protection. In recent years, studies have been carried out in Belize, Bhutan, Bolivia, Botswana, Cambodia, Ecuador, Fiji, Laos, Lesotho, Malta, Namibia, Senegal, Somalia, Uganda and Viet Nam, and proposals have been prepared for projects to strengthen their national capabilities.

Advice on legislation

FAO has assisted developing countries in reviewing and updating their food laws and regulations related to food quality control. Since this work began in the late 1960s, the work of the Codex Alimentarius Commission has been used as the basis for national regulations, and harmonisation of national regulations with the Codex regulations has been promoted. FAO, in collaboration with WHO, has elaborated a model food law which several developing countries have adapted to create food control legislation relevant to their conditions.

Training and human resources development

Training of government and food industry personnel in all areas related to food quality and safety is a major aspect of FAO's work. Importance has been placed on food inspection, food analysis, certification requirements and procedures for export, and management of food control programs at various levels. In Asia, a regional training network has been established for food inspectors, emphasising such topics as food export/import inspection, inspection of food processing industries and sampling techniques. Five training centres, one each in China, India, Indonesia, Malaysia and Thailand, have been established at existing institutions, which are organising the courses. Similar training networks for Latin America, the Near East and Africa are planned and will be implemented when financial resources are available.

Export food and international trade

Special emphasis is being given to improvement of national export food inspection and certification programs, and projects to this end have been established in Costa Rica, Indonesia and Thailand. In India, assistance has been provided in training of export food inspectors. In Senegal, a national workshop was organised recently to assess the export food control situation and define future strategies. Regional workshops were held in Costa Rica, Egypt and Indonesia to define export/import food control needs.

A global study to identify food contaminants affecting international trade was carried out by FAO with funding by the Government of Finland. Thirty-five countries from all regions of the world participated in this one-year study. Food export/import systems were reviewed and data were collected on major contaminants found in foods. A technical meeting held in Bangkok in early 1990 reviewed the study findings and recommended a series of actions to control and monitor the level of food contaminants in the concerned countries.

Street foods

The rapid growth of urban populations and the increased demands for the supply of food to cities have led to the burgeoning of the street-food industry. In many developing countries, a wide variety of raw, cooked, semi-processed, hot and cold foods and beverages are sold by itinerant pedlars or from open-air food stalls. FAO has conducted several studies in Africa, Asia and the Pacific, Latin America and the Caribbean and the Near East to assess the importance of this informal food service in urban nutrition; to evaluate the socio-economic conditions of vendors and users; to identify problems encountered by operators in following proper food-handling practices; and to determine measures needed to ensure adequate consumer protection. These studies led to the formulation and execution of projects to assist local authorities in improving infrastructure (e.g. provision of potable water, garbage disposal facilities and areas for personal hygiene of vendors), strengthening official control over the quality and safety of street foods and training food handlers in basic hygienic practices. Such projects have been implemented in Belize, Colombia, Côte d'Ivoire, Ecuador, Ghana, Guatemala, Honduras, India, Indonesia, Mexico, the Philippines, Thailand and Zaire.

FUTURE ORIENTATION

Future activities will strengthen FAO's leading role in gathering, disseminating and analysing information on food quality, consumer protection and food contaminants. The program will provide a forum for professional debate and policy dialogue on scientific and technical issues related to food quality and safety. It will continue to provide technical advice and assistance to member countries to help them strengthen the various elements of their food control systems, including institutional development, food standards and regulations, food inspection, food analysis and the overall management of food control programs. The program will continue to provide expert advice to governments, the Codex Alimentarius Commission and other international and regional bodies on the quality and safety of food, the safe use of food additives and maximum residue levels of food contaminants and chemicals used in veterinary medicines.

Emphasis will be given to the establishment of regional and subregional centres of excellence in various disciplines related to food control and to the promotion of Technical Cooperation among Developing Countries and Technical Cooperation among Countries in Transition in the operation of these centres. Particular attention will be given to the use of these centres for training of food control professionals at all levels and for applied research and studies on pertinent issues.

The Food Control and Consumer Protection program will give special consideration to promoting food export and to the harmonisation of food import/export inspection and certification procedures among trading partners through the development of prototype systems for determining equivalence in food control systems. These activities will require enhanced collaboration with the World Trade Organisation (WTO), the Office of International Epizootics, WHO and other organisations in the implementation of WTO agreements on sanitary and phytosanitary measures and on technical barriers to trade.

FOOD AND DRUG ADMINISTRATION

The Food and Drug Administration (FDA or USFDA) is an agency of the United States Department of Health and Human Services, one of the United States federal executive departments. The FDA is responsible for protecting and promoting public health through the regulation and supervision of food safety, tobacco products, dietary supplements, prescription and over-the-counter pharmaceutical drugs (medications), vaccines, biopharmaceuticals, blood transfusions, medical devices, electromagnetic radiation emitting devices (ERED), veterinary products, and cosmetics.

The FDA also enforces other laws, notably Section 361 of the Public Health Service Act and associated regulations, many of which are not directly related to food or drugs. These include sanitation requirements on interstate travel and control of disease on products ranging from certain household pets to sperm donation for assisted reproduction.

Glossary

Abiogenesis	:	Abiogenesis is the theory of spontaneous generation of living cells from nonliving material.
ABPA	:	Allergic bronchopulmonary aspergillosis.
Absorption	:	Absorption, in chemistry, is a physical or chemical phenomenon or a process in which atoms, molecules or ions enter some bulk phase—gas, liquid and solid material.
Abundance class	:	Refers to the relative abundance of different mRNA molecules in a cell at any given time.
Acanthamoeba	:	Protozoan; freel-living amoebae commonly found in natural waters.
Accession number	:	Sequential numbering of specimens according to the order in which they are obtained; also used for nucleic acid sequences in a database such as GenBank.
Acellular	:	Without a cell structure.
Acetobacter	:	Acetobacter is a bacterial genus; acid tolerant, aerobic, Gram-negative bacilli, an acetic acid bacterium that ferments ethanol to acetic acid but also has the needed enzymes to complete the cycle by oxidising acetic acid to CO_2 and water; commonly used in the commercial production of vinegar.
Acetogenesis	:	Acetogenesis is the formation of acetate from CO_2 as the result of the metabolic processes of certain bacteria, in contrast to methanogenesis; three recognised processes are the acetyl-CoA pathway, the glycine synthase-dependent pathway, and the reductive citric acid cycle.
Acetogenic bacteria	:	Acetogenic bacteria are approximately 40 recognised species isolated from diverse anaerobic habitats that conduct acetogenesis using the acetyl-CoA pathway for the conservation of energy and growth; a variety of bacillus and coccoid-shaped Gram-negative and Gram-positive bacteria that are mostly mesophilic, although some psychrophilic and thermophilic species have been isolated.
Acidophile	:	Acidophile is a micro-organism that preferentially grows at an acidic pH; cells that have an affinity for acidic dye.
Acid rock drainage (ARD)	:	The bacterial mediated leachate resulting from the oxidation of sulphide minerals exposed to air and water, and the products of the interaction of alkaline rock and water with acidic metal-containing solutions.
Acinetobacter baumannii	:	These are bacterial species; isolated from air samples associated with waste-water treatment operations.
Actinomycetes	:	Bacteria in which species are characterised by the formation of branching and/or true filaments.
Activated sludge process	:	Biological waste-water treatment process in which a mixture of the waste-water and activated sludge is aerated in a reactor basin or aeration tank. Active

515

biological solids bio-oxidise the waste matter and the biological solids are removed by secondary clarification or final settling.

Acute bronchitis	:	Disease that presents with cough productive of sputum that is often secondary to a viral or bacterial infection and the inhalation route of exposure to high concentrations of bioaerosols in agriculture facilities.
Adeno-associated virus	:	Virus used in gene therapy delivery methods.
Adenovirus	:	Virus that can infect through nasal passages, used in gene therapy delivery methods.
Aerated lagoon	:	Waste-water treatment pond in which mechanical or diffused air aeration is used to supplement oxygen supply.
Aerobes	:	Group of organisms that require air or oxygen for their survival and growth.
Aerobic	:	Presence of free molecular oxygen is required.
Aerobic bacteria	:	Bacteria requiring free molecular oxygen for their life processes.
Aerobic digestion	:	Digestion of suspended organic matter by aerobic microbes.
Aerobic respiration	:	Respiration that occurs in an oxygen-rich environment.
Agar	:	A derivative of marine seaweed used as a solidifying agent in many microbiological media.
Agrobacterium tumefaciens	:	Bacterium that infects plants arid causes crown gall disease. Carries a plasmid (the Ti plasmid) used for gene manipulation in plants.
Algae	:	Primitive plant-like organisms, single or multicellular, usually aquatic and capable of utilising food materials through photosynthesis.
Allele	:	One of two or more variants of a particular gene.
Anaerobes	:	Group of organisms that cannot tolerate the presence of air or oxygen, or survive in the absence of air or oxygen.
Anaerobic	:	Without air or oxygen.
Anaerobic bacteria	:	Bacteria that require combined oxygen and the absence of free molecular oxygen.
Anaerobic digestion	:	Digestion of suspended organic matter by anaerobic microbial action.
Anthropogenic	:	Originating in human activity.
Antibody	:	An immunoglobulin that specifically recognises and binds to an antigenic determinant on an antigen.
Archaebacteria	:	Most primitive type of micro-organism among prokaryotes.
Autotrophic bacteria	:	Bacteria that use inorganic materials for energy and growth.
Auxotroph	:	A cell that requires nutritional supplements for growth.
Bacilli	:	Rod-shaped or cylindrical bacterial cells.
Bacillus cereus	:	Bacterial species; associated with both diarrheal food poisoning and emetic food poisoning; endospores survive normal cooking procedures and germinate during improper storage after cooking.
Bacillus thuringiensis	:	Bacterium used in crop protection, and in the generation of *Bt* plants that are resistant to insect attack. The bacterium produces a toxin that affects the insect.
Bacteria	:	These are ubiquitous, single celled prokaryotic micro-organisms; the domain level of taxonomy of micro-organisms that are distinctly different from prokaryotes in the domain Archaea and the eukaryotes in the domain Eukarya.
Bacterial lawn	:	Confluent, uniform distribution of bacterial cells across the surface of an agar medium.
Bacteriocins	:	A group of bacterial proteins toxic to other bacteria.

Batch reactor	:	A reactor that does not have continuous streams entering or leaving. The reactants are added, reaction occurs, then the products are discharged.
Binary fission	:	The manner in which most bacteria multiply. The parent cell divides, usually into two daughter cells.
Bioassay	:	Bioassay is a biological-based analysis.
Biochemical oxidation	:	Oxidation caused by biological activity resulting in a chemical combination of oxygen with organic matter to produce relatively stable end-products.
Biochemical pathway	:	Various steps involved in any bioconversion process.
Bioconversion	:	A biocatalyst-mediated conversion of one substance to another.
Biodegradation	:	The process of chemical breakdown of a substance to smaller products caused by micro-organisms or their enzymes.
Biodeterioration	:	The chemical or physical alteration of a product that decreases the usefulness of that product for its intended purpose, caused by micro-organisms or their enzymes.
Biohazard	:	Biological material that is likely to cause a risk to human health.
Bioleaching	:	Process of using micro-organisms to recover metals from their ores.
Biological oxidation	:	An oxidation caused by biological activity resulting in a chemical combination of oxygen with organic matter to produce stable end-products known as both biochemical oxidation and bio-oxidation.
Bioluminescence	:	Bioluminescence is the generation of visible light by micro-organisms.
Biomarker	:	Biochemical that quantitatively measures the effects of exposure to xenobiotic substances on a biological system.
Biomass	:	The amount of living material present; a measurement of the quantity of energy being stored in a segment of the biological community expressed in units of weight.
Biopreservation	:	The use of micro-organisms or microbial by-products to prevent spoilage and extend the shelf-life of foods.
Bioreactor	:	Apparatus used to carry out biological reactions or processes, especially on an industrial scale.
Bioremediation	:	Process of using organisms to consume or otherwise help remove pollutants from the environment.
Biotransformation	:	Enzyme-catalysed conversion of one chemical, other than the normal body constituents of live organisms, into another. Normal metabolism refers to such conversions restricted to carbohydrates, fats, proteins, etc. taking place inside the body.
Brownian movement	:	Random zig-zag movement of microscopic particles in a gaseous system or suspended in a liquid medium.
Brush aerator	:	A surface aerator consisting of a rotating horizontal axle with protruding steel bristles partially submerged in the still water surface. Oxygen is transferred by air entrainment in the vicinity of the rotating bristles and also by the spray and impingement area.
Buffer action	:	Action of certain ions in solution to oppose a change in pH.
Bulking sludge	:	Activated sludge that settles poorly because of a floc with a low-bulk density.
Campylobacter	:	Bacterial genus; Gram-negative, microaerophilic, chemoorganotrophic, motile with a corkscrew motion, spiral-shaped curved bacteria; many species are

pathogenic to humans and animals; isolated from the intestinal tract, oral cavity and reproductive organs of humans and animals.

Capsomere	:	It is a protein subunit in a viral capsid; the cluster of viral proteins or protomers.
Carbohydrates	:	Class of carbon-hydrogen-oxygen compounds usually represented chemically by the formula $(CH_2O)_n$, where, $n = 3$.
Carboxydotrophic bacteria	:	Bacteria that aerobically utilise carbon monoxide as both a carbon source and as an energy source, for example, *Pseudomonas carboxidoflava* and *Pseudomonas carboxidohydrogena*.
Carcinogen	:	Cancer-causing agent.
Carrier	:	An individual that transmits an infectious agent to others, but does not show any symptoms of the disease.
Catabolism	:	Breakdown of complex biological molecules into simpler ones, usually accompanied with the release of energy in the form of ATP.
CBOD	:	Carbonaceous biological oxygen demand.
CDC	:	Centres for Disease Control and Prevention.
CDFF	:	Constant-depth film fermenter.
cDNA	:	Complementary DNA.
Chemical coagulation	:	The destabilisation and initial aggregation of colloidal and finely suspended matter by the addition of a floc-forming chemical coagulant.
Chemical oxygen demand (COD)	:	The amount of oxygen required to chemically oxidise the organic and sometimes inorganic matter in water or waste-water. Usually expressed in mg/l. COD test does not measure the oxygen required to convert ammonia to nitrites and nitrites to nitrates. COD is frequently assumed to be equal to the ultimate first-stage biochemical oxygen demand.
Chemical sludge	:	Sludge produced by chemical coagulation or chemical precipitation.
Chemically treated secondary effluent	:	Secondary effluent that has been chemically treated, usually by coagulation, along with other processes or operations.
Chronic	:	Continuous, over an extended period of time.
Chronic health effect	:	It is a long-term adverse reaction.
Citrobacter	:	Member of the family Enterobacteriaceae; human pathogen with potential environmental exposure via aerosols generated during waste-water treatment practices; member of the total coliform group.
Coagulant	:	A compound that causes coagulation or a floc-forming agent.
Coagulation	:	In water or waste-water treatment, the destabilisation and initial aggregation of colloidal and finely divided suspended solids by the addition of floc-forming chemicals.
Coliform bacteria	:	A group of bacteria predominately living in the intestines of humans and warm-blooded animals but also found elsewhere, such as in soils. Includes all aerobic and facultative anaerobic, Gram-negative, non-spore forming bacilli that ferment lactose with gas production.
Coliforms	:	Gram-negative, lactose-fermenting, enteric rods as *E. coli*.
Coliphage	:	A virus pathogenic to coliforms.
Complete treatment	:	Waste-water treatment that uses both primary and secondary treatment.
Completely mixed activated sludge	:	An activated sludge process with a completely mixed reactor basin. Usual basin is square, circular or slightly rectangular in plan view, and the influent, on entering, is almost immediately dispersed throughout the reactor basin.

Cosmid	:	Phage-plasmid artificial hybrids.
Cyanogen bromide	:	Chemical used to cleave a fusion protein product from the N-terminal vector-encoded sequence after synthesis.
Dauxie	:	The utilisation of one substance at a given rate before the utilisation of another substance at a different rate.
DBP	:	Disinfection by-product.
DBT	:	Dibenzothiophene.
Death phase	:	Final period of a growth curve of a microbial culture in which the number of organisms decreases over time.
Decussate	:	It is arranged in pairs at right angles to the subsequent pair.
Deep agar	:	Test tube with medium solidified without a slant that is generally inoculated with a needle in a single stab.
Demineralisation	:	Removal of all salts from a water.
Denaturation	:	The separation of double-stranded DNA into two single strands by manipulation of the ionic conditions of the solution; in contrast to melting for separation; in contrast of hybridisation for the construction; also refers to the breaking of hydrogen bonds to alter tertiary structure of proteins.
Dewatered sludge	:	Sludge that has had some of its water content removed.
Diazotroph	:	An organism that is capable of nitrogen fixation.
DIC	:	Differential interference contrast microscopy.
Diffused air aeration	:	Aeration produced in a liquid by the use of compressed air passed through air diffusers.
Digested sludge	:	Sludge digested by aerobic or anaerobic action to the degree that the volatile content is low enough for the sludge to be stable.
Diphasic fungi	:	Characterisation of some fungal genera in which there is a filamentous phase and a yeast phase.
Disinfect	:	Disinfect is to treat a surface or a liquid with a substance that will kill micro-organisms.
Disinfectant	:	A chemical used on surfaces or in water to kill micro-organisms; may cause harm to host tissue.
Dispersed plug-flow activated sludge	:	Activated sludge process with a dispersed plug-flow reactor basin. The basin is rectangular in plan view and has significant longitudinal or axial dispersion of fluid elements throughout its length.
Dispersed plug-flow reactor	:	Reactor that is rectangular in plan view and has significant longitudinal mixing of fluid elements throughout its length.
Dose	:	The amount of a substance, generally that ingested or applied at one time.
Dot-blot	:	Technique in which small spots or dots, of nucleic acid are immobilised on a nitrocellulose or nylon membrane for hybridisation.
Downstream processing	:	Refers to the procedures used to purify products (usually proteins) after they have been expressed in bacterial, fungal or mammalian cells.
Droplets	:	Airborne particles of mucus and sputum from the respiratory tract that contain disease organisms.
Dry suspended solids	:	The suspended matter in water and, in particular, waste-water, which is removed by laboratory filtration and is dried for one hour at 103°C.
Eccentric	:	Asymmetrical in growth.
E. coli	:	*Escherichia coli.*

Ecology	:	The study of the relationships between organisms and the environment; derived from the Greek *oikos* (dwelling) and *logos* (law).
Ecosystem	:	A community of organisms in their natural environment.
Ectopic	:	Occurring in an unusual place or in an unusual form or manner.
Effluent	:	The liquid discharge from sewage treatment and industrial plants.
EFM	:	Epifluorescent microscopy.
Electrophoresis	:	Technique for separating molecules based on the differential mobility in an electric field.
Encrusted	:	Covered with a layer of mineral.
Endogenous	:	Developed or living within an organism.
Endolithic	:	Micro-organisms that live within the rock matrix; in contrast to lithobiotic.
Endotoxin	:	A metabolic poison produced chiefly by Gram-negative bacteria, endotoxins are part of the bacterial cell wall and consequently, are released on cell disintegration, they are composed of lipid polysaccharide-peptide complexes.
Enteric bacteria	:	Bacteria that inhabit the intestines of humans and animals.
Enterovirus	:	A virus that infects intestinal cells.
Enzymes	:	Proteins specialised to trigger biological reactions, e.g. the conversion of certain organic substances into different ones.
Episome	:	A plasmid attached to the chromosome of a bacterium.
Escherichia coli (E. coli)	:	A species of bacteria in the coliform group. Its presence is considered indicative of fresh fecal contamination.
Excess activated sludge	:	Waste-activated sludge.
Exotoxin	:	A metabolic poison produced chiefly by Gram-positive bacteria, exotoxins are released to the environment; they are composed of protein and affect various organs and systems of the body.
Expressivity	:	The degree to which a particular genotype generates its effect in the phenotype.
Extended aeration activated sludge process	:	Activated sludge process with a detention time long enough to allow the amount of cells synthesised to be endogenously decayed.
Ex vivo	:	Outside the body. Usually used to describe gene therapy procedure in which the manipulations are performed outside the body, and the altered cells returned after processing.
Facultative	:	Capable of growth in the presence or absence of an environmental factor.
Facultative anaerobic bacteria	:	Bacteria that use either free molecular oxygen, if available, or combined oxygen. Also known as facultative bacteria.
False negative	:	Result that incorrectly identifies the absence of the analyte of interest when it is actually present in the sample; in contrast to a false positive.
False positive	:	Result that incorrectly identifies the presence of the analyte of interest when it is absent from the sample; in contrast to a true positive.
FAME analysis	:	Fatty acid methyl ester analysis.
Fastidious	:	Having very specific nutritional and environmental requirements.
Fermentation	:	Process by which enzymes, usually coming from micro-organisms, cause desired changes in taste, smell and texture.

Fermenter	:	A micro-organism that uses organic compounds as both primary electron donor and the ultimate electron acceptor.
Fibrobacter	:	Bacterial genus; many species are present in the complex of micro-organisms isolated from the rumen.
Filtration	:	Unit operation that consists of passing a liquid through a granular medium for the removal of suspended and colloidal matter.
Fimbriae	:	Short, hairlike structures used by bacteria for attachment, sometimes used as an alternative expression for pili.
Final clarifier	:	Last settling basin or settling tank at a waste-water treatment plant. In the activated sludge process, it separates the biological solids from the final effluent. In the trickling filter process, it separates the trickling filter humus, that is, sloughed growths from the final effluent.
First-stage biochemical oxygen demand	:	That part of the biochemical oxygen demand that results from the biological oxidation of carbonaceous materials, as distinct from nitrogenous materials. Generally, the major portion of carbonaceous materials are bio-oxidised before the bio-oxidation of nitrogenous materials, or the second-stage biochemical oxygen, demand begins.
Five-day biochemical oxygen demand (BOD_5)	:	Oxygen required by microbes in the stabilisation of a decomposable waste under aerobic conditions for a period of five days at 20°C and under specified conditions. It represents the breakdown of carbonaceous materials as distinct from nitrogenous materials.
Fixed-bed	:	In carbon adsorption or ion exchange treatments using columns or open beds, this refers to a bed that is stationary in the column or in the structure for the open bed.
Fixed factor	:	Statistical term to denote that a condition either exists or it does not; in contrast to a random factor.
Floc	:	The small, gelatinous masses formed in the water by the adding of coagulant. In waste-water treatment, the small, gelatinous biological solids formed at an activated sludge treatment plant.
Flocculation	:	Slow stirring of a coagulated water or waste-water to aggregate the destabilised particles and form a rapid-settling floc. In biological waste-water treatment where a coagulant is not used, aggregation may be accomplished biologically.
Fluidised bed	:	Refers to a bed in which the particles are not in continuous contact due to the upward flow of the water or waste-water.
Fomites	:	Inanimate objects such as clothing or utensils that carry disease organisms.
Fungemia	:	Dissemination of fungi through the circulatory system.
Gel electrophoresis	:	Technique for separating nucleic acid molecules on the basis of their movement through a gel matrix under the influence of an electric field.
Gel electrophoresis	:	Technique for separating nucleic acid molecules on the basis of their movement through a gel matrix under the influence of an electric field.
Gene	:	The unit of inheritance, located on a chromosome. In molecular terms, usually taken to mean a region of DNA that encodes one function. Broadly, therefore, one gene encodes one protein.
Genetic code	:	The triplet codons that determine the types of amino acid that are inserted into a polypeptide during translation. There are 61 codons for 20 amino acids (plus three stop codons), and the code is therefore referred to as degenerate.

Genetic engineering	:	The *in vitro* manipulation of gene sequences.
Genome	:	Used to describe the complete genetic complement of a virus, cell or organism.
Genomics	:	The study of genomes, particularly genome sequencing.
Genomic library	:	A collection of clones which together represent the entire genome of an organism.
Glycolysis	:	Metabolic process in which sugars are broken down into smaller compounds along with the release of energy.
GM	:	Geometric mean.
GMOs	:	Genetically-modified organisms; genetically engineered micro-organisms.
Gravity filters	:	Filters that have gravity flow of the water through the filter bed.
Green bacteria	:	Anoxygenic phototrophic bacteria that conduct photophosphorylation using Bchl *c* and Bchl *d* chlorophyll pigments that are located within chlorosomes, in contrast to the purple bacteria.
Green fluorescent protein (GFP)	:	Protein produced by some bacteria due to the introduced *gfp* gene that is used as a biosensor for the discrimination of bacteria from background matrix.
Grit	:	Dense, mineral, suspended matter present in a water or waste-water, such as silt and sand.
Growth	:	An increase in the number of micro-organisms.
Growth curve	:	Depiction of the cycle of a microbial population in culture in which the population increases, stabilises, and decreases; defined for each microbial population with a lag phase, an exponential phase, a stationary phase, and a death phase.
Halobacteria	:	Generalised term to describe members of the Archaea that are extreme halophiles.
Halophiles	:	Organisms requiring NaCl for growth; extreme halophiles grow in concentrated brines.
Halorespiring	:	The coupling of reductive dehalogenation and electron transport-coupled phosphorylation catalysed by specific enzymes in some bacterial species that results in degradation of haloorganic compounds in anoxic polluted soils, aquifers, and sediments; in contrast to use of metal-containing cofactor for reductive dehalogenation by many anaerobic bacteria.
Harvest	:	In cell culture, describes the collecting of cells or the growth medium in which cells exposed to a sample were grown, so that the cells or medium can be analysed or the cells can be used as a seed for further propagation of the cell culture.
Haemagglutinin	:	An enzyme on the surface spikes of certain influenza viruses that allows the virus to bind to red blood cells.
Haemolysins	:	Enzymes that dissolve red blood cells, produced by streptococci, staphylococci, gas gangrene bacilli, and other micro-organisms.
Hepatotoxin	:	A compound that is toxic to the liver.
Heterotrophic potential	:	The ability of microbial populations to utilise an organic substrate.
Hierarchical stepwise regression	:	Statistical analysis in which a single variable or cluster of variables are examined by stepwise regression but the order of the introduced variables is predetermined.
High-rate digester	:	Anaerobic digester with continuous mixing, continuous feeding and digester heating.
Hirsute	:	Hairy in appearance.
HPC	:	Heterotrophic plate count.
HPLC	:	High performance liquid chromatography.
HSP	:	Heat-shock protein.

HTS	:	High throughput screening.
Humus	:	The organic portion of the soil remaining after microbial decomposition.
Ice-minus bacteria	:	Bacteria engineered to disrupt the normal ice-forming process, used to protect plants from frost damage.
Immobilised enzyme	:	An enzyme bound to a solid support.
IMS	:	Immunomagnetic separation.
Incidence density	:	The number of occurrences within a defined area.
Incidence rate	:	The number of new occurrences of an event (e.g. illness) per population at risk within a defined period of time.
Incubator	:	An enclosed, temperature-regulated chamber for the growth of micro-organisms in culture.
Inducer	:	A substances that may activate the operon of the cell by combining with and negating the repressor protein.
Infect	:	To enter another organism and multiply within it.
Inhibition	:	The prevention of a function; this condition may be temporary.
Inoculating loop	:	A flat, open circle device used to apply micro-organisms to a surface or liquid.
Inoculum	:	The micro-organisms, cells, or other biological material that are added to growth medium to start a culture.
In situ	:	Latin term for the original place; used to denote experiments conducted at the site or on location.
Interferon	:	An antiviral protein produced by body cells on exposure to viruses; interferon triggers production of a second protein that binds to mRNA coded by the virus and thereby inhibits viral replication.
In vitro	:	Latin term 'in glass' used to denote experiments conducted outside of a cell.
In vivo	:	Latin term 'in cell' used to denote experiments conducted in living cell.
Isolation	:	The separation of two or more entities.
Isozymes (isoenzymes)	:	Multiple forms of an enzyme that differ in properties such as substrate specificity and maximum activity.
Japan collection of micro-organisms	:	Culture collection entity located in Wako, Japan that catalogues and sells standard strains of micro-organisms.
Kelly's medium	:	Culture medium for the isolation of *Borrelia* spp.
Kilobase pair	:	A segment containing 1000 base pairs.
Kingdom	:	The second highest taxonomic ranking; the taxonomic ranking below domain.
Klebsiella	:	Bacterial genus, member of the family *Enterobacteriaceae*; nonmotile, gram-negative bacilli some of which are human pathogens while other are commensals in humans and animals, or phytopathogens.
Kogure technique	:	The use of nalidixic acid and yeast extract with acridine orange and light microscopy to enumerate swollen or elongated cells as viable.
Korarchaeota	:	A kingdom of hyperthermophilic Archaea.
K strategists	:	Micro-organisms that depend on physiological adaptations to environmental resources or the carrying capacity of the environment for continued survival within a community so they reproduce slowly and are successful in environments that are limited in nutritional resources.
Lag phase	:	Initial period of time in the growth curve of micro-organisms in which growth does not occur immediately; the period to time prior to exponential growth.
LAL assay	:	*Limulus* amebocyte lysate assay.

Latent virus	:	A virus whose genome is integrated into the host's genome, but is not expressed; upon activation (e.g. by stress or exposure to ultraviolet irradiation), infective virus particles are produced and symptoms of infection appear.
Leaching	:	The removal of metal from ore by chemical or microbial activity; the transport of dissolved materials from upper soil layers deeper into the subsurface.
Legionellaceae	:	Bacterial family; characterised as intracellular parasites or endosymbionts of free-living parasites.
Ligation	:	Formation of a phosphodiester bond to link two adjacent bases separated by a nick in one strand of the double helix of DNA.
Linker	:	A synthetic self-complementary oligonucleotide that contains a restriction enzyme recognition site. Used to add cohesive ends to DNA molecules that have blunt ends.
Lipase	:	Enzyme that hydrolyses fats (lipids).
Lye dip	:	Soaking fruits or vegetables in a lye solution, which makes the product easier to dry and makes the peel easier to remove.
Lyophilisation	:	Process in which cold temperature and air evacuation are used for preservation of micro-organisms; also termed freeze-drying.
MA	:	Muramic acid.
Macromonas	:	Bacterial genus; cylindrical to bean-shaped cells that oxidise sulphur and sulphur compounds; may accumulate calcium carbonate with sulphur globules; found in seawater.
Macromolecules	:	Large molecules, contained within a cell, with molecular weights ranging from a few thousand to hundreds of millions.
Magnetospirillum	:	Bacterial genus; magnetotactic organisms that participate in biomineralisation of magnetosomes.
MCYSTs	:	Microcystins.
Mechanical aeration	:	Transfer of oxygen from the atmosphere into a liquid by the mechanical action of a turbine or other mechanisms. Mixing by mechanical means of the mixed liquor in the reactor basin or aeration tank of an activated sludge treatment plant.
Mesophilic digestion	:	Anaerobic digestion by biological oxidation by anaerobic action at or below 45°C (110°F).
Micro (μ)	:	SI prefix, 10^{-6}.
Microbial activity	:	Chemical changes resulting from biochemical action, the metabolism of living organisms.
Microbial pest control agent (MPCA)	:	A nonpathogenic micro-organism applied to agricultural crops to minimise the colonisation of a microbial phytopathogen.
Microconidia	:	Plural of microconidium.
Microcosm	:	A small-scale experimental model that is designed to reproduce the environmental conditions of interest as closely as possible; used in laboratory experiments to define environmental conditions and test biological populations.
Microenvironment	:	The physical and chemical conditions in the area immediately surrounding an organism.
Microinjection	:	Introduction of DNA into the nucleus or cytoplasm of a cell by insertion of a microcapillary and direct injection.

Micro-organism	:	A microscopic organism that exists as a single cell or in an aggregate of cells, or as an acellular entity (i.e. virus).
Microtubule	:	A structural entity of eukaryotic flagella.
Mixed culture	:	Microbial culture consisting of two or more species.
Monosaccharides	:	Chemical building blocks of carbohydrates with the empirical formula $(CH_2O)_n$.
MPA	:	Microscopic particulate analysis.
MPCA	:	Microbial pest control agent.
Multimedia filtration	:	Filtration of water or waste-water through a granular bed containing two or more filter media.
Mutagenesis	:	The process of inducing mutations in DNA.
Mutant	:	An organism (or gene) carrying a genetic mutation.
Mutation	:	An alteration to the sequence of bases in DNA. May be caused by insertion, deletion or modification of bases.
Neutralisation	:	A type of antigen-antibody reaction in which the activity taking place between reactants is not visible.
Neutralism	:	A relationship of microbial populations in which there is no interaction between the populations; occurs when populations of organisms have different metabolic capabilities, populations are spatially distant from each other, when environmental conditions are unfavourable for active growth or when organisms are in a resting state.
Nitrifying bacteria	:	A group of bacteria that oxidises ammonia to nitrite or nitrite to nitrate.
Node	:	A joint, point of origin of fungal hyphae, or an enlarged area on a fungal hypha.
Nod genes	:	Genetic sequences in nitrogenic fixing bacteria that direct specific steps in the formation of a root nodule.
Nuclease	:	An enzyme that hydrolyses phosphodiester bonds.
Nucleoside	:	A nitrogenous base bound to a sugar.
Nucleotide	:	A nucleoside bound to a phosphate group.
Nucleus	:	Membrane-bound region in a eukaryotic cell that contains the genetic material.
Oligonucleotide	:	A short sequence of nucleotides.
Outlier	:	A value that is inconsistent with the other data obtained during statistical analysis.
PAB	:	Propionic acid bacterium.
PADs	:	Phenolic acid decarboxylases.
Papovavirus	:	Any virus in the family Papovaviridae.
Parasite	:	An organism that lives on or in a host.
Parasitic bacteria	:	Bacteria that require living host organism but do not harm the host.
Passive sampling	:	Collection of material without the use of a mechanical device; gravitational sampling.
Pasteurisation	:	Preservation method in which bottled or canned food is heated at a maximum temperature of 100°C. This process kills most micro-organisms and thereby increases the product's shelf-life up to several weeks, but it is not as effective as sterilisation.
Pathogen/Pathogenic	:	An organism that infects a host and is capable of causing disease.
PBBs	:	Polybrominated biphenyls.
PCA	:	Principal component analysis.
PCBs	:	Polychlorinated biphenyls.
PCP	:	Pentachlorophenol.

Pedigree analysis	:	Determination of the transmission characteristics of a particular gene by examination of family histories.
PFA	:	Polyunsaturated fatty acid.
PFU	:	Plaque-forming unit.
pH	:	Level of acidity.
Phage	:	A short form of the word bacteriophage.
Phagosome	:	A vesicle that contains particles of phagocytised material.
Phenotype	:	The observable characteristics of an organism, determined both by its genotype and its environment.
Photosynthesis	:	Process in green plants of converting carbon dioxide and water into sugar using light as the source of energy.
Pili	:	Physical appendages on bacteria, similar in structure to fimbriae but are longer; generally only one or two are visualised on the bacterial cell when they serve as specific receptors of certain types of virus particles.
Pip	:	A membrane protein that serves as a receptor protein for bacteriophage.
Plaque	:	A cleared area on a bacterial lawn caused by infection by a lytic bacteriophage.
Polynucleotide	:	A polymer made up of nucleotide monomers.
Polypeptide	:	A chain of amino acid residues.
Precipitins	:	Antibodies that participate in precipitation reactions.
Prions	:	Infectious particles of protein, possibly involved in human disease of brain.
Probe	:	A labelled molecule used in hybridisation procedures.
Prokaryotic	:	The property of lacking a membrane-bound nucleus, e.g. bacteria such as *E. coli*.
Prophage	:	A bacteriophage maintained in the lysogenic state in a cell.
Protease	:	Enzyme that hydrolyses polypeptides.
Protein	:	A condensation (dehydration) heteropolymer composed of amino acid residues linked together by peptide bonds to give a polypeptide.
Proteome	:	Refers to the population of proteins produced by a cell.
Protoplast	:	Part of the cell that includes the cell membrane and all intracellular components, except the cell wall.
R	:	Multiple correlation coefficient.
R^2	:	Coefficient of determination.
R2A agar	:	A low nutrient culture medium used for the isolation of oligotrophic bacteria, primarily for isolation of bacteria in water samples.
RAB	:	Rotating annular bioreactor.
Recalcitrant	:	Totally resistant to biodegradation.
Recombinant DNA	:	A segment of DNA that contains nucleic acid from two or more sources.
Redox reaction	:	The oxidation of one compound paired with the reduction of another compound.
Reducing agent	:	Substance that combines with oxygen or loses electrons in a reaction.
Regulatory gene	:	A gene that exerts its effect by controlling the expression of another gene.
Replication	:	Copying the genetic material during the cell cycle. Also refers to the synthesis of new phage DNA during phage multiplication.
Reporter gene	:	A gene used to disclose the function of potential regulatory DNA sequences upstream of the reporter gene.

Repressor protein	:	A protein that inhibits the activity of certain genes, lysogeny is established when repressor protein is produced under direction of a virus.
Retrovirus	:	Any virus in the family Retroviridae; viruses are icosahedral in shape, surrounded by a lipid envelope, contain single-stranded RNA; human pathogens in this family cause different types of cancer, and the human immunodeficiency viruses (causative agent of AIDS) are members of the lentivirus genus in this family.
Reverse transcriptase	:	An enzyme that synthesises a DNA molecule from the code supplied by a RNA molecule.
Rhizobiaceae	:	Bacterial family; characterised by their ability to fix atmospheric nitrogen.
Ribonuclease (RNase)	:	An enzyme that hydrolyses RNA.
Sake	:	A type of rice beer produced primarily in the orient.
Salmonella enterica	:	Bacterial species; foodborne pathogen transmitted via the ingestion route of exposure through the consumption of raw tomatoes.
Salmonella paratyphi	:	Bacterial species; waterborne and foodborne pathogen transmitted via the ingestion route of exposure.
Sanitary landfill	:	Landfill for disposing of solid wastes.
Scotochromogenesis	:	Formation of pigment only when the micro-organism is cultured in dark; used in the classification of some *Mycobacterium* spp.; in contrast of photochromogenesis.
Secondary effluent	:	Effluent leaving the secondary or final clarifier at a waste-water treatment plant.
Secondary sludge	:	Sludge from the final clarifier at waste-water treatment plant. For the activated sludge process, it is the sludge to be recycled. For the trickling filter process, it is the trickle filter growths that have sloughed off—that is, the trickling filter humus.
Sedimentation	:	Removal of settleable suspended solids from water or waste-water by gravity settling in a quiescent tank or basin. Also called clarification or settling.
Selection bias	:	The introduction of a systematic error due to the manner in which the test and control populations are selected in contrast to surveillance bias and mis-classfication bias.
Settled waste-water	:	Waste-water that has been treated by sedimentation. Also called clarified waste-water.
Silencing	:	The process whereby an organism shuts down the expression of a gene.
Sludge conditioning	:	Treatment of sludge, usually by chemical means, to enhance its dewatering characteristics.
Sludge digestion	:	Biological oxidation of organic or volatile matter in sludges to produce more stable substances.
Sludge digestion tank	:	Tank used for the anaerobic digestion of organic sludges.
Somatic cell	:	Body cell, as opposed to germ-line cell.
SOP	:	Standard operating procedure.
Sperm	:	The mature male gamete.
Spore-formers	:	Type of bacteria that carry a certain type of seed that can withstand high temperatures and that grow into bacteria at low temperatures.
Sterilisation	:	Preservation method in which bottled or canned food is heated at a temperature of $100°–121°C$. This process kills all micro-organisms, and extends the product's shelf-life up to a maximum of one year, but it does not kill the spores, which can grow into bacteria once the container is reopened.
Structural gene	:	A gene that encodes a protein product.

Suspended matter	:	Solids in suspension in water or waste-water that can be removed by laboratory filtration techniques, such as membrane filtration.
TEM	:	Transmission electron microscopy.
Temperate	:	Refers to bacteriophages that can undergo lysogenic infection of the host cell.
Tertiary treatment	:	Use of physical, chemical or biological means to upgrade a secondary effluent.
Thermal death point	:	The temperature required to kill an organism in a given length of time.
Toxin	:	A poisonous substance produced by a species of micro-organism, bacterial toxins are classified as exotoxins or endotoxins.
Transcription	:	The synthesis of RNA using a DNA template.
Transduction	:	Genetic recombination process mediated by virus; DNA is incorporated from one cell to another with the assistance of virus by generalised transduction or specialised transduction.
Transfection	:	Introduction of purified phage or virus DNA into cells.
Transformant	:	A cell that has been transformed by exogenous DNA.
Transformation	:	The process of introducing DNA (usually plasmid DNA) into cells. Also used to describe the change in growth characteristics when a cell becomes cancerous.
Transgene	:	The target gene involved in the generation of a transgenic organism.
Transgenic micro-organism	:	A micro-organism with a cloned DNA sequence from another organism.
Trickling filter	:	Biological filter consisting of a bed of coarse material, such as stone, over which waste-water is distributed by a spray from a moving distributor or other device. The waste-water trickles through the bed to the underdrains, giving the microbial slimes an opportunity to absorbed the organic material and clarify the waste-water.
Turbidity	:	Suspended matter in water or waste-water that causes the scattering or absorption of light rays.
Vaccinia	:	The alternative name for cow-pox.
Vacuole	:	A large, fluid-filled sac located in the cytoplasm.
Vector	:	A DNA molecule that is capable of replication in a host organism, and can act as a carrier molecule for the construction of recombinant DNA.
Virus	:	An infectious agent that cannot replicate without a host cell.
VNA	:	Viral nucleic acid.
Waste stabilisation	:	Process of reducing the BOD or COD of organic wastes to render them harmless.
Waste-water analysis	:	The determination of the physical, chemical, and biological characteristics of a waste-water or treatment plant effluent.
Waterborne disease	:	Disease caused by organisms or toxic materials transported by water. The most common waterborne diseases are typhoid fever, cholera, dysentery and other intestinal disturbances.
Water moulds	:	Aquatic fungi that are members of the Oomycetes.
Waterwashed disease	:	Illness caused by organisms that originate in feces and are transmitted through contact because of inadequate sanitation.
WHC	:	Water holding capacity.
Whey	:	A waste liquid of the dairy industry containing lactose and minerals that is used in industrial processes as supplemental carbon.
Xanthomonadins	:	Yellow, membrane-bound, halogenated aryl polyene pigments that are produced by *Xanthomonas* spp. and may provide some protection against photodamage.

Xanthomonas	:	Bacterial genus; member of the family Pseudomonaceae; chemoorganotrophic, Gram-negative, straight, obligate aerobic, bacillus that is motile by a single polar flagellum; many species are phytopathogens.
Xanthomonas campestris	:	Bacterial species; phytopathogen, causative agent of black rot of crucifers.
Xanthomonas oryzae	:	Bacterial species; phytopathogen, causative agent of blight of rice.
Xanthomonas vascularum	:	Bacterial species; phytopathogen, causative agent of gumming of sugar cane.
Xenobiotic	:	Group of chemicals unfamiliar or foreign to micro-organisms and thus not easily degradable by them.
XPS	:	X-ray photoemission spectroscopy.
Yeast	:	Unicellular fungus that reproduces by budding; most are members of the Ascomycetes; some have a filamentous phase; for example, *Saccharomyces cerevisiae* are used extensively in food production for leavening of bread and in beer and wine fermentation.
Yersinia	:	Bacterial genus; member of the family Enterobacteriaceae; facultative, Gram-negative, nonsporulating bacilli with 10 established species, most with simple nutritional requirements; previously classified as the genus *Pasteurella*.
Zonate	:	Arranged in zones or rings radiating from the centre.
Zone of inhibition	:	The area in which an antimicrobial substance prevents growth.
Zooglea	:	The gelatinous material resulting from the attrition of bacterial slime layers. An important constituent of activated sludge floc and trickling filter growths.
Zooglea ramigera	:	Bacterial species; produces extracellular polysaccharide slime matrix during sewage treatment.
Zygomycetes	:	Fungal class; rapid growing non-septate fungi with sporangiospores produced in sporangia and some species have rhizoids and stolons; sexual reproduction produces a dark thick-walled zygospore.
Zymocide	:	A factor present in some yeast cells that is toxic to other yeasts.
Zymomonas	:	Bacterial genus; tolerant of low pH and ethanol concentrations up to 10 per cent; large, Gram-negative bacillus that ferments sugars to ethanol; active in fermentation of plant sap for industrial production (e.g. fermentation of agave in Mexico to produce tequila and palm sap in tropical areas); responsible for spoilage of fruit juices and production of an odour of rotten apples in spoiled beer.

References

Alouf, M., *Biotechnological Innovations in Food Processing*, Butterworths, London.

Alford, A., *Food Chemistry*, John Wiley & Sons, New York.

Anke, K.T., *Food Engineering Operations*, Marcel Dekker Inc., New York.

Berg, V.T., *Dairy Microbiology*, Applied Science Publishers, London.

Batterman, S.A., *Sampling and Analysis of Food Products*, McGraw-Hill, Tokyo.

Benaim Pinto, C., *Sampling and Analysis of Airborne Micro-organisms*, Prentice-Hall, London.

Brown, N.H., *Environmental Microbiology*, Cambridge University Press, Cambridge.

Bradley, S.S., *Food Microbiology*, Academic Press, London.

Budyko, N.I., *Food Processing Waste,* Progress Publishers, Moscow.

Chang, G.D., *Introduction to Environmental Microbiology*, John Wiley & Sons, New York.

Commoner, C., *Food Enzymes*, John Wiley & Sons, New York.

Coolingwood, S.W., *Food Flavours,* John Wiley & Sons, New York.

Cox, C.W., *Food Science*, S.P. Medical and Scientific Books, New York.

Daniel, G.L., *Canned Foods and Their Microbiology*, Pergamon Press, Oxford.

Downe, S.A., *Dairy Microbiology*, John Wiley & Sons, New York.

Dugan, P.R., *Fermentation of Beer*, Plenum Publishing Corporation, London.

Goldman, M., *Treatment of Food Waste*, Gordon and Breach, Science Publishers, New York.

Gould, G.W., *Food Biochemistry*, D. Van Nostrand, New York.

Harding, G., *Transport Processes and Unit Operations*, Prentice-Hall, London.

Krieg, G.M., *Food Engineering and Process Applications,* Heinemann, London.

Lewis, B.B., *Applied Environmental Microbiology*, Elsevier Scientific Publishing Co., Amsterdam.

Miller, M.S., *Food Microbiology*, Prentice-Hall, London.

Riemann, D., *Encyclopedia of Biotechnology and Industrial Microbiology*, Academic Press, London.

Robert, B. and Evison, L., *Principles of Food Science*, John Wiley & Sons, New York.

Sengner, J., *Micro-organisms in Food*, John Wiley & Sons, New York.

Smith, P., *Encyclopedia of Environmental Microbiology*, John Wiley & Sons, New York.

Tanaka, S.K., *Flavonoids: Dietary Occurrence and Biochemical Activity*, Marcel Dekker, New York.

Wilson, W., *Encyclopedia of Food Science*, Academic Press, London.

Index